Defining Mental Disorder

Philosophical Psychopathology

Jennifer Radden and Jeff Poland

Defining Mental Disorder

Jerome Wakefield and His Critics

Edited by Luc Faucher and Denis Forest

The MIT Press
Cambridge, Massachusetts
London, England

The open access edition of this book was made possible by generous funding from Arcadia—a charitable fund of Lisbet Rausing and Peter Baldwin.

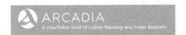

This book was set in Stone Serif and Stone Sans by Westchester Publishing Services. Printed and bound in the United States of America.

Library of Congress Cataloging-in-Publication Data

Names: Faucher, Luc, 1963– editor. | Forest, Denis, editor.
Title: Defining mental disorder : Jerome Wakefield and his critics / edited by Luc Faucher and Denis Forest.
Description: Cambridge, Massachusetts : The MIT Press, [2021] | Series: Philosophical psychopathology | Includes bibliographical references and index.
Identifiers: LCCN 2020016671 | ISBN 9780262045643 (hardcover)
Subjects: LCSH: Wakefield, Jerome C. | Psychiatry--Philosophy. | Mental illness--Philosophy. | Mental illness--Diagnosis. | Mental illness--Classification.
Classification: LCC RC437.5 .D434 2021 | DDC 616.89--dc23
LC record available at https://lccn.loc.gov/2020016671

10 9 8 7 6 5 4 3 2 1

Contents

Introduction

Denis Forest and Luc Faucher

Jerome Wakefield's work is at the center of the contemporary debate as to the nature of mental illness (and the related question of psychiatry's scope and limits), a decades-old debate in both scientific and philosophical literature. His key proposal, the "harmful dysfunction analysis" of mental disorders (HDA thereafter), has been discussed at great length by scientists and philosophers alike. In psychology, discussions of Wakefield's proposal abound in special issues of journals (see, e.g., *Journal of Abnormal Psychology* [1999] and *World Psychiatry* [2007]), but although philosophers have commented on and criticized Wakefield's position on many occasions (see, e.g., Nordenfelt 2003; Bolton 2008; Gold and Kirmayer 2007; Murphy and Woolfolk 2000; Murphy 2006), no book or special issue of a major philosophy journal has been dedicated to the task of offering a survey of these critiques.

With this volume, we propose to remedy that situation, and for the occasion, we have gathered together some of today's most eminent and up-and-coming philosophers of psychiatry to discuss Wakefield's position as well as its theoretical implications and empirical consequences. We hope that the resulting collection of chapters—with extensive replies from Wakefield himself—may be of interest to researchers and students in several related fields ranging from clinical psychiatry to social work, as well as philosophy of mind and philosophy of psychiatry.

HDA: A Presentation

HDA is the claim that "a disorder is a harmful failure of some internal mechanism(s) to perform a naturally selected ('designed') function" (Wakefield 2000, 253). This notion was originally presented by Wakefield in two papers published during the same year (Wakefield 1992a, 1992b). At first sight, each of these papers is quite different: one is a general presentation of HDA, contrasting it with rival conceptions of mental disorders. The other is a critique of the definition of mental disorders as "unexpectable distress or disability" that is used in the revised third edition of the *Diagnostic and Statistical Manual of Mental Disorders* (*DSM-III-R*) (published in 1987). In fact, these two articles offer two different perspectives on the implications of HDA: one is more philosophically oriented and deals with foundational issues; the other is more of a dialogue with medical research and practice and deals with the empirical consequences of theoretical choices, a type of research that the majority of Wakefield's subsequent publications can be grouped into (e.g., the two books coauthored with Allan H. Horwitz; Horwitz and Wakefield 2007, 2012). Since 1992, Wakefield has vindicated his thesis on many occasions, without revising it significantly. Critiques of HDA have tended to focus keenly on the terms "dysfunction" and "harmful," but "analysis" is no less important to understand the nature of his project. HDA is offered as a definition of what a mental disorder is, but it is also the outcome of the application of a method, the method of *conceptual analysis*, and it would be an error to separate the two.

Wakefield characterizes conceptual analysis in the following manner: "In a conceptual analysis, proposed accounts of a concept are tested against relatively uncontroversial and widely shared judgments about what does and does not fall under the concept. To the degree that the analysis explains these uncontroversial judgments, it is considered confirmed, and a sufficiently confirmed analysis may then be used as a guide in thinking about more controversial cases" (Wakefield 1992b, 233). Conceptual analysis is a tool that allows one to judge the merits of competing accounts of what a mental disorder is, HDA being one of the latter. These merits can be evaluated using two criteria. One is that a proper analysis of the concept allows us to correctly specify its extension. The characteristic tone of many of Wakefield's publications derives from the critical use of this method: (1) if analysis A of the concept of mental disorder (C) were sound, then condition X would not be a disorder and condition Y would, (2) but it is uncontroversial that X is recognized as a disorder and that Y is not; (3) accordingly, A is not an adequate analysis of C. For instance, if post-traumatic stress disorder (PTSD) is commonly recognized as a disorder and is quite expected in the context of trauma, then the previously mentioned *DSM-III-R*'s definition of a mental disorder as "a mental condition that causes distress and disability and that is not a statistically expectable response" is not correct (Wakefield 1992b, 233). The other task that an analysis of a given concept must complete is explaining consensus by making explicit what *grounds* the common intuitions of professionals and laymen. An analysis of the concept of mental disorder has to be able to tell us what deserves to be called a mental disorder, to set a standard for the proper use of the concept. As such, the ambition of HDA is not simply to be in harmony with a consensual view.

In the two 1992 articles, Wakefield contrasts the *concept* of mental disorder and a *theory* of disorder (Wakefield 1992a, 374; Wakefield 1992b, 232). The concept defines the proper domain of psychiatry (analyzing it is answering the question, What are mental disorders?), while a theory of mental disorders offers a general strategy for the explanation of such disorders (its purpose is to answer the question, Where do mental disorders come from?). This distinction, as pointed out by Wakefield, is crucial to the

DSM's project: an atheoretical classification of mental disorders, a goal that is only possible if clinicians with divergent theoretical commitments can agree on criteria that enable the diagnosis of mental illnesses in a converging manner. But is it possible to completely disentangle an *analysis* of the concept of mental disorders like HDA and a *theory* of mental disorders? HDA, with its reference to evolutionary biology, natural selection, and design, is obviously theory-laden, and it is in principle possible both to reject (or to ignore) Darwinism and to grasp the usual distinctions between disorders and nondisorders. To address this difficulty, the solution proposed by Wakefield is to argue that the HDA is composed of two distinct claims (Wakefield 1999, 374–375): the first more general claim is that disorders are dysfunctions of mental mechanisms with negative (harmful) consequences. This claim is supposed to articulate what grounds experts' and laymen's shared judgments of what counts (or what does not count) as a disorder in psychiatry. It is not linked to any specific construal of "function," and it would be HDA in its strictest sense. The second claim concerns the meaning of function and dysfunction: the dysfunction of a mental mechanism within the framework proposed by Wakefield is its "failure to perform a natural function for which it was designed by evolution" (Wakefield 1992a, 373). This second claim is derived from the idea that any ascription of mental disorder to an individual involves a factual component and that, to date, our best understanding of biological facts and of biological mechanisms (of which psychological mechanisms are a subtype) comes from evolutionary biology. Thus, HDA is theory-laden because it relies on our best knowledge of natural facts in its understanding of what a dysfunction is.

Once we understand what conceptual analysis is, the next logical question is, "What it is *for*?" The main issue for Wakefield is what he calls "conceptual validity," that is, "discriminating disorder from non-disorder" (Wakefield 1992b, 232), and conceptual validity is what can be achieved through a proper use of conceptual analysis. Of course, one can see that the demarcation between disorder and nondisorder matters for practical reasons—it determines in principle who should be cared for by mental health professionals and who should get reimbursement for treatment. It also matters from an institutional point of view—"'mental disorder' demarcates the special responsibilities of mental health professionals from those of other professionals, such as criminal justice lawyers, teachers, and social welfare workers" (Wakefield 1992a, 373). But conceptual validity matters first of all because we need a theoretical concept of mental disorder to justify the existence of psychiatry as a field of scientific knowledge. The question of justification has a close relationship to the question of boundaries. The question of the boundaries is more important to psychiatry than to other subfields of medicine, because the use of the concept of disorder in this field is surrounded by controversy and suspicion. On one hand, there is the "nihilism" of antipsychiatry, wherein there is no such thing as mental disorders (interestingly, this extremely skeptical view is the first that Wakefield addresses in 1992a). On the other hand, there is what has been called the "medicalization of society," the "process by which nonmedical problems become defined and treated as medical problems" (Conrad 2007, 4). This is a well-known phenomenon in the field of mental health, and it is of much interest for Wakefield as is demonstrated by book titles such as *The Loss of Sadness: How Psychiatry Transformed Normal Sorrow into Depressive Disorder* (Horwitz and Wakefield 2007) or *All We Have to Fear: Psychiatry's Transformation of Natural Anxieties into Mental Disorders* (Horwitz and Wakefield 2012). The rejection of psychiatry as a whole, as well as its overextension, can be understood as two consequences of a same set of difficulties that reinforce each other. According to Wakefield, both derive (at least partly) from a lack of proper understanding of what mental disorders are. In particular, defining mental disorders exclusively through their unhappy consequences (they cause harm and often distress), or by the use of evaluative notions (something being "wrong" with a given individual), has the undesirable consequence of blurring the distinction between genuine disorders and problems in living, unusual, or disapproved behaviors. However, "grieving a lost spouse involves considerable suffering and being in a bad marriage is a problem of living but neither is a disorder" (Wakefield 1992a, 374). It would also be unsatisfying to claim that drapetomania is not a disorder *for us*, just because we do not share the values and beliefs of nineteenth-century advocates of slavery: this would stop us from saying that drapetomania is simply (and has always been) an erroneous category. Similarly, sociology can describe the medicalization of ordinary life, but it is not in a position to justify normative judgments about medical practice. For this reason, it is the specific task of philosophy to adequately address the question of conceptual validity. To define mental disorders as what is taken care of by psychiatry would leave us unable to consider false positives (as in the case of the Rosenhan experiment; Rosenhan 1973), as well as genuine disorders that do not receive proper medical attention.

It is the risk of diluting psychiatry (through relativism, overextension, and lack of legitimacy) that explains why Wakefield holds that the reference to an internal dysfunction, independent from values and social norms, is needed in our analysis of the concept of mental disorder. In his 1992 publications, Wakefield insists on the many disadvantages of the use of the term "dysfunction": (a) the word "dysfunction" in itself is vague and could be taken as a mere synonym of disorder; (b) contrary to the term "harm," dysfunction refers to something that is not directly observable and can only be inferred—we *record* signs of distress, but we *postulate* internal dysfunctions; (c) in the context of psychiatry, speaking of dysfunction obliges us to specify *what* is dysfunctional—cancer is obviously not a *mental* disorder, although organic diseases are both the result of the dysfunction of biological mechanisms and a source of distress and disability, just like mental disorders (Wakefield 1992a, 384); and (d) if we consider that a dysfunction is the basis of a given disorder, this obliges us to specify the norms of functioning that justify our judgment. If we can't provide such a justification, it will always be possible to suspect that what we call a dysfunction is just the product of our negative evaluation of a given context or case.

However, Wakefield holds that these difficulties can be overcome and that the evolutionary view of mental functioning, in particular, is there to solve at least two of these problems.

One of these problems is (c), the question of what is dysfunctional. Thomas Szasz (1974) famously argued that there was no such thing as mental disorder because of an imperfect analogy: organic lesions impair bodily functioning, causing disorders with a causal history that we can describe in medical terms, but in the realm of the mental, there are no organs or lesions to be observed; we are just left with behaviors that are judged abnormal or deviant. He concluded that speaking of a mental "disorder" can only be a metaphorical means of expression hiding some hidden agenda. However, according to an evolutionary view of the mental, mental mechanisms can be inferred from their effects; they can be conceived of as efficient, adaptive tools like other biological mechanisms; and in given circumstances, they may be unable to perform their proper function just like any other evolved features of organisms. Fear responses to a dangerous environment, for instance, can be no less adaptive than any contribution of a bodily part of the organism to its well-being. If so, the breakdown of a mental mechanism is responsible for aberrant fear responses and can cause behaviors that can be considered maladaptive.

The other problem wherein the solution is offered by an evolutionary perspective is (d), the question of the norms of functioning: the proper function of evolved mental mechanisms is what they have been designed to do by evolution, which is independent of our values and preferences. In the case of drapetomania, we agree that there is no mental disorder—not simply because we reject the beliefs and values of advocates of slavery but primarily because to explain the behavior of the fleeing slave, we only need ordinary folk psychology and do not need to postulate anything abnormal within the mind of a slave. In choosing an evolutionary background to define the function of mental mechanisms, Wakefield intends to solve the problem of the normative dimension of the concept of function: "not working as designed" is proposed as a naturalized version of "not working as it should." In this evolutionary approach to the mental, Wakefield is in agreement both with the research program of evolutionary psychology and with the philosophical account of functions suggested by Larry Wright (1973), whom he explicitly references (see Wakefield 1992a). This account was later more fully developed by philosophers of biology such as Karen Neander (1991), and is known as the *etiological* view of functions, where F is a function of a component of type C in an organism O, if by doing F, former tokens of C contributed to the reproductive success of the ancestors of O.

According to HDA, however, the dysfunction of a psychological mechanism is a necessary but nonsufficient condition for the attribution of a mental disorder. To be considered a disorder, the dysfunction must also be *harmful*. In 1992, the harm component of HDA did not receive as much attention as the dysfunction component, but it is equally important, and within the second part of his analysis of the concept, Wakefield distances himself from purely naturalistic accounts of disorder (e.g., Boorse 1976, 1977).

The importance of harm derives from two types of considerations. Considerations of the first type are related to practical aspects of general medicine. According to Wakefield, medicine is not concerned with dysfunction per se but with *significant* dysfunction, that is, dysfunction-producing effects that have some clinical salience (Wakefield 2014). As the breakdown of an internal mechanism or an anatomical anomaly resulting from an atypical developmental path may have no significant impact on the overall functioning of a given individual, we shall only speak of a disorder when the breakdown or the anomaly is detrimental to this individual in terms of well-being and ability.

Considerations of the second type are specific to psychiatry. When it comes to mental functioning and behavior, according to Wakefield, what is detrimental cannot be judged without a context wherein the resulting behavior is valued or disvalued according to established norms. This is why HDA predicts cases where in an individual A, the failure of a mental mechanism to perform a natural function for which it was designed by evolution is not a source of harm or is even advantageous. This possibility results from the difference between the environment in which the effect of the mechanism has been selected because it was advantageous to A's ancestors and the present environment wherein this same effect is no longer adaptive. As the notion of harm is said to have "an intrinsic value component" (Horwitz and Wakefield 2007, 217), the concept of mental disorder, according to HDA, cannot be a purely scientific concept.

In the original presentation of HDA, Wakefield (1992a) pays special attention to the discrepancy between past and present environments. But, perhaps because of the uneasy relations between HDA and cultural psychiatry (Gold and Kirmayer 2007), the roles of harm and values are also reconsidered in a different perspective, above all in more recent writings where Wakefield deals with the issue of cultural relativity. The key question, then, is no longer that of a historical modification of norms of behavior; rather, the question is the context sensitivity of responses to the environment and the distinction between normal and pathological responses. Wakefield recognizes that culture may shape behaviors in such a way that responses to the environment that would be inappropriate in one context may be unproblematic in another. Yet that does not imply that the project of a demarcation between normal and abnormal responses is a chimera. It only means that, for instance, in the case of the distinction between sadness and depression, culture may define what types of loss for which sadness is a normal response (it defines what is, in general, *valuable* to possess) and that we should take this sensitivity to the environment into account to draw the line correctly between disorder and nondisorder (Horwitz and Wakefield 2007).

Worries about HDA

Before introducing the chapters of the present volume, which offer new critical perspectives on HDA, we shall present a brief survey of the debate that has been generated by Wakefield's view of mental disorders since 1992. We will not, however, be able to address every question, such as the relation between the descriptive and the normative dimensions of HDA (Kirmayer and Young 1999) or the role given by HDA to shared intuitions about mental disorders.

One of Wakefield's key claims is that conceptual analysis matters for medical practice, especially because we need a solution to the conceptual validity/demarcation problem. On one hand, Wakefield holds that only a valid definition of what mental disorders are is able to ground our classificatory judgments. On the other hand, symptom-based definitions of mental illnesses too often lead to an unjustified medicalization of normal conditions. Defining mental disorders, then, is of primary importance for the psychiatric community. Yet as we can see from the ongoing debate in the literature, this view is controversial. One issue is the possibility of analyzing the concept of mental disorder in terms of necessary and sufficient conditions that would be identical for all types of syndromes, from schizophrenia to personality disorders (see, in this volume, the contributions of Leen De Vreese and Peter Zachar in chapters 5 and 7, respectively). If there are only family resemblances between kinds of mental disorders, then the quest for an overarching definition (including, through the dysfunction clause, a similar etiology), which would allow us to solve the demarcation problem in a great majority of cases, may prove futile. Another issue is the relevance of theoretical definitions (like that offered by HDA) to medical decisions. Some have argued that when Wakefield is discussing the *DSM*'s criteria and unsubstantiated ascriptions of disorder, he is using, in fact, "folk concepts" and commonsense intuition about what proportionate or appropriate responses to the environment can be in given circumstances and that he does not rely on an evolutionary psychological theory of mental mechanisms (Bolton 2008, 143–145). This retreat could at least partly be explained by our ignorance of the limits of normal variation (Schwartz 2007) and the way we usually infer the existence of a disorder. For instance, in his reply to Lilienfeld and Marino, Wakefield holds that the symptoms "caused by design failures" are "so extreme that they do not significantly overlap with normal functioning" (Wakefield 1999, 387). He adds that "there is a naturally selected range of the sensitivity of fear-response mechanisms, but the spontaneous terrors of panic disorder are not part of that range" (387). We could ask ourselves, however, if "design failures" and "naturally selected range" of a mechanism's sensitivity add anything but adjectival nuance from an evolutionary biology-inspired lexicon of familiar medical categories (disorder and clinical heterogeneity within populations). In this case, deciding which responses are pathological is not based on evolutionary considerations but only on the fact that some clinical phenomena are both statistically rare and harmful. In such contexts, drawing a line between disorder and nondisorder is *compatible* with an evolutionary view of mental functioning, but it does not *depend* on it and it is *not inferred* from a prior knowledge of natural function and design.

Other issues are linked to the dysfunction component of HDA. First, Wakefield's view of the design of the human mind is close to that of evolutionary psychology, which has been criticized on several grounds—in particular, for not meeting the methodological requirements of evolutionary biology (Richardson 2010; see Faucher, chapter 3, this volume). Second, the etiological account of functions is only one among several alternatives, and as a consequence, it is conceivable that one can redefine mental disorders with a different, nonhistorical background. One option is the analysis of causal roles suggested by Robert Cummins (1975). According to Cummins, a function F of a component C in a system S is a contribution of C to the explanation of a given capacity of S. Although it has often been said that this view of functions reflects the use of functional talk in physiology and neuroscience, Cummins himself has linked his view of causal analysis to explanatory practices in psychology (Cummins 1985). Moreover, it is not impossible to derive an account of dysfunctions from this view of functions (Godfrey-Smith 1993), and regarding psychiatry, it has been vindicated as an alternative to HDA, for instance, by McNally (2001) and Murphy (2006; Murphy, chapter 13, this volume). Furthermore, the view of functions and dysfunctions within the biostatistical theory of health offered by Christopher Boorse, which he applies to psychiatry (Boorse 1976), can be understood as a combination of Cummins-style functions with a biological background via the reference to survival and reproduction (Forest and Le Bidan 2016).

Even if we keep Wakefield's evolutionary framework, his historical view of functions, disorders, or problems in living may not come from the dysfunction of an evolutionary mechanism. One alternative is a variant of the idea of evolutionary mismatch evoked in Wakefield (1992a). Instead of a "design failure" that is not harmful, because of the difference between the environment of evolutionary adaptedness (EEA) where the functional effect has been selected and present conditions, we would observe the reverse association (i.e., harmful consequences of normal functioning): in this latter case, the mechanism is working as designed, but its selected effect is no longer beneficial in the given circumstances. If we use Wakefield's example (Wakefield 1992a, 384), high levels of aggression may become grossly inadequate in certain conditions or life. In other cases, evolved mechanisms may be triggered by the "wrong" kind of stimuli in contemporary environments, stimuli for which they have not been designed to respond. Either we should still count the outcome in these kinds of cases as an instance of a genuine mental disorder (on the basis of its negative consequences) and give up HDA, or we should revise psychiatry manuals and shorten the list of mental disorders. Another type of scenario corresponds to what has been called by Nesse (2002) "evolved defenses": evolved defenses may cause pain or discomfort, but they are beneficial nonetheless. Some conditions usually labeled "disorders" would be frequent and heritable because they are, in fact, adaptive; even accompanied by distress, they would not, strictly speaking, be detrimental. Such a hypothesis has been vindicated in the literature, for instance, in the case of depression (for a review, see Faucher 2016). Introducing evolutionary considerations in psychiatry, then, may challenge the traditional understanding of conditions such as depression and block the ascription of an underlying dysfunction instead of supporting it, as is the case within the framework of HDA. It is also worth pointing out that both hypotheses in terms of mismatch and in terms of evolved defenses are concerned with the explanation of the persistence of disorders within human populations rather than with the explanation of individual disorders—a question that is not directly addressed by HDA.

One of Wakefield's key claims with HDA is that we should combine (rather than oppose) two ways of understanding mental disorders: one being biological and objective, the other being social and perspectival, with the idea of harmful consequences that are necessary to the ascription of a mental disorder and open to variation in different contexts of evaluation. As we have seen, the "harm" component of HDA has not received as much attention as the dysfunction component in the original presentation of the theory (Wakefield 1992a). Since then, *how* this process of valuation is supposed to take place, *whose* values are (and should be) taken into account, and *how* conflicts about values are managed have never been completely clarified (Poland 2003). Moreover, choosing a middle ground between naturalism and social constructivism exposes HDA to attacks from both sides. Some researchers may question the role of values and look for purely causal explanations of mental disorders (see Gerrans, chapter 19, this volume). Others criticize HDA either because of a division between facts and values, the natural and the social, that they judge illusory (Bolton 2008), or because of what they perceive as an inadequate vision of the role of social factors in Wakefield's proposal (Kirmayer and Young 1999). In particular, HDA makes a distinction between the (natural) basis of a disorder and the (social) evaluation of the consequences of the underlying dysfunction. Yet social and cultural factors may intervene in the causal chain leading to a disorder (Kendler 2005), and even if we pay attention to the distinction between broad (nonspecific) and narrow (specific) etiology (Wakefield 2014), it seems difficult to restrict the role of society to the evaluation of a preexisting condition whose existence depends solely on the failure of an internal, mental organ to do what it has been designed to do.

Last, HDA was conceived in a context where scientific psychiatry was exemplified by the *DSM*. A key architect of the *DSM* project (like Leo Spitzer) has welcomed HDA as a positive contribution that would help future editions of the *DSM* "make revisions in the diagnostic criteria more valid as true indicators of disorder" (Spitzer 1999, 430). However, in the psychiatric community, there is a growing dissatisfaction with the whole project of an "atheoretical" classification of mental disorders (Demazeux and Singy 2015), and the past decade has been marked by the emergence of the Research Domain Criteria (known as the RDoC) of the National Institute of Mental Health, which has been explicitly presented as an alternative to the *DSM* (at least in psychiatric research context) where mental disorders (more precisely, their symptoms) are linked to their genetics, molecular and neural basis (Insel and Cuthbert 2010; Faucher and Goyer 2015). Wakefield himself has expressed strong reservations as to the RDoC methodology (Wakefield 2014): according to him, the RDoC project as it stands is unable to deal with the key issue of *conceptual validity*, as the description of brain circuits can be linked equally well to disorders or nondisorders; it would be only at the psychological level that we can make the distinctions that allow us to delineate the proper domain of psychiatry. However, the theoretical landscape is quite different today from what it was in 1992, and one wonders if the definition of mental disorders has to be completely divorced from ongoing psychiatric and scientific research.

The Content of the Volume

The present volume is organized in four sections, each reflecting an aspect of Wakefield's analysis of health as "harmful dysfunction." Sections comprise chapters reflecting on HDA's methodology (mostly, conceptual analysis), on its goal (the demarcation between disordered and nondisordered states), or on the elements of the *analysans* proposed by Wakefield ("dysfunction" and "harm"). Each chapter is followed by a reply (which sometimes is also followed by a supplementary reply) from Jerome Wakefield.

Part I: On Conceptual Analysis

In chapter 1, "*DSM* in the Light of HDA (and Conversely)," Steeves Demazeux challenges on historical grounds a claim made by Jerome Wakefield in his defense of his theory—namely, that the HDA is in complete agreement with the spirit of modern psychiatry in general, especially with the conception of mental disorders relied upon by Spitzer and his colleagues in the conception of the *DSM-III*. In fact, Demazeux makes two separate but related claims. The first claim concerns Spitzer's views: in his early, seminal papers, where the criteria of "distress and disability" are essential to the identification of mental disorders, Spitzer does not appear to give a prominent role to the criterion of dysfunction, as it is claimed by Wakefield. The second claim concerns the relationship between HDA and the whole *DSM* project. With his symptom-based approach, the *DSM* could not be easily reconciled with the HDA approach, which involves a very specific type of etiology—a dysfunction of an evolved psychological mechanism. Thus, Wakefield's claim that the *DSM* is contradictory rather reflects his own mischaracterization of the *DSM*'s ambitions rather than being the result of the *DSM*'s failure to be faithful to its own characterization of mental disorder. This chapter is offered not as a rebuttal of HDA but as an attempt to more precisely contextualize the emergence of HDA within the context of psychiatry during the 1980s and 1990s.

In chapter 3, "Facts, Facts, Facts: HD Analysis Goes Factual," Luc Faucher takes on a different task by challenging Wakefield to go "factual" all the way, without reservation, in terms of his theory. Faucher identifies two domains where going factual might prove to be worthy of the effort. First, he reminds us that Wakefield thinks of conceptual analysis as a form of empirical investigation into the structure of our concepts. As the X-Phi (experimental philosophy) movement has shown, conceptual analysis is not devoid of biases, and for this reason, it is better to use various techniques to reveal the content of our concepts. As Faucher observed, Wakefield has already started using some of these techniques and claims that the results of his experiments support his version of HDA. Taking home some of the lessons gleaned from discussions about the methodological limitations of actual X-Phi experiments, as well as identifying some limitations inherent to Wakefield's experiments, Faucher invites Wakefield to more extensively test his theory (with a wider variety of questions and on a variety of groups), in addition to using different methods. As it has been shown via some preliminary studies' results using different methodologies, the concept of mental disorder held by different people might be much more diversified and sensitive to context than Wakefield had originally posited. Second, Faucher considers what has been seen by Wakefield as an "epistemological problem" (i.e., a problem that does not question the validity of his conceptual analysis but only its capacity to be applied in certain contexts): the problem of establishing precisely what is the proper function of a particular mental mechanism. According to Faucher, this problem might indeed demonstrate the limits of Wakefield's analysis. If the dysfunction portion of Wakefield's analysis is supposed to be a prophylactic against the excess of normative theory of mental disorders such as Szasz's, it is important to be able to establish what constitutes the proper function of the mechanisms that are thought to be dysfunctional. If one is not able to do so, there is a risk that values and social norms will sneak back in through the postulation of mental mechanisms that do not exist. Faucher argues that this is precisely the problem in Wakefield's analysis: for many important mental "faculties" or "capacities" (faculties or capacities that play a central role in the explanation of some paradigmatic mental disorders), it might not be possible to establish their proper function, which would leave psychiatry without a scientific image of the properly working mind to which it could refer to, in order to ground its judgments of dysfunction.

Leen De Vreese, in "Against the Disorder/Nondisorder Dichotomy" (chapter 5), argues that "disease" is a multifaceted concept that cannot be captured by HDA (or by any single definition). According to De Vreese, we need a pluralistic approach that would capture the different ways we use the notion of disease, rather than an approach that would aim to capture our intuitions about it. De Vreese analyzes the motivations behind Wakefield's conceptual analysis and observes that Wakefield seems to be moved by contradictory objectives: either to *describe* our intuitions or to *present a revised version* of them (to correct them where they err). Yet De Vreese also shows that whichever objective Wakefield's conceptual analysis is pursuing, it will encounter problems, which will ultimately make HDA difficult to use in practice to demarcate disorders from non-disorders. In and of themselves, these are arguments against the usefulness of conceptual analysis and a reason for the development of new methods to study our different uses (and meanings) of the concept in practice.

In chapter 7, Harold Kincaid begins "Doing without 'Disorder' in the Study of Psychopathology" by identifying what he takes to be three of Wakefield's major contributions. The contributions include (1) maintaining a "healthy" skepticism concerning psychiatric classification, (2) supplying reasons for the belief in a nonarbitrary distinction between disorders and nondisorders, and (3) assessing specific psychiatric categories (depression, phobias, etc.) to determine whether or not they capture (only) disordered conditions (rather than problems in living). Kincaid's main point is that these contributions do not necessitate a conceptual analysis of the concept of disorder. Among the reasons fueling his position are the facts that in science, concepts are usually not strictly defined; that it does not seem to be a good idea to tie the development of a scientific field to commonsense concepts; and that the defense against antipsychiatrist claims of medicalization of normal life can be accomplished without a definition of what disorders are. Kincaid does not believe that Wakefield's particular analysis of disorders in terms of harmful dysfunction of evolved mechanisms is necessary to evaluate the potential overinclusiveness of diagnostic categories (one of Wakefield's major contributions). Rather, according to Kincaid, psychiatric disciplines need objective and explanatory classifications (which need to delineate real distinctions between people that can be used to successfully explain, predict, and control behavior), and such classifications can be achieved without the analysis of the concept of mental disorder and without references to the evolutionary history of mental mechanisms.

Part II: The Demarcation Problem

In chapter 9, "Psychiatric Disorders and the Imperfect Community," Peter Zachar denounces the inherent essentialism (both causal and psychological) behind Wakefield's definition of mental disorder. Zachar posits that, for Wakefield, attributions of disorder are made on the basis of reasoning rather than empirical evidence: basically, it depends on one's concept of "objective natural function," which, despite what Wakefield claims, is not something that is empirically determined. Rather, it seems that one uses a conception about the responses that are to be expected by someone facing a type of situation (e.g., the death of a love one), and from this conception (which is usually not based on science), one infers whether or not the individual's mental mechanism is disordered. If such is the case, as Zachar points out, HDA cannot do what it set out to accomplish (i.e., factually demarcate valid psychiatric diagnostics from invalid ones). Through a discussion of Paul Meehl's notions of "open concept" and "construct validation," Zachar explains how one can reject Wakefield's essentialism and ground psychiatric diagnostic in facts. His argument rests on the observation that what we call disorders are the result of a mix of functional disorders (e.g., intrusive thoughts, impulse control difficulties, or decline in functioning), which form an "imperfect community" in that, if they all have been used to identify disorders (they have this in common), they are different in nature (therefore, they are imperfect because they do not necessarily share any other properties). In the literature, it is posited that from a particular mix or pattern of these functional disorders (what you might want to call the "manifest structure" of a disorder), you can infer a latent variable (i.e., a particular disorder, like depression). Latent variables are either thought of in a realist fashion (i.e., the latent variable is understood as being the thing that causes the observable pattern that defines the disorder) or nonrealist fashion (e.g., the latent variable refers to a stable set of functional disorders resulting from mutual interactions between the elements of the pattern). Zachar argues that the latter way of understanding disorders might prove to be much more fruitful for psychiatry than the essentialist way endorsed by Wakefield.

Part III: The Dysfunction Component

In chapter 11, "Is the Dysfunction Component of the Harmful Dysfunction Analysis Stipulative?" Maël Lemoine argues that in his treatment of the notion of "dysfunction," Wakefield is moving away from a conceptual analysis of the commonsense concept of disorder and entering the realm of stipulation. Relying on Hempel's distinction between various types of definition, Lemoine explains that Wakefield's conceptual analysis has elements of *meaning analysis* and elements of *stipulation*. The principal element of stipulation is the notion of dysfunction. According to Lemoine, the correct analysis of the commonsense concept of disorder is probably what he terms the harmful abnormality analysis (or HAA), where someone has a disorder if (1) they have an abnormality and (2) this abnormality is harmful. Wakefield's HDA can be seen as an explicitation of the HAA, as the concept is made less vague and more powerful empirically. Yet interpreting "abnormality" in terms of "dysfunction of an evolved mechanisms" is not an explicitation of the concept (which consists of arranging and stabilizing the sense of the concept) but rather a stipulation. This is made clear by the fact that there are other ways to interpret "dysfunction," for instance, as per Boorse's argument. There would be no conceptual problem to stipulate that abnormality has to be understood in terms of the dysfunction of an evolved mechanism if Wakefield did not view it as his job to provide a conceptual analysis of the commonsense concept. But this is not the case. Moreover, and this is Lemoine's last point, it is not at all sure that Wakefield's notion of dysfunction is the best one available.

   In chapter 13, "Function and Dysfunction," Dominic Murphy first reminds us that the requirement of the presence of the dysfunction of a psychological mechanism is motivated in Wakefield's analysis by his rebuttal of purely normative accounts of mental disorders. Murphy then questions the relevance of Wakefield's evolutionary understanding of function to the field of psychiatry. As per Murphy, a proper account of function in psychiatry should satisfy the following criteria: first, it should be able to ground our intuition that in some cases, something has gone wrong within the mind of an individual. Second, it should be in accordance with standard scientific practice. Third, it should allow us to handle various cases without adopting a "revisionist" attitude, where we exclude some conditions from the list of disorders just to save the theory we favor. Murphy holds that if we adopt these criteria, the systemic view of functions introduced by Cummins, and then revised in a more naturalistic spirit by his followers, fares at least as well as, and in some cases better than, the evolutionary view advocated by Wakefield. The systemic's perspective of Cummins is no less able to justify our intuitions about dysfunctions than the selectionist's view endorsed by Wakefield. Furthermore, it meshes especially well with biological sciences that are more closely related to research in psychiatry, and it does not lead to a drastic revision of our taxonomy of mental disorders because it does not have to identify each dysfunction with a "design failure."

In chapter 16, "The Developmental Plasticity Challenge to Wakefield's View," Justin Garson challenges Wakefield's idea that a mental disorder necessarily involves a dysfunction of a mental mechanism, where dysfunction is understood in terms of the failure to execute the function for which it has been selected. Indeed, Garson claims that some disorders might be the result of mechanisms in perfect working order. This is the case, he proposes, for some developmental mechanisms for which parameters are set by the environment early on in life. In such cases, there is a possibility of "developmental mismatch"—that is, it is possible that the early environment is not at all like the later environment, and what was adaptive in the first environment is maladaptive in the second one. If such is the case, it is possible that what we judge to be a dysfunctional behavior is caused by the working of a perfectly well-ordered mechanism, whose function is to adapt the organism to its environment by sampling earlier environments and taking this environment as a reliable cue of later environment. Garson argues that this is not only a view from the mind, but that there is an actual current of research in psychiatry that takes this possibility very seriously (the "Developmental Origins of Health and Disease" program). Through a careful discussion of Wakefield's view of dysfunction and his answer to the evolutionary mismatch's argument, Garson also shows that Wakefield is committed to the notion that dysfunctional behavior is caused by a functional mechanism. If Garson is right and some mental disorders are the result of developmental mismatches, then Wakefield's claims that dysfunction of a mental mechanism is a necessary condition for mental disorder are invalidated. Moreover, if the possibility of mental disorders caused by intact mechanisms is taken seriously by psychiatrists, then it seems that Wakefield's conceptual analysis does not perfectly capture the intuition of psychiatrists (at least of some of them and for some psychiatric conditions).

In chapter 19, "Harmful Dysfunction and the Science of Salience," Philip Gerrans holds that the most promising research path in terms of the explanation of mental disorders is not to look for psychological mechanisms that could fail to do what they have been designed to do but rather to focus on lower-level, molecular, and neural mechanisms whose integrity is crucial to our ordinary mental activity, even if they are only indirectly related to it. His key example is the salience system, wherein impaired functioning causes aberrant valuation of stimuli, which, in turn, may cause delusional states. If such is the case, delusions are not caused by the failure of an epistemic system whose task it is to produce true beliefs, because the evolutionary history of a salience system (or dopaminergic system) has little to do with the acquisition of true beliefs. Supporting empirical data for this argument are gathered from a body of fast-growing literature that links key symptoms of schizophrenia with abnormalities in dopamine regulation. Gerrans's idea, then, is to look for explanations of disorders in terms of lower-level relevant neural mechanisms, rather than at the level of psychological mechanisms (as Wakefield has typically done), and to suggest that this might lead one to think of psychiatric conditions in a revisionary way.

In chapter 21, "Autistic Spectrum, Normal Variation, and Harmful Dysfunction," Denis Forest focuses on the example of autism to challenge key components of HDA, namely, the evolutionary background of the function/dysfunction distinction and the link between harm and value. Forest observes that it is true that some psychological theories have tried to explain autism through the malfunction of specific, evolved mental mechanisms or modules, and on this basis, it could be argued that HDA and explanatory theories of autism are in complete harmony. However, autism research is more concerned with the ontogeny of mental mechanisms than with their evolutionary origin. In the context of the neurodiversity movement, which claims that we should consider autism as an instance of normal variation in human populations, it is difficult to see how HDA could tell us when behavioral and cognitive differences should be understood in terms of underlying dysfunction and when they are not. Moreover, confronted with the heterogeneity of cases within the autism spectrum, we want to highlight the difference between autism's harmless and harmful features. But what makes a dysfunction harmful is its intrinsic detrimental consequences, not the fact that it would be disvalued in a given social context. As Forest shows, recent shifts in the representation of high-order autism do not change a disorder into a healthy condition; they unmask abilities that had previously remained undetected. In the context of autism and neurodiversity, we need other criteria of dysfunction and harm than those specified by HDA.

In chapter 23, "Naturalism and Dysfunction," Tim Thornton questions the reductionist, objectivist, naturalist account of dysfunction that is central to HDA. Light can be shed on the prospect of reducing the apparently normative notion of dysfunction by comparing it to two distinct reductionist projects in the philosophy of mental content that stand next to one another as do the contrasting options in the Euthyphro dilemma. A more modest project (Fodor's representational theory of the mind) takes for granted the structure of normative relations between concepts and attempts to solve the engineering problem of how human thought can fit that structure. A more ambitious project (Millikan's teleosemantics) aims to explain that structure itself in naturalistic terms. This ambitious project, however, is undermined by Wittgenstein-Kripke's paradox. Tim Thornton argues that the harmful dysfunction analysis of disorder has to be interpreted as isomorphous with the latter project, as its aim is to explain how disorders are possible within the natural world. It is thus subject to the same objections raised against Millikan's project: if we cannot choose between rival accounts of mental functions, our understanding of mental disorders as natural dysfunctions is also undermined.

Part IV: The Harmful Component
In chapter 25, "Harmless Dysfunction and the Problem of Normal Variation," Andreas De Block and Jonathan Sholl focus on the harm component of HDA, wherein they question the presumed separability of the scientific, objective, factual requirement of a state of dysfunction from the second requirement that concerns harm and value in HDA. First, they point out that clear cases of *harmless* dysfunction are crucial to HDA: it is only because some dysfunctional states are not pathological (because they have no harmful consequences) that we can dissociate a value-free assessment of the loss of functional integrity and a value-laden judgment about the loss of health. Second, they discuss the cases of harmless dysfunction mentioned by Wakefield and offer skeptical counterpoints to his interpretations: one may wonder if fused toes and albinism are genuine cases of harmless dysfunction. Then, in the last and most ambitious part of the chapter, they use the problem of suboptimal variation to directly challenge Wakefield's main thesis. On one hand, if any kind of suboptimal variation is an instance of dysfunction, one departs from the standard use of the term "disorder" and stretches the notion beyond its reasonable limits. On the other hand, if what is suboptimal coincides with what is dysfunctional only when it has detrimental consequences, then we cannot really separate dysfunction from harm and HDA runs into trouble.

In chapter 27, "On Harm," Rachel Cooper expresses both her agreement with Jerome Wakefield (the harm component is crucial to the definition of mental disorders) and her disagreement with him (according to her, harm should not be understood as what is disvalued by a given society). Looking for a different measure of harm, she contrasts what she sees as an overly ambitious goal (grounding a construal of harm on an overall conception of the good life) with a more modest one (defining ways to assess if a given condition is harmful or not). She offers three methods to make progress on this issue: directly assessing the consequences of a given condition, analyzing cases in terms of cost and benefits, and looking for consistency when we use criteria to judge whether something is harmful. Finally, she holds that we should not think in terms of disorder when people are a cause of harm without being harmed themselves; Cooper stresses that in the context of the *DSM-5*, more than ever, the emphasis on harm is linked to a key concern of a reflection on psychiatry: preventing the unwarranted medicalization of ordinary life.

Acknowledgments

This project grew out of a conference organized by one of us (D. F.) on Jerome Wakefield's analysis of mental disorder held in Paris in 2010 and financially supported by the Agence Nationale de Recherche (ANR). We thank Pierre-Henri Castel for teaming us up for this collection of essays and for his support. We are also grateful to Jeffrey Poland for his advice and encouragements about submitting the manuscript to MIT Press. We would like to extend our gratitude to Philip Laughlin, editor at MIT Press, for his help with the project and his incredible patience and to Alex Hoopes, with whom it has been a pleasure to work in preparing the manuscript. L. F. thanks the Faculté des Sciences Humaines (FSH) de l'Université du Québec à Montréal for its financial support of this edition of the book, as well as Evi Amanda Leigh-Cox for the copy editing of this chapter and Cloé Gratton for her work on the formatting of the manuscript.

References

Bolton, D. 2008. *What Is Mental Disorder?* Oxford University Press.

Boorse, C. 1976. What a theory of mental health should be. *Journal of the Theory of Social Behavior* 6(1): 61–84.

Boorse, C. 1977. Health as a theoretical concept. *Philosophy of Science* 44(4): 542–573.

Conrad, P. 2007. *The Medicalization of Society.* Johns Hopkins University Press.

Cummins, R. C. 1975. Functional analysis. *Journal of Philosophy* 72(20): 741–764.

Cummins, R. C. 1985. *The Nature of Psychological Explanation.* MIT Press.

Demazeux, S., and P. Singy, eds. 2015. *The DSM in Perspective: Philosophical Reflections on the Psychiatric Babel.* Springer Verlag.

Faucher, L. 2016. Darwinian blues: Evolutionary psychology and depression. In *Sadness or Depression?* S. Demazeux and J. Wakefield (eds.), 69–94. Springer Verlag.

Faucher, L., and S. Goyer. 2015. RDoC: Thinking outside the *DSM* box without falling into a reductionist trap. In *The DSM in Perspective: Philosophical Reflections on the Psychiatric Babel,* S. Demazeux and P. Singy (eds.), 199–224. Springer Verlag.

Forest, D., and M. Le Bidan. 2016. In search of normal functions: BST, Cummins' functions and Hempel's problem. In *Naturalism in Philosophy of Health: Issues, Limits and Implications*, E. Giroux (ed.), 39–51. Springer Verlag.

Godfrey-Smith, P. 1993. Functions: Consensus without unity. *Pacific Philosophical Quarterly* 74: 196–208.

Gold, I., and L. Kirmayer. 2007. Cultural psychiatry on Wakefield procrustean bed. *World Psychiatry* 6(3): 165–166.

Horwitz, A. V., and J. C. Wakefield. 2007. *The Loss of Sadness: How Psychiatry Transformed Normal Sorrow into Depressive Disorder.* Oxford University Press.

Horwitz, A. V., and J. C. Wakefield. 2012. *All We Have to Fear: Psychiatry's Transformation of Natural Anxieties into Mental Disorders.* Oxford University Press.

Insel, T., and B. Cuthbert. 2010. Research Domain Criteria (RDoC): Toward a new classification framework for research on mental disorders. *American Journal of Psychiatry* 167(7): 748–750.

Kendler, K. S. 2005. Toward a philosophical structure of psychiatry. *American Journal of Psychiatry* 162(3): 433–440.

Kirmayer, L., and A. Young. 1999. Culture and context in the evolutionary concept of mental disorder. *Journal of Abnormal Psychology* 108(3): 446–452.

McNally, R. J. 2001. On Wakefield's harmful dysfunction analysis of mental disorder. *Behavioral Research and Therapy* 39(3): 309–314.

Murphy, D. 2006. *Psychiatry in the Scientific Image.* MIT Press.

Murphy, D., and R. L. Woolfolk. 2000. The harmful dysfunction analysis of mental disorders. *Philosophy, Psychiatry, and Psychology* 7(4): 241–252.

Neander, K. 1991. The teleological notion of 'function.' *Australasian Journal of Philosophy* 69(4): 454–468.

Nesse, R. 2002. Evolutionary biology: A basic science for psychiatry. *World Psychiatry* 1(1): 7–9.

Nordenfelt, L. 2003. On the evolutionary concept of health: Health as natural function. In *Dimensions of Health and Health Promotion*, L. Nordenfelt and P.-E. Liss (eds.), 37–54. Rodopi Press.

Poland, J. 2003. *Whither Mental Disorder.* Unpublished manuscript.

Richardson, R. C. 2010. *Evolutionary Psychology as Maladapted Psychology.* MIT Press.

Rosenhan, D. L. 1973. Being sane in insane places. *Science* 179: 250–258.

Schwartz, P. 2007. Defining dysfunction: Natural selection, design, and drawing a line. *Philosophy of Science* 74(3): 364–385.

Spitzer, L. 1999. Harmful dysfunction and the *DSM* definition of mental disorder. *Journal of Abnormal Psychology* 108(3): 430–432.

Szasz, T. 1974. *The Myth of Mental Illness*. Harper and Row.

Wakefield, J. C. 1992a. The concept of mental disorder: On the boundary between biological facts and social values. *American Psychologist* 47(3): 373–388.

Wakefield, J. C. 1992b. Disorder as harmful dysfunction: A conceptual critique of *DSM-III R*'s definition of mental disorder. *Psychological Review* 99(2): 232–247.

Wakefield, J. C. 1999. Evolutionary versus prototype analyses of the concept of disorder. *Journal of Abnormal Psychology* 108(3): 374–399.

Wakefield, J. C. 2000. Spandrels, vestigial organs, and such: Reply to Murphy and Woolfolk's "The harmful dysfunction analysis of mental disorder." *Philosophy, Psychiatry, and Psychology* 7(4): 253–269.

Wakefield, J. C. 2014. Wittgenstein's nightmare: Why the RDoC grid needs a conceptual dimension. *World Psychiatry* 13(1): 38–40.

Wright, L. 1973. Functions. *Philosophical Review* 82(2): 139–168.

Wakefield Critiques: Introductory Comments

Jerome Wakefield

To the Reader,

Because I eventually chose to answer each of my critics in a separate and detailed reply rather than answering all in one summary essay, there was no natural place for me to offer overarching acknowledgments and caveats. Given the magnitude of this project, that seemed unacceptable. Hence, this "comment" after the editors' introduction that the editors graciously allowed me.

The future role of psychiatry in a free society, including the scope and limits of the application of the concept of mental disorder and its consequences, is a crucial question confronting philosophy of psychiatry. Getting clear about the meaning of psychiatry's foundational concept of mental disorder is an important and highly controversial step in that inquiry. I hope the reader will feel as I do that the extraordinary intellectual power assembled in this unique volume, with contributions by leading philosophers of psychiatry who all focus on the concept of mental disorder, illuminatingly and provocatively advances our understanding of the options and stakes in the debate over the definition of mental disorder.

This volume includes essays by thirteen critics of my harmful dysfunction analysis (HDA) of the concept of medical, including mental, disorder, and my replies. Within the psychiatric and psychological literatures, the HDA is by far the most cited view in researchers' and scholars' discussions of the diagnostic status of various conditions. Within this volume, not only the HDA but also the most important proposed alternatives to the HDA are explored and disputed at a level of detail unavailable elsewhere. Taken together, these essays in my view give as comprehensive and in-depth an introduction to the current status of the philosophy of psychiatry's attempts to understand psychiatry's foundational concept as one is likely to find. For those readers familiar with the HDA, I should mention that the critics' compelling arguments have moved me to alter or amplify or clarify my view on several issues. The HDA survives intact but in a more nuanced and elaborated form.

Now, to the pleasure of acknowledging those to whom I owe a debt of gratitude. I am most exceptionally grateful to Denis Forest and Luc Faucher for undertaking this project and for their superhuman patience in seeing it through to fruition despite so many delays and some major adjustments in its structure. Beyond the editors, my greatest debt of gratitude is to the thirteen critics (which includes the editors) who contributed the fruits of their thinking about the philosophy of psychiatry to this volume. Each of their angles of attack on the HDA was of value to me and provoked me to learn and think in new ways as I engaged intensively with the arguments of each critical essay. I have tried my best but I can scarcely do justice to all of their efforts.

My greatest personal debt is to my research assistant and visiting scholar at the New York University (NYU) Center for Bioethics, Jordan Conrad, who read and provided feedback and editing and reference help on multiple drafts of each reply. His insightful probing and critical feedback, always done in the friendliest of ways, has saved me from many embarrassments and made my replies more measured and focused than they would have been.

I also thank Reinier Schuur for helpful discussions of some of the critics' positions at an early stage of my thinking about this project and for some comments on several of the critics' papers. I am also deeply indebted to my wife, Lisa Peters, and my sons, Joshua and Zachary Wakefield, for not only putting up with the lengthy period of out-of-control workaholism that it took to reply to the thirteen critics and tolerating all the missed or constricted family time that resulted but for actively cheering me on in this task when my spirits flagged.

A few caveats: Given the possibility of downloading individual essays in today's digital world, I have written each of my replies to be relatively self-contained, including references. I have tried to make the essays reasonably accessible to nonphilosophers in the clinical sciences, so I have eschewed some usual philosopher's stylistic choices that are confusing to others, such as the use of single quotation marks to indicate the word versus double quotation marks to indicate the concept and have just used double quotes for both and relied on context for the distinction. Also, to make lengthy quotes more readable, I have freely eliminated citations. Unless otherwise specified, italics are in the original quoted passage.

I have several apologies to make to the critics who so generously contributed their papers. First and foremost is an apology for the exceptionally long time it took to complete my responses and reach publication. As the contributors know, some vicissitudes of life intervened to lengthen the process. More constructively, many of the critics cited various areas of scientific or philosophical scholarship with which I was not sufficiently familiar to feel confident answering. As is evident from my replies, I took these references seriously and often did a deep dive into the relevant literature to understand and evaluate the objection. This enormously enjoyable approach took considerable time.

However, even considering those factors, the delay to the contributors' essays seeing the light of publication was considerable. Despite this, all the contributors hung in there, for which I am grateful. A further caveat on their behalf is only fair. Some of them have probably evolved in their thinking since writing their chapters and might argue their case differently and perhaps more persuasively if writing today; others might take an entirely different position today. So, their critiques, illuminating and intrinsically worthwhile as they are, must be understood as potentially time-stamped and anachronistic from the perspectives of some critics themselves. In such cases, I look forward to an updated interchange in the future.

I also apologize for the limitations of my replies. Even with exceptional freedom as to length generously granted to me by MIT Press and my editors, I could not possibly address every important argument put forward by each critic. So, frustratingly, I picked out what I considered the most compelling and interesting objections to answer and tried to be thorough about those, and other arguments of necessity went unanswered and await future interchanges. These choices are captured in the titles of my replies. However, very often an issue raised in one critic's essay that went unaddressed there is addressed in my reply to another critic who raised a related point, and in my replies, I frequently direct the reader to other replies. The replies are in this sense complementary and together form a comprehensive account of my current thinking about the HDA.

Finally, getting critiqued by thirteen very smart folks is a great privilege and pleasure, but it can also be challenging and try one's emotional fiber. I believe that the HDA amply stands up to the critics' objections—in fact, emerges from this trial considerably strengthened. Nevertheless, allow me to add an apology for anything in my replies that may seem to go beyond argument analysis in tone. Generally, the critics did not hold back in the vigor and bluntness of their arguments, and neither did I. I can only hope that when reading my replies, my critics will not think of me along the lines of what Schopenhauer's mother wrote to her son in a letter: "You have everything that could make you a credit to human society…but you are nevertheless irritating and unbearable.…All of your good qualities…are made useless to the world merely because of your rage at wanting to know everything better than others…no one can tolerate being reproved by you, who also still show so many weaknesses yourself, least of all in your adverse manner, which in oracular tones, proclaims this is so and so, without ever supposing an objection.…If you were less like you, you would only be ridiculous, but thus as you are, you are highly annoying." One thing my critics have taught me for sure: when I henceforth proclaim in oracular tones that the HDA is better than other analyses of "disorder," I will never again suppose that there is no objection! Hopefully, this will allow me to climb from highly annoying to merely ridiculous.

Again, I thank the contributors, the editors, and MIT Press for this opportunity to air what I believe are critically important issues in the philosophy of psychiatry.

I On Conceptual Analysis

1   *DSM* in the Light of HDA (and Conversely)

Steeves Demazeux

According to both the *DSM* definition of mental disorder and my "harmful dysfunction analysis" (HDA) of the concept of disorder, a disorder is an internal dysfunction (meaning a failure of a biologically designed function) that causes harm (as socially evaluated).
—Wakefield (2009, 87)

Introduction

Wakefield's "harmful dysfunction analysis" (HDA) has met with well-deserved success since his seminal 1992 paper. This analysis, according to which there are two main components in the concept of disorder—a harmful and a dysfunctional component—provides us with a means of clarifying the distinction between the normal and the pathological in the mental health field, and of testing the conceptual validity of any diagnostic label. The HDA has proved to be useful in a number of debates, including the one on the recurrent lack of consideration given to the clinical context in many diagnoses (and more specifically the controversial recent decision to eliminate the exclusion of bereavement from the diagnosis of major depressive disorder) and the increasing tendency to pathologize certain natural emotions (e.g., sadness, anxiety) or deviant behaviors (e.g., alcohol use, paraphilias, crime). This approach developed by a philosopher has even managed to convince a number of influential psychiatrists of the American psychiatric institution, among them Robert Spitzer, chair of the third edition of the *Diagnostic and Statistical Manual of Mental Disorders* (*DSM-III*), and Michael First, the editor of Text and Criteria for the *DSM-IV*.

In this chapter, I propose a brief account of the complex historical intertwining of the *DSM* and the HDA. In his work, Jerome Wakefield constantly refers to the *DSM*. From his first presentation of the HDA in 1992 onward, the American classification of mental disorders has played a central role in the philosophical defense of the HDA. Conversely, HDA appears to support, from a philosophical point of view, the general methodological strategy adopted by the *DSM* since 1980.

I do not intend here to "deconstruct" the HDA by means of a historiographical argument: I acknowledge that the philosophical relevance of the HDA should be considered solely in the light of conceptual arguments. Yet, in view of certain historical considerations, I wish to point out some important differences between the HDA and the *DSM*.

I.   Wakefield, an Early Advocate of the *DSM-III*

Wakefield's ambition to capture the essence of the pathological phenomenon can be found early in his work, several years before the official birth of the HDA. It can be traced back to two papers published in 1987 and 1988, interestingly at the time of a debate on the *DSM-III*.

What was at stake? In 1983, three years after the publication of the *DSM-III*, a debate arose in the *American Psychologist* between psychologist Marcie Kaplan and two important architects of the *DSM-III*, namely, Robert Spitzer (chair) and Janet Williams (text editor). With supporting examples, Kaplan (1983) criticized the *DSM-III* for introducing some sexual biases in the diagnostic criteria, which had the faulty consequence of perpetuating sex difference in treatment rates for mental illness. Williams and Spitzer (1983) replied to this accusation by claiming that the *DSM-III* Task Force took all appropriate measures to immunize the classification against all kind of biases, especially sexual biases.

A few years later, Jerome Wakefield (who had defended a social work thesis at Berkeley on "psychosexual disorders" in 1984 and had then worked on the history of concepts of sexual disorder as a postdoctoral fellow at the Pembroke Center for Teaching and Research on Women at Brown University) took part in this particular debate and published two papers, one in the *American Psychologist* and the other in the *Journal of Sex Research*. In these two papers, Wakefield adopts a balanced standpoint that puts him in a conciliatory position in the debate: although he does agree with Kaplan on the existence of potentially damaging sexual biases in many accepted diagnostic labels, he nevertheless takes the defense of the *DSM-III* by arguing that the third edition has efficiently managed to neutralize such biases. His demonstration focuses on the diagnosis of primary orgasmic dysfunction (POD) promoted during the 1970s by the two famous pioneers of American sexology, William H. Masters and Virginia E. Johnson. Wakefield criticizes their influential definition of POD for tending to overpathologize the lack of orgasm in women. The mistake, according to him, lies in the very term of "dysfunction" in the definition, which is much too indeterminate and does not have the same meaning when it applies to women as opposed to men. Indeed, Wakefield demonstrates that a necessary condition for characterizing a condition as pathological in men (e.g., in "ejaculatory incompetence") is the lack of orgasmic "ability." But when it comes to women, the mere absence of orgasm during intercourse is judged sufficient to consider it pathological. This is precisely the case in the definition of POD by Masters and Johnson: their fixation on the many psychosocial factors that impede women's sexuality in North American society has played an important emancipating role, but it led them paradoxically to consider that the mere lack of orgasm in women would in itself be indicative of a pathological condition. Despite its appellation, the diagnosis of "primary orgasmic dysfunction" simply neglects to take into account the very common possibility that a woman may not achieve orgasm during intercourse not because she is ill and has an internal dysfunction but just because she has a poor sexual experience and/or inadequate stimulation.

Does the *DSM-III* rush into the same mistake? Wakefield argues that it does not, thanks to the diagnosis of "inhibited female orgasm" provided in the psychosexual dysfunctions section of the classification. Even if the definition does not refer to the notion of "dysfunction," the term "inhibited" implicitly assumes in the *DSM-III* that the condition is characterized by some internal dysfunction whenever orgasm is not achieved despite sexual stimulation that was adequate "in focus, intensity, and duration" (American Psychiatric Association 1980, 279). The clinical evaluation of this contextual consideration does certainly present many difficulties. Wakefield nevertheless concludes that its appraisal in diagnostic criteria constitutes "substantial progress in diagnostic logic" (Wakefield 1987, 464).

Wakefield reiterated his defense of the *DSM-III* a year later, in 1988. In a paper entitled "Female Primary Orgasmic Dysfunction: Masters and Johnson versus *DSM-III-R* on Diagnosis and Incidence," he emphasizes with even more conviction the contrast between the two approaches and praises the DSM-III for its decision to narrow down the criteria for this specific psychosexual disorder. Wakefield also insists in this paper on the beneficial role that a good conceptual analysis may have in settling many diagnostic quarrels: "My argument is aimed at depathologizing women by highlighting the conceptual flaws in current diagnostic practices" (Wakefield 1988, 364). He then cites three authors—Szasz, Scheff, and Foucault—who have been influential in the past decades for denouncing the misuses of psychiatric labels. But Wakefield immediately differentiates himself from these three skeptical authors: "The critical point is that I accept the legitimacy and coherence of the traditional concept of mental disorder. Roughly and intuitively, a mental disorder, like any other disorder, is a harmful deviation from the way the organism is naturally designed to function" (Wakefield 1988, 364). This quotation encapsulates what can be considered the very first account of the HDA in Wakefield's philosophical career—but not yet with the evolutionary perspective that will be decisive in the 1992 seminal paper. The author insists on the importance of such a "functional conception of disorder" and provides two arguments that he will frequently mobilize in his subsequent work. First, he claims that this account provides a "traditional and reasonable standard" (Wakefield 1988, 364): it does not depart from the long-established use of the concept (the term "traditional" is used twice in the same passage), and it also depends on rational consideration, at least on commonsense intuition. Second, Wakefield is confident that this definition of a mental disorder, despite its roughness and incompleteness, can be fruitful in the psychiatric debate: "No matter how vague or problematic, there is an intuitive functional concept of disorder underlying our judgments, and diagnostic criteria must remain consistent with this conception if they are to be legitimate criteria" (Wakefield 1988, 365).

The reference to the notion of dysfunction is quite useful "no matter how vague and problematic" it is. And the proof of the pudding is in the eating, for this appeal is sufficient here to conclude that the *DSM-III-R* criteria for inhibited female orgasm are "logically superior" (Wakefield 1988, 365) to those developed by Masters and Johnson for POD.

II. *DSM* and the Concept of Mental Disorder

2.1 The Uncanny Familiarity between *DSM* and HDA

Wakefield's most quoted paper is certainly "The Concept of Mental Disorder: On the Boundary between Biological Facts and Social Values" (hereafter CMD), published in 1992 in the *American Psychologist*. This is a philosophical paper in a pure analytical vein, in the wake of Hempel, Putnam, and Searle (of whom Wakefield was a student at Berkeley). It is grounded in the methodological framework of conceptual analysis, which relies on widely shared judgments in order to reveal the ultimate components of a concept (see Aucouturier and Demazeux 2013; Lemoine 2013). Wakefield has never conceded that historical consideration could undermine the credibility of a sound conceptual analysis. This is why he strongly disagrees with Michel Foucault (whom he met when the French philosopher was staying at Berkeley) and Thomas Scheff, since they both attempted "to discredit mental disorder through analysis of the historical processes that led up to the adoption of the concept…or of the sociological processes that influence diagnosis" (Wakefield 1992a, 374). Wakefield, on the contrary, insists on the possibility that a conceptual analysis can be correct even if the concept in question is often misused in practice.

In the CMD paper, Wakefield discusses several definitions of mental disorder and defends the strengths and advantages of his own account. He begins by successively commenting on six alternative proposals, all considered by him to be flawed, albeit for different reasons. The six approaches (respectively, the skeptical antipsychiatric view, the value approach, the disorder as whatever professionals treat, the statistical deviance, the biological disadvantage, and the *DSM*'s definition as "unexpectable distress or disability") are obviously ranked according to their relative closeness to the HDA. In particular, the *DSM-III-R*'s definition—which Wakefield introduces emphatically as the "most influential recent definition of mental disorder" (Wakefield 1992a, 379)—is considered the closest approach to the HDA. Wakefield deliberately makes a connection between the two definitions: "The definition in *DSM-III-R* is inspired by an overall view of disorder very much like the harmful dysfunction approach I propose" (Wakefield 1992a, 380). While the *DSM* definition is thought to be faulty because it concedes too much to the statistical deviance approach, it still relies on the sound intuition that a disorder is essentially a *harmful dysfunction*.

This uncanny familiarity between the *DSM* and the HDA is explored in greater depth in two papers published respectively in 1992 and 1993: "Disorder as Harmful Dysfunction: A Conceptual Critique *of DSM-III-R*'s Definition of Mental Disorder" (hereafter DHD), published in *Psychological Review*, and "Limits of Operationalization: A Critique of Spitzer and Endicott's (1978) Proposed Operational Criteria for Mental Disorder" (hereafter LO), published in the *Abnormal Journal of Psychology*.

In the DHD, Wakefield offers a very detailed critical examination of the official definition of mental disorder provided by the *DSM-III-R* as "unexpectable distress or disability." In the LO, he carefully analyzes and criticizes a previous attempt by Spitzer and Endicott, in 1978. Although this long operational definition never played an official role, it has directly influenced the *DSM* definition. So Wakefield is right to investigate the conceptual strategy put forward by Spitzer back in 1978, because it clearly helps to highlight some implicit assumptions that are still present in the *DSM*. Yet it is quite regretful that he does not push his historical investigation a little bit further: if he went back to the very first definitional attempts by Spitzer in 1973 and by Spitzer and Wilson in 1975, he would had discovered that at the time, there was no hint of any "functional conception" of disorder.

Let's consider the historical sequence of the four attempts where Spitzer was directly involved:

(1) Spitzer's definition provided in the *DSM-II* position statement published in December 1973 on the occasion of the exclusion of homosexuality from the classification,

(2) Spitzer and Wilson's (1975) "elaboration and expansion" of the 1973 definition,

(3) Spitzer and Endicott's long operational definition in 1978, and

(4) finally, the *DSM-III* (American Psychiatric Association 1980) and *DSM-III-R* (American Psychiatric Association 1987) definitions.[1]

Why is it important to trace back this historical sequence? As we shall see, it sheds new light on two important points: (a) the functional account was completely absent from the first two attempts, and (b) it gained a more important—but ambiguous and not decisive—role in the subsequent attempts.

2.2 Mental Disorder before the Rise of the Function Debate

Unlike Wakefield, who starts his investigation with the account of the *DSM-III-R* and goes back to the 1978 attempt to see if it was already relying of the same intuitions,

I provide a chronological reconstruction that highlights the progressive refinement of the four different definitional attempts by Spitzer and his colleagues. In this regard, it is important to note that Spitzer's very first attempt to provide a general definition of mental disorder was made in the middle of the controversy that arose in 1972–1973 around homosexuality (Spitzer and Endicott 1978, 15). The rationale for removing homosexuality from the *DSM-II* is based on a 4-point statement (American Psychiatric Association 1973, 2) that highlights the absence of scientific consensus on the issue among experts. But Spitzer goes further. He justifies the exclusion of homosexuality by saying that this condition, contrary to all the other conditions listed in the official classification, does not fulfill the two general criteria for a mental disorder, namely, "subjective distress" and "generalized impairment." The historian Hannah Decker has reported Spitzer's strong emphasis on the "subjective distress" criterion (Decker 2013, 155). In any case, these two criteria will remain central in all the subsequent attempts.

Of note is the fact that the only occurrences of "function" or "functioning" in this important text are explicitly said to be evaluative and dependent on cultural norms. For instance, it would be misleading to interpret Spitzer's statement that a "significant proportion of homosexuals are apparently satisfied with their sexual orientation, show no significant signs of manifest psychopathology ... and are able to *function* quite effectively" (American Psychiatric Association 1973, 2, my emphasis), as a hint toward a natural model of normal functioning. The same can be said of the few examples that Spitzer provides of other nonoptimal functioning (i.e., celibacy, revolutionary behavior, religious fanaticism, vegetarianism, male chauvinism). This evaluative appreciation of "functioning" is also obvious in a 1974 interview. To a journalist who asks him, "What about the failure to function heterosexually? Is this not a dysfunction and sufficient reason for categorising homosexuality as a disorder?" Spitzer answers,

> No it is not. First of all, many homosexuals can function heterosexually but prefer to function homosexually (in varying degrees). Second, no one would claim that a heterosexual who was unable to function homosexually and had no desire to do so had a homosexual dysfunction. Therefore, homosexuals who have no desire to function heterosexually should not be categorised as suffering from a heterosexual dysfunction. (Spitzer 1974, 17)

In no way can one interpret the term "dysfunction" in this citation as denoting the impairment of a natural function.[2] Homosexuals "function" differently but neither more nor less than do heterosexuals. In Spitzer's mind, it is merely a question of preference. This interpretation explains why Spitzer is prompt to refuse the possibility that the notion of dysfunction may be relevant to resolve the homosexuality controversy. This particular point will also be important to correctly appreciate the introduction of the notion of "organismic dysfunction" in later approaches.

For now, consider the Spitzer and Wilson (1975) definition. It includes three main criteria that we can summarize as follows: (1) a demarcation criterion (between psychiatric and nonpsychiatric disorders), (2) three central defining conditions of a mental disorder, and (3) a criterion of clinical distinctness.

The whole definition embraces what the authors call a "narrow approach" (or European approach) that they contrast with the "broad approach" prevalent in the United States (Spitzer and Wilson 1975, 4). Whereas the broad approach tends to consider any "significant deviation from an ideal state of positive mental health" as the manifestation of a pathological condition, the new approach tries explicitly to be more restrictive. The difficulty, for sure, is to determine how restrictive the narrow approach should be, and this is why some explicit clinical criteria for the definition of mental disorder are needed. Early on, Spitzer felt that the two criteria of "subjective distress" and "generalized impairment" were fundamental but insufficient if one wanted the definition to account for conditions as commonly accepted in the psychiatric tradition as fetishism, exhibitionism, or necrophilia.[3] Retrospectively, Spitzer conceded, "As we considered the many conditions traditionally included in the nomenclature, we realized that although the definition of mental disorder proposed at the time of the controversy regarding homosexuality was suitable for almost all of them, a broader definition seemed necessary" (Spitzer and Endicott 1978, 16).

In 1975, the broadening of the definition was obtained by adding a strange third subcriterion: "Voluntary behavior that the subject wishes he could stop because it is regularly associated with physical disability or illness" (Spitzer and Wilson 1975, 829). This "new concept" aimed at capturing those conditions that did not fulfill the two first criteria but that still deserved clinical attention, such as "compulsive cigarette smoking" or "compulsive eating."

It is worth noting that nowhere in the definition does the idea of a dysfunction appear.[4] Moreover, it is important to stress the fact that the two authors do not envisage that the demarcation problem between the normal and the pathological might be solved by means of an etiological assumption. Their narrow approach, as they state, "also accepts the notion of a continuum of conditions highly desirable (positive mental health) to highly undesirable (mental illness) but places the cut-off point for mental disorder closer to the highly undesirable end of the continuum so that only conditions clearly associated with suffering and disability are designated as illness or disorder" (Spitzer and Wilson 1975, 4).

Elsewhere in the text, they explicitly deny the existence of any etiological consideration in their account: "It should be noted that the criteria for a mental disorder proposed here in no way depends on the etiology of the condition" (Spitzer and Wilson 1975, 9). So far, the contrast with Wakefield's personal account on mental disorder is striking since, according to the HDA, "the condition must be due to an internal dysfunction of some mental mechanism. This is an etiological assumption" (Wakefield 1997, 644; see also Wakefield, 1999b, 966).

2.3   A Divergent Interpretation of Spitzer and Endicott (1978)

From Spitzer and Wilson's (1975) definition to Spitzer and Endicott's (1978) proposed operational criteria for mental disorder, there is clearly some continuity in the basic ideas underlying the two approaches. Yet, for the first time, the expression "organismic dysfunction" is used. How should we interpret this sudden appearance?

According to Wakefield, the HDA is already implicit in the definition provided by Spitzer and Endicott: "The heart of Spitzer and Endicott's (1978) definition of disorder is the insight that a disorder is a harmful dysfunction" (Wakefield 1993, 163). The whole LO paper aims at revealing this core intuition contained in the long and clumsy operational definition. Wakefield patiently analyzes every single passage of the 1978 definition to show that there is extensive redundancy and obscurity in the proposed criteria and that the sole concept of "dysfunction" can efficiently resolve all the ambiguities. Wakefield seems at times to hesitate between hermeneutics (What are the implicit assumptions in the text?) and recommendations (How could we improve the proposed definition?), but his conclusion is univocal: by focusing too exclusively on the reliability of their criteria, the two authors have sacrificed the conceptual validity of the definition.

There is no room here to provide a complete exegesis of the 1978 definition. I will only contradict Wakefield's interpretation concerning the alleged centrality of the "dysfunction requirement" in the text. It is true that the notion of "an inferred or identified organismic dysfunction" is introduced at the beginning of the long twenty-five-page chapter as one of the three "fundamental concepts" in the notion of a medical disorder, alongside "negative consequences of the condition" and "implicit call for action" (Spitzer and Endicott 1978, 17). Furthermore, the "highly abbreviated form" of the definition of medical disorder—provided without much comment at the end of the introduction—integrates these three consensual dimensions of the pathological phenomenon as a medical entity (disease), a personal suffering (illness), and a sick role (sickness).

The abbreviated definition presents an undeniable resemblance with Wakefield's HDA. And this may explain why Wakefield has been unwittingly misled into a faulty reconstruction of the text. He indeed interprets the text as following a "three-step procedure" (Wakefield 1993, 162) where the abbreviated definition of "medical disorder" played a primitive role, before its application to the special case of "mental disorder" (step 2) and the final elimination of the notion of dysfunction in the operational definition (step 3). In this light, Wakefield concludes, while the term "dysfunction" has disappeared, "in effect the third step constituted an analysis of dysfunction" (Wakefield 1993, 162).

I think a more accurate interpretation of the text is to consider that the abbreviated definition came at the end rather than at the beginning of the process. The authors first refined and expanded the Spitzer and Wilson (1975) operational definition and tried in a second step only to summarize the result into a highly abbreviated form. If we accept this interpretation, as we shall see, the "dysfunction requirement" appears to be much less crucial than Wakefield thinks.

To begin with, consider the fact that the operational definition of "medical disorder" by Spitzer and Endicott incorporates all the criteria from the previous definition. Central in the first new criterion (criterion A) are the "three Ds": "Distress," "Disability" (i.e., generalized impairment), and "Disadvantage" (which replaces and broadens the "harmful voluntary behavior" criterion from the 1975 definition—I will comment on this important shift later). The criterion of clinical distinctness (criterion D) remains mostly the same. So the real novelty is the addition of two monothetic criteria: to summarize, a "largely within the organism" criterion (criterion B) and a "necessary price" criterion (criterion C). As it clearly appears through the authors' comments, these two criteria have been introduced in order to immunize the new broader and more ambitious definition against some important common counterexamples: distress or disability that directly results from a noxious environment—like "poverty," "irritable wife" [*sic*], "lack of opportunity in job advancement"—and distress or disability, which appears are the "necessary price for some positive goal" (like in "warranted pregnancy") (Spitzer and Endicott 1978, 28–29). In other words, criteria B and C *complete* the definition in order to exclude conditions that are clearly not pathological. By reconstructing the original intents of the authors behind criterion choice, my ambition is not to deny the growing importance of the notion of internal dysfunction. It is simply to highlight the fact that the notion of dysfunction does not constitute a primitive or a core intuition in the definition.

The latter point becomes even more evident when one focuses on the structure of the first criterion (A). There is indisputably a hierarchy introduced between the three Ds. The first two subcriteria ("distress," always introduced in the first place in all accounts, and "disability," broadly understood as "some impairment in functioning in a wide range of activities"[5]) still do not attach special importance to the notion of dysfunction. Concerning the third new subcriterion, "disadvantage," it is interesting to note that its first consideration by Spitzer can be traced back to 1976. This was not out of a broad reflection on the concept of medical disorder but specifically in order to resolve some special issues raised by the Sexual Disorders Subcommittee during the construction of the *DSM-III* (Decker 2013, 160). It is furthermore crucial for our interpretation to point out that "disadvantage" is explicitly held to be the "most controversial" criterion in the definition (Spitzer and Endicott 1978, 23). In this regard, there is an important concession in the definition that Wakefield fails to report: "It should be noted that if criterion A is met only by virtue of A.3, disadvantage, the designation of the condition as a disorder is *heavily dependent on social definitions of the degree of disadvantage or undesirableness,* as well as other considerations, as to the consequences of considering the condition as a medical disorder" (Spitzer and Endicott 1978, 21, my emphasis). This quotation should be read in conjunction with the following one, where we find the only mention of the notion of "organismic dysfunction"[6] in the operational definition: "The following forms of disadvantage, even when not associated with distress or disability, *are now considered, in our culture*, as suggestive of some type of organismic dysfunction warranting the designation of medical disorder" (Spitzer and Endicott 1978, 20, my emphasis).

Wakefield will interpret a similar phrase in the *DSM-III-R*[7] as a faulty concession to relativism (Wakefield 1992b, 234). I rather interpret this as an argument that "organismic dysfunction" plays a contentious and subaltern role in the definition. This is something like a *last resort* criterion, fragile and value laden, when physicians have to justify the inclusion in the pathological domain of certain contentious conditions without any clear distress or generalized impairment: "There is an extremely small number of conditions generally regarded as medical disorders which are not directly and intrinsically associated with either distress or disability. ... For these reasons, all the conditions considered medical disorders on the basis of the criterion *alone* [i.e., disadvantage] are the ones that are most apt to be a source of intense controversy, particularly those regarded as mental disorders" (Spitzer and Endicott 1978, 24).

If such cases are controversial, it is not because—as a straightforward interpretation of the HDA would suggest—these conditions do not apply to *both* components of the concept (a dysfunction *with* harmful consequences).[8] It is rather because the "organismic dysfunction" reference *by itself* is held to be a fragile criterion. To provide just one proof that dysfunction is not an essential component of the 1978 definition, see how Spitzer, with evident satisfaction, justifies the usefulness of his definition by applying it to "tobacco use disorder." According to him, this is not only a predisposing condition to a medical disorder but a truly mental disorder to be included in the *DSM-III* by virtue of criterion A.1 (distress) or A.3.d ("Atypical and inflexible sexual or other impulse-driven behavior which often leads to painful consequences") of the definition (Spitzer and Endicott 1978, 33). How can we explain that Spitzer is concerned only by the harmful consequences of heavy tobacco use and at no stage of his argumentation by the alleged presence of an "organismic dysfunction"?

To conclude, the supposed centrality of the notion of dysfunction in the 1978 definition does not withstand close examination. Wakefield is wrong when he claims that Spitzer and Endicott "specifically and exhaustively addressed the dysfunction requirement" in their definition (Wakefield 1993, 160). Moreover, I strongly disagree with him when he adds that "there is a hint that the evolutionary model of natural functions is accepted by Spitzer as the basis for attributions of dysfunction" (Wakefield, 1992b, 236; see also Wakefield 1993, 164). Evolution plays strictly no role in any part of the chapter. This is a somewhat excessive interpretation.[9]

What is, however, clear is that the 1978 definition has been deeply influenced by the refinement of the biological arguments defended by such authors as Scadding (1967),

Kendell (1975), and Klein (1978). Slightly perceptible also is the growing influence of arguments from the flourishing field of philosophy of biology. In the mid-1970s, biological function became a hot philosophical topic, to which Larry Wright (1973), Robert Cummins (1975), and Christopher Boorse (1975)[10] were leading contributors. It is not surprising that it progressively infused the psychiatric debate.

III. HDA in the Light of *DSM*

Our brief historical reconstruction has consisted up to now in mitigating Wakefield's strong claim that the notion of "dysfunction" was a central intuition in the definition of Spitzer and Endicott (1978). In this last section, I draw some important conclusions regarding three claims made by Wakefield: (1) the idea that there is a "basic error" in the *DSM*, in the sense of a discrepancy between its general conceptual strategy and the specific solutions it offers; (2) the idea that the concept of mental disorder underpins the "foundation" of the *DSM*'s theory-neutral strategy; and (3) lastly, and more fundamentally, the idea that the HDA exhibits a "widely shared concept, intuitive medical and lay concept" of mental disorder that had already been accepted long before the *DSM* era.

3.1 The "Basic Error" of the *DSM* Concerning the Dysfunction Requirement

The two constant and central criteria in the successive attempts by Spitzer and his colleagues to provide a definition of mental disorder are "subjective distress" and "disability" (i.e., generalized impairment). Even though much complexity developed around the definition, the conceptual strategy remained the same.

This conclusion strongly contrasts with Wakefield perceiving a "dramatic" difference between the 1978 account and the *DSM-III-R* definition.[11] According to him, by focusing on statistical concepts, the *DSM-III-R*'s definition "fails to match the dysfunction requirement that inspired it" (Wakefield 1992a, 381). But actually, it has never inspired it, so it does not go against its main purpose when it puts all the emphasis on "unexpectable distress and disability."

This is a very important consideration for clarifying the whole relation between the HDA and the *DSM*, since Wakefield thinks there is a gap between the (correct) conceptual structure of the *DSM* and its (too frequent) faulty realization. Wondering about the *DSM* system, Wakefield deplored that its "basic error" has been to "pay insufficient attention to the 'dysfunction' requirement" (Wakefield 1997, 652):

> I believe that this conflict within *DSM* is derived from a conflict within the views of the one person who more than anyone else influenced the conceptual structure of *DSM*, Robert Spitzer. The conflict is between Spitzer's sophisticated analysis of the concept of mental disorder (Spitzer & Endicott 1978), from which the *DSM* definition is derived, and his belief that specific disorders must be defined in terms of their symptomatic effects, from which *DSM* diagnostic criteria are derived. (Wakefield 1997, 643)

He thus claims that there is a conflict within the *DSM* and, more precisely, in Spitzer's views. In reality, there has never been any conflict of the sort. Spitzer's main focus, both in his definitional work and in the characterization of specific disorders, has always been the symptomatic effects. And the same can be said for the vast majority of the experts involved in the *DSM* Task Force. Wakefield himself recognizes that the whole classification rests on a strategy that does not pay the slightest attention to the dysfunction requirement:

> We can reason backward from the criteria for specific mental disorders to the definition of mental disorder that would make sense of them. Such an examination reveals that the concept of dysfunction plays no direct role in the formulation of specific diagnostic criteria in *DSM-III-R*. In no criterion do we find, for instance, a clause like "the distress must have been caused by a dysfunction in the person" or any other reference to the existence of a dysfunction. (Wakefield 1992b, 236)

I could not agree more. But this is an argument that reinforces my interpretation that the dysfunction requirement has never been operant in the minds of the *DSM* architects. The diagnostic criteria in the *DSM* have always been consistent with the spirit of the general definition directed toward "unexpectable distress and disability."

3.2   The Foundation of the *DSM* Atheoretical Strategy

Another important consequence of our historical reconstruction concerns the appreciation of the purely descriptive strategy brought forward by the *DSM-III*. Wakefield is right to state that there is a strong congruence between the *DSM* atheoretical strategy and the theoretical neutrality of the HDA. This is perhaps the strongest common point between the *DSM* and the HDA. But whereas I agree with him on the consideration that "philosophy of science supports use of a theory-neutral nosology for now" (Wakefield 1999b, 963), I nevertheless disagree on the idea that the concept of disorder is at the "foundation" of the *DSM*'s theory-neutral nosology (Wakefield 1999c, 1001). Wakefield confounds the "is" and the "ought" when he says that "a theory-neutral manual of mental disorders must rely heavily on the concept of disorder to provide a criterion for inclusion and exclusion of conditions. ... Its use of symptoms and other theory-neutral resources to define disorders is guided only by the requirements of the concept of disorder" (Wakefield 1999c, 1003).

With the noteworthy exception of Robert Spitzer, who was always convinced of the necessity of a general definition of mental disorder and praised its usefulness for certain critical decisions (Spitzer and Endicott 1978, 16; Spitzer et al. 1980, 153), very few psychiatrist experts involved in the *DSM* process have ever been convinced that an overarching definition of mental disorder would be needful or even useful (see, e.g., Frances 2013; American Psychiatric Association 1994, xxi). Historically, the "descriptive approach" was developed in the psychiatric field before and quite independently of the search for a general definition of mental disorder. When, in 1959, Erwin Stengel was already praising the usefulness of operational definitions in psychiatry, he was explicitly encouraging a "frankly practical and utilitarian attitude to psychiatric classification" (Stengel 1959, 612). And it was the same crucial concern (i.e., the improvement of the extremely low reliability of psychiatric diagnoses) that, during the 1970s, guided the development of the Feighner criteria (Feighner et al. 1972) and later the Research Diagnostic Criteria (Spitzer et al. 1978). These historical considerations do not of course invalidate Wakefield's central argument that, in any case, a theory-neutral nosology has to rely on some underlying general notion of mental disorder. But actually, for the most part, professional experts did not—and still simply do not—care about what Wakefield calls "conceptual validity." Furthermore, there is little evidence that they all share the exact same notion of mental disorder. This is indeed deplorable, but it is a fact.

3.3   HDA in the Broad Historical Perspective

Throughout his impressive academic work, there are very few papers where Wakefield does not mention the *DSM* at all. The centrality of the American classification is logical in the sense that since 1980, it has constituted the second most frequently used diagnostic system worldwide, just behind the *International Classification of Diseases* (*ICD*) by the World Health Organization (WHO). Moreover, since 1992 and the publication of the *ICD-10*, the two systems, *DSM* and *ICD*, have shared the same methodological grounds.

However, from a broader historical point of view, it should be noted that the universality of the *DSM* approach in psychiatry is recent and fragile, as attested by the recurrent appeals for a "paradigm shift" and by the enthusiasm for the Research Domain Criteria (RDoC) project launched by the National Institute of Mental Health (NIMH). Wakefield has been repeatedly critical of the many conceptual flaws that taint the *DSM* classification. He has nevertheless defended the *DSM* against radical behaviorists (Wakefield 2003), proponents of dimensional approaches (Wakefield 1997), or RDoC advocates (Wakefield 2014).

Wakefield's HDA is based on the fundamental assumption that the concept of mental disorder is a "widely shared concept, intuitive medical and lay concept" (Wakefield 1999a, 375). As we have seen, there is no evidence that the HDA was implicit from the start in the *DSM*.[12] Might there be more evidence that the HDA was implicit in pre-*DSM* classification systems? Does Wakefield really think that, despite the many hesitations and theoretical reversals in the long run, the concept of mental disorder has retained a fixed meaning? In other words, does the functional account of mental disorder correspond to a traditional view that has remained constant throughout history? Wakefield's "black box essentialism" account suggests that it does: "Disorder is commonly conceived as failure to function (*dysfunction*), so Aristotle's claim that reason is the function of a human being can be considered a progenitor of the common view that mental disorder often consists of a breakdown in the capacity for rational thought and action" (Wakefield 2000, 18). Wakefield thinks that the same broad fixed intuitive meaning runs from Aristotle through Albert Ellis, Sigmund Freud, and the *DSM*. His essentialist account conflicts both with constructivist accounts and with Meehl's conciliatory conception of "open concepts" (Wakefield 2004). For sure, many functional "hints" can be found in the classical psychiatric literature, as in all medical history. We do not have to espouse Foucault's skeptical claim when he says that "the very notion of 'mental illness' is the expression of an attempt doomed from the outset" (Foucault 1976, 76). Still, many historians would acknowledge with Foucault that "in fact, before the nineteenth century, the experience of madness in the Western world was very polymorphic; and its confiscation in our own period in the concept of 'illness' must not deceive us as to its original exuberance" (Foucault 1976, 65–66).

Wakefield's essentialist account takes a charitable view of the scientific intention of psychiatry back to its birth. But the all-embracing ambition of the HDA does not account for all the nonaccidental differences of meaning and contextual variations scattered throughout classical psychiatric literature. For instance, the HDA does not explain why moral depravation modeled so many accounts up to the end of the nineteenth century. It would be a mistake to relativize the importance of such moral considerations that were built into the very conception of madness—and that by the way are still highly associated with the notion of mental disorder nowadays. To try to explain this core importance on the basis of a (wrongful) functional attribution by nineteenth-century alienists would just lead to a huge historical misunderstanding. The risk of the HDA account, from a historiographical point of view, is to fall into what we can call "Whig history" (i.e., the tendency to interpret history as the continuing and inevitable victory of progress over error). Wakefield is obviously right when he writes, "Cultures can be wrong about whether a condition is a disorder or normal, as Victorian physicians were wrong to think that clitoral orgasm was a disorder, ante-bellum confederate U.S. physicians were wrong to think that slaves who ran away from their slavery were disordered" (Wakefield 2007, 155).

It is not a risky claim to say that clitoral orgasm and drapetomania were once wrongly conceived as mental disorders, since the ideological motivations are easy to reconstruct. By contrast, it is a more difficult task to historically investigate conditions such as pathological infantilism (Ribot 1896), childish character (Dupré 1903), or the diagnosis of dependent personality disorder in *DSM-III* (American Psychiatric Association 1980, 324). There is a historical relation in the conceptualization of these three labels that could remain obscure if one looks only at the "conceptual validity" (according to the HDA) of each construct taken separately.

Concluding Remarks

In this chapter, I have shown that Wakefield is somewhat overeager to detect a "dysfunction requirement" central in the *DSM* definition. In his zeal to defend the relevance of his own conceptual approach, he has inadvertently overstated the presence and meaning of the term "dysfunction" in the short *DSM-III* definition of mental disorder. This mistake reveals two important consequences regarding both the *DSM* and the HDA. First, Wakefield appears to be too confident in the overall conceptual validity of the *DSM* atheoretical project. Second, he neglects the fact that the *DSM*, given its historical and ideological background, is far from being able to provide a sound and stable reference for the defense of a universal and ahistorical notion of mental disorder.

It is important to point out that my demonstration does not constitute a direct attack on the conceptual relevance of the harmful dysfunction analysis. I agree with Jerome Wakefield on the fact that psychiatrists should be more concerned by the conceptual validity of the medical entities that they promote. As a philosopher, Wakefield has done a great job in convincing contemporary psychiatrists about this specific importance. Be that as it may, this concern about conceptual validity is quite new in the psychiatric profession and it is not prevalent, even today. This may attest to the still "incredible insecurity of psychiatric nosology" (Kendler and Zachar 2008), rather than the existence of a universally shared pretheoretical notion of mental disorder.

Appendix

1973: *DSM II*

Spitzer position statement for the American Psychiatric Association in "Homosexuality and Sexual Orientation Disturbance: Proposed Change in the *DSM-II*, 6th Printing":

"For a mental or psychiatric condition to be considered a psychiatric disorder, it must either regularly cause subjective distress, or regularly be associated with some generalized impairment in social effectiveness or functioning. With the exception of homosexuality (and perhaps some of the other sexual deviations when in mild form, such as voyeurism), all of the other mental disorders in *DSM-II* fulfill either of these two criteria."

1975: Spitzer and Wilson

(a) Preprint version
  "I. The manifestations of the condition are primarily psychological and involve alterations in behavior. However, it includes conditions which are manifested by somatic changes (e.g., psycho-physiologic reactions) if an understanding of the etiology and course of the condition is largely dependent on the use of psychological concepts, such as personality, motivation, and conflict.

II. The condition in its full blown state is regularly and intrinsically associated with either:
   a. Subjective distress, or
   b. Generalized impairment in social effectiveness or functioning, or
   c. Voluntary behavior that the subject wishes he could stop because it is regularly associated with physical disability or illness
III. The condition is distinct from other conditions in terms of clinical picture, and ideally, follow-up, family studies and response to treatment."

(b) Published version

"1. The manifestations of the condition are primarily psychological and involve alterations in behavior. However, it includes conditions which are manifested by somatic changes, such as psycho-physiologic reactions, if an understanding of the cause and course of the condition is largely dependent on the use of psychological concepts, such as personality, motivation, and conflict.

2. The condition in its full blown state is regularly and intrinsically associated with subjective distress, generalized impairment in social effectiveness or functioning, or voluntary behavior that the subject wishes he could stop because it is regularly associated with physical disability or illness.

3. The condition is distinct from other conditions in terms of clinical picture and, ideally, follow-up, family studies, and response to treatment."

1978: Spitzer and Endicott

(a) Definition of medical and mental disorder in a "highly abbreviated form"

"A medical disorder is a relatively distinct condition resulting from an organismic dysfunction which in its fully developed or extreme form is directly and intrinsically associated with distress, disability, or certain other types of disadvantage. The disadvantage may be of a physical, perceptual, sexual, or interpersonal nature. Implicitly there is a call for action on the part of the person who has the condition, the medical or its allied professions, and society.

A mental disorder is a medical disorder whose manifestations are primarily signs or symptoms of a psychological (behavioral) nature, of if physical, can be understood only using psychological concepts."

(b) Operational definition

"All four criteria, A through D, must be met for a condition to be designated as a medical disorder. It should be noted that if criterion A is met only by virtue of A.3, disadvantage, the designation of the condition as a disorder is heavily dependent on social definitions of the degree of the disadvantage or undesirableness, as well as other considerations, as to the consequences of considering the condition a medical disorder.

A. The condition, in the fully developed or extreme form, in all environments (other than one especially created to compensate for the condition), is directly associated with at least one of the following:
   1. Distress—acknowledged by the individual or manifested,
   2. Disability—some impairment in functioning in a wide range of activities,

3. Disadvantage (not resulting from the above)—certain forms of disadvantage to the individual in interacting with aspects of the physical or social environment because of an identifiable psychological or physical factor.

The following forms of disadvantage, even when not associated with distress or disability, are now considered, in our culture, as suggestive of some type of organismic dysfunction warranting the designation of medical disorder:

a. Impaired ability to make important environmental discriminations.

b. Lack of ability to reproduce.

c. Cosmetically unattractive because of a deviation in kind, rather than degree, from physical structure.

d. Atypical and inflexible sexual or other impulse-driven behavior which often leads to painful consequences.

e. Impairment in the ability to experience sexual pleasure in an interpersonal context.

f. Marked impairment in the ability to form relatively lasting and nonconflictual interpersonal relationships.

B. The controlling variables tend to be attributed to being largely within the organism with regard to either initiating or maintaining the condition.

Therefore, a condition is included only if it meets both of the following criteria:

1. Simple informative or standard educational procedures do not lead to a reversal of the condition.

2. Nontechnical interventions do not bring about a quick reversal of the condition.

C. Conditions are not included if the associated distress, disability, or other disadvantage is apparently the necessary price associated with attaining some positive goal.

D. Distinctness from other conditions in one or more of the following features: clinical phenomenology, course, response to treatment, familial incidence, or etiology."

1980: *DSM-III*

"In *DSM-III* each of the mental disorders is conceptualized as a clinically significant behavioral or psychological syndrome or pattern that occurs in an individual and that is typically associated with either a painful symptom (distress) or impairment in one or more important areas of functioning (disability). In addition, there is an inference that there is a behavioral, psychological, or biological dysfunction, and that the disturbance is not only in the relationship between the individual and society. (When the disturbance is *limited* to a conflict between an individual and society, this may represent social deviance, which may or may not be commendable, but is not by itself a mental disorder.)"

1987: *DSM-III-R*

"In *DSM-III-R* each of the mental disorders is conceptualized as a clinically significant behavioral or psychological syndrome or pattern that occurs in a person and that is associated with present distress (a painful symptom) or disability (impairment in one or more important areas of functioning) or with a significantly increased risk of suffering death, pain, disability, or an important loss of freedom. In addition, this syndrome or pattern must not be merely an expectable response to a particular event, e.g., the death of a loved one. Whatever its original cause, it must currently be considered a manifestation of a behavioral, psychological, or biological dysfunction in the person. Neither deviant behavior, e.g., political, religious, or sexual, nor conflicts that are primarily between the individual and society are mental disorders unless the deviance or conflict is a symptom of a dysfunction in the person, as described above."

1994 and 2000: *DSM-IV* and *DSM-IV-TR*

Same definition than in *DSM-III-R*, but with the preceding mention:

> "Although this manual provides a classification of mental disorders, it must be admitted that no definition adequately specifies precise boundaries for the concept of 'mental disorder.' The concept of mental disorder, like many other concepts in medicine and science, lacks a consistent operational definition that covers all situations. All medical conditions are defined on various levels of abstraction—for example, structural pathology (e.g., ulcerative colitis), symptom presentation (e.g., migraine), deviance from a physiological norm (e.g., hypertension), and etiology (e.g., pneumococcal pneumonia). Mental disorders have also been defined by a variety of concepts (e.g., distress, dysfunction, dyscontrol, disadvantage, disability, inflexibility, irrationality, syndromal pattern, etiology, and statistical deviation). Each is a useful indicator for a mental disorder, but none is equivalent to the concept, and different situations call for different definitions.

Despite these caveats, the definition of *mental disorder* that was included *in DSM-III* and *DSM-III-R* is presented here because it is as useful as any other available definition and has helped to guide decisions regarding which conditions on the boundary between normality and pathology should be included in DSM-IV."

2013: *DSM-5*

"A mental disorder is a syndrome characterized by clinically significant disturbance in an individual's cognition, emotion regulation, or behavior that reflects a dysfunction in the psychological, biological, or developmental processes underlying mental functioning. Mental disorders are usually associated with significant distress or disability in social, occupational, or other important activities. An expectable or culturally approved response to a common stressor or loss, such as the death of a loved one, is not a mental disorder. Socially deviant behavior (e.g., political, religious, or sexual) and conflicts that are primarily between the individual and society are not mental disorders unless the deviance or conflict results from a dysfunction in the individual, as described above."

Notes

1. All these definitions can be found in the appendix at the end of the chapter. The reader is invited to compare them carefully in order to follow our demonstration.

2. In the same way, it would be difficult to find such an account later when Spitzer writes, in 1980, "With this definition (the *DSM-III* definition) it becomes clear (at least to us) that the issue

is not one of *factual* matters about homosexuality, such as whether or not certain familial patterns predispose to the development of the condition, but rather a *value* judgment about the importance of heterosexual functionings" (Spitzer et al. 1980, 154). It is striking that what Spitzer considers "factual matters" here do not refer to any putative internal dysfunction but only to some epidemiological data as evidence of familial predisposition.

3. "Many expected that the logic of the 1973 decision to delete homosexuality from the classification of mental disorders would lead the task force on *DSM-III* to define Necrophilia as a disorder only if the individual complained of the symptom!" (Spitzer et al. 1980, 154).

4. A confirmation of this absence can be found in the rationale that Spitzer provides in 1975 to exclude the possibility, at a time envisaged, that "racism" may constitute a mental disorder: "the racist is not necessarily in either distress or having difficulty with his general functioning, even though he makes others miserable" (from Decker 2013, 157–158).

5. It is important to correctly interpret the "wide range" requisite, which explicitly demands that "there is impairment in more than one area of functioning" (Spitzer and Endicott 1978, 23). Contrary to Wakefield, who considers that "it is not disability but how it is caused that makes it pathological" (Wakefield 2009, 87), Spitzer clearly assumes here that what matters is disability itself (i.e., the general impairment of the patient in his or her daily life). The following passage proves that the emphasis is not put on the causal internal attribution of a dysfunction: "As a consequence of the requirement of generalized impairment, it is possible for a condition to be associated with impairment in a single function but not be classified as a disorder, providing that the condition does not result in any of the other two Ds" (Spitzer and Endicott 1978, 23).

6. Just as Wakefield was right to consider that the mere use of the term "dysfunction" in the diagnosis of POD proposed by Masters and Johnson was not indicative of an underlying theory of natural functions, I think that an accurate interpretation of the term here excludes such an indication. Actually, I believe that the emphasis in "organismic dysfunction" should be placed on *organismic* rather than on *dysfunction*. The difference is subtle but decisive. The term "organismic dysfunction" is taken in the text as a strict synonym of "any disturbance within the organism." As it appears through the examples discussed by Spitzer and Endicott, what matters is to assign a "locus" to the disorder (i.e., "largely within the organism"), not to involve a putative natural function. Retrospectively, Spitzer will concede that his idea that "something is not working in the organism" was not very clear in his mind (Spitzer 1999, 431).

7. "Whatever its original cause, *it must currently be considered* a manifestation of a behavioral, psychological, or biological dysfunction in the person" (American Psychiatric Association 1987, xxii, my emphasis).

8. Contrary to Wakefield's HDA, Spitzer's definition does not rely on the integration of two distinctive components; instead, it is based on a fundamental alternative. As he will explain retrospectively, "It became clear to me that the consequences of a condition, *and not* its etiology, determined whether or not the condition should be considered a disorder...I therefore proposed that the criterion for a mental disorder was either subjective distress or generalized impairment" (Spitzer 1987, 404, my emphasis).

9. Wakefield's argumentation is based on a quotation where Spitzer and Endicott acknowledge that their approach is close to Donald Klein's, proposed in the same volume. But it should be noted that Spitzer disagreed with Klein's insistence that "all legitimate usages [of the term "illness"] imply actual dysfunction" (Klein 1978, 48). It is on the homosexuality issue that this disagreement appears clearly: Spitzer contradicts Klein's argument that homosexuality, even when it is not associated with subjective distress, is a disease since it "demonstrates operationally an intrinsic involuntary incapacity," that is, a natural dysfunction (Klein 1978, 65). In any case, Wakefield's HDA has always been closer to Klein's than to Spitzer's position.

10. Spitzer and Endicott do not reference this influential paper. Boorse specifically addressed the psychiatric debate from the point of view of a philosopher of biology and provided the first clear defense of an objectivist account of disorder based on the notion of biological function.

11. "Despite the historical relation between the two definitions, Spitzer and Endicott's (1978) definition is dramatically different from *DSM-III-R*'s in its conceptual strategy" (Wakefield 1993, 160). Wakefield tends to overestimate the difference between the *DSM-III-R*'s definition summarized by him as "unexpectable distress and disability" and Spitzer and Endicott's definition, which was said to have "eschewed the statistical approach." Actually, exactly the same statistical concerns can be found in the two proposals.

12. But we do not mean that the HDA has not influenced the subsequent editions of the *DSM*. It is interesting to note in the recent definition of mental disorder provided by the *DSM-5* that, for the first time in the history of the manual, "distress" and "disability" are relegated to a subsidiary position, after the presence of a dysfunction. It is very likely that the members of the *DSM-5* Task Force accepted the following specific recommendation made by Wakefield and First to Stein and colleagues (2010): "Because of the centrality of the 'dysfunction' criterion to the logic of the definition, we also suggest moving this criterion up to appear as the second sentence, immediately following criterion A" (First and Wakefield 2010, 1781).

References

American Psychiatric Association. 1973. "Homosexuality and Sexual Orientation Disturbance: Proposed Change in the *DSM-II*, 6th Printing," by R. L. Spitzer. APA Document Reference No. 730008. American Psychiatric Association.

American Psychiatric Association. 1980. *Diagnostic and Statistical Manual of Mental Disorders*. 3rd ed. American Psychiatric Association.

American Psychiatric Association. 1987. *Diagnostic and Statistical Manual of Mental Disorders*. 3rd ed. rev. American Psychiatric Association.

American Psychiatric Association. 1994. *Diagnostic and Statistical Manual of Mental Disorders*. 4th ed. American Psychiatric Association.

American Psychiatric Association. 2013. *Diagnostic and Statistical Manual of Mental Disorders*. 5th ed. American Psychiatric Association.

Aucouturier, V., and S. Demazeux. 2013. The concept of mental disorder. In *Health, Illness and Disease: Philosophical Essays*, H. Carel and R. Cooper (eds.), 77–89. Acumen.

Boorse, C. 1975. On the distinction between disease and illness. *Philosophy and Public Affairs* 5(1): 49–68.

Cummins, R. 1975. Functional analysis. *Journal of Philosophy* 72: 741–760.

Decker, H. 2013. *The Making of DSM-III: A Diagnostic Manual's Conquest of American Psychiatry*. Oxford University Press.

Dupré, E. 1903. Un syndrome psychopathique particulier: le puérilisme mental. *Compte Rendu du Congrès des Aliénistes et neurologistes de France et des pays de langue française*, Bruxelles, 1–8.

Feighner, J. P., E. Robins, S. B. Guze, R. A. Woodruff, G. Winokur, and R. Muñoz. 1972. Diagnostic criteria for use in psychiatric research. *Archives of General Psychiatry* 26: 57–63.

First, M. B., and J. C. Wakefield. 2010. Defining "mental disorder" in *DSM-V*: A commentary on: "What is a mental/psychiatric disorder? From *DSM-IV* to *DSM-V*" by Stein et al. (2010). *Psychological Medicine* 40(11): 1779–1782.

Foucault, M. 1976. *Mental Illness and Psychology*, trans. by A. M. Sheridan-Smith. Harper and Row.

Frances, A. 2013. *DSM* in Philosophyland: Curiouser and curiouser. In *Making the DSM-5*, J. Paris and J. Philips (eds.), 95–103. Springer.

Kaplan, M. 1983. A woman's view of *DSM-III*. *American Psychologist* 38(7): 786–792.

Kendell, R. E. 1975. The concept of disease and its implications for psychiatry. *British Journal of Psychiatry* 127(4): 305–315.

Kendler, K. S., and P. Zachar. 2008. The incredible insecurity of psychiatric nosology. In *Philosophical Issues in Psychiatry: Explanation, Phenomenology, and Nosology*, K. S. Kendler and J. Parnas (eds.), 368–383. Johns Hopkins University Press.

Klein, D. F. 1978. A proposed definition of mental illness. In *Critical Issues in Psychiatric Diagnosis*, R. L. Spitzer and D. F. Klein (eds.), 41–71. Raven Press.

Lemoine, M. 2013. Defining disease beyond conceptual analysis: An analysis of conceptual analysis in philosophy of medicine. *Theoretical Medicine and Bioethics* 34(4): 309–325.

Ribot, T. 1896. *La psychologie des sentiments*. Felix Alcan.

Scadding, J. G. 1967. Diagnosis: The clinician and the computer. *Lancet* 290: 877–882.

Spitzer, R. L. 1974. In defense of the new nomenclature for homosexuality. *Medical Worlds News Review* 1(2): 16–18.

Spitzer R. L. 1987. The diagnostic status of homosexuality in *DSM-III*: A reformulation of the issues. In *Scientific Controversies: Case Studies in the Resolution and Closure of Disputes in Science and Technology*, H. T. Engelhardt and A. L. Caplan (eds.), 401–416. Cambridge University Press.

Spitzer, R. L. 1999. Harmful dysfunction and the *DSM* definition of mental disorder. *Journal of Abnormal Psychology* 108(3): 430–432.

Spitzer, R. L., and J. Endicott. 1978. Medical and mental disorder: Proposed definition and criteria. In *Critical Issues in Psychiatric Diagnosis*, R. L. Spitzer and D. F. Klein (eds.), 15–40. Raven Press.

Spitzer R. L., J. Endicott, and E. Robins. 1978. Research Diagnostic Criteria: Rationale and reliability. *Archives of General Psychiatry* 35(6): 773–782.

Spitzer, R. L., J. B. Williams, and A. E. Skodol. 1980. *DSM-III*: The major achievements and an overview. *American Journal of Psychiatry* 137(2): 151–164.

Spitzer, R. L., and P. T. Wilson. 1975. Nosology and the official psychiatric nomenclature. *Comprehensive Textbook of Psychiatry* 2: 826–845; preprint consultable on http://www.wpic.pitt.edu/research/biometrics/Publications/Biometrics%20Archives%20PDF/581Spitzer&Wilson19750001.pdf.

Stein, D. J., K. A. Phillips, D. Bolton, K. W. M. Fulford, J. Z. Sadler, and K. S. Kendler. 2010. What is a mental/psychiatric disorder? From *DSM-IV* to *DSM-V*. *Psychological Medicine* 40(11): 1759–1765.

Stengel, E. 1959. Classification of mental disorders. *Bulletin of the World Health Organization* 21(4–5): 601–603.

Wakefield, J. C. 1987. Sex bias in the diagnosis of primary orgasmic dysfunction. *American Psychologist* 42(5): 464–471.

Wakefield, J. C. 1988. Female primary orgasmic dysfunction: Masters and Johnson versus *DSM-III-R* on diagnosis and incidence. *Journal of Sex Research* 24(1): 363–377.

Wakefield, J. C. 1992a. The concept of mental disorder: On the boundary between biological facts and social values. *American Psychologist* 47(3): 373–388.

Wakefield, J. C. 1992b. Disorder as harmful dysfunction: A conceptual critique of *DSM-III-R*'s definition of mental disorder. *Psychological Review* 99(2): 232–247.

Wakefield, J. C. 1993. Limits of operationalization: A critique of Spitzer and Endicott's (1978) proposed operational criteria for mental disorder. *Journal of Abnormal Psychology* 102(1): 160–172.

Wakefield, J. C. 1997. Diagnosing *DSM-IV*, Part 2: Eysenck (1986) and the essentialist fallacy. *Behaviour Research and Therapy* 35(7): 651–665.

Wakefield, J. C. 1999a. Evolutionary versus prototype analyses of the concept of disorder. *Journal of Abnormal Psychology* 108: 374–399.

Wakefield, J. C. 1999b. Philosophy of science and the progressiveness of the *DSM*'s theory-neutral nosology: Response to Follette and Houts, Part 1. *Behaviour Research and Therapy* 37(10): 963–999.

Wakefield, J. C. 1999c. The concept of disorder as a foundation for the *DSM*'s theory neutral nosology: Response to Follette and Houts, Part 2. *Behaviour Research and Therapy* 37(10): 1001–1027.

Wakefield, J. C. 2000. Aristotle as sociobiologist: The 'function of a human being' argument, black box essentialism, and the concept of mental disorder. *Philosophy, Psychiatry, and Psychology* 7(1): 17–44.

Wakefield, J. C. 2003. Dysfunction as a factual component of disorder: Reply to Houts, Part 2. *Behaviour Research and Therapy* 41(8): 969–990.

Wakefield, J. C. 2004. The myth of open concepts: Meehl's analysis of construct meaning versus black box essentialism. *Applied & Preventive Psychology* 11: 77–82.

Wakefield, J. C. 2007. The concept of mental disorder: Diagnostic implications of the harmful dysfunction analysis. *World Psychiatry* 6(3): 149–156.

Wakefield, J. C. 2009. Disability and diagnosis: Should role impairment be eliminated from *DSM/ICD* diagnostic criteria? *World Psychiatry* 8(2): 87–88.

Wakefield, J. C. 2014. Wittgenstein's nightmare: Why the RDoC grid needs a conceptual dimension. *World Psychiatry* 13(1): 38–40.

Williams, J. B., and R. L. Spitzer. 1983. The issue of sex bias in *DSM-III*: A critique of "A Woman's View of *DSM-III*" by Marcie Kaplan. *American Psychologist* 38(7): 793–798.

Wright, L. 1973. Function. *Philosophical Review* 82(2): 139–168.

2 From Ribot and Dupré to Spitzer and RDoC: Does the Harmful Dysfunction Analysis Possess Historical Explanatory Power? Reply to Steeves Demazeux

Jerome Wakefield

I thank my dear friend Steeves Demazeux for his challenging critique of the historical validity, from Dupré and Ribot through to Spitzer and Research Domain Criteria (RDoC), of my harmful dysfunction analysis (HDA) of medical, including mental, disorder. The HDA claims that "disorder" refers to "harmful dysfunction," where dysfunction is the failure of some feature to perform a natural function for which it is biologically designed by evolutionary processes and harm is judged in accordance with social values (First and Wakefield 2010, 2013; Spitzer 1997, 1999; Wakefield 1992a, 1992b, 1993, 1995, 1997a, 1997b, 1997c, 1997d, 1998, 1999a, 1999b, 2000a, 2000b, 2001, 2006, 2007a, 2009, 2011, 2014, 2016a, 2016b; Wakefield and First 2003, 2012). Demazeux's systematic presentation in the first part of his paper of Robert Spitzer's successive attempts to define mental disorder immediately becomes an essential source for those reconsidering Spitzer's momentous definitional efforts in the course of his attempts to eliminate homosexuality as a category of disorder and create a new approach to psychiatric diagnosis. I am also grateful to Demazeux for excavating some of my early sexuality papers in which the notions leading to the HDA were gestating. Being reminded of these papers in the context of reconsidering Spitzer's conceptual efforts arouses some emotion. It was Spitzer's reading of one of those sexuality papers evaluating the efforts of the *Diagnostic and Statistical Manual of Mental Disorders* (*DSM*) efforts to define female orgasmic dysfunction (Wakefield 1988) that caused Spitzer to contact me to discuss my work, and this meeting led to our subsequent scholarly collaboration and friendship until his death in late 2015.

Demazeux's goal is not to do history for history's sake. Rather, his analysis of Spitzer's work is aimed at challenging my claim that Spitzer's definition already contained an inchoate version of the HDA's "dysfunction" component and thus denying me a piece of evidence I have presented in support of the widespread nature of HDA-type intuitions. Moreover, in the second part of his paper, Demazeux attempts to parlay the Spitzer analysis into a broader historicist critique of my claim that the HDA captures a widespread historical understanding of the concept of medical disorder by exploring several other historical examples. Demazeux admits that no historical argument like this by itself can refute the HDA, which must ultimately be judged on conceptual grounds ("I acknowledge that the philosophical relevance of the HDA should be considered solely in the light of conceptual arguments"). However, he holds that his argument "impacts significantly on the postulated existence of a 'common pretheoretical concept of mental disorder' shared by professionals," thus paving the way for a broader historicist critique of the HDA. I will consider these two aspects of his paper in turn.

Demazeux versus Wakefield on How to Think about the 1975 Spitzer and Wilson Definition

As Demazeux explains, Spitzer initially made two brief attempts in 1973 and 1975 to formulate a definition of mental disorder in connection with the debate over the diagnostic status of homosexuality. I agree with Demazeux that these definitions were formulated strictly in terms of the negative consequences of a condition, specifically distress or generalized role impairment. I also agree that these early definitions made no use of "function" in the HDA biological design sense. When they did mention "function," it was only in a more general evaluative sense (e.g., as in "I am functioning effectively at work"). Demazeux, considering my choice to focus in my publications on Spitzer's later 1978 definition, laments, "Yet it is quite regretful that he does not push his historical investigation a little bit further: if he went back to the very first definitional attempts by Spitzer in 1973, and by Spitzer and Wilson in 1975, he would had discovered that at the time there was no hint of any 'functional conception' of disorder." There is no reason for regret because I agree with Demazeux's characterization.

The difference is in how we interpret these facts about Spitzer's early negative-consequence definitional attempts. Demazeux sees a basic intuition about the meaning of "disorder" that is divergent from the HDA and was sustained by Spitzer, whereas I see an obviously invalid initial approximation that was gradually corrected. In trying to understand the limitations of the 1973 and 1975 definitions and the subsequent changes in 1978, it is important to keep in mind that Spitzer was not a philosopher by training. He once told me he took no philosophy courses and only one course in logic in college. So, despite his clear natural talent for conceptual analysis, it is not surprising that he commits elementary mistakes in his initial attempts. Moreover, he was focused not on the perspicuity of the analysis but on justifying his decision regarding the elimination of homosexuality from the manual. His rejection of homosexuality as a mental disorder was based on the rationale that homosexuality need not directly (i.e., independently of oppressive social attitudes) give rise to distress or generalized impairment, and this rationale only depends on harmful consequences being a necessary condition for disorder. Thus, like so many of my students when they are learning to do conceptual analysis, he came up with a proposed necessary condition for disorder—negative consequences—that serves his purposes, but he fails to test systematically for counterexamples that would reveal the need for further necessary conditions to comprise a sufficient criterion. It is only in the 1978 definition that Spitzer took a leap forward as a conceptual analyst with his more sophisticated analysis that adds a dysfunction requirement. Demazeux says, "(a) the functional account was completely absent from the first two attempts, and (b) it gained a more important—but ambiguous not decisive—role in the subsequent attempts." I agree with "a," but "b" is manifestly incorrect; the role of dysfunction was decisive in the later definitions, as we shall see.

Indeed, I would hypothesize that Spitzer knew that his early definition of mental disorder in terms of a condition's consequences of distress or generalized impairment was seriously flawed but decided not at that time to open a conceptual-analytic can of worms because the early definition was adequate to accomplish his goal of defending his decision about homosexuality. Why do I say that Spitzer must have been aware of what he later acknowledged, that the harmful-consequences definition was inadequate? Spitzer may have been a neophyte at conceptual analysis, but he was a very sharp neophyte. The Spitzer-Wilson definition is subject to such obvious counterexamples to sufficiency—many nondisordered conditions cause distress, for example—that this must have been apparent to Spitzer. For example, when later, in his 1978 paper with Endicott, Spitzer mentions counterexamples to the 1975 definition, they include distress entailed by marital conflict. However, that obvious "distress" counterexample was already mentioned as a nondisorder—but not raised as a problem for the definition—in the 1975 paper. An entire category newly added to *DSM-II* by Spitzer himself, "conditions without manifest psychiatric disorder and nonspecific conditions," is described in the 1975 paper and is characterized as follows: "This category, not present in *DSM-I*, performs the function of encompassing the 'conditions of individuals who are psychiatrically normal but who nevertheless have severe enough problems to warrant examination by a psychiatrist.' These conditions are therefore not mental disorders" (1975, 844). One of the groups of conditions that are specified as falling under this category is "social maladjustment without manifest psychiatric disorder, such as marital or occupational maladjustment" (1975, 844). In writing those words, Spitzer could not be unaware that this posed a problem for his definition of mental disorder, although he did not face the problem until 1978.

Another piece of evidence lies in the definition of medical disorder that Spitzer and Wilson (1975) provide in passing. They are addressing the possible challenge that there is no formal definition of medical disorder in medical diagnostic manuals, so why does psychiatry need a definition of mental disorder? Their answer is that in physical medicine, there is good consensus over what determines disorder: "No definition is needed. Medical (nonpsychiatric) disorders are conditions associated with physical pain, disability, or death. ... Consequently, persons with migraine headaches or painful, swollen, rheumatoid joints never insist that these conditions are normal and should not be classified as illnesses" (1975, 827). However, this "negative consequences" definition of physical disorder is manifestly invalid. The excruciating pain of childbirth, the discomfort of teething pain, and the painfulness of fatigue after extreme exercise do not make the respective conditions disorders. It is a conceptual-analytic neophyte's error to offer confirming instances (e.g., migraine, arthritis) as support for a conceptual claim rather than hunting for disconfirming instances. But surely Spitzer could not have failed to notice the obvious problem—which he does notice and address in 1978—even if he was not ready to alter his definitional approach at the time and did not need to do so in the context of the homosexuality debate because his argument there depended only on negative consequences being a necessary condition of disorder.

Demazeux versus Wakefield on How to Think about the Role of "Organismic Dysfunction" in the 1978 Spitzer and Endicott Definition and the *DSM-III* (1980) Definition

Spitzer and Endicott (1978) published a pivotal analysis in the run-up to *DSM-III* that at much greater length formulated the definition of mental disorder specifically as a form of medical disorder. In that analysis, they introduced the requirement that a condition must involve an "organismic dysfunction" to qualify as a disorder. The 1978 definition was the precursor for the much shorter definition of mental disorder that appears in Spitzer's (1980) introduction to the third edition of the American Psychiatric Association's *Diagnostic and Statistical Manual of Mental Disorders* (*DSM-III*; American Psychiatric Association 1980). In slightly varying forms, it appears in all subsequent editions of the *DSM*, including *DSM-5*.

In two papers (Wakefield 1992b, 1993) that I published at about the same time as the paper in which I initially proposed the HDA (Wakefield 1992a), I analyzed and critiqued Spitzer's 1978 and 1980 definitions. I observed that although Spitzer and Endicott did not yet have an evolutionary understanding of dysfunction—Spitzer later admitted that he was quite baffled by the problem of how to explicate the idea that something has gone wrong inside the organism—they did make clear that "organismic dysfunction," which they intuitively expressed as "something has gone wrong with the organism," is a necessary condition for disorder. I interpreted their inclusion of the organismic dysfunction requirement as an inchoate precursor of the HDA's evolutionary dysfunction criterion and cited it in support of my claim that there are widespread intuitions consistent with the HDA.

Demazeux vigorously disputes my claim that an intuitive version of the HDA's "dysfunction" criterion played a role in the 1978 and 1980 definitions. He states that he will "contradict Wakefield's interpretation concerning the alleged centrality of the 'dysfunction requirement' in the text" and "highlight the fact that the notion of dysfunction does not constitute a primitive or a core intuition in the definition." His interpretation is that Spitzer's 1978 introduction of "organismic dysfunction" as a requirement for disorder is merely terminological window dressing, substantively continuous with earlier "negative consequence" definitions: "The two constant and central criteria in the successive attempts by Spitzer and his colleagues to provide a definition of mental disorder are 'subjective distress' and 'disability' (i.e., generalized impairment). Even though much complexity developed around the definition, the conceptual strategy remained the same." He acknowledges that the term "dysfunction" is introduced in 1978 for the first time into Spitzer's definitional attempts: "It is true that the notion of 'an inferred or identified organismic dysfunction' is introduced...as one of the three 'fundamental concepts' in the notion of a medical disorder, alongside 'negative consequences of the condition.'" He nevertheless argues that, despite the explicit "dysfunction" language, rather than inaugurating the inclusion of a novel dysfunction criterion, the 1978 paper and the subsequent *DSM-III* definition based on it have no affinity whatever to the HDA in this respect and that the dysfunction criterion is not intended in the sense I interpreted it. Rather, he claims, these definitions are simply using the language of dysfunction as a shorthand for harms like distress or impairment and are basically terminological variants of the 1973 and 1975 negative-consequence definitions.

Demazeux admits that the definition of medical disorder Spitzer and Endicott present has an uncanny structural resemblance to the HDA: "The abbreviated definition [of medical disorder] presents an undeniable resemblance with Wakefield's HDA." But, rather than accepting this fact as support for an affinity between the 1978 definition and the HDA, Demazeux interprets them as the explanation for why my interpretation so easily goes astray in my eagerness to see a connection: "This may explain why Wakefield has been unwittingly misled into a faulty reconstruction of the text.... Wakefield is somewhat overeager to detect a 'dysfunction requirement' central in the *DSM* definition." It seems worth mentioning that Spitzer himself seems to have been similarly misled, because he later endorsed the HDA and explained that the HDA captured what he was after but could not explicate when he used "dysfunction" to indicate that something has gone wrong with the organism (Spitzer 1997, 1999).

Understanding the Introduction of "Organismic Dysfunction" into the 1978 and 1980 Definitions as an Attempt to Eliminate Counterexamples to the 1975 Definition

It seems to have become clear to Spitzer after the *DSM-III* Task Force was formed in 1975 from criticisms by psychiatric colleagues that the definition of mental disorder must make clear why it is a subcategory of medical disorder if the definition was to accomplish the crucial task of legitimizing psychiatry as part of medicine. This in turn was critical for rebutting the arguments of the antipsychiatry movement that psychiatry illegitimately uses medical terminology in service of social control. The attempt to explain why "mental disorder" is best understood as a subcategory of "medical disorder" leads inexorably to a dysfunction requirement because, as we have seen (and will consider further below), the negative-consequence criterion obviously doesn't work as a stand-alone definition of physical disorder due to the many painful conditions that are not medical disorders.

The introduction of the "organismic dysfunction" requirement into the 1978 definition is in fact part of a coordinated introduction of three closely related novel elements aimed at addressing accumulating problems that made the earlier definitions inadequate to the demanding *DSM-III* context: (1) for the first time, there is a decision to analyze the more general concept of "medical disorder" and subsume mental disorder under the broader category as simply one type of medical disorder. (2) There is the introduction of "organismic dysfunction" as a fundamental requirement of medical and mental disorder. It is only causation by a dysfunction that is able to provide the needed distinction between true medical problems and other nondisordered causes of pain or disability. (3) For the first time, there is the use of the explanatory phrase that, in a disorder, unlike in problematic normal variation, "something has gone wrong" with the organism, which serves as a useful intuitive explication of the notion of dysfunction that Spitzer was unable to explicate more clearly; that is part of the HDA's contribution. These three features go together to yield a fundamentally new approach to the essence of medical and mental disorder and to address the counterexamples to the earlier negative-consequence definitions.

Demazeux interprets the 1978 and 1980 definitions with their reference to organismic dysfunction as essentially minor verbal variations on the 1975 analysis. However, the record indicates that Spitzer recognized, correctly, that the earlier definition was just plain wrong and the 1978 definition was aimed at correcting it. The fact that the 1978 analysis is a genuinely novel attempt and not just a verbal variation on the earlier definition is made clear in the paper itself. Spitzer and Endicott tell us that, far from simply repeating the essence of the earlier definitions, they are changing the definition in response to criticisms and deficiencies in the earlier definition: "We have continued to modify the definition to meet some of the criticisms received" (17); "We...hope that many of the deficiencies of the initial attempt have been corrected" (17). They explain that the impetus for reconsidering the definition of disorder is that the challenges of *DSM-III* require a more perspicuous definition than the one that sufficed for addressing the homosexuality debate: "As we considered the many conditions traditionally included in the nomenclature, we realized that...a broader definition seemed necessary" (1978, 16).

An impetus for the introduction of the organismic dysfunction criterion was the growing awareness and explicit recognition of many counterexamples to the negative-consequence definition. This concern is manifested throughout the 1978 paper. For example, at the outset of the 1978 paper, Spitzer and Endicott observe that there are obvious counterexamples to the simple definition of medical disorder as any condition that causes pain or certain other negative consequences, such as the pain of childbirth and the impairments of pregnancy: "Physicians rarely concern themselves with defining what is a medical disorder. . . . If questioned, they readily acknowledge that much of their work actually involves conditions which are generally not considered medical disorders, such as pregnancy or childbirth" (1978, 15). Again, after introducing "relative disadvantage" as an additional form of negative consequence that can sometimes indicate disorder, Spitzer and Endicott observe that there are many counterexamples to any attempt to use the disadvantage criterion as a stand-alone criterion because not all disadvantage is due to something being wrong with the organism: "Many conditions which place an individual at a relative disadvantage are not usually considered medical disorders, for example, short stature, tone deafness, greediness, poor sense of humor, unattractive appearance, and limited intelligence (but not mental retardation). Conditions such as these are usually regarded as the inevitable consequence of 'normal variation' rather than a result of 'something having gone wrong'" (24). Note that all of these negative conditions are "in the individual" and yet are not considered to be "something going wrong." The implication of these counterexamples is that the existence of negative consequences is one dimension of disorder and something going wrong as opposed to normal variation is another dimension, and both are requirements that must be fulfilled in order to have a disorder. So, contra Demazeux, "something is going wrong" must mean more than just "a condition in the individual has negative consequences" if it is to play its role of eliminating the counterexamples. The precise nature of that additional crucial meaning is not further elaborated by Spitzer and is explicated by the HDA's interpretation of dysfunction.

Demazeux's discussion suggests two ways that one might try to assimilate the novel phrase "organismic dysfunction" to something from past definitions that is not dysfunction in anything like an HDA sense. First, one might interpret "organismic dysfunction" with an emphasis on "organismic," as simply requiring that the problem be in the individual. Second, one might interpret "organismic dysfunction" as using "dysfunction" as a value term (e.g., "this marriage is dysfunctional") that just restates the fact that there are negative consequences.

There is a simple but strong argument against either of these interpretations. In carefully paring down the lengthy 1978 definition to yield the brief *DSM-III* definition, Spitzer, Williams, and Skodol (1980) note that "every word and comma was carefully examined" (153) in formulating the much-compressed *DSM-III* definition, which reads as follows:

> In *DSM-III*, a mental disorder is conceptualized as a clinically significant behavioral or psychologic syndrome or pattern that occurs in an individual and that is typically associated with either a painful symptom (distress) or impairment in one or more important areas of functioning (disability). In addition, there is an inference that there is a behavioral, psychologic or biologic dysfunction and that the disturbance is not only in the relationship between the individual and society. (Spitzer 1980, 6)

If, as Demazeux suggests, "organismic dysfunction" is not very important and was essentially redundant with "impairment of function," then in the radical shortening of the definition for *DSM-III*, one would not have expected the notion of dysfunction to survive the pruning. Yet, it not only survived but warranted its very own sentence, on a par with impairment of functioning. Indeed, "function" appears twice in this definition, first in the phrase "important areas of functioning (disability)," which is possibly a matter of negative consequences, and again in the phrase "behavioral, psychologic or biologic dysfunction," which has no apparent link to negative consequences. Given how carefully this definition reportedly was crafted, the two occurrences of "function" are unlikely to be mere sloppy redundancy; the second use presumably introduces a new idea. Moreover, the *DSM-III* definition states that to be a disorder, the condition must be "in the individual" and that it must cause distress or impairment, and then it states that "in addition, there is an inference that there is a behavioral, psychological, or biological dysfunction" (Spitzer 1980, 6). The phrase "in addition" indicates that the organismic dysfunction is different from either the harm or the location in the individual that is specified earlier in the definition. Finally, the harm and the location in the individual are manifest features "typically associated" with the condition, whereas the dysfunction is described as arrived at by inference, placing it in a different epistemological category. In any event, we have seen that by 1978, Spitzer understood that an internal condition with negative consequences is necessary but not sufficient for disorder and subject to counterexamples (e.g., grief, childbirth pain) because both normal and disordered distress and impairment are consequences that are in the individual. So, he understood that reiterating the in-the-individual or negative-consequence requirements would not address the definition's problems.

A close look at the 1978 paper reveals that Demazeux's central thesis that the notion of dysfunction is introduced as a superficial add-on with no intended important conceptual definitional role simply does not fit the paper's text. Spitzer and Endicott are quite explicit about the fundamental importance of the organismic dysfunction requirement, placing it on an equal footing with negative consequences, and make clear that it is introduced not as a stylistic variant but to address problems with the previous negative-consequence attempts. This is expressed quite clearly in an early section of the 1978 paper labeled "key concepts in the definition of medical disorder"—medical, not mental—and it begins:

> We believe that there are several fundamental concepts in the notion of a medical disorder: negative consequences of the condition, an inferred or identified organismic dysfunction, and an implicit call for action. There is no assumption that the organismic dysfunction or its negative consequences are of a physical nature. (1978, 17)

In analyzing the overarching concept of medical disorder, Spitzer and Endicott (1978) delineate "several fundamental concepts" in this notion—"fundamental," not superficial or redundant or unimportant. (I ignore the call to action as in fact redundant with negative consequences and in any event questionable on other grounds and later omitted by Spitzer in *DSM-III* and eventually explicitly disavowed [Spitzer, 1998].) The first fundamental concept is negative consequences, which includes distress, impairment, and disadvantage. Demazeux, implausibly, insists that this exhausts the essential meaning. The second fundamental concept, which is stated separately and distinguished from negative consequences, is organismic dysfunction. The next sentence, "There is no assumption that the organismic dysfunction or its negative consequences are of a physical nature," allows pluralism of etiological theory. It also makes clear that the pathological condition itself that has the negative consequences is in fact the organismic dysfunction and implies that the relationship between the organismic dysfunction and the negative consequences is a causal relationship, which, contra Demazeux, eliminates the possibility that the organismic dysfunction is just another way of specifying the negative consequences.

Relation of *DSM* Criteria to the Dysfunction Requirement

To buttress his case that dysfunction plays no role in *DSM* nosology, Demazeux calls me as a witness in my own prosecution, claiming that I assert that dysfunction plays no role in the formulation of specific diagnostic criteria:

> Wakefield himself recognizes that the whole classification rests on a strategy that does not pay the slightest attention to the dysfunction requirement: "…we can reason backward from the criteria for specific mental disorders to the definition of mental disorder that would make sense of them. Such an examination reveals that the concept of dysfunction plays no direct role in the formulation of specific diagnostic criteria in *DSM-III-R*. In no criterion do we find, for instance, a clause like 'the distress must have been caused by a dysfunction in the person' or any other reference to the existence of a dysfunction." (Wakefield 1992, 236)

This is a misreading. Rather than stating that the *DSM* "does not pay the slightest attention to the dysfunction requirement," I state quite clearly that "the concept of dysfunction plays no *direct* role in the *formulation* of specific diagnostic criteria in *DSM-III-R*." I then go on to explain what I mean, namely, that unlike the definition that refers to dysfunction explicitly, in no diagnostic criterion do we find a direct and *explicit* reference to dysfunction, such as "the distress must have been caused by a dysfunction." Rather, the criteria capture dysfunction indirectly through the way the criteria are selected to reflect that something has gone wrong with the organism and to provide adequate grounds for inferring a dysfunction (First and Wakefield 2013), much as Spitzer and Endicott's operational criteria for mental disorder do in the 1978 paper.

This approach is understandable. Given the *DSM*'s goals of increasing reliability while retaining validity in diagnoses by working clinicians, simply referring to the abstract notion of dysfunction is a less attractive strategy than providing operationalized criteria sufficient for inferring the likely presence of a dysfunction. Every feature of the criteria, including durational requirements, symptom thresholds, the specific nature of the symptoms, and even contextual exclusions—for example, you don't have a sexual dysfunction if the reason you've never had an orgasm is lack of adequate stimulation (Wakefield and First 2012)—are all best understood as attempts to operationalize the distinction between dysfunction and nondysfunction (First and Wakefield 2013; Wakefield and First 2012). The many nuanced decisions about such criteria can best be explained as attempts to formulate criteria that indicate dysfunction in the HDA's sense.

Is RDoC a Threat to the HDA?

Despite having argued at length that the *DSM-III*'s definition of mental disorder and the HDA are conceptually unrelated, Demazeux nonetheless goes on to argue that the HDA's plausibility is in doubt because it is dependent on a link to the *DSM* approach, and the *DSM* approach itself is threatened as evidenced by calls for a *DSM-5* "paradigm shift" and the recent inauguration of the National Institute of Mental Health's (NIMH's) RDoC program seeking the brain etiologies of mental disorders: "The universality of the *DSM* approach in psychiatry is recent and fragile, as attested by the recurrent appeals for a 'paradigm shift' and by the recent enthusiasm for the RDoC project launched by the NIMH."

In fact, the HDA has no special dependence on *DSM*'s current theory-neutral approach to diagnosis. That approach is a pragmatic necessity thrust upon psychiatry by the lack of knowledge of etiology. The notion, raised in the revision process that led to *DSM-5*, of a "paradigm shift" that would incorporate pathophysiology and biomarkers into diagnostic criteria turned out to be premature and evaporated in the course of revising *DSM-5*. However, there was nothing in it antagonistic to the HDA. Indeed, such progress toward etiological criteria that explicitly identified the dysfunction in a disorder rather than using etiology-neutral symptom-based criteria to indirectly indicate dysfunction had been envisioned by Spitzer from the beginning. He states as much in the introduction to *DSM-III* that also contains the definition of disorder:

> The approach taken in *DSM-III* is atheoretical with regard to etiology or pathophysiological process except for those disorders for which this is well established and therefore included in the definition of the disorder. Undoubtedly, with time, some of the disorders of unknown etiology will be found to have specific biological etiologies, others to have specific psychological causes, and still others to result mainly from a particular interplay of psychological, social and biological factors. (Spitzer 1980, 7)

The *DSM-5* "paradigm shift" language was misleading and displayed a lack of understanding that theory-neutral criteria were created merely as a stop-gap against unreliability and invalidity given ignorance of the etiological essences of disorders. It is scientific progress, not a paradigm shift, to finally identify the long-sought essence of a phenomenon one has been studying.

In any event, the potential "paradigm shift" has now become the task of RDoC. Given the reality of the lack of understanding of the hypothesized brain dysfunctions underlying mental disorders, even the RDoC website now disavows any intention of replacing standard diagnostic systems any time soon. We just don't know enough to do so. However, is Demazeux correct that in principle, the RDoC program's potential dethronement of the *DSM* etiology-neutral approach to diagnosis presents a basic challenge to the HDA?

Contrary to Demazeux's analysis, the *DSM* and RDoC approaches are equally consistent with the HDA. Nothing more clearly illustrates Demazeux's misunderstanding of the situation than the fact that leaders of the RDoC initiative themselves credit the HDA for being part of the inspiration for the initiative. One of the RDoC's primary developers and defenders, Bruce Cuthbert, includes in his standard PowerPoint slide set presenting the RDoC program the following slide: "RDoC: Conceptual Approach. Try to understand mental disorders in terms of deviations from normal functioning of psychological and neurobiological mechanisms. Cf. Wakefield, 'harmful dysfunction'" (Bruce Cuthbert, personal communication, May 27, 2015). Both the failed paradigm shift toward explicit pathophysiological underpinnings attempted in *DSM-5* and the current RDoC program's attempt to identify brain dysfunctions underlying mental disorders are entirely consistent with and indeed presuppose something like the HDA's account of disorder.

Demazeux seems to have been misled by the fact that in some sense, the RDoC program is (or was, as initially presented) "opposed" to *DSM*, and because the HDA explains *DSM*'s approach, the HDA must also be opposed by RDoC. Things don't work that way. Opposed views, if they are both views of disorder, will both be committed to an HDA conceptualization but opposed on other aspects of diagnosis. The ill-fated aspiration to a *DSM* "paradigm shift" as well as the current RDoC program has nothing to do with the concept of disorder per se and a lot to do with different approaches to identifying the dysfunctions required for disorder by the HDA.

The Historicist Challenge: Three Proposed Counterexamples to the HDA

Once Demazeux thinks he has established conceptual daylight between the core of Spitzer's 1978 and 1980 definitions and the HDA, this opens the historicist spigot and emboldens him to engage in a wider search for historical counterexamples to the HDA. Indeed, through his historicist-colored lens, Demazeux finds it beyond comprehension that I claim that human beings can share salient concepts across historical episodes, asking incredulously, "Does Wakefield really think that, despite the many hesitations and theoretical reversals in the long run, the concept of mental disorder has retained a fixed meaning?" The answer is "yes"; I believe the notion of disorder has been more or less constant since Hippocrates.

Of course, theories of disorder and judgments about specific instances of disorder and nondisorder change over time for a variety of reasons, but the conceptual understanding of disorder—that is, the conceptual understanding of what is being asserted when one says that a given instance is or is not a disorder—can still remain constant over time. It is also true that in the history of views of mental pathology, there is much nonsense, and terms like "pathology" and its cognates are often used loosely and incorrectly as terms of abuse, exploiting the value component of disorder or denied as a means of liberation from medical categorization. However, the HDA implies that one can generally discern a harmful dysfunction structure behind such claims and counterclaims in serious discussions. There is no reason why one should see anything like such a correlation on Demazeux's ecumenical approach that allows sheer harm, which is everywhere, to determine disorder. I have offered examples: for example, conservative Victorian physicians claimed that female clitoral orgasm during intercourse is a disorder, whereas Masters and Johnson (1966) claim that lack of clitoral orgasm during intercourse is a disorder, and, as the HDA predicts, one finds that these opposite views represent not merely a relativistic historicist conceptual divide but two different theories of biological design that determine the opinion of what is a dysfunction. Similarly, the diagnosis of runaway slaves as having the disorder of drapetomania was not justified by an alternative account of disorder but through theories, common in the antebellum South, that those enslaved were naturally designed to be subservient.

Demazeux dismisses these examples in which mistaken diagnoses were justified by mistaken accounts of natural function and dysfunction and challenges me with his own examples that are supposed to illustrate the historical limitations of the HDA:

> It is not a risky claim to say that clitoral orgasm and drapetomania were once wrongly conceived as mental disorders, since the ideological motivations are easy to reconstruct. By contrast, it is a more difficult task to historically investigate such conditions as pathological infantilism (Ribot 1896), childish character (Dupré 1903), or the diagnosis of dependent personality disorder in *DSM-III* (American Psychiatric Association 1980, 324). There is a historical relation in the conceptualization of these three labels that could remain obscure if one looks only at the "conceptual validity" (according to the HDA) of each construct taken separately.

Demazeux appears here to take it as a criticism of the HDA that it does not cover various sociohistorical aspects of mental disorder judgments. However, the HDA is not designed to address such problems. Of course, I agree with Demazeux that there are endless historical insights and hidden influences and motives one might discover about disorder attributions that have nothing to do with conceptual validity or other conceptual issues related to the HDA. For example, social values and ideologies regularly determine what people think is natural functioning and dysfunction and can lead them to judge, often incorrectly, that various behaviors are disordered. The HDA is an account of the meaning of claims about disorder, not a theory of why such claims are made. Without an understanding of the concept of disorder of the kind provided by the HDA, sociological studies of shifting views of conditions as disorders or nondisorders are likely to be quite confused.

The relevant question is: Are the categories selected by Demazeux, two of which long antedate the *DSM*, counterexamples to the HDA, as he claims? I accept Demazeux's historicist challenge and examine whether the proposed counterexamples display an HDA structure that plausibly implies the presence of a dysfunction.

First, then, Ribot (1897/1903), writing of "the pathology of the moral sense," notes that one theory of criminality is "infantilism, which has recourse, not to heredity, but to arrested development, and alleges that the perversion which is permanent in the criminal is normal, but transient, in the child" (300). "Arrested development" in which what is transient in the child becomes fixated in the adult clearly refers to something going wrong with the natural design of the organism's development, that is, developmental dysfunction (cf. Wakefield 1997). If one has any doubt about this, consider Ribot's further descriptions of the general category of moral pathology as follows:

> "Moral insanity is a form of mental derangement in which the intellectual faculties appear to have sustained little or no injury, while the disorder is manifested principally or alone in the state of the feelings, temper, or habit." Such is the formula of Prichard...it signifies: a complete absence or perversion of the altruistic feelings, insensibility to the representation of the happiness or suffering of others, absolute egoism, with all its consequences. By a self-evident analogy, this state has been called one of moral blindness; and, like physical blindness, it has various degrees. It has also been compared to idiocy. (301)

> The character is an un-coordinated bundle of appetites and wishes, each of which, in turn, drives out the rest. Then there is weakness or total absence of will under its higher inhibitory form, which rules and coordinates. Are they impulsive for want of inhibition, or incapable of controlling themselves through the excess of their impulses? Both these cases are met with, and the result is the same. The formula of their character...is the same as that of the unstable—i.e., there is no constituted character.

> The term *infantilism* is equally applicable to the congenital and the acquired forms. The former have never left their childhood behind, the latter return to it....In the one case we have arrested development, in the other retrogression. In short,...character has either not come into being or has ceased to exist. (422)

These descriptions are clear attempts to identify psychological dysfunctions of the kind that we too would currently recognize. Arrested development and atavistic return to a childlike state are standard views of dysfunction, and when Ribot characterizes infantilism as the failure of adult personality to develop, this suggests what today we would call a personality disorder. Note further that Ribot's views of the emotions were shaped by the James-Lange theory: "The doctrine which I have called physiological (Bain, Spencer, Maudsley, James, Lange) connects all states of feeling with biological conditions....It is the thesis which has been adopted, without any restriction, in this work" (1903, vii). The James-Lange theory was itself explicitly an outgrowth of a Darwinian evolutionary functionalist analysis, as is Ribot's approach.

Turning now to Dupré, I was unable to locate a translation of Dupré's work cited by Demazeux, but here is how Wikipedia summarizes his theory:

> Ernest Dupré developed a biopsychological theory of the origin of crime: the theory of instinctive perversions. For him, there are three instincts in man: the instinct of reproduction, the instinct of preservation and the instinct of association. In the criminal, these instincts are the object of abnormalities which can be excesses, atrophies or even inversions like suicide attempts for the instinct of preservation. According to Dupré, these anomalies can lead to perversions that may lead to the commission of offenses. (Ernest Dupré n.d.)

There is no question that Dupré's account, like Ribot's, falls within the HDA's conceptual umbrella. Dupré follows the standard classical schema of the triad of ways that biological functions can go wrong and become medical pathology. Relative to its natural normal-range level and target, a mechanism's functioning can go wrong by being hyperactive (higher than normal range), hypoactive (lower than normal range), or perverse (directed at a biologically unnatural target). Behind this triad is an implicit understanding of natural functions and how they can go wrong that makes Dupré's analysis consistent with an HDA-type schema.

Demazeux focuses on the harmful moral deviation that marked many early (and current) mental disorder categories, suggesting that somehow this focus on morality is in tension with the HDA. However, first, one must keep in mind the fact that at the time, "moral" was used broadly for mental and emotional conditions (Shorter 1993; Weiner 1990); for example, during this period, economics and sociology are described as "moral sciences." Demazeux emphasizes the "importance of such moral considerations which were built into the very conception of madness," but other historians insist that in this literature, "the fact that something is 'moral' in the psychological sense should not be taken to imply that it is also 'moral' in the ethical sense" (Charland 2008, 16). In any event, the above examination of Demazeux's examples reveals that it is not simply the moral or emotional deviance as such that warrants attribution of disorder in Ribot's or Dupré's accounts. Rather, it is the fact that the moral or emotional depravity is taken to reveal the presence of a dysfunction in the HDA sense, in which normal functioning of some internal mechanisms has gone awry to cause the moral symptoms.

Regarding Demazeux's example of *DSM-III* dependent personality disorder, it must first be said that the entire category of personality disorders and its diagnosis was quite controversial at the time of *DSM-III*. As discussed in Spitzer and Endicott's 1978 paper, a distinction was drawn between personality traits that are problematic but part of normal variation versus failure of personality organization to perform its hypothesized functions such as "the ability to form relatively stable and nonconflictual relationships" (1978, 34). *DSM-III* distinguished personality disorders from undesirable personality traits as follows: "Personality *traits* are enduring patterns of perceiving, relating to, and thinking about the environment and oneself, and are exhibited in a wide range of important social and personal contexts. It is only when *personality traits* are inflexible and maladaptive and cause either significant impairment in social or occupational functioning or subjective distress that they constitute *Personality Disorders*" (American Psychiatric Association 1980, 305). Whether or not one accepts the validity of *DSM-III*'s general characterization of personality disorders (I do not; e.g., Wakefield 2008), the requirement that pathological traits be "inflexible" and "maladaptive" are plausibly understood as an attempt to suggest a dysfunction of personality organization that causes the consequent harms.

Turning to Demazeux's specific example, to warrant diagnosis of *DSM-III* dependent personality disorder, the following characteristics of the individual's long-term functioning must cause impaired social or occupational functioning or subjective distress:

A. Passively allows others to assume responsibility for major areas of life because of inability to function independently (e.g., lets spouse decide what kind of job he or she should have).

B. Subordinates own needs to those of persons on whom he or she depends in order to avoid any possibility of having to rely on self, e.g., tolerates abusive spouse.

C. Lacks self-confidence, e.g., sees self as helpless, stupid. (American Psychiatric Association 1980, 325–326)

The description of an individual who is unable to function independently and is dependent on someone else to the degree of subordinating all his or her needs to those of the other is surely aimed at suggesting a problem that goes beyond undesirable normal variation to constitute some sort of dysfunction, as the 1978 discussion indicates. Nonetheless, one can easily see why this category has been quite controversial. The HDA can explain the nature of the controversy, whereas Demazeux's focus exclusively on harms like distress and impairment cannot. Credible questions arose as to whether these criteria, which were generally agreed to pick out characteristics that are negative and harmful in our modern society, do in fact pick out a dysfunction-caused disorder or merely label undesirable but normal-range functioning that is socially shaped. Feminist critics pointed out was that there was an alternative explanation to dysfunction for the inflexible and seemingly maladaptive maintenance of these submissive and often self-destructive patterns, namely, adoption of the traditional gender role model in our culture of ideal feminine behavior as passive and submissive to a partner's needs. Feminists argued that, given that women were traditionally socialized to be unassertive, this category pathologized those who most firmly embraced those traditional social values that were in conflict with newly emerging vision of more assertive and egalitarian female behavior. In such cases, there might be distress or impairment, but there was no genuine dysfunction, just social conformity. Opponents in the dependent personality debate agreed that the described degree of submissiveness is harmful and negative and should be the target of efforts at change, yet, contrary to a sheer harm-based approach, they still vigorously disagreed about its pathological status. What, then, were they disagreeing about? The HDA offers an answer; they were disagreeing about whether there is a dysfunction.

Incidentally, despite the objections, the category has survived thus far and appears in *DSM-5*. This is perhaps because the claim that the diagnosis is undergirded by a dysfunction has been indirectly buttressed by the theory, disputable but widely accepted, that such dependent behavior represents an insecure form of attachment in childhood as described in John Bowlby's popular attachment theory and that such variants of attachment are inherently dysfunctions and pathological. Finally, regarding the relationship of the HDA to the personality disorders, it may be worth mentioning that in the run-up to *DSM-5*, there was explicit mention of the HDA and the citation of HDA articles in the work group's discussion of revisions to personality disorder categories.

Regarding the above examples, Demazeux states, "There is a historical relation in the conceptualization of these three labels that could remain obscure if one looks only at the 'conceptual validity' (according to the HDA) of each construct taken separately." This may well be correct. The HDA, which is a theory of conceptual validity, does not address these or many, many other questions. It only addresses the one question of the logical structure of disorder attributions.

I conclude that, despite having centuries of examples from which to choose to prove his historicist point, Demazeux's handpicked categories fail to provide clear counterexamples to the HDA. The failure of Demazeux's historical excursion offers unexpected support for my hypothesis that "the concept of mental disorder has retained a fixed meaning" across a broad domain of times and places.

What about Foucault?

My thesis that the HDA has broad cross-temporal applicability requires further comment. I have argued that a full conceptual/sociohistorical analysis would include both a conceptual component and a "Foucaultian" archeological/genealogical component that analyzes why a particular concept came to have social power and how the details of its deployment reflect strategies of power (Wakefield 2002). However, a meaningful historical sociology of concept deployment depends on a prior conceptual analysis to understand what concept was being deployed and what features made it attractive. Ignoring the necessary conceptual step was, I think, a central weakness of some of Foucault's analyses.

Demazeux sees a contradiction between the universal pretensions of the HDA and Foucault's statement that "in fact, before the nineteenth century, the experience of madness in the Western world was very polymorphic; and its confiscation in our own period in the concept of 'illness' must not deceive us as to its original exuberance" (Foucault 1976, 65–66). In my view, there is no contradiction. For Foucault, the shift he describes matters because "madness" is not (and was not) the same concept as "mental disorder"; otherwise, there was a mere terminological change with no substantive implications. Foucault's point is that earlier, there were various ways of understanding a certain set of phenomena as "madness," but those phenomena were recategorized under a single concept, "mental disorder," and thus understood differently. To understand the shift and evaluate Foucault's claim, one must ask what it entails conceptually to categorize a condition as a mental disorder. The HDA explains what it means to label a phenomenon as a disorder and thus explains the meaning of Foucault's claim that madness was reclassified as disorder.

Foucault is no doubt correct that, for example, the Enlightenment's emphasis on the desirability of reason led to a new view of some forms of irrationality, including those formerly vaguely categorized as "madness." The excessive pathologization of irrationality following acceptance of Enlightenment ideals of human functioning was a typical elevation of social values into a mistaken view of functional normality, analogous to Victorian pathologization of socially disapproved sexual pleasures. Foucault was not the only one to notice this aspect of the reaction to the Enlightenment. Consider, for example, the following statement published in 1885 by Carl Lange, the co-originator of the classic James-Lange theory of emotion inspired by Darwin's book on emotion, in which Lange explains his motivation in exploring the evolutionary theory of emotions:

> Kant, in a passage in his *Anthropologie*, qualifies the affections [i.e., emotions] as diseases of the mind. He considers the mind normal only as long as it is under the incontrovertible and absolute control of reason. Anything that causes it to be disturbed seems to him to be abnormal and harmful to the individual. To a more realistic school of psychology, which knows no abstract "Ideal" man, but rather "takes men as they are," such a doctrine of the soul must appear strange....Such a theory will consider the imperturbable arithmetic teacher, to whom every impression is merely an impulse to draw rational conclusions, as the only normal, healthy individual. (Lange 1885/1922, 33)

As Foucault and many others have made clear, the same conditions may be conceptualized in different ways at different times or places. Indeed, in our own time, there are heated debates about whether to understand various conditions, from depressive feelings during grief and fidgeting in school to the more provocative actions of President Trump, as normal-range features or disorders. The HDA does not attempt to explain the cultural history of thinking about the conditions that are now considered mental disorders or why the same conditions might be considered disorders at one time or place and nondisorders at another time or place. That is Foucault's domain. So, it is of course to be expected that there are endless points that "could remain obscure if one looks only at the 'conceptual validity' (according to the HDA) of each construct taken separately." The HDA is limited to attempting to explain the logic of what is being affirmed or denied when such attributions occur. One might add what I hope is clear by now: that there are equally many points that remain obscure if one looks only at the Foucaultian historicist claims without conceptual analysis.

From a Foucaultian perspective, the potential value of the HDA can easily be underrated. The HDA provides a framework for understanding how society can exploit medical concepts for social control purposes by relabeling as natural and unnatural socially desirable and undesirable behavior, respectively. Any serious attempt to explain medical disorder judgments, which have, to an amazing extent, been shared across epochs does lead one to the functional view, as documented in detail for the history of the category of depression in *The Loss of Sadness* (Horwitz and Wakefield 2007). In sum, with regard to historical understanding and explanation, the HDA provides illumination that explains much but not (as Demazeux unreasonably demands) more than an analysis of one concept can explain.

References

American Psychiatric Association. 1980. *Diagnostic and Statistical Manual of Mental Disorders*. 3rd ed. American Psychiatric Association.

Charland, L. C. 2008. A moral line in the sand. In *Fact and Value in Emotion*, L. C. Charland and P. Zachar (eds.), 15–33. John Benjamins.

Dupré, E. n.d. https://fr.wikipedia.org/wiki/Ernest_Dupr%C3%A9. August 2, 2018.

First, M. B., and J. C. Wakefield. 2010. Defining 'mental disorder' in *DSM-V*. *Psychological Medicine* 40(11): 1779–1782.

First, M. B., and J. C. Wakefield. 2013. Diagnostic criteria as dysfunction indicators: Bridging the chasm between the definition of mental disorder and diagnostic criteria for specific disorders. *Canadian Journal of Psychiatry* 58(12): 663–669.

Foucault, M. 1976. *Mental Illness and Psychology*. University of California Press.

Horwitz, A. V., and J. C. Wakefield. 2007. *The Loss of Sadness: How Psychiatry Transformed Normal Sorrow into Depressive Disorder*. Oxford University Press.

Lange, C. G. 1855/1922. The emotions: A psychophysiological study (I. A. Haupt, trans.). In *The Emotions*, K. Dunlap (ed.), 33–90. Williams & Wilkins.

Masters, W. H., and V. E. Johnson. 1966. *Human Sexual Response*. Little, Brown.

Ribot, T. 1897/1903. *The Psychology of the Emotions*. Walter Scott Publishing Co.

Shorter, E. 1993. *A Short History of Psychiatry*. John Wiley.

Spitzer, R. L. 1980. Introduction. In *Diagnostic and Statistical Manual of Mental Disorders*, 1–12. 3rd ed. American Psychiatric Association.

Spitzer, R. L. 1981. The diagnostic status of homosexuality in *DSM-III*: A reformulation of the issues. *American Journal of Psychiatry* 138(2): 210–215.

Spitzer, R. L. 1997. Brief comments from a psychiatric nosologist weary from his own attempts to define mental disorder: Why Ossorio's definition muddles and Wakefield's "harmful dysfunction" illuminates the issues. *Clinical Psychology: Science and Practice* 4(3): 259–261.

Spitzer, R. L. 1998. Diagnosis and need for treatment are not the same. *Archives of General Psychiatry* 55(2): 120.

Spitzer, R. L. 1999. Harmful dysfunction and the *DSM* definition of mental disorder. *Journal of Abnormal Psychology* 108(3): 430–432.

Spitzer, R. L., and J. Endicott. 1978. Medical and mental disorder: Proposed definition and criteria. In *Critical Issues in Psychiatric Diagnosis*, R. L. Spitzer and D. F. Klein (eds.), 15–39. Raven Press.

Spitzer, R. L., and J. B. W. Williams. 1982. The definition and diagnosis of mental disorder. In *Deviance and Mental Illness*, W. R. Gove (ed.), 15–31. Sage.

Spitzer, R. L., J. B. W. Williams, and A. E. Skodol. 1980. *DSM-III*: The major achievements and an overview. *American Journal of Psychiatry* 137(2): 151–164.

Spitzer, R. L., and P. T. Wilson. 1975. Nosology and the official psychiatric nomenclature. In *Comprehensive Textbook of Psychiatry*, A. M. Freedman, H. I. Kaplan, and B. J. Sadock (eds.), 826–845. Vol. 2. Williams & Wilkins.

Wakefield, J. C. 1988. Female primary orgasmic dysfunction: Masters and Johnson versus *DSM-III-R* on diagnosis and incidence. *Journal of Sex Research* 24: 363–377.

Wakefield, J. C. 1992a. The concept of mental disorder: On the boundary between biological facts and social values. *American Psychologist* 47: 373–388.

Wakefield, J. C. 1992b. Disorder as harmful dysfunction: A conceptual critique of *DSM-III-R*'s definition of mental disorder. *Psychological Review* 99: 232–247.

Wakefield, J. C. 1993. Limits of operationalization: A critique of Spitzer and Endicott's (1978) proposed operational criteria of mental disorder. *Journal of Abnormal Psychology* 102: 160–172.

Wakefield, J. C. 1995. Dysfunction as a value-free concept: A reply to Sadler and Agich. *Philosophy, Psychiatry, and Psychology* 2: 233–46.

Wakefield, J. C. 1997a. Diagnosing *DSM-IV*, part 1: *DSM-IV* and the concept of mental disorder. *Behaviour Research and Therapy* 35: 633–650.

Wakefield, J. C. 1997b. Diagnosing *DSM-IV*, part 2: Eysenck (1986) and the essentialist fallacy. *Behaviour Research and Therapy*: 35: 651–666.

Wakefield, J. C. 1997c. Normal inability versus pathological disability: Why Ossorio's (1985) definition of mental disorder is not sufficient. *Clinical Psychology: Science and Practice* 4: 249–258.

Wakefield, J. C. 1997d. When is development disordered? Developmental psychopathology and the harmful dysfunction analysis of mental disorder. *Development and Psychopathology* 9: 269–290.

Wakefield, J. C. 1998. The *DSM*'s theory-neutral nosology is scientifically progressive: Response to Follette and Houts. *Journal of Consulting and Clinical Psychology* 66: 846–852.

Wakefield, J. C. 1999a. Evolutionary versus prototype analyses of the concept of disorder. *Journal of Abnormal Psychology* 108: 374–399.

Wakefield, J. C. 1999b. Mental disorder as a black box essentialist concept. *Journal of Abnormal Psychology* 108: 465–472.

Wakefield, J. C. 2000a. Aristotle as sociobiologist: The "function of a human being" argument, black box essentialism, and the concept of mental disorder. *Philosophy, Psychiatry, and Psychology* 7: 17–44.

Wakefield, J. C. 2000b. Spandrels, vestigial organs, and such: Reply to Murphy and Woolfolk's "The harmful dysfunction analysis of mental disorder." *Philosophy, Psychiatry, and Psychology* 7: 253–269.

Wakefield, J. C. 2001. Evolutionary history versus current causal role in the definition of disorder: Reply to McNally. *Behaviour Research and Therapy* 39: 347–366.

Wakefield, J. C. 2002. Fixing a Foucault sandwich: Cognitive universals and cultural particulars in the concept of mental disorder. In *Culture in Mind: Toward a Sociology of Culture and Cognition*, K. A. Cerulo (ed.), 245–266. Routledge.

Wakefield, J. C. 2006. What makes a mental disorder mental? *Philosophy, Psychiatry, and Psychology* 13: 123–131.

Wakefield, J. C. 2007. The concept of mental disorder: Diagnostic implications of the harmful dysfunction analysis. *World Psychiatry* 6: 149–156.

Wakefield, J. C. 2009. Mental disorder and moral responsibility: Disorders of personhood as harmful dysfunctions, with special reference to alcoholism. *Philosophy, Psychiatry, and Psychology* 16: 91–99.

Wakefield, J. C. 2011. Darwin, functional explanation, and the philosophy of psychiatry. In *Maladapting Minds: Philosophy, Psychiatry, and Evolutionary Theory*, P. R. Andriaens and A. De Block (eds.), 143–172. Oxford University Press.

Wakefield, J. C. 2014. The biostatistical theory versus the harmful dysfunction analysis, part 1: Is part-dysfunction a sufficient condition for medical disorder? *Journal of Medicine and Philosophy* 39: 648–682.

Wakefield, J. C. 2016a. The concepts of biological function and dysfunction: Toward a conceptual foundation for evolutionary psychopathology. In *Handbook of Evolutionary Psychology*, D. Buss (ed.), 2nd ed., vol. 2, 988–1006. Oxford University Press.

Wakefield, J. C. 2016b. Diagnostic issues and controversies in *DSM-5*: Return of the false positives problem. *Annual Review of Clinical Psychology* 12: 105–132.

Wakefield, J. C. Forthcoming. *Robert Spitzer and the Definition of Mental Disorder*. Oxford University Press.

Wakefield, J. C., and M. B. First. 2003. Clarifying the distinction between disorder and nondisorder: Confronting the overdiagnosis ("false positives") problem in *DSM-V*. In *Advancing DSM: Dilemmas in Psychiatric Diagnosis*, K. A. Phillips, M. B. First, and H. A. Pincus (eds.), 23–56. American Psychiatric Press.

Wakefield, J. C., and M. B. First. 2012. Placing symptoms in context: The role of contextual criteria in reducing false positives in *DSM* diagnosis. *Comprehensive Psychiatry* 53: 130–139.

Weiner, D. B. 1990. Mind and body in the clinic: Phillippe Pinel, Alexander Chrichton, Dominque Esquirol, and the birth of psychiatry. In *The Languages of Psyche: Mind and Body in Enlightenment Thought*, G. S. Rousseau (ed.), 331–402. University of California Press.

3 Facts, Facts, Facts: HD Analysis Goes Factual

Luc Faucher

Wakefield's harmful dysfunction (henceforth HD in what follows) analysis has received well-deserved attention in psychiatry and philosophy. Although many commentators have considered Wakefield's analysis to be correct (or at least on the right track), there is also no shortage of criticism as to his position. I want my contribution to be of a different "flavor" than what is usually found in literature on Wakefield (with the exception of De Block 2008). In fact, I want to indicate a few places where his analysis could make fruitful contact with empirical research. To be more specific, I want to accomplish two things in this chapter. First, I hope to show that "going factual" might reveal why disputes about which analysis of the concept of mental disorder is the right analysis are so endemic in both psychiatry and philosophy. Indeed, Wakefield claims that his analysis is the result of a conceptual analysis. After the recent wave of X-Philosophy investigations, one becomes suspicious of what is presented as an armchair analysis of a concept. I want to suggest that we might want to "go X" in the case of the concept(s) used in psychiatry too and conduct empirical investigations of the concept of mental disorder that ordinary individuals and specialists have (as I will demonstrate, Wakefield is aware of the limits of conceptual analysis and has "gone X"). I want to propose a few experiments that should be performed in order to probe our concepts about mental disorders, but I also want to present different techniques available to the X-Philosopher and suggest that some techniques might be more adequate to investigate our concept of mental disorder. These techniques might reveal a diversity of ways to conceptualize mental disorders that explain why discussions on this topic have endured. Second, I want to argue that an empirical attitude might make the dysfunction component of the analysis more speculative (but not entirely so) than Wakefield seems to think. Indeed, Wakefield has suggested that hope for a more "factual" psychiatry lies in the development of evolutionary psychiatry. I want to show that, at least for some disorders, prospects are not promising in terms of arriving at something other than speculation about mechanisms that are malfunctioning. This does not put into question Wakefield's conceptual analysis, but shows that it might be of limited use in certain cases.

Before discussing these points of contact, let me briefly summarize Wakefield's analysis.

I. HD Analysis

In a series of papers (1992a, 1992b, 1993, 1999, 2000, 2007a), Jerome Wakefield proposes a definition of the concept of "mental disorder" that he hopes will provide psychiatry with an objective criterion for declaring a mental condition a disorder. His definition is presented as an "explicitation" of the intuitive concept of disorder used not only by health professionals (in medicine in general and in psychiatry) but also by the general public (e.g., Wakefield et al. 2006, 212; Wakefield 2007a, 150). Wakefield has also argued that his HD analysis "has proven useful for thinking about the validity of diagnostic criteria; in particular, explicitly formulating issues in terms of function and dysfunction seems to help identify false positives and limit undue diagnostic expansiveness" (2006, 159).[1] As Jeffrey Poland (2003) puts it, Wakefield's HD analysis has two distinct aspects: a descriptive one (which consists of adequately capturing and reconstructing our shared concept of mental disorders) and a normative one (which consists of using the shared concept to evaluate current diagnostic criteria).

Wakefield believes that we can analyze the intuitive concept of "mental disorder" underlying the field of psychiatry (and our ordinary judgments about who's disordered and who's not) by saying that it is the result of a "dysfunction" of a psychological or mental mechanism[2] that is judged "harmful" (e.g., 1993, 163). This definition is a hybrid account of disorder for it has both a purely scientific and factual component (the notion of dysfunction) and a value component (the notion of harm). According to Wakefield, both of these components are jointly necessary to capture our intuitive concept of mental illness (1992a, 374). Wakefield has little to say about the "value" component of his definition[3]; he is far more interested in the notion of dysfunction that, he expects, will provide psychiatry the objective foundations it needs.

Although the notions of "function" and "dysfunction" or "malfunction" have been used in medicine and psychiatry for a long time, according to Wakefield, only evolutionary theory can analyze these in causal and scientific terms. Thus, he proposes understanding previous uses of function as cases of what he calls "black-box essentialism." This theory is an extension of Putnam's theory of reference that asserts that we use concepts on the basis of defeasible stereotypical properties (e.g., using "water," the fact of being transparent, liquid, drinkable, etc.) before the underlying essence of what we refer to is scientifically discovered (e.g., the concept of "water" existed long before we finally discovered its underlying essence, in this case, its molecular structure). Wakefield's idea is that the notion of function (and malfunction) used by Aristotle, Harvey, and others has been based on prototypical instances of "non-accidentally beneficial effects like sight [in the case of the eyes] and on the idea that some common underlying process must be responsible for such remarkable phenomena" (2000, 39). However, the process responsible for such phenomena was unknown until the advent of Darwinian theory. Since then, though, one must make reference to evolutionary biology in order to determine the "real" function of mental mechanisms that are supposed to be dysfunctional. As Wakefield puts it, "[If] the HD analysis is at least roughly correct, however, then validly distinguishing disorder from non-disorder depends on an evolutionary-functional analysis" (2006, 158; see also 1993, 170). One can thus understand that Wakefield is making two separate claims: (1) the correct analysis of our concept of mental disorder has to be made in terms of harm and dysfunction of a mental mechanism, and (2) the correct understanding of the concept of dysfunction is in terms of evolutionary function. For this reason, some (e.g., Poland 2003) distinguish HD analysis from HDW analysis because one could agree with (1) and not with (2) (see, e.g., Woolfolk 1999; Roe and Murphy 2011).

I will say a few words about the evolutionary analysis of function. According to evolutionary theory, the presence of certain traits (including psychological mechanisms responsible for behaviors) is explained by the fact that these traits (or mechanisms) performed certain functions in the organisms' ancestors, the effects of which had been beneficial enough for the organisms' ancestors to preserve them in their species through natural selection. The function for which a trait (or a mechanism) had been selected is what has been called in philosophical literature the "normal function" or "proper function" of that trait (or mechanism) (Millikan 2002; Neander 1991). In other words, the normal or proper function of mechanism X is to do what it has been designed to do by natural selection. It follows that there is a dysfunction or a malfunction when a trait (or a mechanism) is not able to properly accomplish its normal function. It should be noted that the notion of "normal function" is independent of the current adaptivity of the trait (or of the mechanism). Thus, the fact that a trait (or mechanism) is maladaptive in a current environment is not necessarily a sign of a dysfunction. To use one of Wakefield's examples, the fact that we are not capable of breathing under water is not an indication of a malfunction of the lungs, but rather of the fact that lungs can't perform their function in environments for which they have not been designed.[4] It should also be noted that the notion of function is presumed to be independent of our values.[5] For instance, imagine that killing and rape have been found to be produced by mechanisms that have been selected for (as some would argue; for references to killing, see, e.g., Buss 2006; for rape, see Thornhill and Palmer 2000). If such were the case, we would have to judge that, when the mechanisms responsible for these behaviors are in good working order, these behaviors are adaptive, even though we abhor them.

II. Conceptual Analysis as a Form of Empirical Psychology

As mentioned earlier, Wakefield sees his analysis as the result of a form of conceptual analysis of concepts used not only by those working in the psychiatric field but also by ordinary people when they are judging a condition to be disordered or not. Conceptual analysis is a philosopher's tool and seeks to provide the set of necessary and sufficient conditions for the application of a concept. Proposed analyses are usually tested against the philosopher's intuitions or against what philosophers think individuals' intuitions are (see, e.g., Horwitz and Wakefield 2012, 79). Indeed, generally, philosophers use imagined cases where one condition deemed to be necessary for the application of a concept would be missing, or where all conditions would be present, and see if the concept is judged to apply in those circumstances or if it generates counterintuitive consequences and is judged not to apply. For instance, Aristotle famously proposed an analysis of the concept of responsibility in which someone is said to be responsible if and only if they meet two conditions: the knowledge condition (someone has to know what they are doing) and the control condition (someone has to be in control of what they are doing). A philosopher could test this analysis by imagining cases where someone does not know what they are doing (e.g., someone becomes entangled in an argument and forgets that they left their dog in the car) or where that person knows what they are doing but has no control over it. An analysis is said to be valid if it agrees with one's intuition and invalid if it disagrees with intuition (at least when applied to clear cases). Thus, intuitions—more specifically, the philosopher's intuitions—are considered "evidence" in determining the adequacy of a conceptual analysis.

Wakefield rightly sees this kind of investigation as a form of empirical psychology. As he puts it, "Our conceptual enterprise is also an empirical enterprise aimed at discovering a certain fact about the world, namely what conceptual criterion or definition in the heads of people in our linguistic community ultimately determines and explains their judgments about whatever conditions are mental disorders" (1997, 257).[6] He also identifies quite well one of the premises on which conceptual analysis relies when he writes that "the process of conceptual analysis does not look empirical because one generally uses one's own intuitions about the clear cases rather than going out and collecting data. However, *this oddity results from the presupposition that one is dealing with a culturally shared concept, and the confidence that one's clear intuitions about the application of the term are likely to be shared*" (1997, 257, my emphasis).

But, one might wonder, what are the grounds for such a presupposition? After all, the individual performing the analysis (in our case, Wakefield or another philosopher of psychiatry) might not be representative of others' intuitions about a concept. His intuition might be idiosyncratic or group or culture relative. Moreover, the method of conceptual analysis (which usually describes rather abstract cases and seeks to describe explicit concepts) might not be able to unveil certain aspects of our conceptual knowledge (e.g., implicit aspects of our knowledge) or the variability of our concepts in different contexts.[7]

These kinds of shortcomings in conceptual analysis inspired a new movement in philosophy: experimental philosophy (or X-Phi in what follows). As one of the early advocates of this form of philosophy claims, "Experimental philosophy focuses on many of the same types of intuitions that have long been at the center of philosophical study, but it examines those intuitions using the methods associated with contemporary cognitive science—systematic experimentation and statistical analysis" (Knobe 2007, 81). Such methods have been used in philosophy of mind, epistemology, ethics, aesthetics, philosophy of race, philosophy of science, philosophy of language, and many more areas of philosophy, leading to many unexpected results. Allow me to briefly describe to you what Knobe has in mind when he talks about X-Phi using two examples.

The first example comes from the work of Nichols and colleagues (2003) on epistemic intuitions. They wanted to test the classical conceptual analysis of the concept of knowledge as justified true beliefs (so in order to have knowledge, it is not sufficient to have a true belief, you must have a *justified* true belief). In order to test this analysis, Nichols et al. submitted the following vignettes to members of different ethnic communities: "Bob is a friend to Jill, who has driven a Buick for many years. Bob therefore thinks that Jill drives an American car. He is not aware, however, that her Buick has recently been stolen, and he is not aware that Jill has replaced it with a Pontiac, which is a different kind of American car. Does Bob really know that Jill drives an American car, or does he only believe it?" (234). They then asked subjects the following question: "Does Bob really know or does he only believe that Jill drives an American car?" The results were quite surprising as 74% Western-heritage subjects said that Bob *only believes* that Jill drives an American car while 57% of subjects from East Asia and 61% of subjects from India said that he *really knows* that Jill drives an American car. If the results of this study were to generalize, it would prove that the concept of knowledge is understood differently in different cultures and that one cannot extend their conceptual analysis to other cultures.[8]

My second example involves the concept of responsibility. Intrigued by results from Nahmias (2006; Nahmias et al. 2005) that demonstrate that, contrary to philosophers' expectations, people judged an agent as morally blameworthy even if they have performed their immoral action in a deterministic universe, Nichols and Knobe (2007) designed a series of experiments to test people's intuitions about moral responsibility. They probed the intuitions of subjects by presenting them randomly one of two vignettes concerning a universe (Universe A) in which every event unfolds according to deterministic laws. Subjects in the "abstract condition" were given the following question:

In Universe A, is it possible for a person to be fully morally responsible for their action?

Subjects in the "concrete condition" were given the following question:

In Universe A, a man named Bill has become attracted to his secretary, and he decides that the only way to be with her is to kill his wife and 3 children. He knows that it is impossible to escape from his house in the event of a fire. Before he leaves on a business trip, he sets up a device in his basement that burns down the house and kills his family. Is Bill fully morally responsible for killing his wife and children?

The results were that only 5% of subjects in the abstract condition said that the agent (Bill) was fully morally responsible, while 72% of subjects in the concrete condition said he was fully morally responsible.

Experiments such as the following have led Knobe and Doris (2010) to argue that recent work in experimental philosophy about moral responsibility shows that our attribution of moral responsibility depends on and changes as a function of certain contextual variables. They call this idea "variantism," as opposed to "invariantism." They argue that invariantism has dominated philosophical discussions up to now and consists of the idea "that people should apply the *same* criteria in *all* of their moral responsibility judgments. In other words, it is supposed to be possible to come up with a single basic set of criteria that can account for all moral responsibility judgments in all cases" (322). However, they observe that "it seems that people do not make moral responsibility judgments by applying invariant principles. Instead, it appears that people tend to apply quite different criteria in different kinds of cases. Thus if one wants to understand why people make the judgments they do, it is no use looking for a single basic set of criteria that fits all people's ordinary judgments. A more promising approach would be to look at how and why people may adopt different criteria in different cases, depending on the way an issue is framed, whether an agent is a friend or a stranger, and so on" (322).

Thus, as these two examples show, X-Phi takes seriously the idea of empirically probing the intuition of ordinary people (but also of scientific communities; see, e.g., Griffiths and Stotz 2008) and does so by applying methods inspired by psychology and the social sciences to do it. By so doing, it has revealed surprising and puzzling facts about people's intuitions. So great is the success of X-Phi that one could even argue that it's now the only way to probe people's intuitions. Given this, it is natural to propose that Wakefield should go the way of X-Phi. Given the limits of traditional conceptual analysis, Wakefield should apply X-Phi methods to his topic of interest. Interestingly, this is precisely what the *Research Agenda* (Kupfer et al. 2002) suggested back at the beginning of the process that was to lead to the *Diagnostic and Statistical Manual of Mental Disorders* (*DSM-5*). As the authors of the agenda stated, the question of what is the concept of mental illness used by clinicians could be addressed by

conduct[ing] surveys…to elucidate the concepts of disease or of mental illness or disorder used, explicitly or implicitly, by psychiatrists, other physicians, clinical psychologists, research workers, patients, health care providers, and members of different social and ethnic groups. This could be done either by exploring the meaning they attribute to such terms or by asking them to decide which of a list of contentious conditions they themselves regarded as disease or mental disorders. (7)

One will probably be surprised to learn (as I was initially) that Wakefield actually went X! In a pilot study (Kirk et al. 1999) and another study (2002), Wakefield and his colleagues tested social workers' judgments of mental disorders. More precisely, they tried to determine "to what extent do social workers use contextual information to distinguish between disordered and non-disordered adolescent antisocial behaviour?" (Kirk et al. 1999, 84). The question that Wakefield was interested in was the following: are social workers making the distinction between someone whose symptoms are normal reactions to their social environment (and therefore is not disordered) and someone whose symptoms are not explained by their social environment but by internal dysfunction (and who therefore are suffering from a disorder), or are they "reluctant to pathologize deviant and nonconforming behaviours and would instead have a tendency to see them as normal responses by people in stressful or oppressive social environments" (Kirk et al. 1999, 85)?

In order to answer this question, Wakefield and his colleagues asked subjects to read three kinds of vignettes that they identify as "neutral," "environmental reaction," and "internal disorder." "Neutral" just describes a case where one youth, "Carlos," has three key symptoms of antisocial personality disorder. "Environmental reaction" asserts that environmental factors might explain why it was rational and adaptive to behave that way. Finally, "internal disorder" suggests that his reactions are the result of neither a rational nor an adaptive strategy. Here's an example of a vignette (for the sake of space, I am presenting an abridged version; for a complete description, see Kirk et al. 1999, 91):

> Carlos' family appears to be stable and caring. Carlos attends a respected public junior high school that has very little violence and provides a secure learning environment. However, Carlos reacts to the slightest perception of provocation with severe anger. Once he gets angry he often escalates fights from fists to weapons like bats and bricks even when the other boy wants to stop. Carlos consistently ignores his teachers' requests and discipline seems to only exacerbate his problematic behaviour. Even with those he hangs out with, Carlos is easily irritated and frequently initiates fights.

They then asked subjects (master's students in psychology or social work programs) if they agree or disagree with the following item[9] (they had to reply using a Likert scale ranging from 1 = "I strongly agree" to 6 = "I strongly disagree"): "According to my own view, this youth has a mental has a mental/psychiatric disorder."

The results were quite univocal: when the symptoms could be explained by the social context, only 2.9% of the subjects thought that the youth had a mental disorder; when the symptoms were not explained by the social context and could indicate an internal disorder (condition "internal disorder"), 95.2% agreed that he was suffering from a mental disorder. In a similar experiment, performed on nonprofessionals (non-psychiatric nurses, nonclinical social workers, undergraduates), they received somewhat similar results: with 7.9% of undergraduates saying that Carlos had a disorder in the environmental reaction vignette and 73.9% stating he had a disorder in the internal disorder vignette. Wakefield and colleagues conclude from these studies that "as predicted, identical behavioural symptoms meeting the *DSM-IV* criteria for conduct disorder are judged as less indicative of the presence of mental or psychiatric disorder in the environmental reaction context than they are in the internal dysfunction context" (Kirk et al. 1999, 92).

If these results are suggestive that Wakefield's analysis is valid, I want to argue that they might not be decisive for three different reasons (some of them recognized by Wakefield and his colleagues). First, the sample being tested is composed of students in psychology and social work, nonpsychiatric nurses, nonpsychiatric social workers, and undergraduates. This sample might be representative of the professional community and share its concepts of disorders, but it is not at all obvious that it allows the probing of the layperson's concept (after all, students in psychiatry or social work are being trained to think about disorders in a certain way, while nurses and social workers have also been taught, even if their subject matter concerns physical disorders). Studying American undergraduates, even if they never did psychiatry classes, is not necessarily a better way to probe the layperson's mind. Indeed, the idea that studying students' intuitions or cognition is a way to study the layperson's intuitions or cognition has been contested by many. In a now famous paper, Heinrich and his colleagues (2010) reviewed reasons why researchers should "worry about the representativeness of prevalent undergraduate samples in behavioural sciences … [because, as studies show] the sample of contemporary Western undergraduates … is frequently a distinct outlier vis-à-vis other global samples" (22). According to Heinrich et al., undergraduates are not only different from people from other cultures (e.g., Westerners are more likely to explain behavior in decontextualized terms and allude to internal causes, more so than East Asians, who explain behavior in more holistic terms[10]) but also from members of their own culture: for instance, from people belonging to different social classes or generations. Therefore, Wakefield's studies might suffer from a sampling bias.[11] Second, Wakefield proposed a version of HD (HDW) according to which disorders are identified by a default of their designed or proper function (whoever or whatever gave them that function). The previous experiment tested only HD. To conclude that it tested HDW, one would need to assume that the only interpretation of "function" possible is some kind of designed function. Yet there are many different interpretations of function, for instance, in terms of system-function (Cummins-Function), propensity function, and so on. Finally, in the experiment, subjects have to react to an abstract situation described by vignettes and are forced to choose an answer (there is no option to abstain). One might wonder if this kind of reaction is representative of all aspects of their conceptual representations or even if it captures concepts that are used or that are more operative in practice. Many philosophers (Cullen 2010; Kauppinen 2007; Woolfolk 2013) have criticized X-Phi for its exclusive reliance on self-report methods based on questionnaires of the sort used by Wakefield. According to these researchers, questionnaires are open to numerous distortions due to wording, framing of questions, question order, and so on. For instance, Cullen (2010) provided subjects vignettes that Nichols and colleagues (2003, 288) used but framed the questions differently. Instead of asking "Does X really knows" or "Does X only believes," he asked "Does X know" or "Does X not know." Instead of having a majority of individuals saying that X "only believes," as was the case with the Nichols et al. experiment, Cullen's results were that a majority of people stated that X "knows." This is not to say that vignettes and self-reporting are not good tools for probing concepts, but rather that a more comprehensive view that would include naturalistic clinic data, surveys, and structured interviews may be more desirable.

In order to overcome these shortcomings, I propose two things.

First, I would test a representative sample of the general American population but also people belonging to different cultures, using vignettes seeking to verify how the two components of HDW fare with them. I would therefore use a series of vignettes where a trait has a designed function (for simplicity's sake, below I am using natural selection as the "designer" of the function, but it can be replaced by "God" or by "Nature," if needed), but where the function is now maladaptive (so I would try to see if something can be judged functional but considered disordered). I would also create vignettes where someone would have a disorder with a designed function but that causes no harm to the subject (I would suppose that if subjects say that someone is disordered even if there is no harm done to them, that goes against HD analysis). I would then test the intuitions of my sample.

Here are a few examples of the kind of questions I would ask. In the group of designed function now considered maladaptive, I would for instance offer subjects an "internal disorder" vignette like Wakefield used to describe Carlos, to which I would add the following:

> Psychologists have found that it has been adaptive in the environment of our ancestors, for a small fraction of the population, to show a high level of aggressiveness and to have a very short fuse. Therefore, natural selection has conserved this trait in the population by selecting the genes responsible for it. Carlos is known to have such genes.

Then I would ask, "Is Carlos suffering from a mental/psychiatric disorder?"

I would also try the same sort of vignette with a disorder such as attention-deficit/hyperactivity disorder (ADHD). For instance (following a suggestion made by Panksepp 2007), I would propose vignettes describing children with typical symptoms of ADHD to which I would add the following:

> In the environments of our ancestors, it was adaptive for some children to move a lot and to have a very short attention span in order to be able to respond to ever-changing environmental conditions. These children were, biologically speaking, identical to children suffering from ADHD.

Then I would ask, "Are these children (who are similar to our ancestors) suffering from a mental/psychiatric disorder?"

I would also offer subjects more intricate vignettes, like the following inspired from De Block (2008):

> Seasonal affective disorder (SAD) is an adaptive pattern of responses that contributes to the individual's reproductive success in higher latitude regions.
>
> Heidi is born is Sweden. Mild SAD was part of her ancestors' phenotype. At one point, Heidi moved to Africa. Like every winter in Sweden, she experienced mild symptoms of SAD, even if it was not adaptive. These symptoms caused her great pain.

Then I would ask, "When in Africa, is Heidi suffering from a mental/psychiatric disorder?"

For the second set of vignettes, those testing the harmful component, I would propose vignettes such as what follows where someone has a disorder, but it is not seen as harmful (inspired by Sacks 1997):

> There are some people living on an isolated Micronesian island who are incapable of identifying or recognizing human faces and emotional responses from faces, and for that reason, they cannot form friendships or interact with people. On the other hand, they are better than anyone else at identifying comestible varieties of plants and mushrooms. Until now, this state has been beneficial to them in allowing them to occupy a niche (they are exceptional gatherers) in which they are now thriving. For instance, because of their capacity to identify plants and mushrooms, they turn out to be the most prosperous inhabitants of the island. It appears that, despite their difficulty in forming friendships, they haven't suffered from loneliness or isolation because they are so absorbed by their work.

Then I would ask, "Are people on this island suffering from a mental disorder/ psychiatric disorder?"

I'll stop here with my suggestion of vignettes, but it seems plain to me that not only Wakefield but also philosophers, psychiatrists, cultural anthropologists, and sociologists should engage in that kind of enterprise. I'll explain why after my second suggestion.

My second suggestion is inspired by Colombo and colleagues' (2003; Fulford and Colombo 2004) series of studies. In these studies, they used a different technique than Wakefield and his colleagues. As Wakefield did, they gave vignettes to subjects from distinct groups (psychiatrists, psychiatric nurses, patients, informal careers, social workers, etc.) to read. These vignettes are longer and describe someone who shows symptoms of schizophrenia, with their background (life situation, childhood, etc.). Then, instead of asking subjects to make a choice between stated options as in Wakefield's experiment, researchers conduct interviews in which they ask this group of people about possible etiology, the individual's level of responsibility, how the individual should be treated, and so on. Researchers then code responses according to six models they constructed and that are supposed to reflect current conceptualizations of mental disorders: for instance, the biomedical model, the social model (the disorder is within society), the family model (the whole family is sick, not just the patient), and so on. Colombo et al. used this method because they adopted a "linguistic-analysis model" of concept (inspired by Wittgenstein) where the content of a concept is not exhausted by what one says about it but rather by what does with it, how it is used. According to them,

> Asking people, whether professionals or users, directly about mental disorders will elicit, mainly, their explicit views. The most familiar explicit model, nowadays, is perhaps the so-called "biopsychosocial" [medical] model. … If the linguistic-analytic insight is right, on the other hand, if such concepts use is a surer guide to meaning than explicit definition, then … how they actually respond to … mental disorders, will be driven by their implicit models of disorder. (Fulford and Colombo 2004, 136)

Their results show a quite different picture from Wakefield's; for instance, while 91.3% of psychiatrists agreed with the medical model, only 8.8% of social workers agreed with it, instead showing preference for the social model (47.5%).

What this set of studies reveals is that different people (and different professional groups) seem to use different models of mental illness. Even worse (for Wakefield), according to some other studies (Harland et al. 2009), different disorders seem to activate different models. If these studies are on the right track, then there is a more complex picture (different groups have different concepts, at different times, for different types of patient, etc.) than the unified and universal picture that Wakefield proposed. This makes it even more important that we also use and offer subjects the kinds of vignettes I have proposed (varying different aspects of them—like wording, framing, part of the context, or even mood) and apply different kinds of methods to different kinds of people (professional groups/culture/social classes, etc.). It is possible that, after performing such research, Wakefield would find that laypeople's intuitions and/or some professional people's intuitions are incompatible with his particular brand of harmful dysfunction analysis (HDW). He could discover that laypeople's intuitions are not compatible with HDW (or not always compatible with it), while professionals' intuitions are. If such were the case (I am not claiming that it is, but it is a possibility and until we have run more experiments and probed more deeply the minds of different kinds of people, it is hazardous to claim that there is only one concept shared by everyone), which concept should be preferred? Should one be preferred? On which basis should we decide on one or another? In replying to these questions, one would not be able to avoid normative considerations. I think these that these considerations would have to be invoked even if at the end of the day Wakefield was right and that there was only one concept of mental disorder shared by everyone. If such were the case, one would need to explain the origin of the consensus somehow. For instance, one might invoke psychological dispositions that inclined us to think about mental illness the same way. But why should we assume that our natural way to think about mental disorder is the right one? Our natural inclinations to think about physical phenomena in a way that goes against our best science (McCloskey 1983) and our natural essentialism about species are an obstacle to a correct understanding of biology (Gelman 2010). What this shows is that even if Wakefield's description of our concept was correct, he would still have to invoke normative considerations to explain why we should adopt this concept in psychiatry.

III.   Evolutionary Psychology to the Rescue

In this section, I want to return to an objection that has been previously made to Wakefield's analysis: the so-called epistemic objection. According to this objection, "because the harmful dysfunction analysis holds that whether one has a disorder depends on facts about internal mechanisms and their evolutionary history, and we are largely ignorant of these facts, therefore the analysis implies that it is impossible to know at this time whether conditions are disorders or non-disorders" (Bergner 1997, 255). Wakefield rightly points out that this objection does not target his conceptual analysis (see also his reply to McNally 2001, 349). Indeed, those who endorsed the epistemic objection could grant that Wakefield's HDW analysis is correct, but they would point out that the adoption of an evolutionary framework would be impracticable for psychiatry. So the epistemological objection is important because it is hard to see how Wakefield's analysis could play its normative role without a picture of the normal mind.[12] Indeed, if one is to criticize the *DSM*'s criteria of depression or anxiety because it includes cases of normal sadness or normal fear (i.e., of nondysfunctional reactions to some stimuli), one should have a means to tell what is normal from what is disordered. But where would that knowledge come from? It is thus important that Wakefield provides an answer to the epistemic objection, even if it does not touch upon the core of his conceptual analysis.

One can find three different replies to the epistemic objection through Wakefield's writing: (1) we have intuitions about what is and what is not functioning correctly, (2) sometimes the function of a mechanism is obvious, and finally (3) sometimes we need help from evolutionary psychology to identify the function of known components of our mind or to identify these very components.[13] In this section, I want to argue that there are problems with (1) and (2) and that we should thus rely on (3). However, I will also show that for a class of mechanisms, reply (3) won't be able to deliver the expected results to us. If such is the case, there will be a hole in the middle of our nosology concerning mechanisms that might be crucial to understanding some disorders.

Let start with answer (1). Wakefield writes that the fact that we do not know about the precise design of an artifact does impinge our judgment that we are facing a dysfunction. For instance, he writes that "I do know almost nothing about the design of automobiles, but I am perfectly capable of recognizing many cases of automobile

malfunction and regularly discriminate such cases from proper automotive functioning" (1997, 256; see also 2001, 349). That is, I can discriminate cases where the car
doesn't start because the tank is empty (in which case, the car is not broken) from cases
where it does not start because something is broken. Basically, I can recognize that
something is disordered or malfunctioning even if I know next to nothing about its
exact function. But I see two problems with this answer. First, while I can sometimes
distinguish cases of malfunction from proper functioning, my understanding of what
went wrong is still very rudimentary—I still need to go to the garage to know what is
wrong with my car. The fact that my car sometimes still has problems even when exiting
the garage proves that it is not necessarily easy to identify these problems. Likely, I might
have intuition that this behavior is not normal, that it must be produced by a malfunctioning mechanism, but without a precise knowledge of which mechanism, it is hard to
develop or apply adequate treatment. What I mean to say (and I am sure Wakefield will
agree) is that for psychiatry to fulfill its role(s) (identifying disorders for diagnosis and
prognosis, guiding research, providing indications as to which treatments will work better, etc.), the discipline will have to move away from intuitions to a more scientific basis.
At best, intuitions can be a starting point for scientific inquiries into the mechanisms
responsible for disorders. Second, relying on intuitions to distinguish malfunctioning
from proper functioning is a dangerous game. This is why cars are often equipped with
an indicator on the dashboard to signal problems with the engine. Often times, we have
no clue that something is going wrong with the engine. Now take an artifact that you do
not know very well. For instance, when I got my first iPod years ago, I tried to use it while
running. Yet as soon as I was running, the iPod would skip from song to song. I thought
there was a problem with the iPod and was ready to throw the thing away (or to go back
to the store) until I finally discovered that I had to shut the screen off before starting off
on my run. In that case, I was thinking that there was something wrong with my iPod
because I did not know its proper functioning. The human mind might be more like the
new gadget for which you haven't taken the time to read the instruction book than to a
car, as we don't know much about how it is supposed to be functioning (this is a claim
that evolutionary psychologists frequently make; see, e.g., Cosmides and Tooby [1994],
who discuss the power of evolutionary psychology to go beyond intuition and instinct
blindness). Therefore, we should beware that we have a natural inclination to make
essentialist inferences based on the fact that certain behaviors are deviant to the presence
of dysfunction, yet that does not guarantee that we are in presence of a dysfunction. Our
intuitions have no special evidentiary status, quite the contrary. In the past, our inclinations or intuitions have shown to be insufficient guides to dysfunction, as the cases
of masturbation, female orgasm, drapetomenia, and so on have proven. As Wakefield
himself claimed, ignorance of the facts about the functions of mental mechanisms has
left the door open to the use of social norms or values and leads to classifying behaviors
that were normal as pathological.[14]

So let's turn to reply (2). Wakefield writes that sometimes, the function of a mechanism is obvious. For instance, in his first book with Horwitz (Horwitz and Wakefield 2007), he writes that "in some cases, a mechanism's biological function is immediately obvious: for example, it cannot be accidental that the eyes see, the hands grasps, the feet walk, or the teeth chew, and it is clear that these beneficial effects explain the existence via natural selection of the respective mechanisms," and he continues, "Sadness is somewhat like sleep; the function is not obvious, yet the designed nature is" (47). This claim deserves a few remarks. First, the fact that the function of a mechanism seems obvious to us is not a good guide to the evolutionary function of the mechanism or even to its designed nature. Take the case of sutures in the skulls of mammals. As Darwin observed long ago, "The sutures of the skulls of young mammals have been advanced as a beautiful adaptation for aiding parturition and not doubt the facilitate, or may be indispensable for this act; but as sutures occur in the skulls of young birds and reptiles, which have only to escape from a broken egg, we may infer that this structure has arisen from the laws of growth, and has been taken advantage of in the parturition of the higher animals" (quoted by Gould and Vrba 1982, 5). To use another example, take Dennett's claim that it is obvious that the *Archaeopteryx* was designed for flight: "Did Archaeopteryx, the extinct birdlike creature that some have called a winged dinosaur, ever really get off the ground? …*An analysis of the claw curvature*, supplemented by aerodynamic analysis of Archaeopteryx wing structure, *makes it quite plain that the creature was well designed for flight*" (1995, 233, my emphasis). Unfortunately, things are not that simple. Some (Nudds and Dyke 2010) have argued that *Archaeopteryx* was not designed to fly. For instance, they suggest that the central shaft of the feathers is thinner and weaker than required by modern birds to fly.[15] Moreover, as Naish observed, "Claims that Archaeopteryx possesses a claw geometry indicating an arboreal lifestyle (Feduccia 1993) are contradicted by newer analyses (Hopson 2001; Glen and Bennett 2007), and virtually all non-avian maniraptorans lack features indicative of a climbing lifestyle" (Naish 2011, 435[16]). If such is the case, *Archaeopteryx* would more resemble birds that stay on the ground (ground dwellers) and sometimes climb on trees (maybe assisted by their wings) to evade predators (like chickens) than flying birds (Richardson 2007, 49).

So obviousness of design does not fare better than intuition: it is not a reliable guide to adaptation. Wakefield agrees with this as he writes, "Obviously, one can go wrong in such explanatory attempts; what seems non-accidental may turn out to be accidental," but he adds that "often one is right" (1992a, 383). But one might ask, where is the evidence that we are often right? How do we know we are right? If there is no such evidence, we would again be relying on our intuition, which can be misleading.

So it seems that the only way to answer the epistemological objection is to turn to a discipline able to identify the mental mechanisms that our mind comprises and describe their functions, as well as their normal environment of functioning: evolutionary psychology (henceforth EP; this is reply (3)). According to Wakefield, only EP is able to reveal our "human species-typical biological design" (Horwitz and Wakefield 2007, 38). That's why Wakefield thinks that "the destiny of the professions of mental health in regard to theoretical and scientific process in the comprehension of the etiology, the diagnostic and the treatment of mental disorder might depend in a large part from the progress in evolutionary psychology" (2005, 900). As I will show, reply (3) is not without problems of its own.

Evolutionary psychology's central commitment, which allows the use of both of its paradigmatic methods (i.e., adaptive thinking and reverse engineering[17]), is the existence of a strong relationship between biological form and adaptive forces. Without such a relationship, there would be no reason to expect that isolating adaptive problems would be of any help in discovering the architecture of the mind or that starting with known mechanisms will lead to the reliable discovery of adaptive pressures that have acted on them in the past. But, as Griffiths (1996) observed (this is what he called the "historical turn in the study of adaptation"), "adaptive generalizations...cannot explain form except in conjunction with a rich set of historical initial conditions" (515). According to Griffiths, the reason why historical initial conditions are important is that they act as constraints on the two aforementioned modes of reasoning. For instance, adaptive problems depend on the biological features of the organism (e.g., in what kind of ecological niche ancestors of that creature were living), features of the environment of evolution adaptation, and the variations available for natural selection. To put it differently, knowledge of initial historical conditions is crucial to the identification of adaptation, given that an adaptation is relative to

(1) traits or mechanisms that were present at the moment of selection,

(2) a particular selective regime at the time (the selective pressures that existed at the time).

So in order to establish that something is an adaptation, one needs information about at least three things: (1) the traits that were present at the same time as the moment of selection, (2) the traits possessed by immediate ancestors of the bearer of the studied trait, and (3) the particular selective regime under which selection has taken place. Because of this, Griffiths suggests (1996; also Richardson 2007) that adaptations are best identified using the comparative method, which consists of comparing a trait to those of phylogenetic ancestors and to prevalent environmental conditions. To give just one example of the kind of surprise one can get from using this method, take the case of the descended larynx that has been hypothesized (using the reverse engineering method; Lieberman 1998) to be a uniquely human adaptation to speech. Fitch and Reby (2001) have shown that many other species have a descended larynx, including some deer species (*Cervus elaphus* and *Dama dama*), but also roaring cats and some bird species. According to them, "these comparative data suggest that vocal-tract elongation is a relatively widespread response to ubiquitous constraints imposed by basic physics intersecting with the physiology of vertebrate vocal production," and they go on to conclude that "it suggests that a descent of the larynx serving simply to exaggerate size could have pre-dated, and perhaps served as a preadaptation for, speech- or language-specific functions of the descended larynx" (173–174). Another surprising example concerns human hands. It has long been thought that the particular shape of human hands (the fact that we have a relatively long thumb and shorter fingers than other primates) was a typically human adaptation. But recent results (Almécija et al. 2015) suggest that the shape of human hands might not be an adaptation to tool use as has long been thought but rather that the shape is primitive rather than derived—that is, that the common ancestor of chimps and humans had hands more like humans than chimps and that it is the chimps' hand with its elongated finger that is a derived trait (an adaptation). These two cases show why the use of history is necessary both to go beyond intuition and to constrain adaptationist explanations.

In principle, the historization of adaptationist explanations should not bother Wakefield greatly; after all, one cannot be against virtue. But the problem is the following: sometimes we have the information needed to establish that a human trait is an adaptation. For instance, we have access to traits that were present in our nonhuman primate ancestors or to traits that vary according to certain features of the evolutionary environment of adaptation (as in the case of malaria resistance, AIDS resistance, skin color, or lactose tolerance). But for many specifically universal human adaptations, the evidence necessary to establish that a trait is an adaptation does not exist. As Kaplan put it, "Such evidence is rarely available in the case of purported 'universal' human psychological adaptations. The very limited information available on the environments which key aspects of human evolution took place makes optimization techniques difficult to apply here. Further, while in some cases phylogenetic information about *Hominidea* may provide evidence relevant to adaptive hypotheses in humans, nature and history have 'conspired' to make the task more difficult with humans than it is in many other species" (2002, 297; for a similar conclusion, see Alden-Smith 2007, 253–254 and Thornhill 2007, 32). What Kaplan means by the latter is that our closest living relatives are the great apes (and we are not that close to them, as we diverged from a common ancestor about 6 million years ago). Because there is no other hominid alive, we cannot compare the fitness consequences of a trait that would have appeared somewhere in hominids' evolution. Was that trait giving an adaptive advantage over others who did not have it (or did have it to a lesser degree)? We cannot answer this question for many universal human traits (like language). Therefore, it seems to be impossible to establish the designed function of these putative adaptive traits.

What this means for evolutionary psychiatry is that is possible to establish evolutionary functional criteria for some mechanisms that evolved before the *Homo* genus. For instance, if Price and colleagues (1994) are right about depression, that is, if it is the result of an adaptation to life in social groups (a form of de-escalation strategy) that we inherited from group-living ancestors common to primates, we should be able to use the comparative method and establish that the mechanism is indeed an adaptation. Similarly, in principle, it should be possible to establish the adaptive character of traits that vary inside the human population too. But for some mechanisms (the number of which has to be empirically determined but might include language, reasoning, inhibitory control, some forms of learning, imagination, and many others), we might just never know the facts necessary to establish that they are adaptations (for similar claims, see Richardson 2007, 38). Therefore, judgments about their dysfunction will be based on hunches about what is normal or abnormal, and as we saw, the past demonstrates that hunches such as these are unreliable, as they are especially open to the influence of values and norms.

What is there to conclude from this? Surely not that the epistemological objection cannot be met for some of the mental mechanisms that populate our mind. For instance, Stephen Downes (2009) recently observed that there is no reason to think that our species-typical mechanisms (if we understand "species-typical" mechanisms as meaning the mechanisms that are possessed by members of our species and not those that are exclusive to our species) were all produced in the Pleistocene. Some might predate that period, and some might be more recent. For both groups of mechanism, there is hope that we could find the facts necessary to establish with certainty that they are adaptations.[18] But as Kaplan and others have observed, for the mechanisms that are supposed to have appeared in the Pleistocene, the task might be forever beyond our reach. If such is the case, the picture of the normal mind on which psychiatry is supposed to lean will be forever incomplete.

Conclusion

I have shown that HD analysis could take advantage of X-Phi methods. It could turn out that HDA is not what laypeople or professionals have in mind. If this is the case, Wakefield might want to argue that it is what they should have in mind, and thus in that case, his argument would be a normative argument. It could also turn out that people's concepts of disorder vary as a function of different cues. In that case, it would be important to identify these cues in order to understand and prevent misunderstandings caused by these different concepts. Finally, Wakefield could be right on with his analysis. In that case, using X-Phi will only strengthen his position.

I also proposed a version of the epistemic objection. As I demonstrated, it applies only for a subclass of mental capacities, those that are human specific and universal. For these, the prospects of establishing that they are adaptations are slim. If such is the case, and depending on the number of mental capacities belonging to that subclass, some of the attributions of mental disorder might be desperately speculative. The epistemic objection can thus become an objection to HDA. Not that it is not a good description of the concept that we are using, but given that it will leave a (large?) part of our mental attribution subject to value judgments or norms, it cannot play a normative role.

Notes

1. As Wakefield writes elsewhere, "A manual will be coherent and conceptually valid (i.e., valid in discriminating disorder from non disorder) only if its construction is guided by an adequate definition of disorder. In addition to determining which conditions are identified as disorders, such definition provides a framework for constructing diagnostic criteria for specific disorders" (1993, 160).

2. Recently, Wakefield has defined the "mental" in "mental disorder" a bit more precisely: "Mental dysfunctions are not specific mental states but rather dysfunctions in the brain mechanisms designed to produce or regulate mental states, and the dysfunction emerges in irregularities in the production and the regulation of mental states" (2007b, 127). This definition has important implications for psychiatry that I am not sure Wakefield endorsed. For instance, one can suppose that one psychological function of vision is to produce "mental representations" of the visual scene. If such is the case, then blindness should be considered a mental dysfunction, which is not the case. To which extent would Wakefield would want to reform psychiatry based on this definition is an unanswered question (see Murphy 2006 for a reformative position on the matter).

3. This surely does not mean that it is without problems (see Cooper, this volume; De Block and Sholl, this volume). For instance, it is not clear for whom the dysfunction has to be harmful to for it to be judged a full-fledged disorder. Does it have to be harmful for an individual, their genes, family, or society in general?

4. As Wakefield puts it, "Mechanisms are naturally selected because they confer greater fitness on the organism *in a particular range of environments*. It is not the sheer number of environments in which there is harm, *but whether there is harm in the kinds of environments for which the organism was designed to operate harm free, that determines whether there is a dysfunction*" (1993, 166, my emphasis).

5. Neander (1995) rightly notes that this notion of normativity that is associated with evolutionary function or normal function is not evaluative. She writes, "Teenage fertility is biologically normal, but it does not follow that teenage fertility is a good thing; on the contrary, if we could induce (temporary and reversible) infertility in all girls under the age of twenty, that would probably be better [Boorse, 1975]. *Judging that something is functioning properly is not the same as judging that its functioning is good*" (111, my emphasis).

6. Wakefield makes such claims throughout his papers. For instance, he recently wrote that "every claim about a concept can be considered *an implicit empirical claim* about how individuals in some linguistic community use a term, so it is possible to empirically study whether the proposed conceptual analysis accurately portrays the community's linguistic practices" (2007c, 41, my emphasis).

7. Poland (2003) makes similar criticisms to Wakefield's method: "there is good reason to be suspicious of just exactly how reliable such intuitions are, what they do and do not tap, and hence just how indicative they are of the actual employment of the concept of mental disorder in mental health practice. Regarding reliability, it is an important area of inquiry to determine just what kinds of factors influence and shape intuitive judgments, and what kinds of factors can support or undermine consistency of intuitive judgment across individuals or context.... there are serious concerns that consultation of linguistic intuitions is far too impoverished an evidential basis for inferring the conceptual commitments of mental practitioners. Mental health practice takes place in a variety of very different contexts, and it concerns more than just talk.... *Information about the actual diagnostic decisions that are made in clinical contexts, the ways in which the concept of mental disorder is reflected in relevant scientific research, as well as the role of the concept in other practical contexts (e.g., legal, public policy) is very likely a far more accurate and probative measure of conceptual commitments of practitioners than their intuitive response to hypothetical cases*" (34, my emphasis). I will return later to the latter idea in this chapter.

8. Nichols and colleagues take the results of this experiment and others as showing that some epistemic intuitions are not universal, as they vary with culture, socioeconomical status, and educational background. They take this as motivating a form of skepticism concerning the possibility of providing a conceptual analysis that would be accepted in every culture.

9. Some other items were also tested, for instance, the need for professional assistance or the possible duration of the condition, but for the sake of space, I will mention the results only briefly. In short, clinicians think that individuals meeting *DSM-IV* criteria for antisocial personality disorder while not being disordered should still be treated by a professional and believe that their problems could continue into their adult life (see Wakefield et al. 2002).

10. A difference that might show up in the understanding of mental disorders.

11. Studies from Pottick and colleagues (2007) suggest that certain features of the situation (occupation of the professional, race or ethnicity of the patient, etc.) might affect judgments of mental disorder. It seems that Wakefield considers these effects as performance distortions (following Chomsky's distinction, someone can be a competent user of a concept, even if they err in applying it to a situation or a thing, due to fatigue, for instance) or difference due to various particular theories about the same concept. An alternative account could be that people have (sometimes slightly) different concepts of mental disorders.

12. Wakefield recognizes this: for instance, he writes that "an evolutionary approach to natural versus disordered anxiety can offer a conceptual basis to help restrain such excesses [which consist in pathologizing natural emotions]" (Horwitz and Wakefield 2012, 19).

13. In his reply to McNally, Wakefield (2001) is making an additional point. As he says, "Often the evolutionary conclusions are themselves so speculative and unreliable that they can distort rather than solidify the evidential process. So, as an epistemological necessity, of course inquiry into function and dysfunction will continue to rely mainly on the study of current causal relationships—with the critical proviso...that current causal relationships are often taken as proxies for past design" (350). I am not convinced at all by this line of argument. Take your

standard paper in cognitive science; for instance, Munakata et al. (2011) describe two different pathways that are responsible for the inhibition of thoughts, actions, or emotions. The phenomenon of interest is cognitive inhibition, and what researchers want to know is how inhibition is produced. Researchers are making no assumptions concerning the evolutionary origin of the phenomenon nor would they think that the phenomenon is less in need of explanation if it was learned that inhibition is a spandrel or is not the result of natural selection.

14. Wakefield writes that, as it is clearly shown from historical and anthropological accounts of psychopathology, "values, norms and ideologies deeply influence what people take to be natural functions, in particular when scientific understanding of what is functional and dysfunctional is lacking (as it is the case for numerous aspects of the mental life)" (2006, my translation).

15. There is still a debate about this question, but the fact that the debate even exists proves that it is far from obvious that the dinosaur had wings designed for flying.

16. On the basis of an analysis of claw curvature, Naish (2011) remarks that different *Archaeopteryx* species might have a different behavioral lifestyle.

17. *Adaptive thinking* starts with a consideration of the adaptive problems (say choosing a place to live) that a creature has to solve in its evolutionary environment of adaptation to infer or to hypothesize the presence of mechanisms that are designed to solve them (e.g., aesthetics preferences for certain types of habitat; Orians and Heerwagen 1992). *Reverse engineering* starts with the presence of a mechanism (e.g., color vision) and tries to infer the problem it is designed to solve (e.g., making fruit more perceptually salient in a darker foliage background; Mollon 1996). In other words, "reverse engineering infers the adaptive problem from the solution which was adopted. Adaptive thinking infers the solution from the adaptive problem" (Griffiths 1996, 514).

18. This is if the human cultural environment does not profoundly modify the functioning of these older structures (Buller 2009, 79). For instance, work by Dehaene and colleagues (2010) shows that learning to read profoundly modifies the organization of the cortex. According to these researchers, "during education, reading processes must invade and 'recycle' cortical space devoted to evolutionary older functions, opening the possibility that these functions suffer as reading expertise sets in" (1359).

References

Alden-Smith, E. 2007. Reconstructing the evolution of the human mind. In *The Evolution of the Mind: Fundamental Questions and Controversies*, S. W. Gangestad and J. A. Simpson (eds.), 53–59. Guilford.

Almécija, S., J. B. Smaers, and W. L. Jungers. 2015. The evolution of human and ape hand proportions. *Nature Communications* (6): 7717.

Bergner, R. M. 1997. What is psychopathology? And so what? *Clinical Psychology: Science and Practice* 4(3): 235–248.

Boorse, C. 1975. On the distinction between disease and illness. *Philosophy and Public Affairs* 5(1): 49–68.

Buller, D. 2009. Four fallacies of pop evolutionary psychology. *Scientific American,* January, 74–81.

Buss, D. 2006. *The Murder Next Door: Why the Mind Is Designed to Kill.* Penguin Books.

Colombo, A., G. Bendelow, B. Fulford, and S. Williams. 2003. Evaluating the influence of implicit models of mental disorder on processes of shared decision making within community-based multi-disciplinary teams. *Social Science and Medicine* 56(7): 1557–1570.

Cosmides, L., and J. Tooby. 1994. Beyond intuition and instinct blindness: Toward an evolutionary rigorous cognitive science. *Cognition* 50(1–3): 41–77.

Cullen, S. 2010. Survey-driven romanticism. *Review of Philosophy and Psychology* 1(2): 275–296.

De Block, A. 2008. Why mental disorders are just mental dysfunctions (and nothing more): Some Darwinian arguments. *Studies in History and Philosophy of Science Part C* 39(3): 338–346.

Dehaene, S., F. Pegado, L. W. Braga, P. Ventura, G. Nunes Filho, A. Jobert, G. Dehaene-Lambertz, R. Kolinski, J. Morais, and L. Cohen. 2010. How learning to read changes the cortical networks for vision and language. *Science* 330(6009): 1359–1364.

Dennett, D. C. 1995. *Darwin's Dangerous Idea: Evolution and the Meaning of Life.* Simon & Schuster.

Downes, S. M. 2009. The basic components of the human mind were not solidified during the Pleistocene Epoch. In *Contemporary Debates in Philosophy of Biology,* F. Ayala and R. Arp (eds.), 243–252. Blackwell.

Fitch, W. T., and D. Reby. 2001. The descended larynx is not uniquely human. *Proceedings of the Royal Society B* 268: 1669–1675.

Fulford, K. W. M., and A. Colombo. 2004. Six models of mental disorder: A study combining linguistic-analytic and empirical methods. *Philosophy, Psychiatry, and Psychology* 11(2): 129–144.

Gelman, S. 2010. Modules, theories, or islands of expertise? Domain-specificity in socialization. *Child Development* 81(3): 715–719.

Gould, S. J., and E. S. Vrba. 1982. Exaptation: A missing term in the science of form. *Paleaobiology* 8(1): 4–15.

Griffiths, P. E. 1996. The historical turn in the study of adaptation. *British Journal for the Philosophy of Science* 47(4): 511–532.

Griffiths, P. E., and K. Stotz. 2008. Experimental philosophy of science. *Philosophy Compass* 3(3): 507–521.

Harland, R., E. Antonova, G. S. Owen, M. Broome, S. Landau, Q. Deeley, and R. Murray. 2009. A study of psychiatrist's concepts of mental illness. *Psychological Medicine* 39(6): 967–976.

Heinrich, J., S. J. Heine, and A. Norenzayan. 2010. The weirdest people in the world. *Behavioral and Brain Sciences* 33(2–3): 1–23.

Horwitz, A. V., and J. C. Wakefield. 2007. *The Loss of Sadness: How Psychiatry Transformed Normal Sorrow into Depressive Disorder.* Oxford University Press.

Horwitz, A. V., and J. C. Wakefield. 2012. *All We Have to Fear: Psychiatry's Transformation of Natural Anxieties into Mental Disorders*. Oxford University Press.

Kaplan, J. M. 2002. Historical evidence and human adaptations. *Philosophy of Science* 69(53): S294–S304.

Kauppinen, A. 2007. The rise and fall of experimental philosophy. *Philosophical Explorations* 10(2): 95–118.

Kirk, S. A., J. C. Wakefield, D. Hsieh, and K. Pottick. 1999. Social context and social workers' judgment of mental disorder. *Social Service Review* 73(1): 82–104.

Knobe, J. 2007. Experimental philosophy. *Philosophy Compass* 2(1): 81–92.

Knobe, J., and J. Doris. 2010. Responsibility. In *The Moral Psychology Handbook*, J. Doris and the Moral Psychology Research Group (dir. publ.), 321–354. Oxford University Press.

Kupfer, D. J., M. B. First, and D. A. Regier, eds. 2002. A *Research Agenda for the DSM-V*. Washington Press Association.

Lieberman, P. 1998. *Eve Spoke: Human Language and Human Evolution*. Norton.

McCloskey, M. 1983. Intuitive physics. *Scientific American* 248(4): 122–130.

McNally, R. J. 2001. On Wakefield's harmful dysfunction analysis of mental disorder. *Behaviour Research and Therapy* 39(3): 309–314.

Millikan, R. 2002. Biofunctions: Two paradigms. In *Functions: New Essays in the Philosophy of Psychology and Biology*, A. Ariew, R. Cummins, and M. Perlman (eds.), 113–143. Clarendon.

Mollon, J. D. 1996. The evolution of trichromacy: An essay to mark the bicentennial of Thomas Young's graduation in Göttingen. In *Brain and Evolution*, N. Elsner and H.-U. Schnitzler (eds.), 125–139. Springer.

Munakata, Y., S. A. Herd, C. H. Chatham, B. E. Depue, M. T. Banich, and R. C. O'Reilly. 2011. A unified framework for inhibitory control. *Trends in Cognitive Sciences* 15(10): 453–459.

Murphy, D. 2006. *Psychiatry in the Scientific Image*. MIT Press.

Nahmias, E. 2006. Is incompatibilism intuitive? *Philosophy and Phenomenological Research* 73(1): 28–53.

Nahmias, E., S. G. Morris, T. Nadelhoffer, and J. Turner. 2005. Surveying freedom: Folk intuitions about free will and moral responsibility. *Philosophical Psychology* 18(5): 561–584.

Naish, D. 2011. [Review of] Glorified dinosaurs: The origin and evolution of birds. *Historical Biology* 23: 435–438.

Neander, K. 1991. Functions as selected effects: The conceptual analyst's defense. *Philosophy of Science* 58(2): 168–184.

Neander, K. 1995. Misrepresenting and malfunctioning. *Philosophical Studies* 79(2): 109–141.

Nichols, S., and J. Knobe. 2007. Moral responsibility and determinism: The cognitive science of folk intuitions. *Noûs* 41(4): 663–685.

Nichols, S., S. Stich, and J. M. Weinberg. 2003. Metaskepticism: Meditations in ethnoepistemology. In *The Skeptics*, S. Luper (ed.), 227–247. Ashgate.

Nudds, R. L., and G. J. Dyke. 2010. Narrow primary feather rachises in Confuciusornis and Archaeopteryx suggest poor flight ability. *Science* 328(5980): 887–889.

Orians, G. H. and J. H. Heerwagen. 1992. Evolved responses to landscapes. In *The Adapted Mind: Evolutionary Psychology and the Generation of Culture*. J. H. Barkow, L. Cosmides, and J. Tooby (eds.), 555–579. Oxford University Press.

Panksepp, J. 2007. Can PLAY diminish ADHD and facilitate the construction of the social brain? *Journal of the Canadian Academia of Adolescent Psychiatry* 16(2): 57–66.

Poland, J. 2003. *Whither Mental Disorder."* Unpublished manuscript.

Pottick, K. J., S. A. Kirk, D. K. Hsieh, and X. Tian. 2007. Judging mental disorder: Effects of client, clinician, and contextual differences. *Journal of Consulting and Clinical Psychology* 75(1): 1–8.

Price, J., L. Sloman, R. Gardner, P. Gilbert, and P. Rohde. 1994. The social competition hypothesis of depression. *British Journal of Psychiatry* 164(3): 309–315.

Richardson, R. 2007. *Evolutionary Psychology as Maladapted Psychology*. MIT Press.

Roe, K., and D. Murphy. 2011. Function, dysfunction, and adaptation? In *Maladapting Minds: Philosophy, Psychiatry, and Evolutionary Theory*, P. R. Adriaens and A. De Block (eds.), 216–237. Oxford University Press.

Sacks, O. 1997. *The Island of the Colorblind*. Vintage.

Thornhill, R. 2007. Comprehensive knowledge of human evolutionary history requires both adaptationism and phylogenetics. In *The Evolution of the Mind: Fundamental Questions and Controversies*, S. W. Gangestad and J. A. Simpson (eds.), 31–37. Guilford.

Thornhill, R., and C. T. Palmer. 2000. *A Natural History of Rape: Biological Bases of Sexual Coercion*. MIT Press.

Wakefield, J. C. 1992a. The concept of mental disorder: On the boundary between biological facts and social values. *American Psychologist* 47(3): 373–388.

Wakefield, J. C. 1992b. Disorder as harmful dysfunction: A conceptual critique of *DSM-III-R*'s definition of mental disorder. *Psychological Review* 99(2): 232–247.

Wakefield, J. C. 1993. Limits of operationalization: A critique of Spitzer and Endicott's (1978) proposed operational criteria for mental disorder. *Journal of Abnormal Psychology* 102(1): 160–172.

Wakefield, J. C. 1997. Normal inability versus pathological disability: Why Ossorio's (1985) definition of mental disorder is not sufficient. *Clinical Psychology: Science and Practice* 4: 249–258.

Wakefield, J. C. 1999. Evolutionary versus prototype analyses of the concept of disorder. *Journal of Abnormal Psychology* 108(3): 374–399.

Wakefield, J. C. 2000. Aristotle as sociobiologist: The 'Function of a human being' argument, black box essentialism, and the concept of mental Disorder. *Philosophy, Psychiatry, and Psychology* 7(1): 17–44.

Wakefield, J. C. 2001. Evolutionary history versus current causal role in the definition of disorder: Reply to McNally. *Behavior Research and Therapy* 39(3): 347–366.

Wakefield, J. C. 2005. Biological function and dysfunction. In *Handbook of Evolutionary Psychology*, D. Buss (ed.), 878–902. Oxford University Press.

Wakefield, J. C. 2006. Fait et valeur dans le concept de trouble mental: le trouble en tant que dysfonction préjudiciable. *Philosophiques* 33(1): 37–64.

Wakefield, J. C. 2007a. The concept of mental disorder: Diagnostic implications of the harmful dysfunction analysis. *World Psychiatry* 6(3): 149–156.

Wakefield, J. C. 2007b. What makes a mental disorder *mental*? *Philosophy, Psychiatry, and Psychology* 13(2): 123–131.

Wakefield, J. C. 2007c. Why psychology needs conceptual analysts: Wachtel's 'discontents' revisited. *Applied and Preventive Psychology* 12(1): 39–43.

Wakefield, J. C., S. A. Kirk, K. J. Pottick, X. Tian, and D. K. Hsieh. 2006. The lay concept of conduct disorder: Do non-professional use syndromal symptoms or internal dysfunction to distinguish disorder from delinquency? *Canadian Journal of Psychiatry* 51(4): 210–217.

Wakefield, J. C., K. J. Pottick, and S. A. Kirk. 2002. Should the *DSM-IV* diagnostic criteria for conduct disorder consider social context? *American Journal of Psychiatry* 159(3): 380–386.

Woolfolk, R. L. 1999. Malfunction and mental illness. *The Monist* 82(4): 658–670.

Woolfolk, R. L. 2013. Experimental philosophy: A methodological critique. *Metaphilosophy* 44(1–2): 79–87.

4 Do the Empirical Facts Support the Harmful Dysfunction Analysis? Reply to Luc Faucher

Jerome Wakefield

I have long appreciated Luc Faucher's provocative interweaving of conceptual and empirical arguments (e.g., Faucher and Blanchette 2011), and I am delighted that he brings the discussion in this volume around to the implications of empirical studies for the conceptual analysis of "disorder." In particular, his contribution offers an opportunity to consider the empirical testing of my harmful dysfunction analysis (HDA) of medical, including mental, disorder. The HDA claims that "disorder" refers to "harmful dysfunction," where dysfunction is the failure of some feature to perform a natural function for which it is biologically designed by evolutionary processes and harm is judged in accordance with social values (First and Wakefield 2010, 2013; Spitzer 1997, 1999; Wakefield 1992a, 1992b, 1993, 1995, 1997a, 1997b, 1997c, 1997d, 1998, 1999a, 1999b, 2000a, 2000b, 2001, 2006, 2007, 2009, 2011, 2014, 2016a, 2016b; Wakefield and First 2003, 2012). I am also extremely grateful to him for his role as an editor of this volume.

Faucher urges philosophers of psychiatry to "go factual" with empirical studies. Not only do I agree, but as Faucher notices, I early did so myself in a series of studies of clinical judgment about adolescent conduct disorder. In those days, I was listed as doing X-Phi on the empirical philosophy website. However, "the facts" always need interpretation, and any hope that going factual will in some simple way resolve conceptual disputes is overly optimistic. As a case in point, despite my basic agreement with Faucher as to the value of empirical work on the concept of mental disorder, I disagree with the anti-HDA interpretations Faucher offers of some extant studies of models of mental disorder, and I also disagree with his speculations about what empirical studies with varying outcomes are likely to mean. I thus respond to Faucher's points as a cautionary tale about the potential pitfalls that face such empirical work. I will also revisit my own HDA-related empirical studies of clinical judgments about conduct disorder (CD), considering not only Faucher's critique of them in his paper but also previous critiques by Dominic Murphy and Robert Woolfolk as well as by Arthur Houts. Finally, I comment briefly at the end on Faucher's additional comments regarding supposed epistemological challenges facing the HDA's application.

Do the Colombo et al. and Harland et al. Studies Challenge the HDA?

I start by considering Faucher's claims that two clinical-judgment type empirical studies pose significant problems for the HDA. Specifically, Faucher claims that because different groups have different judgments, that must mean that there are multiple concepts of disorder. I am going to closely examine the studies that Faucher claims are problematic for the HDA and explain how he misconstrues their results and how the different judgments by different groups of subjects have no implications at all for the concept of disorder.

Faucher describes the first study and how it supposedly diverges from the HDA as follows:

> Colombo and colleagues (2003a)...give vignettes to subjects from distinct groups (psychiatrists, psychiatric nurses, patients, informal carers, social workers, etc.) [that]...describe someone who shows symptoms of schizophrenia, with their background (life situation, childhood, etc.)....Researchers then code responses according to six models they constructed and that are supposed to reflect current conceptualizations of mental disorders: for instance, the biomedical model, the social model (the disorder is within society), the family model (the whole family is sick, not just the patient), and so on....Their results show a quite different picture from Wakefield's; for instance, while 91.3% of psychiatrists agreed with the medical model, only 8.8% of social worker agreed with it, instead showing preference for the social model (47.5%).

Faucher concludes, "What this set of studies reveals is that different people (and different professional groups) seem to use different models of mental illness." He presents this as a challenge to the HDA, suggesting that it shows that there are variant concepts of mental disorder.

In fact, the cited statistics are irrelevant to the HDA and to the concept of disorder. In the Colombo et al. (2003) study, the respondents started by reading a vignette about a 30-year-old male whose behavior, including social withdrawal and strange ideas such as that a religious group is putting thoughts into his mind, suggests the onset of schizophrenia, but the vignette also mentions various social stressors both early (a death in the family) and recent (business failure) in the man's life and notes that there was no previous history of psychiatric problems. After reading the case vignette, participants, twenty each of the psychiatrists and social workers on whom I will focus, responded to twelve open-ended interview questions about the nature of the individual's problem and its treatment. The questions fell into categories including, for example, diagnosis/definition, interpretation of behavior, labels, etiology, treatment, and prognosis. For example, the question concerning etiology was "what do you think caused Tom to behave like this?" (2003, 1558). The transcribed open-ended answers to the questions were then qualitatively scored by raters for agreement with one or more of six models of disorder: medical-organic, social-stresses, cognitive-behavioral, psycho-therapeutic, family interactions, and conspiratorial-myth. Guidelines for when answers fit each model were provided by the researchers (see below). Although generally a response fit one model, raters could score agreement with from zero to three models.

Now, regarding the Colombo et al. report's summary differences in psychiatry's and social work's endorsed models noted by Faucher, those percentages lump together many different indicators, most of which are irrelevant to judgments of disorder. Fortunately, detailed data are presented on the psychiatrists' and social workers' responses to specific study questions, allowing a look past the summary statistics. (Colombo et al. appear to use endorsement of a model by at least half of respondents as the threshold for attributing that model to the group, and I will follow this metric in my discussion.)

Surveying the responses to some specific questions most relevant to disorder attribution, we find that, despite their general sympathy with the social model, none of the social workers (0%; n = 0) agreed with the social model's definition of diagnosis that implied health versus illness (described in the guidelines as "Health/low stress—illness/high stress continuum"), and none endorsed the medical model ("physical health—illness continuum"), which 100% of the psychiatrists endorsed. Half of the social workers (50%; n = 10) agreed with the "labels" social model item that asserts explicitly that the person's condition is not a disorder ("person is seen as a victim of social forces and not as ill"), whereas none (0%) of the psychiatrists did so. Most social workers (75%; n = 15) agreed with the social model of etiology ("social and economic stress, cultural conflict, marginal status, etc."), while few psychiatrists did so (15%; n = 3), and correspondingly, the social workers agreed that, other than long-term individual psychotherapy, treatment should be "social change to reduce stress" (50%; n = 10), which does not directly address internal states at all, whereas 0% of psychiatrists endorsed that answer. All this is consistent with the sharp divergence in prognosis, for which by far the most frequent social worker's answer (80%; n = 16) was the social model's, "Good if changes made at the social level"; 0% of psychiatrist's agreed with this outlook.

It thus seems that a number of social workers rejected the label of mental disorder for the described individual in this study because they judged that the individual was having a problematic reaction to a stressful environment and that there was no internal dysfunction sustaining the symptoms independent of the social stressors. The study is aimed at exploring potential issues on professional teams due to different ways of modeling disorder, and one issue pointed to by the study is the potential for confusing caregivers by their getting caught in the crossfire between professionals who believe there is a mental disorder and those who do not, as in the following report by a caregiver: "my daughter had some problems and got schizophrenia and that's an illness so I was told…I started to do things for her because she was sick…she got annoyed and said she wasn't sick. The social worker told me to give her space and said she was just depressed because of her problems…I mean what is going on?" (1567).

However, none of this suggests that psychiatrists and social workers have different concepts of mental disorder. Rather, the pattern of answers reveals that the psychiatrists' and social workers' different views of whether the described individual has a disorder track their respective beliefs about whether the individual has a dysfunction, as the HDA predicts.

The basic problem here is that Faucher fails to distinguish *theories* of mental disorder from the *concept* of mental disorder. To construct a credible scientific theory of mental disorder, one must understand the target phenomenon, so one must already possess the concept of mental disorder. Colombo et al. do at one point refer to what they are examining as "conceptions of mental disorder" (1565), but this is misleading; their results have nothing to do with the *concept* of mental disorder and rather address different *theories* or *models* of the nature of mental disorder. The mental health professions entertain many models or theories of mental disorder ranging from brain disease, repressed conflict, and cognitive distortion to family dynamics, behavioral reinforcement, and social stress. To some degree, members of different professions—particularly psychiatrists versus social workers versus psychologists—tend to be trained in and to embrace different models that are distinctively relevant to their profession's expertise and focus. The *Diagnostic and Statistical Manual of Mental Disorders* (*DSM*) recognizes that it is essential that its diagnostic criteria be designed in a theory-neutral way precisely because a single disorder, say depression, may be explained by rival theories in different ways. The HDA, like the *DSM*, provides a theory-neutral formulation of what constitutes a mental disorder, independent of theoretical orientations. Thus, differences over theories of mental disorder, and even differences over whether specific conditions are mental disorders, do not imply differences over the concept of mental disorder.

Turning to the second study cited by Faucher as challenging the HDA, Faucher says the following about Harland et al.'s (2009) "A Study of Psychiatrists' Concepts of Mental Illness": "Even worse (for Wakefield), according to some other studies (Harland et al. 2009), different disorders seem to activate different models. If these studies are on the right track, then there is a more complex picture (different groups have different concepts, at different times, for different types of patient, etc.) than the unified and universal picture that Wakefield proposed."

In fact, despite its promising title, the Harland et al. study is irrelevant to testing the HDA and to illuminating the concept of disorder. The title is an instance of how researchers often use "concept" not for concepts in the philosopher's sense but for models and theories of what falls under the concept.

Harland et al. (2009) is a study of "how a group of trainee psychiatrists understand familiar mental illnesses in terms of propositions drawn from different models" (967). Despite the study's promising title and the fact that Harland et al. call the models "conceptual paradigms" (968), the "models" are *not* competing analyses of the concept of "mental disorder" but in fact mostly competing theories of the etiology of mental disorder (biological, cognitive, behavioral, psychodynamic, social realist, and spiritualist) along with a couple of views that question whether standard categories really are mental disorders (social constructivist, nihilist). The study's questionnaire asked four Likert-scale "agree-disagree" questions about each of the eight models for each of four standard psychiatric disorders (schizophrenia, major depressive disorder, generalized anxiety disorder [GAD], and antisocial personality disorder).

In regard to the six etiological theories, the question most pertinent to the concept of mental disorder is the etiology question, and all of these questions presuppose that the condition is a disorder and ask about what causes it ("The disorder results from brain dysfunction"; "Maladaptive thoughts and beliefs are normally distributed in the population and it is the extreme ends of this distribution that account for the disorder"; "The disorder results from maladapted associative learning"; "The disorder results from the failure to successfully complete developmental psychic stages"; "Social factors such as prejudice, poor housing, and unemployment are the main causes of the disorder"; "Neglecting the spiritual or moral dimension of life leads to the disorder"). The fact that that every question uses the term "disorder" to describe the condition is a fatal problem for drawing any conclusions regarding the distinction between disorder and nondisorder because there is no "nondisorder" option. The etiological questions for the skeptical social constructivist and nihilist models do seem to imply nondisorder ("The disorder is a culturally determined construction that reflects the interests and ideology of socially dominant groups"; "All classifications and 'treatments' of the disorder are myths," respectively), but there is nothing in the study that shows what other beliefs are correlated with them, so there is no information about what the distinction between disorder and nondisorder means to the participants. Moreover, few endorsed those categories, and there are no questions that explore associated beliefs about dysfunction or whether something has gone wrong with psychological functioning. The point is not whether the respondent has a certain view of a condition as being a disorder versus nondisorder but why the respondent has that view of the condition, and for that you need to test for correlated variations in other potentially related beliefs.

Note that the judgment that a condition is or is not a disorder says nothing in itself about the nature of the concept of mental disorder, which is supposed to offer an explanation for why people judge disorder versus nondisorder. In the mental health field, some think that virtually no standard disorder categories are really disorders, and others think that virtually all are, and many think some are and some aren't, and the HDA predicts the basis for such judgments but says nothing about which judgments people will actually make.

So, to return to Faucher's claim, these studies' results are decidedly *not* "even worse (for Wakefield)." Faucher claims there is a problem for the HDA because, he says, Harland et al. show that "different disorders seem to activate different models." But this has nothing at all to do with the *concept* of mental disorder; it has to do with different theoretical views of the etiology of specific mental disorders. It is entirely consistent with the HDA to hold various different theoretical positions about the nature and causes of dysfunction. For example, it is consistent with the HDA to believe that schizophrenia and GAD are both harmful dysfunctions in which something has gone wrong with biologically designed functioning but believe that schizophrenia is caused primarily by a genetic or brain dysfunction, whereas GAD is primarily the result of cognitive issues. Faucher says, "If these studies are on the right track, then there is a more complex picture (different groups have different concepts, at different times, for different types of patient, etc.) than the unified and universal picture that Wakefield proposed." That is not what the study shows. The study shows not that the concept of mental disorder varies with group, time, or condition but, at most, that different groups may have different theories of the etiology of mental disorders. To address the HDA, at a minimum you would need to allow respondents to judge whether a described condition is or is not a mental disorder and then correlate that judgment with indicators of harm and dysfunction. The Harland et al. study lacks these minimal requirements because it was never meant to address the conceptual issue, in the philosophers' sense of the term.

In sum, in citing the Colombo et al. and Harland et al. studies as addressing the concept of disorder and having implications for the HDA, Faucher confuses theories of the nature and etiology of mental disorder (which in the literature are often referred to as "models" of mental disorder) with disputes about the concept of mental disorder itself. Obviously, there are many competing theories of mental disorder, some of which tend to break down along professional disciplinary lines but many of which vary from individual clinician to clinician. One can disagree about how the dysfunctions in various mental disorders are caused and even disagree over whether a certain condition is caused by a dysfunction, while having exactly the same concept of mental disorder.

Conceptual analysis is in my view a form of psychological theorizing about shared cognitive structures underlying shared classificatory judgments. Conceptual analysis generates hypotheses and identifies evidential support but should be continuous with empirical work to evaluate claims about both the existence and the nature of the hypothesized shared representational structure in a target linguistic community of interest. Empirical studies thus have an important role as an adjunct to conceptual analysis if designed, executed, and interpreted with care. However, isolated studies almost never prove anything taken individually; they must be part of a research program in which alternative hypotheses about the meaning of the results of a study are generated and progressively tested, as occurs in any science. Moreover, empirical study of conceptual issues is challenging, especially when it comes to designing the experimental manipulation for testing rival hypotheses to yield relatively unambiguous outcomes. This is because concepts interact in a variety of ways with the background web of beliefs to yield classificatory judgments, so judgments in response to a target vignette can represent many different things. For example, one time when I was testing vignettes on graduate students in clinical social work, I noticed that if I specified that the individual described in a vignette had been sexually abused as a child, then that enormously increased the percentage of responses agreeing that the individual has a mental disorder, irrespective of the environmental-context versus internal-causation manipulation. The reason was not divergent concepts of disorder but rather that at that time, it was an article of deeply held theory among mental health professionals that anyone who is sexually abused almost certainly will develop a mental disorder, a belief that has been called into question to much controversy (Rind et al. 1998). There are many such alternative hypotheses available to explain most judgments, and the art of vignette and questionnaire construction is largely the art of narrowing the range of plausible interpretations.

Faucher, in being concerned about variations in individual uses of "mental disorder," seems to me to have lost track of the primary motivation for the conceptual analysis of "mental disorder." It is not a linguistic exercise or conceptual fishing expedition to discover all the various ways people use the term "disorder" and argue for one. Surely, like almost all interesting abstract and theoretical terms, "disorder" has a large range of subtle variations in usage. It is rather an attempt to address specific foundational challenges to psychiatry as a science raised by the antipsychiatry movement and some Foucaultian and postmodernist theorists. The question is whether there is a widely shared meaning of "disorder" in our professional/lay linguistic community that simultaneously (a) is consistent with psychiatry being a medical specialty, in the sense that "disorder" in "mental disorder" is used in the same sense as "disorder" in "physical disorder" and "medical disorder" and thus locates mental disorders within the "medical model" of conditions that are medical disorders, and (b) offers at least an in principle distinction between genuine mental disorders and various normal-range problems in living, emotional distress, social deviance, disapproved and undesirable behavior, and other acknowledged misapplications of "disorder" that are not true medical conditions. Many researchers, theoreticians, and clinicians clearly believe that "mental disorder" has such a meaning despite the many antipsychiatric challenges. The analysis of "mental disorder" in my view is first and foremost an attempt to resolve this issue and show that "mental disorder" does have a widely understood meaning with both of the aforementioned properties, thus securing the conceptual and scientific foundations of psychiatry as a medical discipline.

Conduct Disorder Studies

I now turn to my series of conduct disorder studies (Kirk et al. 1999; Pottick et al. 2003; Wakefield et al. 1999; Wakefield et al. 2002; Wakefield et al. 2006) that Faucher discusses, in which subjects judged mental disorder in a described youth engaging in antisocial behavior that satisfied *DSM-IV*'s criteria for conduct disorder. I will focus on the data, reported and unreported, from the 2006 study in which we compared four samples: three lay samples (nonclinical social work graduate students who had not taken a *DSM* course and generally had no mental health experience; nonpsychiatric general or pediatric nursing graduate students, with most having nursing experience but no mental health experience; and undergraduates in sociology courses reporting no mental health experience [for details, see Wakefield et al. 2006]), and the clinician sample reported earlier in the 2002 study consisting of 117 graduate students in clinical psychology and clinical social work with an average of four years of clinical experience (the two clinical groups were pooled when initial analyses showed that their responses were extremely similar). (As an aside, these studies yielded results of interest regarding the concept of disorder that are not here pursued. Notably, for example, contrary to what some philosophers have suggested, neither clinicians nor laypeople equate treatment with disorder status [see Wakefield et al. 2002].)

The *DSM-IV* diagnostic criteria for CD are stated purely in terms of symptomatic behaviors, for example: "often bullies, threatens, or intimidates others"; "often initiates physical fights"; "has used a weapon that can cause serious physical harm to others (e.g., a bat, brick, broken bottle, knife, gun)"; "often stays out at night despite parental prohibitions, beginning before age 13 years"; "is often truant from school, beginning before age 13 years"; "has broken into someone else's house, building, or car"; "often lies to obtain goods or favors or to avoid obligations"; "has stolen items of nontrivial value without confronting a victim (e.g., shoplifting…),," and so on. It is also required that "the disturbance in behavior causes clinically significant impairment in social, academic, or occupational functioning."

In many of its diagnostic categories, the *DSM* uses contextual exclusions to discriminate genuine disorders from normal-range responses to problematic environments (Wakefield and First 2012). However, it does not do so in the CD category. Contrary to the *DSM*, the HDA predicts that whether CD symptoms are interpreted as indicators of mental disorder will depend on what the diagnostician infers about the explanation of the symptoms. Specifically, if the symptoms are seen as likely due to an internal dysfunction, they would tend to be seen as psychopathology, but if they are seen as a reasonable response to environmental circumstances, the same symptoms would tend to be understood as not pathological. Thus, to test whether the HDA or *DSM* more accurately reflects intuitions about disorder, we constructed vignettes with the same symptoms satisfying *DSM* criteria for CD but added additional contextual information designed to trigger causal attributions either to the environmental context or to an internal dysfunction (without using those or related labels so as not to bias the subjects' reactions) and evaluated whether subjects judged the symptoms to indicate a disorder.

In these studies, for each of two described youths (Carlos, Judy), there were three vignettes: "symptom only," "environmental context," and "internal dysfunction." Each subject responded to one version for each youth. The symptom-only vignettes included some demographic and history information of a kind common in case descriptions and described the youth's symptoms, which were formulated to satisfy

DSM-IV CD diagnostic criteria (i.e., three or more symptoms from the *DSM*'s list plus resulting role impairment), as follows:

> Judy is a 13 year old white junior high school student who has been in trouble with school authorities for over a year for frequent truancy, which has markedly impaired her academic performance. She has also been caught shoplifting. Recently, an incident in which she was arrested for breaking into a car brought her into court.…She often lied to escape from her responsibilities around the house, she often stayed out until late at night despite their prohibitions.

> Because of many disciplinary actions initiated by his teachers, [Carlos] was referred to the school social worker for an evaluation. In addition to his often being truant, teachers have reported that Carlos often bullies or threatens his classmates and often initiates physical fights, which has seriously limited his social relationships. He was recently caught using a baseball bat as a weapon in a schoolyard fight.

These symptom-only vignettes formed the first paragraph of the other two vignette conditions, which each added a paragraph of contextual information to the symptom description. The environmental-context vignette offered background information that tended to explain the symptoms as understandable reactions to environmental circumstances, specifically as Judy's reaction to attempted sexual abuse by her stepfather and Carlos's self-protective reaction to a gang violence–infested school environment, as in these excerpts:

> When Carlos first arrived at the school, he was terrified by the violence. Eventually, to avoid being preyed on, he and many of his classmates joined one of the rival gangs. Gang fights at the school often involve weapons like bats and bricks on both sides…Carlos learned over time that the most effective defense…was to be highly aggressive and intimidating to others. However, within his gang and outside in the community, he has close relationships and a keen sense of loyalty. Last summer, when Carlos returned to Mexico for his first extended visit with his grandparents,…he got into no trouble.…But, once he returned to Los Angeles, his problematic behavior began again.

> [Judy's] troubles began shortly after her stepfather started attempting to sexually abuse her when she was 12. After that, Judy often made up excuses to get out of the house, stayed out late, and even ran away overnight to avoid him.…She became truant partly to avoid her stepfather, who often waited to pick her up at the end of the school day.…Because she had no money for food when out of the house, Judy began shoplifting and once she broke into a car to get some change she saw on the dashboard, even though she felt bad about doing so.

The "internal-dysfunction" vignettes provided information that suggested an internal source of the symptoms that seemed beyond normal range, as these excerpts illustrate:

> Judy's schoolmates…reported that she was often unreliable and dishonest with them.…Her problematic behavior was not confined to home and school; in the residential facility, Judy did not obey the house rules and lied in order to get out of her assigned chores, and she tried to run away on her third night there.

Carlos reacts to the slightest perception of provocation with severe anger.... He often escalates fights from fists to weapons.... Discipline seems to only exacerbate his problematic behaviour. Even with those he hangs out with, Carlos is easily irritated and frequently initiates fights. Last summer, when Carlos returned to Mexico for his first extended visit with his grandparents, he got into trouble.

As Faucher explains, each vignette was followed by a set of questions asking the subject to rate their agreement or disagreement (recorded on a Likert scale ranging from 1 = "I strongly agree" to 6 = "I strongly disagree") with several items, among which was the following: "*According to my own view, this youth has a mental/psychiatric disorder.*" As Faucher also explains, "the results were quite univocal," with the symptoms judged as less indicative of the presence of mental or psychiatric disorder in the environmental-context condition than in the internal-dysfunction condition, thus strongly supporting the HDA over the *DSM* as a better predictor of judgments of mental disorder.

Having explained the nature of the CD studies at some length, I now turn to Faucher's critical comments on the CD studies. First, Faucher cautions, "If these results are suggestive that Wakefield's analysis is valid, I want to argue that they might not be decisive." Of course the CD studies are not *decisive* proof of the HDA, because decisive support is not what they—or almost any other empirical studies in psychology—are designed to provide. The studies do provide solid evidence that the HDA is superior to the *DSM* diagnostic criteria as an account of disorder intuitions. However, as for any successful study, there are likely multiple alternative hypotheses that suggest that further studies would be useful.

Faucher offers one general and three specific reasons for concern about the CD studies. The general reason is a standard concern about "armchair" conceptual analysis. Faucher quotes my (Wakefield 1999c) comment explaining why, despite appearances to the contrary, conceptual analysis is a quasi-empirical process that relies on a confidence that one shares certain judgments with others in the linguistic community and objects, "But, one might wonder what are the grounds for such a presupposition? ... After the recent wave of X-Philosophy investigations, one becomes suspicious of what is presented as an armchair analysis of a concept." Perhaps, but the "armchair" concern can be overdone in the case of mental disorder. There is a world of difference between the situation in this regard in philosophy of psychiatry versus most other areas of philosophy where "armchair analyses" often involve bewildering counterfactuals that no one has ever considered outside of the philosophical context. Unlike, say, the nuances of the "justified true belief" account of knowledge or the variations in judgments of moral responsibility under various scenarios of determinism (these are examples of X-Phi that Faucher presents), the area of psychiatric and medical diagnosis has been subject to exhaustive scholarly and public analysis and debate over the distinction between disorders and nondisordered problems in living. This has been not only in response to the antipsychiatric challenge but also as part of the vigorous airing of disputes during the revision process leading to each new edition of the *DSM*. Thus, the concept of mental disorder has a plentiful and well-elaborated professional and lay public history of discussion. Consequently, in this area, "armchair" methodology need not be a matter of idiosyncratic and untethered intuitions of the individual philosopher about esoteric counterfactual cases but rather a matter of evidential judgment informed and constrained by a broad base of public data about usage and the reasons that emerge in disagreements. This is not "armchair" philosophy in the usual sense. In some areas of philosophy, the armchair—unless one goes with X-Phi—is all there is, but in philosophy of psychiatry, one can simultaneously be a philosopher and a member of the mental health community who can inform on community linguistic practices.

Faucher asks what the basis is for the presupposition that one's judgments are not idiosyncratic and that one shares judgments with a community. Here is Robert Spitzer, the leading psychiatric nosologist of the past century, answering that question: "What is remarkable—and is in keeping with Wakefield's analysis of the problem—is the great degree of consensus that exists about whether particular psychological or physical conditions are or are not disordered in the absence of a definition of disorder in general. Neither physician, psychologist, nor the public have any problem in agreeing that childbirth (painful), being in love (overevaluation of the loved object), and normal grief (marked distress) are not disorders and that unprovoked panic attacks (dysfunction of the anxiety system), severe depression (dysfunction of mood regulation), and schizophrenia (dysfunction of reality testing and motivation) are disorders" (Spitzer 1999, 430).

Turning to Faucher's concerns specifically about the CD studies, he writes that the sample, which is deliberately heterogeneous, still might be biased in some unknown way. This is a very speculative concern that appears to be based on no immediate weakness identified in the research. It is of course legitimate, but it could be applied to all such studies, even those that, like mine, purposely used heterogenous samples.

Faucher's second concern is that the CD studies did not specifically test the evolutionary component of the HDA and that they "tested only HD [i.e., harmful internal dysfunction but without the evolutionary interpretation]. To conclude that it tested [the evolutionary component as well], one would need to assume that the only interpretation of "function" possible is some kind of designed function. Yet there are many different interpretations of function, for instance, in terms of system-function (Cummins-Function), propensity function, and so on."

These studies did not attempt to test the evolutionary component because, as I have repeatedly explained (see, for example, my response to Lemoine in this volume), the evolutionary component is a theoretical scientific discovery about what constitutes biological design and not part of the conceptual-analytic understanding of "disorder," and thus the HDA makes no simple prediction about general lay judgments on this technical scientific matter. People can understand the concept of "disorder" as "harmful dysfunction" without understanding or agreeing with or even knowing about the evolutionary account of function and dysfunction (e.g., Hippocrates did not know about it and Christian fundamentalists reject it, yet both make mostly the same judgments of disorder as contemporary medical professionals do). So, it makes no sense to test evolutionary beliefs as part of a study of "disorder" unless it is a specially selected sample with that specific issue in mind.

Moreover, it is questionable whether there is really a need for empirical studies comparing the sorts of philosophical views of function that Faucher mentions. It is a fallacious argument to reason, as Faucher does, from the correct premise that within philosophy of biology, "there are many different interpretations of function" (e.g., propensity, systems, biological design) to the implicit conclusion that there are many different interpretations of function potentially relevant to understanding the concept of medical or psychiatric disorder. This is where philosophy has a role in helping to identify what are prima facie plausible hypotheses worthy of empirical effort. If one accepts that there are several possible meanings of "function" in biology, the question for philosophy of medicine is which of those accounts of "function" provide a corresponding account of "dysfunction" as failure of function that is prima facie plausible as the specific sense of "dysfunction" that explains medical judgments of disorder. This is where many critics of the HDA go awry. They note that evolutionary function is just one of several competing philosophical analyses of the use of "biological function" and leap from there to the objection that my choice of evolutionary function is arbitrary (e.g., see Murphy's chapter in this volume). However, my use of evolutionary function is based on an analysis of which biological meaning or meanings of "function" are prima facie plausible candidates to undergird medical notions of function and dysfunction. The step missing from such objections is the systematic testing of the proposed alternative accounts of "function" against common medical judgments to establish whether they are plausible accounts of function and dysfunction in the medical sense.

In fact, the alternative analyses of "function" mentioned by Faucher, even if they explain some judgments about "biological function," do not work as accounts of function and dysfunction in the senses relevant to judgments of medical disorder and thus can be safely ignored in the context of philosophy of medicine. For example, the "propensity theory" (which holds that the effect of a condition on current reproductive fitness is the criterion for function and dysfunction) cannot even explain why, say, dyslexia is considered a disorder but illiteracy due to lack of education is not, supposing that these conditions with similar effects have similar negative impacts on reproductive fitness in our modern social environment. Similarly, the endless dispute about attention-deficit/hyperactivity disorder's (ADHD's) diagnostic status is over whether normal-range rambunctious children are being misdiagnosed, yet even if such rambunctious children suffer a fitness-propensity insult the same size as those with true ADHD (due, perhaps, to their unfortunate interaction with our constrictive school environments), they are still not considered disordered. Do physicians or patients really think that if broken legs or blindness or chronic pain are shown not to influence reproductive fitness in our modern environment, they are no longer disorders? Certainly, according to the propensity account, deciding not to have children would be a dysfunction. Moreover, the propensity theory opens psychiatry up to uses for social control, because social rules can be designed to influence fitness. The propensity theory thus fails the test of answering the antipsychiatric challenge.

The systems view (which holds that the effect of any part on the capacities or properties of a larger containing system is a function of the part) is even less applicable to diagnosis. Everyone, including Cummins (Cummins and Roth 2009), agrees that the systems view makes no distinction between health versus medical disorder as "functions" of whatever internal structures bring them about in the organism. If you are interested in understanding the etiology of CD, then CD is a function of its causes, and an internal state that prevents the development of conduct disorder is a "dysfunction" in that context, according to this view. In biological research, where one is trying to understand how things work, this usage of "function" does often occur. However, the systems account is so inclusive of functions that it is not clear how one would actually formulate an empirical test within the medical context. (For an exhaustive analysis of why the systems view does not work in the medical context, see my reply to Murphy in this volume.) Granted that the understanding of "internal dysfunction" in the sense relevant to diagnosis could use additional empirical exploration (indeed, see below for some unpublished results on this from my CD studies), the types of alternatives mentioned by Faucher can be dismissed out of hand.

Third, Faucher objects that the experimental situation may not represent what happens in actual clinical practice: "subjects have to react to an abstract situation described by vignettes. ... One might wonder if this kind of reaction ... captures concepts that are used or that are more operative in practice." It is possible that the experimental results don't represent what people would do in some clinical situations, but this is just a speculation, and contrary to Faucher's assumption, even if it were so, this does not imply that what people do in practice involves a different concept. Practice involves many compromises with considerations other than the concept of mental disorder. What we want here is not just abstract generic worries but alternative hypotheses with some basis in theory or empiricism. (See my reply to De Vreese in this volume for further discussion of the way that excessive focus on what is done in practice can confuse the conceptual investigation.)

Faucher also notes that some philosophers have argued that self-report and forced-choice instruments of the kind I used in the CD studies "are open to numerous distortions due to wording, framing of questions, question order, and so on." These are routine concerns in experimental work, and addressing them is the art and skill of vignette and questionnaire construction and experimental methodology. The point is to test predictions that distinguish rival hypotheses, and methodology aims to eliminate as many extraneous explanations for the outcome as possible. The precise nature of wording, the balanced ordering of stimuli across subjects, the nonbiasing framing of questions, and so on take months of focused attention to get as close to right as possible, and Faucher offers no reason to think the CD studies suffered from this sort of defect in a way that could jeopardize the meaning of the results. And, of course, it is good to use multiple methodologies, as I have in pursuing epidemiological analyses of HDA-related hypotheses (e.g., Wakefield 2013; Wakefield et al. 2017; Wakefield and Schmitz 2013; 2014; Wakefield et al. 2007). As objections to the CD studies, these concerns are too abstract and generic to be credible.

Replies to Murphy and Woolfolk's and Houts's Critiques of the Conduct Disorder Studies

Faucher's concerns stay at too abstract a level to cast any serious doubt on my CD studies as support for the HDA. However, others have been more targeted and empirically grounded in their criticisms, and I take this opportunity to answer the two most salient objections.

First, Arthur Houts (2001), defending a symptom-based behaviorist account of disorder that denies any inference to internal dysfunction, argued that the CD studies' results do not support the HDA because there is no evidence that subjects in the "internal-dysfunction" vignette condition actually inferred a dysfunction or anything else about the described individuals' minds. Houts observed that, whereas environmental-context vignettes described environmental circumstances that triggered antisocial behavior, the "internal-dysfunction" vignettes did not specify or mention internal dysfunctions but only described behavior without any environmental explanation. Houts thus in effect challenged the validity of the study's fundamental experimental manipulation: how do we know that the internal-dysfunction vignettes actually triggered a dysfunction inference about the described youth and the environmental-reaction vignettes did not? Houts argues that the subjects may have instead attributed disorder simply based on lack of any information about environmental contingencies:

> These outcomes were interpreted as supporting Wakefield's claim that people infer there is a mental disorder when they infer a dysfunction, but in fact, the investigators did not report what inferences led to the differential frequency of seeing a mental disorder when antisocial behaviors were presented under different collateral information conditions. Based on the information provided in this study, a more consistent conclusion is that the social work students attributed antisocial behavior to a mental disorder when they could not otherwise explain it based on current environmental conditions. In other words, the inference to mental disorder is an inference based not on knowledge of function or dysfunction, but an inference based on ignorance. (Houts 2001, 1122–1123)

It always strengthens a study to test for the success of the experimental manipulation, and fortunately, we anticipated Houts's type of concern and added some additional questions to address what if anything the subjects inferred about the described youth. So, I can report analyses that directly address Houts's objection. Due to word limitations, we did not include these analyses in the published versions, so keep in mind that these are un-peer-reviewed results. However, the relevant analyses were done at the time of the publication of the studies using the same methodology and analytic techniques that were peer-reviewed in other analyses.

The most direct way to test Houts's hypothesis is to establish whether subjects did in fact infer internal dysfunction versus no internal dysfunction or related properties from the internal-dysfunction versus environmental-context experimental manipulations, respectively, contrary to his claim. We collected two kinds of data aimed precisely at this point. First, we presented the following item to the psychologist and nurse samples: *"This youth's problematic behaviors likely result from a dysfunction of some cognitive, affective, or other mental mechanism in the youth."* This item explicitly identifies the cause of the problem specifically as a dysfunction of a mental mechanism inside the individual.

The results decisively falsified Houts's hypothesis. For both psychology and nurse samples, in both youth conditions (i.e., Judy and Carlos vignette sets), as the HDA predicted, internal-dysfunction vignettes generally caused subjects to infer dysfunction, and environmental-reaction vignettes did not. Averaging across the four cells (two samples, two youths), the average percentages agreeing with "dysfunction" in the internal-dysfunction versus environmental-context conditions were 81.6% versus 24.0%, respectively (one-tailed Fisher's exact test, $p < .01$ in each of the four cases). These large differences disconfirm Houts's hypothesis that subjects did not infer internal dysfunction and confirm the validity of the study's context manipulation.

However, Houts might argue that the "dysfunction" item in isolation remains potentially ambiguous. Fortunately, we went further. The "dysfunction" item seemed to us a bit technical for nonclinical samples and so was presented only to the two professional samples mentioned earlier. To test for inferences to dysfunction in all of our lay and professional samples, we used a less technical item: *"It seems likely that something is wrong with this youth's mind."* Many theorists (e.g., Klein 1978; Spitzer and Endicott 1978) state that a person has a mental dysfunction when "something has gone wrong with" the person's mind, and this language seemed the closest we could get to colloquial, nontechnical usage for dysfunction in the HDA sense.

All samples answered the "something wrong with the mind" item, and professional and lay responses were similar. In all groups, the percentage agreeing with "something wrong" was substantially and significantly greater in the internal-dysfunction than environmental-reaction context (average percentage agreeing to "something wrong" across all groups and both youths was 76.2% versus 16.9%, respectively; one-tailed

Fisher's exact test, $p < .001$ in all cases). Thus, the results support the initial results for the "dysfunction" item and again strongly disconfirm Houts's hypothesis that subjects did not infer anything wrong internally with the described youths in the internal dysfunction experimental condition.

Second, in a similar vein, Murphy and Woolfolk (2000) lodged the following objection to taking the CD studies as evidence for the HDA: "A careful analysis of the experimental materials employed suggests that the study confounded severity of the anti-social behavior presented in vignettes with the ostensible and intended independent variable manipulation: whether or not the anti-social behavior was readily attributable to external circumstances" (289). That is, perhaps subjects judged disorder in the internal-dysfunction context and nondisorder in the environmental-reaction context based not on inferences to dysfunction versus nondysfunction but based on the severity versus nonseverity of the symptoms portrayed in the respective vignettes.

The suggestion that disorder was distinguished from nondisorder on the basis of symptom severity immediately runs into some problems. This hypothesis implies that the severity level of the symptoms in the environmental-context vignettes was so low that, despite fully satisfying *DSM-IV* diagnostic criteria, they nonetheless fell below the minimal threshold of severity for intuitive disorder attribution. Yet, there is nothing incoherent about a mild disorder, and people judge that they have mild disorders (e.g., colds, rashes) all the time. Moreover, as noted, all of the study's CD vignettes were designed to fully satisfy *DSM* standards for diagnosis, including the *DSM*'s clinical significance criterion requiring that the symptoms cause impairment in some area of role functioning (e.g., school, family, or job problems), which would seem to place them over any reasonable minimal severity threshold for disorder.

Nonetheless, the objection that the case vignettes confound severity with dysfunction has prima facie merit and cannot be dismissed out of hand. As noted, all case vignettes for a given youth started with the same symptom description, which by itself constituted the symptoms-only vignette, and the internal-dysfunction and environmental-context versions were obtained by adding a paragraph of contextual information to the symptom description. This procedure that separated symptom description from contextual information was designed to control for symptom severity. However, it was flawed, and in retrospect, the additional contextual information aimed at indicating internal dysfunction versus reaction to the environmental context did create potential confounds with symptom severity because the contextual information indicated differential intensity, duration, and generality of symptoms. For example, in the vignette excerpts reproduced above, it is clear that the internal-dysfunction vignettes implied in multiple ways that symptoms occurred across a broader domain of circumstances than in the environment-context vignettes (e.g., with close associates and strangers as well as rival gang members; in the facility versus only at home; in Mexico visiting the grandparents as well as at home), and this could be interpreted as greater severity. This confound is exceedingly difficult to avoid because indicators of dysfunction, such as situational nonspecificity, irrationality, and disproportionality, are interpretable as indicators of severity. Of course, severity itself might be interpreted merely as an indicator of dysfunction, and if so, the severity hypothesis is not inconsistent with the HDA. However, Murphy and Woolfolk's hypothesis is that it is severity itself, unmediated by internal dysfunction, that could be the basis for disorder attributions, and the published analyses do not address this possibility. So, the "severity" objection needs to be addressed.

The most compelling test of the Murphy and Woolfolk hypothesis would be to hold severity constant and evaluate whether judgments of disorder and dysfunction still go together within the constant severity condition. In theory, one could look within any one vignette condition to hold severity constant, but in fact, the robust responses to the internal-dysfunction and environmental-context vignettes created rather homogeneous response sets (but see below). Consequently, the best way to test the severity hypothesis is to examine the results within the symptom-only vignette condition, which due to its minimal information triggered diverse "disorder" responses and also has the simplest symptom descriptions.

The severity account predicts no particular relationship between disorder and dysfunction when severity is constant, whereas the HDA predicts that disorder and dysfunction judgments should tend to go together even when severity is constant. The point here is not whether subjects judged disorder versus nondisorder but whether their disorder versus nondisorder judgments, whatever they were, went together with dysfunction versus nondysfunction judgments, respectively. To do this test, we defined "congruent" responses to disorder and dysfunction items as follows: a congruent combined judgment was defined as either (1) agree that there is a disorder *and* agree that there is a dysfunction (or something wrong) or (2) disagree that there is a disorder *and* disagree that there is a dysfunction (or something wrong).

The results are that within the symptom-only context, psychologists and nurses responded congruently to "disorder" and "dysfunction" items 80.5% and 74.4% of the time, respectively, both significantly greater than incongruent rates (one-tailed large sample test, $z = 3.90$, $p < .001$; $z = 3.20$, $p < .001$). Clinical and lay "disorder" and "something wrong" responses were congruent 71.4% and 73.2% of the time, respectively, both significant (one-tailed large sample test, $z = 3.93$, $p < .001$; $z = 4.20$, $p < .001$). These results are unexplained by the severity account and make it unlikely that symptom severity independent of dysfunction inference played the sole or dominant role in disorder response.

One might still ask: not just in the symptom-only condition, but in the other vignette conditions as well, did "dysfunction" or "something wrong" judgments tend to go along with disorder judgments, as predicted by the HDA? To answer this question, we reanalyzed the data for the internal-dysfunction and environmental-context vignettes using as our "items" congruent versus incongruent combined disorder-dysfunction judgments. The results confirm the HDA predictions. Combining internal-dysfunction and environmental-context replies, there was high overall congruence between "disorder" and "dysfunction" items, with nurses' responses congruent 79% of the time, the mental health (clinical social workers and clinical psychology graduate students) sample's responses to "disorder" and "something wrong with the mind" congruent 86% of the time, and the lay sample's responses congruent 84% of the time.

I conclude that these attempts to cast doubt on the CD studies' supportiveness of the HDA fail. The alternative hypotheses proposed by Houts and by Murphy and Wolfolk are inconsistent with the relationships found among both professional and lay subjects' judgments of "disorder," "dysfunction," and "something wrong with the mind."

Epistemology

I now turn briefly to Faucher's discussion of epistemological obstacles to the application of the HDA to psychiatry. Faucher acknowledges at the outset that epistemological concerns have no bearing on whether the HDA is a correct analysis of what we mean by mental disorder and thus are not a critique of the HDA itself. Nonetheless, Faucher points out that to the degree that epistemological obstacles block our ability to distinguish disorders from nondisorders, that will limit how effectively the HDA can accomplish its "normative" role of providing an intellectual justification for reining in diagnostic abuse. The HDA might then meet the antipsychiatric challenge in principle but not in practice.

Faucher focuses on epistemological challenges in establishing evolutionary hypotheses and the fallibility of our judgments about biological design and function. There are indeed limits to our current ability to distinguish disorder from nondisorder due to limitations in our understanding of what is evolved psychological functioning. Like every empirical domain, judgments of biological design and function are fallible and must be subjected to continued scrutiny and testing against alternative theories.

However, the extreme skepticism expressed by Faucher is unwarranted. Faucher objects to the claimed obviousness of many instances of design and function: "the fact that the function of a mechanism seems obvious to us is not a good guide to the evolutionary function of the mechanism or even to its designed nature." This blanket claim is bewildering and itself begs for epistemic support. What percentage of hypotheses that a system is biologically designed have been proven wrong in the history of biology and medicine? Was Aristotle wrong to take acorns growing into oak trees as an obvious example of biological design requiring a special "final cause" explanation? Despite their ignorance of evolution, Hippocrates and Galen surely had adequate grounds for hypothesizing that, say, psychotic delusions, profound melancholia, mania, social phobia, and hysterical paroxysms—all recognized disorders in their time and still so recognized over two millennia later in ours—were failures of human biological design, whereas erotic love and grief—highly disruptive and often distressing mental states—were not in themselves disorders (although they might trigger disorders). Most historical hypotheses identifying conditions as disordered, of the kind that fill the pages of Hippocrates and Galen, have not been overturned even as our scientific understanding has grown. How is that possible if judgments of design and failure of design are not at least a reasonably good prima facie guide to design and failure of design? Is the *DSM* generally wrong to assume that human thought and perception; human emotional systems such as fear and sadness; human biopsychological systems such as sleep, sex, and eating; and human developmental mechanisms are part of our biological design and thus their failure warrants disorder status? The categories of disorder in the *DSM* are by and large not subtle categories; does Faucher dispute that it is prima facie plausible that such conditions as autism, schizophrenia, bipolar disorder, panic disorder, reactive attachment disorder, conversion disorder, anorexia nervosa, erectile disorder (primary impotence), and many others are likely failures of human biological design? Yes, these judgments can be challenged, as in the case of the "neurodiversity" movement that argues that autism (or at least certain forms higher up on the "autistic spectrum") is a normal variation of cognitive functioning (Wakefield et al. 2020) or in R. D. Laing's (1967) arguments that schizophrenia is a normal response to an abnormal family situation. However, like all scientific disputes, these disputes about whether there is in fact a dysfunction are subject to argumentation on evidential grounds and not epistemically untouchable, despite the limits of our knowledge.

Faucher's claims about great epistemic difficulties afflicting the HDA are based on overly pessimistic assumptions about the intractability of our ignorance. For example, how can you possibly empirically address the debate over whether some children labeled ADHD due to their behavior in school are in fact normally rambunctious or disordered? Here are some indirect ways. First, it has been found that within a class, the youngest students consistently get diagnosed with ADHD more frequently, and the only explanation that makes sense is that relatively younger developmental age is being mistaken for disorder. Also, one can study brain development and see whether there are any abnormalities in those labeled ADHD, and it turns out there are not—but there is slower maturation, consistent with the school-age finding. Also, you can see whether ADHD is associated with an enduring impairment, as is generally assumed, or is transient and would then be better explained as normal variation in developmental rates—as we see in every area of physical and mental development—that is interacting badly with our age-specified educational system. Then, if you are really ambitious, you can examine whether children with a specific genetic variation known to be associated with ADHD are indeed impaired in more nomadic cultures that do not have the lock-step educational system we do (because the main alternative hypothesis to failure of designed attentional systems is that normal children are being overly constrained by our school environments), and perhaps you find that the very same genetic variation appears adaptive in nomadic groups but maladaptive in settled groups with constricting educational environments—even where the groups are from the same genetic and cultural population otherwise. Such work has a real impact on whether such children are considered disordered or nondisordered (see my reply to De Vreese in this volume for references and details). Scientists are far from helpless; formulating tests that distinguish hypotheses that seem difficult to distinguish is what scientists do for a living.

Moreover, what is epistemically challenging can change radically and relatively quickly (think of longtime impossibilities like being able to see the back of the moon or tell the sex of a child before birth), making it additionally important to keep epistemic and conceptual/ontological issues separate. Actually, this is already happening in the area of biological design. Enormous and dramatic progress has recently been made in evaluating hypotheses about what has been naturally selected in our species. This is because of the remarkable fact that our evolutionary history is largely preserved in our genetic heritage, which only recently has become accessible to detailed analysis. There are now scientific methods that did not exist a few years ago for examining the patterns of genetic loci near a target locus and determining whether it is likely that the target locus was the result of positive selection pressures or not. These methods have been applied to variety of loci, some potentially related to disorder pathogenesis (e.g., Ding et al. 2002; Lind et al. 2019; Polimanti and Gelernter 2017). Such methods of genetic analysis of selective pressures offer a degree of ability to enter into evolutionary inquiry without need for a time machine, in a way unimaginable a few years ago.

Faucher says, "We should beware that we have a natural inclination to make essentialist inferences based on the fact that certain behaviors are deviant to the presence of dysfunction, yet *that does not guarantee* that we are in presence of a dysfunction" (emphasis added). True, we are essentializing fallibly causal-theorizing creatures, and that is one of our major strengths as a species. Faucher is of course correct that such a hypothesis "does not guarantee" that there is a dysfunction, and the correction of such incorrect hypotheses about nondisordered deviance is enhanced by the HDA's analysis of the concepts being deployed. However, one cannot leap from the modest "does not guarantee" point to the claim: "Our intuitions have no special evidentiary status, quite the contrary. In the past, our inclinations or intuitions have shown to be insufficient guides to dysfunction, as cases of masturbation, female orgasm, drapetomania, and so on have proven." If some past mistakes and abuses were sufficient to show "no special evidentiary status," then a parallel argument would wipe away medicine in general and science altogether, for there are similar occasional errors and abuses there. Fortunately, the fact that Victorians allowed their morals to be confused with medical judgments does not reduce the prima facie likelihood that eyes that can't see, hands that can't grasp, thoughts that lack coherence, anxiety unrelated to any threat, and so on are dysfunctions in systems that are biologically designed. Faucher cites my statement that "one can go wrong in such explanatory attempts," but the fact that one can go wrong using a method does not imply that a method is generally unreliable or that it cannot be used as a beginning for successful bootstrapping to the truth: the fact that there are hallucinations and dreams does not mean that we cannot generally rely on perception for knowledge of the world, and the fact that there are diagnostic errors and abuses does not imply that we are generally wrong about design and function.

Faucher offers two examples of how functions and dysfunctions are not obvious, but his examples also show that they are not beyond our ability to study scientifically. The first is Darwin's own wonderful example of how one can be misled by the unfused skull sutures in the infant, which "have been advanced as a beautiful adaptation for aiding parturition" because they allow the bones of the skull to move and adjust during the birth process and thus allow movement of the baby's large skull through the constrictive birth canal and fuse solidly only at around the age of two years. Darwin observed, however, that, even though the sutures may be "indispensible" to human birth, "as sutures occur in the skulls of young birds and reptiles, which have only to escape from a broken egg, we may infer that this structure has arisen from the laws of growth, and has been taken advantage of in the parturition of the higher animals" (Darwin, as quoted by Gould and Vrba, as quoted by Faucher, this volume). Gould and Vrba use this example to support their distinction between adaptation, which they limit to the original selective pressure that brought about a feature, and what they label "exaptation," which includes subsequent selective pressures that co-opt an already existing feature for new functions. However, structures are routinely exploited for new purposes in evolution, and later selective pressures that maintain a feature are still "adaptations" and instances of "design" or at least "biological functions" in the modern evolutionary sense.

This example does not support Faucher's case. First, the intuition that the sutures are biologically designed is correct. Second, the "obvious" function of the unfused sutures of allowing noninjurious birth is indeed a function, and almost certainly the suture-skull-deformation/birth-canal interaction has been shaped by natural selection and so is biologically designed. Darwin's point is that there is another earlier evolved function of the sutures of allowing unencumbered spherical brain growth. Given these functions, early fusing is a genuine dysfunction and disorder (craniosynostosis). If anything, this example shows that it is possible to identify scientific evidence, including comparative evidence, allowing one to correct false intuitive hypotheses about the evolutionary history of a clearly designed feature.

Faucher's second example concerns the debate over whether *Archaeopteryx* could fly. *Archaeopteryx* was a winged creature that lived about 150 million years ago and had features of both dinosaurs and birds, including feathered wings. It initially seemed obvious by a simple analogy to modern birds that *Archaeopteryx*'s feathered wings as well as its claw and wing structure showed that it was well designed for flight and that it could fly—indeed, its German name was *urvogel* ("first bird"). Faucher points to the fact that such intuitions are fallible and are open to debate. Contrary structural arguments concerning claw structure, wing structure, and feather structure have been put forward suggesting *Archaeopteryx* was not designed to fly but was more likely a ground-dweller that may sometimes have climbed on trees to evade predators, perhaps assisted by the wings for short-distance soaring. For example, *Archaeopteryx* has a long, heavy unfeathered tail and a flat sternum unlike living birds, which, except for flightless birds, have a keeled sternum to which their large, powerful flight muscles attach—although it has been argued that the *Archaeopteryx*'s large collar bone might have served as such an anchor for flight muscles. It is also generally accepted that feathers initially evolved for thermoregulation, not flying, and so it is arguable whether one or both functions were served by *Archaeopteryx*'s transitional feathered wings.

Based on this dispute, Faucher concludes, "So obviousness of design does not fare better than intuition: it is not a reliable guide to adaptation." This does not follow. Both sides in the dispute over *Archaeopteryx* agree that its feathers are the result of design and have some function. The disagreement is about the precise function. Faucher emphasizes that the function is not necessarily the initially obvious one, and that is often true. Indeed, the functions of even familiar clearly designed processes, such as sleep or grief, may be unclear. In the case of *Archaeopteryx*, it is an extinct creature and so of necessity, the evidence about how its wings functioned is a matter of inference open to dispute. Presumably, Faucher would not have similar doubts that a robin's wings have the biological function of enabling flight. The details of the *Archaeopteryx* debate illustrate the amazing power of scientific method to tackle even remarkably difficult questions of function and design.

In no way do I intend to minimize the very substantial obstacles that exist in many cases to establishing biologically designed human psychological nature, and Faucher points to some of these obstacles. Yet, I see no reason to think that the situation is more dire than that occurring in the initial stages of many other areas of science, including the beginnings of physical medicine 2,500 years ago. The need to take the distinction between biological design and dysfunction seriously is underscored by the fact that it is regularly through bogus attributions of this distinction that socially oppressive uses of medical power are justified. Serious attention to this difficult distinction is thus in the long run a corrective to such exploitation. In sum, Faucher's concerns are real, but they are precisely the sorts of concerns that science is designed to confront and overcome in the long run and is in the process of doing so.

References

Colombo, A., G. Bendelow, B. Fulford, and S. Williams. 2003. Evaluating the influence of implicit models of mental disorder on process of shared decision making within community-based multidisciplinary teams. *Social Science and Medicine* 56: 1557–1570.

Cummins, R., and M. Roth. 2009. Traits have not evolved to function the way they do because of a past advantage. In *Contemporary Debates in Philosophy of Biology*, F. Ayala and R. Arp (eds.), 72–86. Blackwell.

Ding, Y. C., H. C. Chi, D. L. Grady, A. Morishima, J. R. Kidd, K. K. Kidd, et al. 2002. Evidence of positive selection acting at the human dopamine receptor D4 gene locus. *Proceedings of the National Academy of Sciences of the United States of America* 99(1): 309–314.

Faucher, L., and I. Blanchette. 2011. Fearing new dangers: Phobias and the cognitive complexity of human emotions. In *Maladapting Minds: Philosophy, Psychiatry, and Evolutionary Theory*, P. R. Adriaens and A. De Block (eds.), 33–64. Oxford University Press.

First, M. B., and J. C. Wakefield. 2010. Defining 'mental disorder' in *DSM-V*. *Psychological Medicine* 40(11): 1779–1782.

First, M. B., and J. C. Wakefield. 2013. Diagnostic criteria as dysfunction indicators: Bridging the chasm between the definition of mental disorder and diagnostic criteria for specific disorders. *Canadian Journal of Psychiatry* 58(12): 663–669.

Harland, R., E. Antonova, G. S. Owen, M. Broome, S. Landau, Q. Deeley, and R. Murray. 2009. A study of psychiatrists' concepts of mental illness. *Psychological Medicine* 39: 967–976.

Houts, A. C. 2001. Harmful dysfunction and the search for value neutrality in the definition of mental disorder: Response to Wakefield (part 2). *Behaviour Research and Therapy* 39: 1099–1132.

Kirk, S. A., J. C. Wakefield, D. Hsieh, and K. Pottick. 1999. Social context and social workers' judgment of mental disorder. *Social Service Review* 73: 82–104.

Klein, D. F. 1978. A proposed definition of mental illness. In *Critical Issues in Psychiatric Diagnosis*, R. L. Spitzer and D. F. Klein (eds.), 41–71. Raven Press.

Laing, R. D. 1967. *The Politics of Experience*. Penguin Books.

Lind, A. L., Y. Y. Y. Lai, Y. Mostovoy, A. K. Holloway, A. Iannucci, A. C. Y. Mak, et al. 2019. Genome of the Komodo dragon reveals adaptations in the cardiovascular and chemosensory systems of monitor lizards. *Nature Ecology & Evolution* 3(8): 1241–1252.

Murphy, D., and R. L. Woolfolk. 2000. The harmful dysfunction analysis of mental disorder *Philosophy, Psychiatry, and Psychology* 7: 241–252.

Polimanti, R., and J. Gelernter. 2017. Widespread signatures of positive selection in common risk alleles associated to autism spectrum disorder. *PLoS Genetics* 13(2): e1006618.

Pottick, K. J., J. C. Wakefield, S. A. Kirk, and X. Tian. 2003. Influence of social workers' characteristics on the perception of mental disorder in youths. *Social Service Review* 77: 431–454.

Rind, B., P. Tromovitch, and R. Bauserman. 1998. A meta-analytic examination of assumed properties of child sexual abuse using college samples. *Psychological Bulletin* 124(1): 22–53.

Spitzer, R. L. 1997. Brief comments from a psychiatric nosologist weary from his own attempts to define mental disorder: Why Ossorio's definition muddles and Wakefield's "harmful dysfunction" illuminates the issues. *Clinical Psychology: Science and Practice* 4(3): 259–261.

Spitzer, R. L. 1999. Harmful dysfunction and the *DSM* definition of mental disorder. *Journal of Abnormal Psychology* 108(3): 430–432.

Spitzer, R. L., and J. Endicott. 1978. Medical and mental disorder: Proposed definition and criteria. In *Critical Issues in Psychiatric Diagnosis*, R. L. Spitzer and D. F. Klein (eds.), 15–39. Raven Press.

Wakefield, J. C. 1992a. The concept of mental disorder: On the boundary between biological facts and social values. *American Psychologist* 47: 373–388.

Wakefield, J. C. 1992b. Disorder as harmful dysfunction: A conceptual critique of *DSM-III-R*'s definition of mental disorder. *Psychological Review* 99: 232–247.

Wakefield, J. C. 1993. Limits of operationalization: A critique of Spitzer and Endicott's (1978) proposed operational criteria of mental disorder. *Journal of Abnormal Psychology* 102: 160–172.

Wakefield, J. C. 1995. Dysfunction as a value-free concept: A reply to Sadler and Agich. *Philosophy, Psychiatry, and Psychology* 2: 233–46.

Wakefield, J. C. 1997a. Diagnosing *DSM-IV*, part 1: *DSM-IV* and the concept of mental disorder. *Behaviour Research and Therapy* 35: 633–650.

Wakefield, J. C. 1997b. Diagnosing *DSM-IV*, part 2: Eysenck (1986) and the essentialist fallacy. *Behaviour Research and Therapy* 35: 651–666.

Wakefield, J. C. 1997c. Normal inability versus pathological disability: Why Ossorio's (1985) definition of mental disorder is not sufficient. *Clinical Psychology: Science and Practice* 4: 249–258.

Wakefield, J. C. 1997d. When is development disordered? Developmental psychopathology and the harmful dysfunction analysis of mental disorder. *Development and Psychopathology* 9: 269–290.

Wakefield, J. C. 1998. *The DSM*'s theory-neutral nosology is scientifically progressive: Response to Follette and Houts. *Journal of Consulting and Clinical Psychology* 66: 846–852.

Wakefield, J. C. 1999a. Evolutionary versus prototype analyses of the concept of disorder. *Journal of Abnormal Psychology* 108: 374–399.

Wakefield, J. C. 1999b. Mental disorder as a black box essentialist concept. *Journal of Abnormal Psychology* 108: 465–472.

Wakefield, J. C. 2000a. Aristotle as sociobiologist: The "function of a human being" argument, black box essentialism, and the concept of mental disorder. *Philosophy, Psychiatry, and Psychology* 7: 17–44.

Wakefield, J. C. 2000b. Spandrels, vestigial organs, and such: Reply to Murphy and Woolfolk's "The harmful dysfunction analysis of mental disorder." *Philosophy, Psychiatry, and Psychology* 7: 253–269.

Wakefield, J. C. 2001. Evolutionary history versus current causal role in the definition of disorder: Reply to McNally. *Behaviour Research and Therapy* 39: 347–366.

Wakefield, J. C. 2006. What makes a mental disorder mental? *Philosophy, Psychiatry, and Psychology* 13: 123–131.

Wakefield, J. C. 2007. The concept of mental disorder: Diagnostic implications of the harmful dysfunction analysis. *World Psychiatry* 6: 149–156.

Wakefield, J. C. 2009. Mental disorder and moral responsibility: Disorders of personhood as harmful dysfunctions, with special reference to alcoholism. *Philosophy, Psychiatry and Psychology* 16: 91–99.

Wakefield, J. C. 2011. Darwin, functional explanation, and the philosophy of psychiatry. In *Maladapting Minds: Philosophy, Psychiatry, and Evolutionary Theory*, P. R. Andriaens and A. De Block (eds.), 143–172. Oxford University Press.

Wakefield, J. C. 2013. The *DSM-5* debate over the bereavement exclusion: Psychiatric diagnosis and the future of empirically supported practice. *Clinical Psychology Review* 33: 825–845.

Wakefield, J. C. 2014. The biostatistical theory versus the harmful dysfunction analysis, part 1: Is part-dysfunction a sufficient condition for medical disorder? *Journal of Medicine and Philosophy* 39: 648–682.

Wakefield, J. C. 2016a. The concepts of biological function and dysfunction: Toward a conceptual foundation for evolutionary psychopathology. In *Handbook of Evolutionary Psychology*, D. Buss (ed.), 2nd ed., vol. 2, 988–1006. Oxford University Press.

Wakefield, J. C. 2016b. Diagnostic issues and controversies in *DSM-5*: Return of the false positives problem. *Annual Review of Clinical Psychology* 12: 105–132.

Wakefield, J. C., and M. B. First. 2003. Clarifying the distinction between disorder and nondisorder: Confronting the overdiagnosis ("false positives") problem in *DSM-V*. In *Advancing DSM: Dilemmas in Psychiatric Diagnosis*, K. A. Phillips, M. B. First, and H. A. Pincus (eds.), 23–56. American Psychiatric Press.

Wakefield, J. C., and M. B. First. 2012. Placing symptoms in context: The role of contextual criteria in reducing false positives in *DSM* diagnosis. *Comprehensive Psychiatry* 53: 130–139.

Wakefield, J. C., A. V. Horwitz, and L. Lorenzo-Luaces. 2017. Uncomplicated depression as normal sadness: Rethinking the boundary between normal and disordered depression. In *Oxford Handbook of Mood Disorders*, R. J. DeRubeis and D. R. Strunk (eds.), 83–94. Oxford University Press.

Wakefield, J. C., S. A. Kirk, K. Pottick, and D. Hsieh. 1999. Disorder attribution and clinical judgment in the assessment of adolescent antisocial behavior. *Social Work Research* 23: 227–241.

Wakefield, J. C., S. A. Kirk, K. J. Pottick, X. Tian, and D. K. Hsieh. 2006. The lay concept of conduct disorder: Do non-professionals use syndromal symptoms or internal dysfunction to distinguish disorder from delinquency? *Canadian Journal of Psychiatry* 51: 210–217.

Wakefield, J. C., K. J. Pottick, and S. A. Kirk. 2002. Should the *DSM-IV* diagnostic criteria for conduct disorder consider social context? *American Journal of Psychiatry* 159: 380–386.

Wakefield, J. C., and M. F. Schmitz. 2013. When does depression become a disorder? Using recurrence rates to evaluate the validity of proposed changes in major depression diagnostic thresholds. *World Psychiatry* 12: 44–52.

Wakefield, J. C., and M. F. Schmitz. 2014. Predictive validation of single-episode uncomplicated depression as a benign subtype of unipolar major depression. *Acta Psychiatrica Scandinavica* 129: 445–457.

Wakefield, J. C., M. F. Schmitz, M. B. First, and A. V. Horwitz. 2007. Extending the bereavement exclusion for major depression to other losses: Evidence from the National Comorbidity Survey. *Archives of General Psychiatry* 64: 433–440.

Wakefield, J. C., D. Wasserman, and J. A. Conrad. 2020. Neurodiversity, autism, and psychiatric disability: The harmful dysfunction perspective. In *Oxford Handbook of Philosophy and Disability*, A. Cureton and D. Wasserman (eds.), 501–521. Oxford University Press.

5   Against the Disorder/Nondisorder Dichotomy

Leen De Vreese

Introduction

In this chapter, I do not comment on Jerome Wakefield's harmful dysfunction analysis (HDA) as such but rather perform a meta-analysis of HDA's goals and aims, as well as evaluate the methods that are used in order to reach these goals. This means that I will focus on methodological and epistemological issues underlying the HDA approach, rather than on problems with the harm or dysfunction aspect of the HDA per se, counter-examples that can be raised against the HDA, or the like. Actually, I think Jerome Wakefield's approach is one of the best attempts to capture the meaning of the notion disorder. The goal of the HDA is nonetheless—as is the case for any traditional analysis of the disorder[1] concept—to provide a single description that can delineate what is and what is not a (mental) disorder. Now, the question that I will raise is whether any attempt at providing a universal definition of the notion disorder—no matter how valuable it is—can ever succeed in clearly delineating (mental) disorders. While I agree with Jerome Wakefield that the meaning of our notion disorder comprises both an evaluative and a factual component, I will argue that it cannot convincingly be argued that the harmful dysfunction analysis forms a basis for delineating disorder and non-disorder in a uniform way. I will argue that disorder is a multifaceted concept, for which a single definition making a straightforward dichotomy between disorder and nondisorder is not justifiable, not necessary, and not useful for practice. We rather need a pluralistic approach, which approves of both the normative and the factual component in the meaning of the concept but also recognizes the diversity in the practical application of the notion. This does not imply that the harmful dysfunction analysis is useless but rather that a reconsideration of how to conceive of it (and of its alternatives) is necessary.

In section I, I will focus on the methodology that has been used to develop the HDA (i.e., conceptual analysis) and on the presuppositions underlying the choice for this methodology. Further, I will clarify the aims of conceptual analysis in general and of Wakefield's HDA more specifically. In section II, I will analyze whether the HDA can best be conceived of as a descriptive or revisionist conceptual approach. I will also argue that the HDA is problematic on both interpretations. In section III, I go a bit deeper into the problem of the vague boundaries of the disorder concept and of Wakefield's view on this. In section IV, I argue for an alternative way of analyzing the disorder concept, which is grounded in practice rather than intuitions. I will make a sketch of how such an approach might be developed and look at the implications for Wakefield's HDA. I come to final conclusions in the last section.

I. HDA as a Conceptual Analysis: Characteristics and Goals

Wakefield's approach fits in with the traditional philosophical approach using conceptual analysis as a tool to find *the* best definition of a certain concept. A conceptual analysis is concerned with our everyday causal intuitions, the way we think and reason about disorders in commonsense situations, and the way the concept is used when making everyday causal judgments. The following quote confirms that Wakefield has consciously chosen this tool in developing the HDA:

> The method used is conceptual analysis, in which proposed analyses are tested against shared judgments about which conditions do an do not fall under the concept of disorder. Consensual judgments are used to test the explanatory power of proposed analyses much as linguists use sentences commonly accepted as grammatical to test hypotheses about grammar. It is not assumed that consensual judgments are always correct.... In such cases, a good analysis will explain why background beliefs interacting with the concept of disorder produced the incorrect classificatory judgment. (Wakefield 1999, 376)

In this section, I look at the underlying motivations and aims for giving a conceptual analysis. In section 1.1, I will first analyze the general characteristics and presuppositions of a conceptual analysis of disorder. In section 1.2, I take a closer look at Wakefield's own motivations for analyzing the concept.

1.1   Characteristics and Presuppositions

Conceptual analyses of the concept disorder share some characteristics and presuppositions. This is not different for Wakefield's approach, as I will illustrate in this section using citations from his own work. First, all conceptual analyses of disorder try to give an account of the concept that is preferably valid for both physical and mental disorders. This is also the case for Wakefield's HDA, which is primarily meant as an analysis of mental disorders but about which Wakefield further states, "First, at issue is the concept of disorder as applied throughout physical and mental medicine. Therefore, the debate draws freely on physical and mental examples in testing proposed analyses. This generality is essential to one of the points of the HD analysis, which is to show that mental conditions can be disorders in the strict medical sense" (Wakefield 1999, 376).

Nevertheless, none of the traditional definitions can live upon its promise of giving the final definition of disorder. All kinds of definitions have been refuted in the literature on the basis of counterexamples, showing that the accounts offered are too broad to exclude nondiseases or too narrow to cover all diseases. Actually, the whole debate about the "right" definition of the concept is driven by a game of giving examples and counterexamples. A single counterexample is thereby supposed to suffice to refute a whole analysis. Further, new approaches presented in the literature are supposed to avoid any counterexamples. Wakefield is well aware of this:

> A classical conceptual analysis, such as the HD analysis, specifies features that are claimed to determine classificatory judgments for a category and its complement, thus taking a substantial risk of falsification. To refute a classical analysis, one simply has to present a clear counterexample in which the concept (as expressed in shared, intuitive judgments) and the proposed analysis of the concept yield divergent classificatory judgments. (Wakefield 1999, 377)

Wakefield is convinced that his own conceptual analysis in terms of harmful dysfunctions is superior to the rival analyses and does possess "the adequate explanatory power to account for common classificatory judgments regarding disorder and non-disorder" (Wakefield 1999, 374). However, it cannot be denied that Wakefield's approach has also been refuted in the literature on the basis of counterexamples demonstrating that people's intuitions are not always in accordance with the HDA. It is not the goal of this chapter to go into details about the shortcomings of, and counterexamples to, the HDA. These can be found in the literature (see, e.g., Cooper 2007; Schwartz 2007) and in other chapters of this book. Admittedly, one should not forget that Jerome Wakefield has put a great deal of work in defending his approach and refuting these counterarguments throughout his writings. It can be debated to what extent his counterarguments to the counterexamples are convincing.[2] But anyhow, it is not the case that the HDA is meanwhile accepted as the "agreed on and adequate analysis of this concept" (Wakefield 1992, 373), which is what Wakefield aimed for. In fact, the debate is still ongoing, and several new approaches have been brought to the fore more recently (see, e.g., Cooper 2007; Schwartz 2007).

And so the story goes on: authors in the field (among which Wakefield himself) keep arguing and counterarguing about the right definition of disorder. The way they do suggests the presence of a number of related, underlying presuppositions. First, that it is possible to find a single, delineating definition of what a "disorder" is. Second, that it is also necessary to search for such a single account that offers *the* necessary and sufficient criteria for disorder. Third, that on the basis of such a definition, one would afterward be able to discern disorders from nondisorders. And lastly, that all human conditions gathered under this definition will be of a single, uniform kind (or have a single, uniform essence). All this seems too much to expect from a single, monolithic definition. This is not surprising, but results from general problems for conceptual analysis. Schwartz extensively argued for this:

As scientists have acquired better and better understanding of diseases and their causes, they find not a unifying microstructure, as for gold or water, but variation. While many have sought an essence that all and only diseases share, this quest has been blocked at every step by variability and heterogeneity. Any definition that would draw a sharp line through all conditions, determining for each whether it is a disease or not, looks like the imposition of a decision, rather than the application of a discovery.

This means adopting any precise account will impose at least some changes on our currently non-reflective and relatively unprincipled way of distinguishing disease for health. Choosing a definition will partly involve deciding which changes from current practice are acceptable. (Schwartz 2007, 59)

It must be said that Wakefield partially acknowledges these problems for conceptual analyses at some points in his work. He seems to think nonetheless that they do not apply to the HDA approach, as he conceives of it. While he is convinced that the essence of disorder is harmful dysfunction, he allows for vagueness and continuity between disorder and nondisorder on the basis that what is harm and what is dysfunction themselves is sometimes vague and debatable. Hence, where there is vagueness and uncertainty about whether or not to conceive of a certain state as disordered on the basis of the HDA, this would not result from the definition of disorder as harmful dysfunction itself but from the vagueness that is characteristic for the defining notions of harm and dysfunction. However, this seems only to shift the problem to another plane, rather than solving it. I will come back to this later (see section 3.1 and section 4). In any case, this weakening of Wakefield of what can be expected from his conceptual analysis does not change the fact that he subscribes to the traditional aim of finding a *single, overall* definition that should (at least largely) cover the use of the concept on the whole.

1.2 Contradictory Motivations

Let us have a closer look at the motivations that Wakefield himself puts forward for his conceptual analysis. At different places in his work, Jerome Wakefield gives two major justifications for the development and adoption of the HDA. These reflect nonetheless two contrary goals.

On one hand, Wakefield states that the goal is *only to explain clear classificatory judgments* and not to impose decisions in unclear cases. The analysis of the clear cases should only demonstrate why there is ambiguity in some unclear cases without resolving them. This motivation is most clearly present in Evolutionary versus Prototype Analyses of the Concept of Disorder (Wakefield 1999):

The analysis was aimed at explaining shared judgments about a range of important cases that clearly fall on one side or the other of the boundary. (379)

Perhaps they are here once again confusing the task of setting a precise boundary for a concept, which does often depend on arbitrary conventions and value considerations, with the analysis of the concept's meaning, which is an attempt to explain clear classificatory judgments and is certainly not purely evaluative in the case of disorder. (397)

It should also be cautioned that the status of a condition as disordered or nondisordered from the HD or any other perspective has no necessary implication for the priority the condition deserves with respect to treatment, prevention, or policy. Such issues require independent consideration not attempted here. (374)

The theory is, on the other hand, motivated on the basis that a clear concept is *necessary for solving controversies and correcting false positives*. This goal is brought to the fore in papers such as "The Concept of Mental Disorder" (Wakefield 1992), "When Is Development Disordered?" (Wakefield 1997), and "False Positives in Psychiatric Diagnosis" (Wakefield 2010). The following quotes are testament to this fact:

Lack of a valid concept of disorder is not just conceptually and methodologically problematic, it is potentially ethically problematic as well. Classification of a condition as disordered has ramifications ranging from those of labeling a child or adult as disordered to determinations of whether it is appropriate to treat the condition with drugs. (Wakefield 1997, 271)

Thus, if the symptom-based approach to diagnostic criteria and disorder, whatever its other merits, is potentially prone to false positives as I have argued, it is essential to reconsider the concept of disorder and what is supposed to fall under this core category. (Wakefield 2010, 12)

Hence, Wakefield seems to hesitate on whether he wants to passively analyze the concept for purely theoretical reasons or whether his analysis should also have practical implications. This ambiguity in Wakefield's goals seems to go hand in hand with mixing up of two kinds of possible but different goals of conceptual analysis, as I will further explain in the next section.

II. HDA as a Conceptual Analysis: Which of Two Flavors?

2.1 Descriptive versus Revisionist Conceptual Analysis

Traditionally, a conceptual analysis can have two goals: it aims for a descriptive account that tries to line up nicely with our intuitions, or it aims for a revisionist account that urges for a revision of the concept in order to clear out the inconsistencies in our intuitions. What concerns Wakefield's HDA, the question now becomes whether we should understand it as a descriptive conceptual analysis or as a revisionist one. Wakefield's contrary motivations for his theory seem to imply that he cannot choose between both. On one hand, he seems to interpret the HDA as a purely descriptive approach. According to his first motivation cited above, his analysis is based on "shared judgments about clear cases." Insofar as it is unclear whether a certain condition holds as a disorder or not, this would then reflect our unclearness on whether or not there is any harm involved and/or whether or not one can rightly speak of a dysfunction (in line with Wakefield's descriptions of these terms). This would imply that the HDA is a descriptive conceptual analysis only of "the clear cases" of disorder. Further, it would imply that we have shared intuitions about what are the unclear cases. However, the fact that authors disagree with Wakefield as to what are the clear and unclear cases (see, e.g., Lilienfeld and Marino 1995) demonstrates that this weakened descriptive view does not solve the problem of ambiguities. When reading through Wakefield's papers, it also becomes clear that he does not just accept conflicting intuitions about counterexamples as illustrative of shared ambiguities surrounding the notions of harm and dysfunction. He rather tries to refute the counterexamples that are brought up against his theory by turning them into examples confirming his approach, that is, by fine-tuning how to interpret the notions of harm and dysfunction such that they are in line with the intuitions of his critics. In other terms: he gives arguments on the basis of which his opponents are directed to revise their intuitions as actually being in line with the HDA. Still in other terms: instead of urging the critics to revise their intuitions on whether or not their counterexamples are real disorders—which would be the most straightforward revisionist approach—he urges them to revise their view on whether or not the criteria of harm and/or dysfunction are fulfilled. This means that examples of clear cases of (non)disorders that, according to the critics, cannot be interpreted as such in terms of the HDA are then claimed by Wakefield to be clear cases of (non)disorders in line with the HDA, given certain more specific interpretations of what is a harm or dysfunction. Hence, from this reading, one can argue that Wakefield pleas for a partial revision of our everyday use of the concept. We do not just have shared ambiguous intuitions that can be understood on the basis of the vagueness of harm and dysfunction. We should have the same intuitions if we all interpreted harm and dysfunction in the way that Wakefield defends. Hence, Wakefield does not only shift the problem to another plane, as I stated earlier. He also enforces a solution by way of imposing certain interpretations of the notions of harm and dysfunction. These specific understandings of harm and dysfunction are nonetheless only necessary in function of resolving the controversies surrounding unclear cases.

To conclude, Wakefield's revisionary talk follows from the way in which he tries to solve controversies on the basis of his own theory. This is in line with Wakefield's second motivation that I brought up in the previous section.

I hope to have convinced the reader by now that it is unclear what kind of conceptual analysis Wakefield aims for or how he wants to combine the two kinds of conceptual analysis (that are, in fact, inherently contradictory in their aims). However, no matter which of two flavors he eventually chooses, both of them have further problems, as I will show in the next two sections.

2.2 Problems for the Descriptive Aspect: Intuitions

Intuitions about "clear cases" form the basis for the HDA. Nevertheless, what are "clear cases" can be discussed. Whose intuitions do we need to follow on this point? Those of the author? Those of medical doctors? Those of the general public? In fact, intuitions might differ more than we are aware of (see, e.g., Smith 2002). Further, one can never start from scratch. Intuitions always rely on value-laden and/or theory-laden presuppositions about what is and what is not a disorder. This brings us to an unavoidable circularity: someone's thoughts about whether or not something is a "clear case" is already determined by his or her underlying theoretical presuppositions beforehand. What concerns the dysfunction aspect, Wakefield nonetheless argues in defense of his own approach: "However, the fact is that when one asks people for their judgments about disorder and non-disorder, their judgments go against the 'current mismatch' approach and in favor of the evolutionary approach" (Wakefield 2010, 15).[3]

Can such claims be justified? Is it really true that all people (all people, in all situations) really reason about disorder and nondisorder on the basis of "a breakdown in a mechanism x, that is not in line with how humans are designed" in combination with some kind of harm? Or how should we interpret this kind of defense of the HDA as a superior approach? The real test would be to, first, collect all judgments on "clear cases of disorders" on which all people agree and that are based in the same and justified background knowledge. The proof of the pudding would lie then in answering whether all these judgments are justified by the HDA, while they cannot be captured by alternative approaches.[4]

Is it not much more plausible that intuitions will vary widely (across people, across situations), according to varying presuppositions, that might be explicated by various conceptual approaches? If so, choosing for the HDA as the best analysis of disorder already automatically implies a revision (in light of the preferred theory) of how we conceive of disorder/nondisorder, even in "clear cases." This would also imply that choosing for the HDA as the best descriptive conceptual analysis among alternatives is arbitrary.

2.3   Problems for the Revisionist Aspect: Generalization

What about the HDA as a revisionist approach? Interpreting the HDA as a revisionist approach raises additional problems. Even if the HDA would form the best approach to clear cases of disorder, one can argue that those judgments on disorder that all people with justified background knowledge share might concern too little cases to justify a generalization of the HDA to all diseases.

What would then justify the generalization of the HDA from "the clear cases" to "all cases"? Won't we narrow down the scope of what it means to be disordered to only these kinds of diseases about which we have "clear intuitions"? Further, what justifies that contrary intuitions are not a problem once we are applying the HDA to "unclear cases," while such intuitions form the basis on which alternative approaches were first rejected? And on which basis can we justify the selection of this single theory to all others as the basis for revisions? All these questions remain unanswered.

The problems for a conceptual analysis of "disorder" along traditional lines are clear. We seem unable to discover the essence of what it means to be disordered. This implies that deciding to pick out just one or another definition as *the* definition will automatically result in a revision of the everyday use and meaning of the concept in light of this decision. In other words, any conceptual analysis of disease resulting in a monolithic definition seems to lead to a revisionist account instead of a descriptive one. The question that follows is whether we really want to revise the concept or whether we prefer a description of the concept's actual use. When considering this, we should recognize that it is unclear on what basis one can privilege one account above the others as *the* single, true one. The only possible justification seems to be the intuitions one already had beforehand about whether or not certain example diseases are "true" cases of disease or not. The choice for any final definition on the basis of which we should revise our intuitions will therefore be arbitrary.

III. Boundaries

In this section, I would like to make some final remarks concerning boundaries and the vagueness of the concept disorder. Wakefield gives two justifications for vague boundaries (Wakefield 1999, 378). First, what appears to be a vague boundary can result from a lack of knowledge about factors that would provide a precise boundary if known. This kind of vagueness seems to me to be the least problematic for a conceptual analysis of disorder, since it implies that there is a clear distinction in principle. The other kind of vagueness is the vagueness from vague boundaries of the defining criteria themselves. This is the kind of vagueness that Wakefield most explicitly defends as unproblematic for the HDA. As I stated before, Wakefield allows for vagueness of boundaries of the disorder concept (and hence for some kind of continuity between disorder and non-disorder) on the basis of the vague boundaries of the concepts of harm and dysfunction: "The concept of disorder is analyzable as harmful dysfunction, but harm and dysfunction themselves may contain vagueness and indeterminacies that give a degree of imprecision to the overarching concept" (Wakefield 1999, 378).

Wakefield does not perceive of this as a problem for his conceptual analysis: "analyzing a concept's meaning or definition, which is what the HD analysis aims to do, is different from setting a precise boundary for the concept. Most meaningful concepts, like red and tall, do not have precise boundaries but are useful for classifying clear cases" (Wakefield 1999, 378). Nonetheless, I am convinced that such vagueness subverts the power of his conceptual analysis. This kind of vagueness seems to lead to one of the following implications for the HDA:

Either (1) one is in the end really limited to describing only the clear cases using the HDA. This would imply that the HDA is a descriptive conceptual analysis which has no significant practical implications at all. This is in line with Wakefield's quotation above. However, this seems also in contradiction with Wakefield's second motivation for the HDA (cf. section 2.2) and would really impoverish the usefulness of the HDA. Is it not a pity that after providing a conceptual analysis which is aimed at clarifying what are disorders, and what not, Wakefield has to conclude regarding some medical conditions: "In none of these cases is there a precise boundary between dysfunction and nondysfunction, yet for practical medical purposes physicians are able to 'adequately distinguish disorder from nondisorder'" (Wakefield 1999, 380)?

Or, (2) one might in fact end up with three kinds of disorders: harm and dysfunction-related disorders (where you have a clear case of harmful dysfunction), primarily dysfunction-related disorders (where you have a clear dysfunction and vague reasons also to suspect harm), primarily harm-related disorders (where you have a clear case of harm and vague reasons also to accept the presence of a dysfunctional mechanism). This would lead us to a pluralist definition, which is clearly in contradiction with Wakefield's goal of finding an overarching definition and with Wakefield's first motivation for the HDA (cf. section 2.2).

IV. Relation with (Medical) Practice

The previous sections make clear that the combination of Wakefield's method, motivations, and goals brings him into a difficult position. Although he made a very reasonable attempt to give an analysis of the concept disorder, it turns out that his HDA as such has little bearing in practice. This is a pity and should not have been the case if he would have had a wider view on how an analysis of the concept disorder could look like.

Looking back at my analysis of the HDA in this chapter, the following questions (and answers) arise:

What is problematic about the possibility that there are different kinds of disorders that might need (partially) different analyses? (I think nothing is.)

Is vagueness not rather the result of the fact that our concept cannot be simply defined because disorder is a multifaceted concept? (I think it is.)

Is it useful to keep on searching for analyses that aim at clarifying the concept but nonetheless do not have practical implications? (I do not think so.)

Is it not much more fruitful to try to offer an approach that can form a basis for critical reflection in practice, instead of holding on to the traditional methodology of conceptual analysis and the traditional aim of a unifying approach? (Yes, I think it is.)

Is it not better to recognize and analyze the diversity in our use of the concept disorder, instead of trying to lump all instances as much as possible together in a single, overarching approach? (Yes, I think this makes much more sense.)

In general, I think the problem can be brought back to the starting point of our traditional analyses. Why do we not just admit that presuppositions cannot be excluded and start in the development of an approach from the use of the concept in *practice?* Would this not be much better than acting as if one can start from scratch in making a traditional philosophical conceptual analysis on the basis of armchair intuitions?

Clearly, no single physician will change his or her mind on whether, for example, attention-deficit/hyperactivity disorder is a "real" disease on the basis of a conceptual analysis of disorder according to which it is not. Therefore, it seems better to recognize the diversity in the meanings we put on the concept disorder in practice. This will also make the resulting framework much more useful for reflection in medical practice. Actually, one can assume that practitioners are very well aware of the diversity in diseases and disease kinds and therefore suppose that "for practical medical purposes physicians are able to 'adequately distinguish disorder from nondisorder'" (Wakefield 1999, 380). But on the other hand, practitioners might tend to classify people's problems too often as diseases, given that they were trained and work in a strictly scientific-medical setting. Therefore, a practice-related, pluralist framework might not only provide us with a more realistic descriptive account of the meaning of disorder but also be very useful for practitioners as a basis for reflection and comparison.

Hence, we should find a way to get a grip on how the notion of disorder is used in practice, even when this use is not uniform. Instead of aiming for an overarching approach, it seems therefore much more useful to aim for a pluralist conceptual approach that is based in, and can be critically evaluated in relation to, practice. Within such a framework, different (aspects of different) traditional approaches can be used as an analyzing tool rather than as final definitions. This would imply that the HDA remains very useful but should no longer be defended as the only superior approach. What we primarily need is a basis for reflection, not a basis for arbitrary decisions. A conceptual approach to disorder should keep us reflecting instead of relaxing. Within a pragmatic, pluralist approach, "counter-examples" will no longer form a reason to reject or revise everything, but they will help us in further reflection, further comparison, and further nuancing of disorder labeling. This is probably the best an analysis of the concept disorder can do for us all.[5]

Conclusion

An analysis of the HDA from a methodological and epistemological point of view demonstrates that it cannot convincingly be argued that the HDA should be accepted as a superior conceptual analysis of disorder. Disorder rather seems to be a multifaceted concept for which a single definition that hopes to make a straightforward dichotomy between disorders and nondisorders is not justifiable, not necessary, and not useful for practice. This does not imply that the HDA is useless but rather that a reconsideration of how to conceive of it (and of its alternatives) seems necessary.

Notes

1. An important preliminary remark needs to be made. I am well aware of the slight differences in meaning and use of the concepts of disease, disorder, illness, and related terms—at least in the

English language. The differences between these are also discussed in the philosophical literature. I will nonetheless sidestep this discussion and use the terms "disorder" and "disease" as broad, general terms referring to all those things people usually refer to as a disease, disorder, illness, injury, sickness, and suchlike. Herein I follow Wakefield, among others, in his discussion of the concept (see Wakefield 1992, 374).

2. At least, I can attest that some of his arguments go against my intuitions and against my intuitions about what are "common classificatory judgments."

3. According to the current mismatch approach, we should focus on how well we are adapted to our current environment and not on how we have been biologically designed in the past. The latter is what the HDA focuses on. The discussion itself is not important for my argument here. I use this quote only to demonstrate how Wakefield reasons from intuitions on how people would usually reason about disorder.

4. If so, one should ideally also be able to explain all the "unclear cases" that remain on the basis of ambiguities in the concepts of harm and dysfunction.

5. It is not the aim of this chapter to describe in more detail how such an approach might look like, but a more concrete outline of such an approach can be found in De Vreese (2014).

References

Cooper, R. 2007. *Psychiatry and the Philosophy of Science*. Acumen.

De Vreese, L. 2014. The concept of disease and our responsibility for children. In *Philosophical Perspectives on Classification and Diagnosis in Child and Adolescent Psychiatry*, Lloyd Wells and Christian Perring (eds.), 35–55. Oxford University Press.

Lilienfeld, S. O., and L. Marino. 1995. Mental disorder as a Roschian concept: A critique of Wakefield's "Harmful Dysfunction Analysis." *Journal of Abnormal Psychology* 104(3): 411–420.

Schwartz, P. H. 2007. Decision and discovery in defining 'disease'. In *Establishing Medical Reality: Essays in the Metaphysics and Epistemology of Biomedical Science*, H. Kincaid and J. McKitrick (eds.), 47–63. Springer.

Smith, R. 2002. In search of "non-disease." *British Medical Journal* 324(7342): 883–885.

Wakefield, J. C. 1992. The concept of mental disorder: On the boundary between biological facts and social values. *American Psychologist* 47(3): 373–388.

Wakefield, J. C. 1997. When is development disordered? Developmental psychopathology and the harmful dysfunction analysis of mental disorder. *Development and Psychopathology* 9(2): 269–290.

Wakefield, J. C. 1999. Evolutionary versus prototype analysis of the concept of disorder. *Journal of Abnormal Psychology* 108(3): 374–399.

Wakefield, J. C. 2010. False positives in psychiatric diagnosis: Implications for human freedom. *Theoretical Medicine and Bioethics* 31(1): 5–17.

6   Do Clinicians Understand the Harmful Dysfunction Analysis of Mental Disorder? Reply to Leen De Vreese

Jerome Wakefield

I thank Leen De Vreese for continuing, via her essay, our interaction begun in person some years ago during my very enjoyable visit to Leuven and for her thoughtful challenge to the viability for illuminating medical practice of my harmful dysfunction analysis (HDA) of medical, including mental, disorder. The HDA claims that "disorder" refers to "harmful dysfunction," where dysfunction is the failure of some feature to perform a natural function for which it is biologically designed by evolutionary processes and harm is judged in accordance with social values (First and Wakefield 2010, 2013; Spitzer 1997, 1999; Wakefield 1992a, 1992b, 1993, 1995, 1997a, 1997b, 1997c, 1997d, 1998, 1999a, 1999b, 1999c, 2000a, 2000b, 2001, 2006, 2007, 2009, 2011, 2014, 2016a, 2016b; Wakefield and First 2003, 2012). Like the classic answer to the question of how a musician gets to Carnegie Hall, De Vreese thinks that the way a philosopher gets to an account of disorder is *practice, practice, practice*—that is, immersion in the study of clinical practice in all its diversity and contextual anchoring. She argues for an analysis of "disorder" that "is grounded in practice rather than [conceptual] intuitions." Clinical judgments are based on the clinician's varying presuppositions, thus best understood within a pluralistic approach, she argues, whereas conceptual analysis arrogantly imposes one univocal meaning of "disorder" on clinical diversity and should be abandoned.

I agree that understanding clinical practice in all its rich detail independent of conceptual analysis is an interesting and important undertaking, albeit one that arguably might be better undertaken by social scientists than philosophers. However, rather than seeing the study of disorder judgments in practice as being *opposed* to an HDA-like conceptual analytic approach to "disorder," I understand the two approaches as importantly complementary given that the concept of disorder is one influence on clinical judgment. A symbiosis of the two is especially necessary for recognizing and correcting misdiagnosis, a crucial goal for which a grounded view that accepts clinical labeling at face value and simply tries to describe and understand it provides no help. Only an analysis of the concept of disorder provides a way to evaluate whether what a clinician judges in practice in a given context is correct or an instance of the overpathologizing of normal distress or social deviance. In effect, De Vreese's uncritical practice-descriptive approach suggests that a disorder is whatever each psychiatrist chooses to label a disorder, which leaves the antipsychiatric critique of diagnosis unanswered. Elevating the clinician to a position of such privileged classificatory authority involves its own form of arrogance.

Before considering De Vreese's specific objections to conceptual analysis, an oddity of her argument—and consequently of my reply as well—needs to be mentioned. In undertaking to explain the methodological reasons for the HDA's failure, De Vreese does not argue but simply *presupposes* that the HDA in fact fails to explain disorder judgments and is subject to decisive counterexamples. However, De Vreese herself presents no such counterexamples. Instead, she in effect outsources the HDA's refutation to others, citing two sources for the HDA's refutation:

> It cannot be denied that Wakefield's approach has also been refuted in the literature on the basis of counterexamples demonstrating that people's intuitions are not always in accordance with the HDA. It is not the goal of this chapter to go into details about the shortcomings of, and counterexamples to, the HDA. These can be found in the literature (see, e.g., Cooper 2007; Schwartz 2007).

I consider De Vreese's methodological objections to conceptual analysis on their own merits, below. However, to fully answer De Vreese, I also need to address the two cited philosophers' critiques of the HDA that according to her "cannot be denied" and that form a presupposition of her methodological critique. Rather than going that far afield in this reply, I focus here on De Vreese's methodological claims and address Cooper's and Schwartz's proposed counterexamples to the HDA in a supplementary reply to Cooper in this volume.

De Vreese's Methodological Objections to Conceptual Analysis

I now turn to De Vreese's criticisms of the conceptual analytic methodology I use to support the HDA. First, De Vreese argues that it is arrogant to claim that one can get *the* right answer to what a concept means, so one should remain more modestly pluralist. However, it is presumably not arrogant to be open to *the* most explanatory account, whether univocal or pluralist. One may wonder at the consistency of an avowed pluralist who, observing the complementary methods of grounded description of practice and conceptual analysis, sees a zero-sum competition and insists that *the* right method is the study of practice, thus endorsing a methodological monism (albeit one that embraces a pluralism across clinicians and situations) when one can perfectly well do both.

Second, De Vreese expresses impatience with the slow and contentious process of formulating and testing theories of classificatory judgments; "the whole debate about the 'right' definition of the concept is driven by a game of giving examples and counterexamples"; "And so the story goes on: authors…keep arguing and counterarguing about the right definition of disorder." Granted, evaluating explanatory power and evidential support in a contentious field is often lengthy and tedious, but these "games" are the best available technique we have for gaining clarity and improving explanatory power over time. De Vreese offers no reason to think that theorizing about clinical practice rather than concepts would yield any less contentious or lengthy disputes. Indeed, one cannot help but wonder whether there is any area of philosophy that would remain standing if subjected to De Vreese's impatient gaze. One recalls here the joke: "Question: What is the difference between philosophers and Rottweilers? Answer: Rottweilers eventually let go."

Third, De Vreese argues that there are many types of disorders that do not fit one mold: "I will argue that disease is a multifaceted concept, for which a single definition making a straightforward dichotomy between disorder and nondisorder is not justifiable, not necessary, and not useful for practice." However, from the fact that disorders themselves are diverse, it does not follow that there is no univocal conceptual definition that subsumes them all. (On this issue, see also my reply to Zachar in this volume.) Great diversity exists among chairs (bean bag versus leather recliners), elements (helium versus gold), animals (snails versus chimpanzees), water (steam, ice, and liquid water), and stars (neutron stars versus red dwarf stars), yet one can give decent univocal accounts of the features that explain why something falls under each of these categories. De Vreese confuses multiplicity of *kinds of disorders* with the idea that there is no univocal *concept of disorder* that unites the multiplicity.

Fourth, De Vreese argues that individual clinicians' intuitions about how to classify conditions are anchored in the varying contexts in which they make those judgments, and this implies lack of a univocal concept, so a one-size-fits-all conceptual analysis is misguided and hopelessly prescriptive. Yet, precisely the opposite is true. A survey and analysis of the contextual features in the *Diagnostic and Statistical Manual of Mental Disorders* (*DSM*) diagnostic criteria revealed that taking into account contextual variation when diagnosing superficially similar conditions is actually a strategy for distinguishing internal dysfunctions from normal responses and so determining whether a condition satisfies the univocal concept of disorder (Wakefield and First 2012). The contextual information provides information about whether core features of the univocal disorder concept hold in that context. For example, intense chronic anxiety usually implies an anxiety disorder *unless* there is a chronic contextual threat that explains such anxiety as a normal response. The HDA thus potentially explains *why* varying contexts yield the varying judgments they do.

Perhaps De Vreese can be interpreted here as claiming more strongly that the *intuitive judgments of category membership of one and the same condition in one and the same context* vary, thus casting doubt on the existence of an evidential base of shared classificatory judgments of disorder and nondisorder that are needed for a conceptual analysis.

The problem with this argument is that there is a remarkable degree of prima facie agreement about many conditions' normality or pathology among a large number of observers, providing an ample target for explanation. Robert Spitzer, the most eminent psychodiagnostician of the twentieth century and someone who, from his experience editing *DSM-III* and *DSM-III-R*, knew a thing or two about agreement and disagreement among psychiatrists and laypeople about diagnosis, put it this way:

> What is remarkable—and is in keeping with Wakefield's analysis of the problem—is the great degree of consensus that exists about whether particular psychological or physical conditions are or are not disordered in the absence of a definition of disorder in general. Neither physician, psychologist, nor the public have any problem in agreeing that childbirth (painful), being in love (overevaluation of the loved object), and normal grief (marked distress) are not disorders and that unprovoked panic attacks (dysfunction of the anxiety system), severe depression (dysfunction of mood regulation), and schizophrenia (dysfunction of reality testing and motivation) are disorders. (Spitzer 1999, 430)

Fifth, above all, De Vreese argues that individual clinicians' intuitions about how to classify conditions are based on their varying presuppositions about values and facts, so that analyzing the concept of disorder in a one-size-fits-all way is futile: "Why do we not just admit that presuppositions cannot be excluded and start in the development of an approach from the use of the concept in *practice*. Would this not be much better than acting as if one can start from scratch in making a traditional philosophical conceptual analysis on the basis of armchair intuitions?"

The problem here is that De Vreese's pluralist proposal simply accepts such divergent judgments based on varying presuppositions at face value, providing no understanding of why certain presupposed beliefs and values nonrandomly tend to yield certain judgments of disorder. The concept of disorder is an explanatory construct explaining these links. De Vreese's "presupposition" argument reveals a misunderstanding of the role of conceptual analysis in an account of practice. She writes as if a conceptual analysis by itself determines whether a certain condition is or is not a disorder, but in fact a conceptual analysis *explains why certain background presuppositions lead to the disorder judgments* that they do. The fact that different presuppositions lead people to different disorder judgments is consistent with there being one shared concept of disorder that mediates the relationship between presupposition and judgment.

Concepts by themselves do not determine classificatory judgments. You and a friend can totally agree on the meaning of the term "bachelor" and totally disagree about whether a specific individual you met at a party is or is not a bachelor based on different observations, beliefs, and inferences. Concepts only set the conditions under which something falls within a category, and one's beliefs about whether those conditions are satisfied provide the presuppositions that determine one's category judgment. The concept and the presuppositions are jointly necessary for explaining classificatory judgments.

A sixth objection by De Vreese is that the HD emerges from armchair intuitions and that such analyses "do not have practical implications." These claims are inaccurate. The HDA emerged from my attempts to grapple with clinical intuitions taken from clinical practice and empirical research results concerning conditions as varied as major depression and female orgasmic disorder (see Steeves Demazeux's chapter in this volume for a discussion of my early sexual disorder papers). It has since been applied to many disorders (e.g., Wakefield 2011b, 2016, 2019; Wakefield, Horwitz, and Schmitz 2005; Wakefield and Schmitz 2017a) and been the basis for two research programs, one on clinical judgment (e.g., Wakefield et al. 2002; Wakefield et al. 2006) and the other on epidemiological estimates of prevalence (e.g., Wakefield et al. 2007; Wakefield and Schmitz 2015, 2017b; Wakefield, Horwitz, and Lorenzo-Luaces 2017; Wakefield, Schmitz, and Baer 2010). As opposed to, for example, Boorse's biostatistical theory of disorder, which is generally cited by philosophers but not by clinicians and clinical researchers, the HDA is heavily cited in the mental health literature. In contrast, De Vreese fails to provide even one example of how the study of practice in the way she suggests yields fruitful philosophical or diagnostic understanding. (I comment below on the example of attention-deficit/hyperactivity disorder [ADHD] that she develops in another paper.) The reality is that the HDA is the most clinically anchored—and clinically cited—analysis of the concept of mental disorder of those currently available and has been extensively deployed by non-armchair mental health clinicians and researchers in discussions of the validity of diagnosis and in debates over revisions to diagnostic criteria more than any other approach.

Finally, although De Vreese is generally allergic to the notion of "dysfunction," she suggests at one point that according to her pluralistic approach, *dimensions* of dysfunction and harm should replace the HDA's categories:

> One might in fact end up with three kinds of disorders: harm and dysfunction-related disorders (where you have a clear case of harmful dysfunction), primarily dysfunction-related disorders (where you have a clear dysfunction and vague reasons also to suspect harm), and primarily harm-related disorders (where you have a clear case of harm and vague reasons also to accept the presence of a dysfunctional mechanism). This would lead us to a pluralist definition, which is clearly in contradiction with Wakefield's goal of finding an overarching definition.

Rather than being "clearly in contradiction," the switch to dimensions is entirely consistent with the HDA. I have argued that dysfunction and harm are both fuzzy concepts, so of course there will be clear cases of dysfunction in which harm is debatable and clear cases of harm in which dysfunction is debatable. The HDA would predict, however, that the less clear the dysfunction or harm judgments, the less clear the disorder judgment, and in the extreme case of dysfunction with no harm or harm with no dysfunction, there would tend to be a nondisorder judgment. That is perhaps a prediction on which De Vreese and I would disagree and thus a useful test. (See my reply to De Block and Sholl in this volume, as well as Wakefield 2014, for examples of how lack of harm yields lack of disorder status.)

Why Haslam's (2002) "Kinds of Kinds" Fails to Support De Vreese's Disorder Pluralism

De Vreese (2014) states that her pluralistic anti-HDA view of uses of "disorder" is "based on the view of Nick Haslam (2002)" (37). I believe there are many who similarly interpreted Haslam's analysis in that paper to be in conflict with the HDA. Haslam is an exceptionally thoughtful scholar and one of the few researchers engaged in both empirical and conceptual exploration of the foundations of diagnosis. However, the Haslam paper referenced by De Vreese provides no legitimate rationale for rejecting the HDA in favor of pluralism about "disorder," for reasons I will now explain.

Haslam (2002) argues for a pluralistic taxonomy of types of disorder constructs. He appropriately laments the unjustifiably constricted ideological views that permeate psychiatry according to which all psychiatric categories must refer to one kind of construct, whether the neo-Kraepelinian's biological essentialism, Zachar's "practical kinds," currently fashionable dimensional constructs, or social constructivist notions: "Psychiatric disorders are presented as being uniformly of one kind. ... The possibility that different structural models might capture different forms of psychopathology goes unrecognized" (2002, 209). Haslam reasonably argues that it is more likely that science will reveal various kinds of constructs underlying disorder categories and that there are probably a variety of kinds of constructs underlying current provisional categories. Haslam's corrective to dogmatic construct monism is to formulate a taxonomy of possible types of disorder constructs that offers "a pluralistic view of psychiatric classification ... according to which psychiatric categories take a variety of structural forms ... —non-kinds, practical kinds, fuzzy kinds, discrete kinds, and natural kinds" (2002, 203), organized as a hierarchy of progressively more structurally demanding types of constructs, analogous to the hierarchy of measurement scales from nominal to ratio, "with each successive structure meeting a requirement that the preceding one does not" (2002, 204). Haslam argues that our current set of psychiatric categories can be plausibly interpreted as encompassing constructs of these various forms, and he offers examples of psychiatric categories that may provisionally be understood as fitting each of the proposed types of constructs.

Regarding the relation between Haslam's paper and the HDA, nothing Haslam says in his paper about construct pluralism addresses, let alone answers, the question addressed by the HDA: what qualifies a category (of whatever kind of construct) as a category of psychiatric disorder? All of Haslam's types of constructs apply to normal as well as disordered conditions, so one needs an additional conceptual level of analysis not addressed in Haslam's paper to determine which constructs are disorders and which are not. Pluralism of disorder *constructs* does not imply pluralism of disorder *concepts*. Haslam argues only that various conditions already recognized independently as disorders fall into various different levels of his construct typology. He never argues for the absurdity that being an instance of one or another of his types of constructs is sufficient for being a disorder because he understands that his various constructs can exist on both sides of the disorder-nondisorder divide. To use Haslam's analogy, the fact that something is measurable at one or another level of the typology of scales from nominal to ratio tells you nothing about whether it is a disorder or nondisorder because both disorder and nondisorder categories can be measurable in various ways. Haslam's pluralistic typology of constructs is neutral on what constitutes a disorder and thus provides no support whatever for De Vreese's anti-HDA position.

Two concerns I have about Haslam's analysis are worth brief mention. The first is that he tends to take an overly blinkered psychometrician's view. For example, Haslam's discussion of his example of depression as a dimensional construct is problematic because the symptom-severity continuum on which depressive disorder is commonly claimed to fall and which Haslam embraces as the framework for his discussion is in fact orthogonal to the defensible common distinction between normal versus disordered sadness, in which severity is one dimension and dysfunction is another. Thus, normal grief and other clear cases of normal sadness in response to life events can be more severe than some mild cases of pathological depression. A second and related concern is that Haslam emphasizes that any smoothly distributed dimensional continuum along which individuals differ by degrees of a given variable is excluded from being divided into a categorical kind and is thus a nonkind because "although a binary distinction can be imposed on such a continuum, its placement is purely arbitrary; there is no correct location where the line should be drawn, and any such line creates a discontinuity that is merely artificial" (2002, 204). Of course, if you assume that you are limited in your considerations to only the dimensional continuum and have no other facts at your disposal, then by definition, Haslam's point is correct. But in real life, nosologists and scientists are never that limited. There is always the question of whether there are ways of understanding superficially continuous distributions in terms of deeper processes so that there are theory-driven nonarbitrary cut-points. The reason for such an inference could be as abstract as a belief about which part of the dimension was likely responsible for the natural selection of the mechanisms generating the dimension versus which part was not. (See my reply to De Block and Sholl in this volume for an extended example of this sort of inferential division of a continuous symptom-severity dimension.)

The Example of Attention-Deficit/Hyperactivity Disorder (ADHD)

I now consider De Vreese's comments on ADHD, first in her chapter in this volume and then in another paper of hers (De Vreese 2014) to which she refers the reader that makes clearer her own approach to the concept of disorder. In her present chapter, De Vreese is skeptical that the conceptual meaning of "disorder" actually shapes clinical judgments: "Clearly, no single physician will change his or her mind on whether, for example, attention-deficit/hyperactivity disorder is a 'real' disease on the basis of a conceptual analysis of disorder according to which it is not. Therefore, it seems better to recognize the diversity in the meanings we put on the concept disorder in practice." De Vreese's notion that clinicians are unaware of disparities between disorder diagnoses in practice and conceptually correct disorder attributions, or that they do not change their minds about disorder diagnoses when evidence conflicts with the concept of disorder, is dramatically out of touch with the realities of practice. In the United States, the need to use a diagnosis to justify insurance reimbursement means that clinicians are constantly confronted with conditions that they do not believe are disorders based on their conceptual understanding but that they diagnose as disorders anyway to justify treatment reimbursement. As *New York Times* articles have documented (e.g., Schwartz 2012), it is common for clinicians to diagnose school-challenged children with ADHD and prescribe medication whether or not they are believed to be disordered. I have asked New York psychiatrists who have exclusively ADHD practices what percentage of the children that they diagnose with ADHD do they believe are having difficulty in school but do not actually have a disorder, and invariably they estimate that more than half of their diagnosed patients are not really disordered. Clinicians are quite aware of disparities between a diagnosis they give *in practice* for a variety of pragmatic reasons versus whether a condition really satisfies the conceptual requirements for being a disorder.

This phenomenon goes well beyond ADHD. Many diagnoses such as adjustment disorder, depression, and anxiety categories are routinely applied to individuals in distress who, clinicians will tell you in private, are suffering from normal emotional reactions but will benefit from therapeutic support. Typically, reimbursement for treatment of marital problems, which is not itself reimbursable, is obtained by classifying the normal reactions of distress to marital discord as depressive or anxiety disorders in each partner. The category of substance abuse was not believed to be a category of genuine disorder by many nosologists and substance addiction specialists and it was rejected by the *International Classification of Diseases* (ICD), yet for decades, the pragmatic pressure to justify insurance reimbursement to help all those with substance use problems caused *DSM* committees to retain it as a diagnostic category (it was finally eliminated in *DSM-5*). Similarly, *DSM-5* shrank the category of autism spectrum disorder to eliminate some milder cases formerly classified as Asperger's disorder that critics argued are normal-range eccentricity rather than mental disorder, but the implications for special education funding were so controversial that *DSM-5* added a clause that overrides the revision and allows diagnosis of anyone who qualified for *a DSM-IV* Asperger's diagnosis. In the other direction, at the time that homosexuality per se was eliminated from *DSM-II*, many psychiatrists who voted for that momentous change in fact believed that homosexuality does represent a form of psychopathology but felt that this consideration was overridden by the need to help end the unjust oppression of homosexual individuals by declaring the condition a nondisorder. In sum, studying *diagnostic practice* is not quite the same as studying *disorder judgments*, and understanding the concept of disorder is necessary to understand how diagnostic practice and conceptual understanding can diverge.

What about De Vreese's denial that the concept of disorder has the power to explain changes of mind about disorder status? A conceptual analysis alone would not convince someone to change their mind about a condition's disorder status, but that plus changes in beliefs about a condition that imply that the condition does not satisfy the conceptual requirements for disorder could cause a change. In this way, research casting doubt on the existence of dysfunction in the HDA's sense regularly changes clinicians' and researchers' views of ADHD's disorder status. For example, recent research showing that it is disproportionately the youngest children in a class that get diagnosed with ADHD (e.g., Elder 2010; Evans et al. 2010; Holland and Sayal 2019; Zoega et al. 2012) has convinced many experts that normal variation in developmental rate is being confused with dysfunction, so that these younger children are likely being misdiagnosed. The behavior is the same, and it does the same harm to the child's school performance, but if there is no dysfunction, it is inferred that there is no disorder. Recent findings in genetic research (Eisenberg et al. 2008) have similarly convinced experts that some children currently diagnosed with ADHD do not have a dysfunction and so are not disordered. For example, *New York Times* psychiatric reporter Richard Friedman introduced an article reporting his change of mind as follows:

> Recent neuroscience research shows that people with A.D.H.D. are actually hard-wired for novelty-seeking—a trait that had, until relatively recently, a distinct evolutionary advantage. Compared with the rest of us, they have sluggish and underfed brain reward circuits, so much of everyday life feels routine and understimulating. To compensate, they are drawn to new and exciting experiences and get famously impatient and restless with the regimented structure that characterizes our modern world. In short, people with A.D.H.D. may not have a disease, so much as a set of behavioral traits that don't match the expectations of our contemporary culture. (2014, 1)

De Vreese allows that both value and factual elements enter into the notion of disease but does not spell out her own view in her chapter in this volume. She is more explicit in a recent paper to which she refers the reader (De Vreese 2014), in which she asserts that a prototypical disease is a disvalued condition with an identified and medically manipulable cause:

> I argue that our use of the term is determined by two interacting factors. One of these is value-laden considerations about the (un)desirability of certain physiological and/or psychological states. The other is the discovery of bodily and/or psychological causes which are explanatorily relevant in view of possible medical interventions to prevent, cure, or at least improve the undesired state. (De Vreese 2014, 38)

In terms of evidential support and explanatory power, De Vreese's account is at odds with the history of medical and psychiatric practice and fails both as a necessary and a sufficient criterion for disease. Regarding necessity, the causes of even those conditions that are considered the clearest cases of disease are often entirely unknown and thus should not fall on the clear end of the perceived disease continuum according to De Vreese's account. Before Pasteur, no one knew what caused most infectious diseases, yet bubonic plague, smallpox, and cholera were prototypical cases of disease. Today, many diseases—for example, many of the most horrific neurological diseases—remain unknown as to etiology, yet are considered crystal-clear cases of disease. Moreover, there is not even one major mental disorder for which we have a good theory of causation, yet some of them, such as schizophrenia, are generally considered prototypical cases of mental disorder. It is clear that a disorder judgment can be based on a justified inference that there is a certain kind of cause—namely, a dysfunction—and no actual knowledge of the cause is needed. The same evidence goes against the necessity of De Vreese's manipulability requirement. Many cases of disease fall on the consensually clear end of the disease continuum but for which there is no known treatment. Indeed, due to unique financial incentives, an entire industry exists to find treatments for rare diseases for which there is no effective treatment.

Regarding sufficiency, De Vreese's account is subject to massive numbers of counterexamples because there are endless disvalued, causally understood, and medically manipulable conditions (e.g., pain in childbirth, grief, homeliness) that are predicted by her account to be high on "diseaseness" but are not considered disorders. Notably, all of the above disconfirmations disappear if one replaces the "known manipulable cause" criterion with a "dysfunction" criterion, whether the dysfunction is known or merely inferred to exist and whether the dysfunction is treatable and manipulable or not.

De Vreese considers the question, "Is attention deficit hyperactivity disorder (ADHD) in children a real disease?" (2014, 35). She observes that those who argue that ADHD is not a real disease "are convinced that these children's behavior merely demonstrates the differences in character that can always be found among children. Additionally, they argue, performance standards in our modern society are too demanding for the more active and impulsive children" (35). One would think that these rationales for refusing to label ADHD a disease would offer valuable clues to the concept. Instead, oddly ignoring the ground-level judgments and presuppositions that she claims to be privileged data, De Vreese dismisses such considerations, saying that they cannot "directly guarantee or refute the appropriateness of the disease label for ADHD" (35). The problem here for De Vreese's account is that both sides in these disputes agree that the disputed conditions are disvalued, internally caused, and medically manipulable (via well-tested medications), so her account predicts that everyone should agree that ADHD is a disorder. Yet, in fact, there is prominent and heated disagreement that her analysis can't explain and that she chooses to ignore. What does explain the two sides' differences in judgments is crystal clear from the literature: they disagree about whether the disputed conditions are in fact due to internal dysfunctions or rather result from normal-range internal variation mismatched to current social demands. This crucial test of explanatory power between De Vreese's versus the HDA's perspective on ADHD falls squarely on the side of the HDA.

De Vreese also suggests a more pragmatic approach:

> All this does not answer the question of whether ADHD is *really* a disease. But according to the pragmatic framework developed here, that is a misguided question. It is not a matter of simply identifying it as a real or an unreal disease (whatever the latter might be). It is a matter of reflecting on why we actually are inclined to interpret ADHD as a real disease. What is the basis for this. (2014, 51)

This perspective in which we accept that ADHD is a disorder because some doctors label it so and simply explore why they so label it brings us back to a central problem with De Vreese's pragmatic approach; it has no conceptual place to stand to be critical of the practice it studies and so cannot address the deep problems that the analysis of "disorder" aims to address. One might wonder about drapetomania in the antebellum South, clitoral orgasm in Victorian England, and the Soviet political dissidents seeking liberty, all labeled as disorders. Given that medical treatment was available and effective in addressing these problematic conditions—runaway slaves could be medically sedated, women who experienced orgasms in Victorian England could have surgical clitoridectomies, and Soviet dissidents could be "cured" of their social protesting by psychiatric institutionalization and antipsychotic medication—De Vreese's position seems to entail that we take these conditions at face value and merely reflect on *why* they were considered diseases rather than subjecting them to conceptual scrutiny as to whether they were in fact real disorders. Her skepticism about the very notion of real versus bogus disorder implies that her view fails a crucial transcendental test of a fruitful analysis, namely, providing a basis for critiquing oppressive practice based on invalid application of the concept of disorder.

References

De Vreese, L. 2014. The concept of disease and our responsibility for children. In *Philosophical Perspectives on Classification and Diagnosis in Child and Adolescent Psychiatry*, L. Wells and C. Perring (eds.), 35–55. Oxford University Press.

Eisenberg, D. T. A., B. Campbell, P. B. Gray, and M. D. Sorenson. 2008. Dopamine receptor genetic polymorphisms and body composition in undernourished pastoralists: An exploration of nutrition indices among nomadic and recently settled Ariaal men of northern Kenya. *BMC Evolutionary Biology* 8: 173.

Elder, T. E. 2010. The importance of relative standards in ADHD diagnoses: Evidence based on exact birth dates. *Journal of Health Economics* 29: 641–656.

Evans, W. N., M. S. Morrill, and S. T. Parente. 2010. Measuring inappropriate medical diagnosis and treatment in survey data: The case of ADHD among school-age children. *Journal of Health Economics* 29: 657–673.

First, M. B., and J. C. Wakefield. 2010. Defining 'mental disorder' in *DSM-V*. *Psychological Medicine* 40(11): 1779–1782.

First, M. B., and J. C. Wakefield. 2013. Diagnostic criteria as dysfunction indicators: Bridging the chasm between the definition of mental disorder and diagnostic criteria for specific disorders. *Canadian Journal of Psychiatry* 58(12): 663–669.

Friedman, R. A. 2014. A natural fix for A.D.H.D. *New York Times*, October 31. https://www.nytimes.com/2014/11/02/opinion/sunday/a-natural-fix-for-adhd.html.

Haslam, N. 2002. Kinds of kinds: A taxonomy of psychiatric categories. *Philosophy, Psychiatry, and Psychology* 9(3): 203–217.

Holland, J., and K. Sayal. 2019. Relative age and ADHD symptoms, diagnosis and medication: A systematic review. *European Child & Adolescent Psychiatry 28(11): 1417–1429.*

Kirk, S. A., J. C. Wakefield, D. Hsieh, and K. Pottick. 1999. Social context and social workers' judgment of mental disorder. *Social Service Review* 73: 82–104.

Schwartz, A. 2012. Attention disorder or not, pills to help in school. *New York Times*, October 9. https://www.nytimes.com/2012/10/09/health/attention-disorder-or-not-children-prescribed-pills-to-help-in-school.html.

Spitzer, R. L. 1997. Brief comments from a psychiatric nosologist weary from his own attempts to define mental disorder: Why Ossorio's definition muddles and Wakefield's "harmful dysfunction" illuminates the issues. *Clinical Psychology: Science and Practice* 4(3): 259–261.

Spitzer, R. L. 1999. Harmful dysfunction and the *DSM* definition of mental disorder. *Journal of Abnormal Psychology* 108(3): 430–432.

Wakefield, J. C. 1992a. The concept of mental disorder: On the boundary between biological facts and social values. *American Psychologist* 47: 373–388.

Wakefield, J. C. 1992b. Disorder as harmful dysfunction: A conceptual critique of *DSM-III-R*'s definition of mental disorder. *Psychological Review* 99: 232–247.

Wakefield, J. C. 1993. Limits of operationalization: A critique of Spitzer and Endicott's (1978) proposed operational criteria of mental disorder. *Journal of Abnormal Psychology* 102: 160–172.

Wakefield, J. C. 1995. Dysfunction as a value-free concept: A reply to Sadler and Agich. *Philosophy, Psychiatry, and Psychology* 2: 233–46.

Wakefield, J. C. 1997a. Diagnosing *DSM-IV*, part 1: *DSM-IV* and the concept of mental disorder. *Behaviour Research and Therapy* 35: 633–650.

Wakefield, J. C. 1997b. Diagnosing *DSM-IV*, part 2: Eysenck (1986) and the essentialist fallacy. *Behaviour Research and Therapy*: 35: 651–666.

Wakefield, J. C. 1997c. Normal inability versus pathological disability: Why Ossorio's (1985) definition of mental disorder is not sufficient. *Clinical Psychology: Science and Practice* 4: 249–258.

Wakefield, J. C. 1997d. When is development disordered? Developmental psychopathology and the harmful dysfunction analysis of mental disorder. *Development and Psychopathology* 9: 269–290.

Wakefield, J. C. 1998. The *DSM*'s theory-neutral nosology is scientifically progressive: Response to Follette and Houts. *Journal of Consulting and Clinical Psychology* 66: 846–852.

Wakefield, J. C. 1999a. Evolutionary versus prototype analyses of the concept of disorder. *Journal of Abnormal Psychology* 108: 374–399.

Wakefield, J. C. 1999b. Mental disorder as a black box essentialist concept. *Journal of Abnormal Psychology* 108: 465–472.

Wakefield, J. C. 1999c. The concept of mental disorder as a foundation for the *DSM*'s theory-neutral nosology: Response to Follette and Houts, Part 2. *Behaviour Research and Therapy* 37: 1001–1027.

Wakefield, J. C. 2000a. Aristotle as sociobiologist: The "function of a human being" argument, black box essentialism, and the concept of mental disorder. *Philosophy, Psychiatry, and Psychology* 7: 17–44.

Wakefield, J. C. 2000b. Spandrels, vestigial organs, and such: Reply to Murphy and Woolfolk's "The harmful dysfunction analysis of mental disorder." *Philosophy, Psychiatry, and Psychology* 7: 253–269.

Wakefield, J. C. 2001. Evolutionary history versus current causal role in the definition of disorder: Reply to McNally. *Behaviour Research and Therapy* 39: 347–366.

Wakefield, J. C. 2006. What makes a mental disorder mental? *Philosophy, Psychiatry, and Psychology* 13: 123–131.

Wakefield, J. C. 2007. The concept of mental disorder: Diagnostic implications of the harmful dysfunction analysis. *World Psychiatry* 6: 149–156.

Wakefield, J. C. 2009. Mental disorder and moral responsibility: Disorders of personhood as harmful dysfunctions, with special reference to alcoholism. *Philosophy, Psychiatry, and Psychology* 16: 91–99.

Wakefield, J. C. 2011. Darwin, functional explanation, and the philosophy of psychiatry. In *Maladapting Minds: Philosophy, Psychiatry, and Evolutionary Theory*, P. R. Andriaens and A. De Block (eds.), 143–172. Oxford University Press.

Wakefield, J. C. 2014. The biostatistical theory versus the harmful dysfunction analysis, part 1: Is part-dysfunction a sufficient condition for medical disorder? *Journal of Medicine and Philosophy* 39: 648–682.

Wakefield, J. C. 2016a. The concepts of biological function and dysfunction: Toward a conceptual foundation for evolutionary psychopathology. In *Handbook of Evolutionary Psychology*, D. Buss (ed.), 2nd ed., vol. 2, 988–1006. Oxford University Press.

Wakefield, J. C. 2016b. Diagnostic issues and controversies in *DSM-5*: Return of the false positives problem. *Annual Review of Clinical Psychology* 12: 105–132.

Wakefield, J. C., and M. B. First. 2003. Clarifying the distinction between disorder and nondisorder: Confronting the overdiagnosis ("false positives") problem in *DSM-V*. In *Advancing DSM: Dilemmas in Psychiatric Diagnosis*, K. A. Phillips, M. B. First, and H. A. Pincus (eds.), 23–56. American Psychiatric Press.

Wakefield, J. C., and M. B. First. 2012. Placing symptoms in context: The role of contextual criteria in reducing false positives in *DSM* diagnosis. *Comprehensive Psychiatry* 53: 130–139.

Wakefield, J. C., A. V. Horwitz, and L. Lorenzo-Luaces. 2017. Uncomplicated depression as normal sadness: Rethinking the boundary between normal and disordered depression. In *Oxford Handbook of Mood Disorders*, R. J. DeRubeis and D. R. Strunk (eds.), 83–94. Oxford University Press.

Wakefield, J. C., A. V. Horwitz, and M. Schmitz. 2005. Are we overpathologizing social anxiety? Social phobia from a harmful dysfunction perspective. *Canadian Journal of Psychiatry* 50: 317–319.

Wakefield, J. C., S. A. Kirk, K. J. Pottick, X. Tian, and D. K. Hsieh. 2006. The lay concept of conduct disorder: Do non-professionals use syndromal symptoms or internal dysfunction to distinguish disorder from delinquency? *Canadian Journal of Psychiatry* 51: 210–217.

Wakefield, J. C., K. J. Pottick, and S. A. Kirk. 2002. Should the *DSM-IV* diagnostic criteria for conduct disorder consider social context? *American Journal of Psychiatry* 159: 380–386.

Wakefield, J. C., and M. F. Schmitz. 2015. The harmful dysfunction model of alcohol use disorder: Revised criteria to improve the validity of diagnosis and prevalence estimates. *Addiction* 110(6): 931–942.

Wakefield, J. C., and M. F. Schmitz. 2017a. The measurement of mental disorder. In *A Handbook for the Study of Mental Health: Social Contexts, Theories, and Systems*, T. Scheid and T. Brown (eds.), 3rd ed., 20–44. Cambridge University Press.

Wakefield, J. C., and M. F. Schmitz. 2017b. Symptom quality versus quantity in judging prognosis: Using NESARC predictive validators to locate uncomplicated major depression on the number-of-symptoms severity continuum. *Journal of Affective Disorders* 208: 325–329.

Wakefield, J. C., M. F. Schmitz, and J. C. Baer. 2010. Does the *DSM-IV* clinical significance criterion for major depression reduce false positives? Evidence from the NCS-R. *American Journal of Psychiatry* 167: 298–304.

Wakefield, J. C., M. F. Schmitz, M. B. First, and A. V. Horwitz. 2007. Extending the bereavement exclusion for major depression to other losses: Evidence from the National Comorbidity Survey. *Archives of General Psychiatry* 64: 433–440.

Zoega, H., U. A. Valdimarsdottir, and S. Hernandez-Diaz. 2012. Age, academic performance, and stimulant prescribing for ADHD: A nationwide cohort study. *Pediatrics* 130: 1012–1018.

7   Doing without "Disorder" in the Study of Psychopathology

Harold Kincaid

Jerome Wakefield has made major contributions to thinking about psychiatric classification, contributions that have important ramifications for the practice of psychiatry and related disciplines.[1] I argue in this chapter that those contributions are independent of his own views about the nature of psychopathology. Wakefield's picture of psychopathology on my view relies on dubious assumptions about the methods, aims, and abilities of philosophy; his account of psychopathology and the disciplines that study and treat it oversimplifies a complex reality. Nonetheless, these criticisms do not undermine Wakefield's contributions because those contributions do not depend on his specific account of psychopathology, and moreover, his oversimplifications point to a fruitful research agenda.

In section I, I outline some of what I take to be some of Wakefield's main contributions. Those contributions center on the recognition that the behaviors that get labeled as psychopathology are a heterogeneous lot, with important theoretical and practical consequences following. Section II argues that psychiatry does not need a foundation in a conceptual analysis of mental disorder and that searching for such an analysis rests on a mistaken philosophical project. Using evolutionary considerations to identify mental disorders is the topic of section III. Wakefield's actual points about the different behaviors that get labeled psychopathological are not actually supported by evolutionary accounts of mental disorders, and the prospects and uses for such accounts are limited. Section IV sketches an alternative pluralist view of psychopathology that makes the search for objective explanatory classifications of psychopathology paramount, a goal inspired by and consistent with Wakefield's insightful critique of psychiatric practice.

I.   Contributions

Wakefield's overriding concern is the proper application of psychiatric diagnostic categories. He (and his sometimes coauthor Horwitz) defends the view that some specific disorders are mistakenly applied. Unlike the antipsychiatry tradition, he does not argue that psychiatric classification and practice rest on a mistake tout court and/or are entirely social constructions. Nor does he fall into the trap of arguing—as do some philosophers—that there is something about the nature of the mental or of folk psychological concepts that precludes the naturalistic study of psychopathology or renders current psychiatric classifications unscientific. Rather than making such blanket assessments, he argues case by case, looking at the application of specific diagnostic categories—a procedure that is a vast improvement over the practice of much antipsychiatry criticism. Wakefield finds that some alleged psychiatric disorders such as grief are not disorders at all. Yet his arguments for this blanket skepticism about particular disorders are compatible with a more limited skepticism about other psychiatric classifications such as depression. There are clear cases of behavior that are legitimately labeled as depressive disorders. Yet that is compatible with the psychiatric professions misapplying the diagnosis in some or even a great many cases and in a way that does not just rely on the measurement error that is unavoidable in the social behavioral sciences. Instead, some psychiatric categories are systematically misapplied in identifiable ways.

So contribution number 1 is promoting a healthy skepticism of psychiatric classification practices but one that does not throw the baby out with the bathwater. Contribution number 2 is supplying an imminently plausible justification for that skepticism and for the accompanying optimism about psychiatry's scientific possibilities. That justification is in the form of an empirical claim about the range of human behaviors. For some types of symptoms and behaviors, there are qualitative differences that we can reasonably identify and defend. The qualitative differences are between behavioral symptoms that result from more or less enduring abnormal psychological mechanisms or processes largely inside the individual and those that result from situational and time-bound circumstances that are part of the vicissitudes of life. Wakefield asserts that there are objective facts of the matter about which types of behavior are present and that we can sometimes make reasonable well-confirmed judgments about them. This claim is nontrivial. It goes against the popular grain of psychometric approaches to psychopathology that see psychopathology as a continuous and not categorical phenomenon and thus conclude that there is no nonarbitrary distinction between the normal and the pathological.[2] Contribution number 2 is important and interesting.

A third contribution from Wakefield instantiates the above points by providing compelling assessments of various putative psychopathological categories. His work with Horwitz on depression is perhaps the most substantial. There the argument is that the application of the current *Diagnostic and Statistical Manual of Mental Disorders* (*DSM-IV*) criteria for depression leads to enormous numbers of false positives. If the *DSM* criteria are applied without taking into account situational factors, then a large number of individuals will be classified as suffering from a psychiatric depressive disorder when they are in fact only experiencing predictable and normal problems in living. Depressive symptoms can, Wakefield thinks, indicate a real psychological disorder when the symptoms are not the result of normal reactions to problems in living, so he is not a skeptic about the category itself, only its misapplication. For other putative disorders, however, he provides compelling evidence that no disorder whatsoever is picked out. For example, he argues convincingly that the criteria for the category "prolonged grief disorder," which was considered for the *DSM-5*, describes what are normal reactions to loss, with understandable individual variation in the intensity and duration of those reactions. This conclusion is supported by recent work on the grief process. Because the proposed criteria would label normal behavior pathological and there is no prospect for building in situational exclusions as there is with depression, Wakefield (2012) thinks that the category as it stands does not pick out a mental disorder and argues against its inclusion in the *DSM*. It was not included.

II. Unneeded Grounds

All the points made above were done so without appeal to a key component in Wakefield's writings: the harmful dysfunction analysis of the concept of mental disorder. Wakefield thinks that much rests on getting the correct analysis of the concept of a mental disorder. So he says, "What do we mean when we say that a mental condition is a medical disorder rather than a normal form of human suffering or a problem in living? The status of psychiatry as a medical discipline depends on a persuasive answer to this question" (2007, 149). This assertion that the status of psychiatry depends on having a proper analysis of disorder is repeated frequently across his substantial corpus of writings.

Wakefield also believes that having a correct account of mental disorder *in general* is necessary for having correct accounts of *specific* disorders. We can identify the sets of symptoms that make a specific disorder by showing that they reflect a malfunction in what some psychological mechanism was designed to do by natural selection. Where symptoms do not reflect the failed functions of evolutionarily selected mechanisms, mental disorder does not exist.

On my view the fact that the contributions cited in the first section do not mention Wakefield's conceptual analysis is a virtue, for I do not think the harmful dysfunction analysis is needed or generally helpful. In this section, I explain why I do not think we need an analysis of the concept of mental disorder and in the next why evolutionary notions of disorder are not generally helpful in understanding specific psychopathologies.

My qualms about the project of providing an account of "mental disorder" have their roots in a Quinian naturalism about philosophy and science. That naturalism doubts that there are conceptual truths that can be tested by intuition about possible counterexamples and by reports on what we would say. My naturalism also leads to doubts that philosophical analysis of concepts can provide results that allow us to rule on the epistemic standing of scientific disciplines. These doubts are grounded in skepticism about the analytic/synthetic distinction and the coherence of substantial a priori knowledge. They are reinforced by work in the history, philosophy, and social studies of science showing that successful science does not first start with getting a definition in terms of necessary and sufficient conditions and then proceeding; instead, science often muddles along with concepts that are undefined or that are prototypes (like most human concepts) or that have competing but useful definitions depending on the application (see Wilson's [2006] wonderful detailed account of concepts in the applied physical sciences). The concept of a gene still has not precise analytic definition (Moss 2004), and thermodynamics made great strides despite having an only partially explicated and not entirely coherent concept of temperature (Chang 2004).

Let me concretize these general results from philosophy and philosophy of science with some questions about Wakefield's project defining disorder. We should first ask, who gets to vote in the game of definition and counterexample that is to define "mental disorder"? We should then ask how we are to tally the results. Do the intuitions of those outside the psychiatric professions count as much as those inside? What do we do when reasonable people report different intuitions about defining disorder? (This is not just a hypothetical question—there are perfectly reasonable people who think that being a disorder is a matter of deviations from playing a standard role in complex systems.) We can also ask what we would do with a conceptual analysis produced by such methods. Suppose there was a consensus among all those who participated in public debates about defining "mental disorder" about the correct definition. Would we really want then to use that sociological fact to tell psychiatric researchers what they should be studying and how they should be studying it? I don't think so.

So my argument contra Wakefield is that the disciplines that study and treat psychopathology do not need and can get along without a philosophically satisfying (i.e., necessary and sufficient condition) definition of mental disorder. In this respect, I think they are no different from the rest of medicine. As I have argued elsewhere (Kincaid 2008), there are no clear individually necessary and jointly sufficient conditions for being a cancer, but that does not mean oncology is based on a mistake and that its "status as a medical discipline" is at stake.[3] Oncology, like the rest of medicine, studies and treats conditions that it can objectively and reliably identify and conditions where it can predict and alter the course of development in ways that people perceive to improve their lives. Psychiatry presumably has the same pretensions if unfortunately not the same prospects. This alternative picture of psychiatry freed from any deep ties to disease concepts will be elaborated in the final section of the chapter.

I want to answer two likely objections, given Wakefield's published arguments. One is that we are being incoherent if we talk about psychopathology without a worked-out account of the concept of disorder, and the other is that we need an account if we are to avoid a nihilist social constructivism about mental disorders.

Don't we need an analysis of disorder to talk about psychopathology? Nothing prevents us from using the term despite having no strict definition; if we could only use terms strictly defined, we would be in big linguistic trouble. The question is then whether the disease label is doing any useful scientific work (it no doubt has ethical and social consequences). I think it may well be that generally it does not, and thus psychiatric research should get on without the concept of a disorder. If we can find compelling evidence of malfunctioning evolutionarily selected psychological mechanisms, then it would have a role in those cases. I also find it plausible that some behavior that gets labeled pathological involves a breakdown in the normal operation of cognitive and neurobiological systems, the idea promoted by competitors to Wakefield's analysis of function. Here the term "psychopathological" would also have a more delimited and defensible meaning. If we eschew the conceptual analysis project of defining mental disorder, we can allow such a restricted use of "psychopathology" without committing ourselves to the view that a breakdown in normal system functioning captures all and only the ways we use terms like "mental disorder" or "psychopathology." However, I would argue that finding malfunctions in evolutionary mechanisms or breakdown of roles in a complex system are just valuable means to the end of getting objective, explanatory classifications of behavior that psychiatry and related disciplines study and treat.

A second objection by Wakefield to my suggestion that we do not need a conceptual analysis of mental disorder is this: "a central goal of an analysis of 'mental disorder' is to clarify and reveal the degree of legitimacy in psychiatry's claims to be a truly medical discipline rather than, as antipsychiatrists and others have claimed, a social control institution masquerading as a medical discipline." In other words, we need a clear defensible definition of mental disorder if we are to hold off the social constructivist nihilists massing at the gate.

The gate is surely worth defending, although many useful insights have come from the social constructivist camp as I sure Wakefield would agree. Still we can defend the gate quite nicely without a definition of mental disorder. What we need to show is that the psychiatric-related disciplines can produce objective and explanatory categorizations of behavior, ideally ones that lead to successful treatments. Tying those classifications to mechanisms selected by natural selection would be one way to ground them, but surely not the only way as I will argue in more detail in section IV. For example, the Big Five personality classification system relies on reliable and psychometrically validated measures; scores on those measures predict differences in behavior. Here psychological phenomena are classified in objectively grounded ways that refute pure social constructivist stories and do so without any tie to evolutionary functions. So it is quite possible to avoid social constructionist conclusions without the machinery of evolutionarily selected mental mechanisms.

I should finish my rejection of Wakefield's conceptual analysis project by noting that I am not denying that clarifying concepts in the study of psychopathology is a worthwhile effort or that philosophers can contribute to such clarification. My objections are to the grander project of establishing the legitimacy of fields that study psychopathology by providing a conceptual analysis of "mental disorder."

III. Evolutionary Foundations?

Suppose we drop Wakefield's conceptual analysis project. Is it nonetheless still true that Wakefield has shown that the best way or a good way to understand specific psychopathologies is in terms of the failure of evolutionarily selected psychological mechanisms? I consider this part of Wakefield's project in this section.

A look at Wakefield's various discussions of psychopathological concepts such as depression shows that an appeal to evolutionary functions plays little role. In exposing the false-positive rate in diagnoses of depression, Wakefield does not tell a plausible evolutionary story about the origins of the relevant psychological mechanisms and then go on to argue that those mechanisms are functioning properly in the cases where psychopathological concepts are being misapplied. Instead, he argues that the behavior in question is a normal and reasonable response to a life circumstance. Depressive symptoms in the case of a lost job or marital breakup are normal, understandable responses to life events and thus should not be classified as depressive disorders. What we need according to Wakefield are "judgments of proportionality—that is, whether the nature of a triggering stressor is capable of explaining, within the normal range of emotional processing, the severity of the resulting symptoms" (2012, 181). It is the appeal to the normal range, not the proper functioning of a mechanism produced by natural selection, that is doing the work here.

At times, Wakefield talks as if picking out mechanisms can be easily done even if we do not have a good evolutionary story. So he suggests that we know that the eye is designed for seeing and that we can know that without having any good idea about the design process. *Maybe* that is true for biological functions, but is that true of evolutionarily evolved mental mechanisms? I doubt it.

If we look at the work of biologists actually applying detailed evolutionary considerations to psychopathology, then we run into reasons to doubt that evolutionarily based dysfunction accounts fit with the kind of (reasonable) intuitive judgments that Wakefield wants to make about which symptoms constitute disorders and which do not. The problem is that there are plausible evolutionary stories where a wide range of behaviors that we are inclined to call disorders turn out to be the products of evolutionarily selected mechanisms. There are at least three potential facts supporting this conclusion: the likelihood that psychological mechanisms producing false positives would be fitness improving, the prospect that fitness-enhancing psychological mechanisms in the Pleistocene may be invoked in maladaptive ways in complex industrial societies in which they did not evolve, and the general fact that evolution produces traits with a wide reaction norm, raising the prospect that extremes of human behavior that we call pathological are the distributional tails of normal traits.

Success under natural selection requires a trade-off between costly unnecessary responses to threats to reproduction and costly failures to detect such threats. Where the threat to reproductive success is death, it is not hard to imagine that natural selection would err on the side of false positives. A one strike and you are out threat would seemingly produce traits that produce lots of false positives in reacting to such threats, given the extreme consequences of a false negative.

What do such false positives have to do with psychopathology? Two of the most prototypical psychopathologies—various forms of severe anxiety and depression—have natural stories as being evolutionarily selected false positives. Depressive symptoms can be seen as promoting avoidance of, and helping to repair, the breaking of social bonds, something that no doubt had drastic consequences in our evolutionary history. The motivation to avoid depressive pain by behaving in ways to protect social bonds is fairly obvious. The repairing role that depression may play takes more storytelling (see McGuire et al. 1997), but there is compelling evidence from our primate cousins about some of that story in terms of restoring social bonds in changing dominance hierarchies. Similar narratives exist about extreme anxieties, where the threats are both social and environmental. Possible live and let live, laid-back ancestors may have fared badly in ancestral environments where threats to life were ever present and where the cost of social exclusion was deadly as well. In short, significant anxiety and depression may have just been the price our ancestors paid for reproductive success and the price we pay for being their ancestors.

Another just so story—one in principle compatible with the one just told—does not require widespread Pleistocene depression and anxiety but finds the roots of disorder in past evolved mechanisms that have to deal with the complexities of modern society. This is a route familiar in broad outlines from Freud in *Civilization and Its Discontents* (1962). The idea is that modern society provokes in abundance naturally selected mechanisms producing depressive and anxious systems. We can give this just so story a quite concrete guise by thinking, for example, about poverty and psychopathology. A few miles from where I live, there are over a million people cramped into wall-to-wall corrugated metal shacks without running water and sanitation. Most live on less than $2 a day. Probably 50% are unemployed. The murder rate is enormous and sexual assault pervasive. Wakefield argues that depressive symptoms in response to a job loss should not be counted as a disorder. However, what if the job loss is a repeated or a permanent part of life as it is for the residents of these townships and the response is permanent depressive symptoms? Should we deny that they have a depressive disorder? What about crippling anxiety in women subject to ongoing sexual abuse? Since in my view, "only" ethical and social considerations turn on what we *say,* nothing social scientific is at issue in asking these questions and to that extent they can be ignored. Instead, the question is whether these conditions allow for objective, explanatory classifications, a question that makes no essential judgment about evolutionary considerations. But this is not Wakefield's view. Such examples should be a chance for clarification of his views.

A third evolutionary approach arguing that psychopathology is the standard functioning of naturally selected traits points out that biological traits can have a wide reaction norm. Seemingly normal traits in common environments can exhibit extreme deviations from the average, given subtle changes in the developmental environment. The claim thus would be that major depression is just the tail of the expression of a normal, presumably adaptive, trait of sadness. This is the kind of view advocated by the psychometric tradition that wants to treat psychopathology as a continuous trait and replace talk of disorders and psychopathology with talk of abnormal behavior.

Neither of three pictures above is beyond doubt. However, they do suggest some of the kinds of questions we must answer if we want to ground judgments about psychopathology on the idea of properly functioning mental mechanisms. Pursuing Wakefield's general approach thus raises a variety of fruitful research questions, albeit difficult ones.

IV. An Alternative Picture

The alternative approach I favor denies that we must have a clear conceptual analysis of disorder in order to understand the practice of psychopathology research or for that research to form a coherent scientific enterprise (Kincaid 2014). Instead, I think that the ideal for the sciences of psychopathology is to establish the existence of objective, explanatory classifications. Let me explain what I mean by this terminology and then discuss the role of evolutionary and other considerations in identifying these classifications.

"Objective" classifications, as I use the term, are ones that put individuals into classes based on real differences in facts about those individuals.[4] One important way to show that we have real differences is to provide evidence that they can be identified by evidentially independent means. "Explanatory" classifications, as I am using the term, are those that ground regularities and causal relations. We get evidence for regularities and causal relations by showing that our classifications of individuals allow us to make successful predictions about (1) the factors determining who comes to exhibit the behaviors that the classification picks out and (2) the outcomes that the classified individuals undergo.

So, for example, consider the case of major depression (Kincaid 2014). There are multiple sources of evidence that we can pick out a qualitatively distinct set of individuals based on their behavior broadly construed. Taxometric analyses (Ruscio et al. 2006) using diagnostic screens as indicators point to a dichotomous division of individuals into a depressive taxon and a distinct complement group. Tests on cognitive tasks and neurobiological measures such as functional magnetic resonance imaging (fMRI) differences in activation and differences in cortisol secretion provide additional independent lines of evidence in addition to the taxometric analysis of responses to diagnostic screens. So there is evidence that distinct differences between individuals are being picked out by the classification of depression. That classification then allows successful identification of causes and consequences of depression. Belonging to the category is predicted by family history and histories of marital discord, food insecurity, and job stress. Belonging to the category predicts subsequent suicide attempts.

The fields studying psychopathology will be vindicated as scientific endeavors if they can produce for other domains of behavior results like the findings for depression. Such success would be entirely consistent with Wakefield's concern to avoid lumping together problems in living with major psychiatric conditions. It would not, however, require an account of the concept of mental disorder or that specific disorders be identified with evolutionary malfunctions.

On the general picture just sketched, evidence about evolutionary dysfunction would be a useful but not essential ingredient. Accounts of evolutionary function and dysfunction could, for example, motivate the kinds of predictors of psychopathology we should look for. However, none of the evidence I listed about the existence of an objective category picking out depression relied on evolutionary considerations or essentially assumed that the behavior constitutes a disorder in any substantial sense. I should also note that the evidence did not rely strongly on the assumptions that some of Wakefield's critics—those who claim that the true meaning of disorder is the breakdown of roles in complex systems—think essential. Some of the fMRI evidence might be interpreted in these terms, but at the present, the connections are still fairly speculative. As with evolutionary functions, functions in the sense of roles in complex psychological and neurobiological systems might well be of use in picking out the objective, explanatory classifications. Yet, fortunately, researchers can make progress without having anything like a full, well-confirmed theory of cognitive-neurobiological functioning.

Notes

1. It is hard to know how much influence his contributions have had on practice, but it seems clear that their influence is unfortunately not as large as they should be (witness the dropping of the bereavement exclusion from the *DSM-5* criteria for major depressive disorder).

2. The conclusion is unnecessary. Psychopathology might be manifested in continuous rather than categorical traits that in no way are distributed across the entire population. Huntington's disease varies significantly in severity, but it is not the case that everybody has at least a little bit of it.

3. They commissioned a study on whether they should worry about whether obesity is a disease. They concluded that there might be ethical and social reasons to answer the question but that scientifically, the question was irrelevant (Allison et al. 2008).

4. I am setting the issues up here on the assumption that psychopathologies are categorical rather than dimensional. While I think that is true for some prime examples of psychopathology, it is not essential for there to be objective, explanatory categories; they might be dimensional in nature.

References

Allison, D., M. Downey, R. Atkinson, C. Billington, G. Bray, R. Eckel, E. Finkelstein, M. Jensen, and A. Tremblay. 2008. Obesity as a disease: A white paper on evidence and arguments. *Obesity* 16(6): 1161–1177.

Chang, H. 2004. *Inventing Temperature Measurement and Scientific Progress.* Oxford University Press.

Freud, S. 1962. *Civilization and Its Discontents.* New York.

Kincaid, H. 2008. Do we need theory to study disease? Lessons from cancer research and their implications for mental illness. *Perspectives in Biology and Medicine* 51(3): 367–337.

Kincaid, H. 2014. Defensible natural kinds in the study of psychopathology. In *Classifying Psychopathology: Mental Illness and Natural Kinds,* H. Kincaid and J. Sullivan (eds.), 145–173. MIT Press.

McGuire, M., A. Triosi, and M. Raleigh. 1997. Depression in evolutionary context. In *The Maladapted Mind,* S. Baron-Cohen (ed.), 255–278. Psychology Press.

Moss, L. 2004. *What Genes Can't Do.* MIT Press.

Ruscio, J., N. Haslam, and A. Ruscio. 2006. *Introduction to the Taxometric Method: A Practical Guide.* Lawrence Erlbaum.

Wakefield, J. C. 2007. The concept of mental disorder: Diagnostic implications of the harmful dysfunction analysis. *World Psychiatry* 6(3): 149–156.

Wakefield, J. C. 2012. Mapping melancholia: The continuing typological challenge for major depression. *Journal of Affective Disorders* 138(1–2): 180–182.

Wilson, M. 2006. *Wandering Significance: An Essay on Conceptual Behavior.* Oxford University Press.

8 Quinian Qualms, or Does Psychiatry Really Need the Harmful Dysfunction Analysis? Reply to Harold Kincaid

Jerome Wakefield

I have long been an admirer of Harold Kincaid's wide-ranging and sophisticated contributions to philosophy of psychopathology and philosophy of science more generally. I am grateful to him for his challenging commentary on my harmful dysfunction analysis (HDA) of medical, including mental, disorder. The HDA claims that "disorder" refers to "harmful dysfunction," where dysfunction is the failure of some feature to perform a natural function for which it is biologically designed by evolutionary processes and harm is judged in accordance with social values (HDA; First and Wakefield 2010, 2013; Spitzer 1997, 1999; Wakefield 1992a, 1992b 1993, 1995, 1997a, 1997b, 1997c, 1997d, 1998, 1999a, 1999b, 2000a, 2000b, 2001, 2006, 2007, 2009, 2011, 2014, 2016a, 2016b; Wakefield and First 2003, 2012).

In his chapter, Kincaid enumerates some of the contributions of my work but nevertheless wonders how much influence they have actually had given that the *Diagnostic and Statistical Manual of Mental Disorders* (*DSM-5*) (American Psychiatric Association 2013) eliminated the bereavement exclusion despite my vigorous objections. That was indeed a disappointment and an ill-advised change. However, even there a newly introduced "Note" to the major depression diagnostic criteria that was added in response to the debate opens a back door to many of the conclusions I have argued for. It acknowledges that major depression-mimicking normal sadness is not limited to bereavement but can occur in response to a wide range of losses and that earlier criteria were mistaken to use duration thresholds on the order of a few months to mark a shift from normal to pathological sadness, and it allows for clinical judgment in making the discrimination between normal versus pathological depression. Elsewhere, the HDA remains influential and continues to be regularly applied by researchers to nosological disputes on topics ranging from psychopathy (see my reply to Cooper in this volume) to hebephilia (Rind and Yuill 2012).

Psychiatry's Need for a Conceptual Analysis of Mental Disorder

Kincaid proposes "doing without 'disorder' in the study of psychopathology" and offers a variety of arguments against the usefulness of the HDA for psychiatric nosology. (One is of course sorely tempted to ask: the study of *what*? "Psychopathology" is a synonym for "mental disorder," so Kincaid seems to beg the question.) Until I read Kincaid's chapter, I had not realized that he and I are coming from such different philosophical perspectives that for him, even my attempt to conceptually analyze "mental disorder" "relies on dubious assumptions about the methods, aims, and abilities of philosophy." Kincaid thus joins the chorus of philosophers of psychiatry attempting to delegitimize conceptual analysis as a way to explain classificatory judgments. In Kincaid's case, this harsh judgment emerges from his Quinian "doubts that there are conceptual truths that can be tested by intuition about possible counterexamples and by reports on what we would say…grounded in skepticism about the analytic/synthetic distinction and the coherence of substantial a priori knowledge." At this point in post-Quinian philosophical history, deploying all that unnecessary philosophical baggage to preempt a proposed conceptual analysis seems "dubious" to me. In the course of his commentary, Kincaid praises the concrete evidential and differentiating points that I make about specific psychological conditions and suggests those points stand independent of the HDA framework that inspired them. I would suggest that a similar "proof is in the pudding" attitude is appropriate to the HDA itself. Rather than summarily extirpating the HDA in the hallowed name of "Two Dogmas," consider it a hypothesis about shared mental representations underlying classificatory judgments within a target linguistic community, to be tested like all such hypotheses by explanatory power and evidential support.

Beyond Quinian doctrine, Kincaid attempts to support his rejection of the HDA's conceptual analytic methodology with the historical argument that studies of science show that "successful science does not first start with getting a definition in terms of necessary and sufficient conditions and then proceeding; instead, science often muddles along with concepts that are undefined." This is quite true as a broad generalization but irrelevant to the present case. The (absurd) "definitions first, science second" doctrine cannot apply to current attempts to analyze "disorder" because we are hardly at the "start" of psychiatry. Medicine in the Western tradition has been pursuing prescientific and scientific theories and research about mental disorder for going on 2,500 years.

The analysis of "disorder" has instead come into prominence as a way of addressing very specific issues that have arisen from ongoing psychiatric practice and science. For example, Robert Spitzer said that he never thought it was important to define "mental disorder" until the dispute over the diagnostic status of homosexuality broke out precisely on the question of whether homosexuality fits the concept of mental disorder. Similarly, the HDA was undertaken as a response to antipsychiatric attacks on the discipline of psychiatry that challenged psychiatry's coherence and legitimacy as a medical profession. As well, the abuses of psychiatric diagnosis in the Soviet Union, the *DSM-5* quagmire over the issue of whether psychiatric expansiveness is leading to medicalization of normal variation, and accusations that big pharma is redefining normal conditions as disorders are all recent challenges that call for attention to the nature of the concept of mental disorder as a claimed subconcept of medical disorder. Kincaid himself admits elsewhere that his anticonceptual analytic bias does not apply to such situations in which conceptual clarification can be a route to moving a discipline forward: "Philosophical analysis can be useful when it is part of clarifying scientific controversies, but then that is something scientists do all the time" (2008, 678). Scientists "do it all the time" because, far from being some historical or ontological oddity, conceptual analytic exploration is continuous with creative empirical and theoretical exploration. Numerous first-rank scientists have taken on conceptual questions when faced with obstacles to progress that demanded such analysis, from Einstein analyzing the concept of simultaneity and Mach analyzing the nature of the evidence in physics to Hilbert analyzing the nature of mathematical proof and Freud rethinking the nature of mental states.

Kincaid further defends his rejection of conceptual analysis as follows: "So my argument contra Wakefield is that the disciplines that study and treat psychopathology do not need and can get along without a philosophically satisfying (i.e., necessary and sufficient condition) definition of mental disorder." I am not sure what the argument here is supposed to be. "Analysis X is unneeded for discipline Y to get along" does not imply "analysis X is incorrect" or even "analysis X is not valuable and illuminating for discipline Y." For example, science has not needed and gotten along just fine without Quinian philosophy (as Kincaid elsewhere observes, "the full implications [of Quine's work] are still often ignored" [2008, 368]), yet Kincaid nonetheless finds Quinianism valuable and illuminating in understanding the nature of science. Kincaid also argues that conceptual analysis is futile because whether we classify conditions as disorder versus nondisorder does not really matter scientifically; it is merely a matter of *what we say* and has no substantive scientific content, only ethical and social implications: "Nothing social scientific is at issue in asking these questions and to that extent they can be ignored." The HDA explains why he is wrong. Burying one's head in the Quinian sand doesn't change the fact that judging that people are disordered—dissidents in the Soviet Union, runaway slaves in the antebellum U.S. South, females having clitoral orgasms in Victorian England—is not just verbal behavior but makes implicit claims about causal processes and their relation to biological design that interact in complex scientifically significant ways with the "web of belief." At this point in history, when we judge conditions as mental disorders, we generally are doing so on the basis of circumstantial evidence without a knowledge of the specific underlying etiology—just as Hippocrates and Galen did with judgments about physical disorders. However, according to the HDA, disorder versus nondisorder attributions carry with them different presuppositions about the *general domain* in which the etiological explanation for the superficial symptoms lies—very roughly, dysfunctions for disorders versus biologically designed human functioning for nondisorders. Although our intuitions about disorder versus nondisorder based on indirect evidence are fallible, they have generally been surprisingly good indicators of real-world differences in categories of causation.

Consequently, science done without attention to this distinction is likely to be mixing different categories of etiologies, leaving the meaning of one's results ambiguous. Moreover, disorder intuitions, being suggestive guides to divergent causal etiologies, indicate fertile paths for research foci (e.g., see the discussion of hyperemesis gravidarum in my reply to De Block and Sholl in this volume).

Kincaid questions my claim that we are often capable of (fallibly!) inferring biological design and its failures in the domain of mental mechanisms and thus judging mental disorder versus nondisorder according to the HDA, although he allows that this is perhaps possible for physical mechanisms. However, diagnostic manuals from Hippocrates to *DSM-5* illustrate that it is possible to draw some justified inferences about psychological biological design or its failure despite lack of knowledge of specific etiology. For starters, here are ten prominent diagnostic categories each taken from a different chapter of *DSM-5* and thus a different domain of human psychological functioning, each of which in their prototypical presentations appear intuitively incompatible with the biologically designed functioning of a human being: autism spectrum disorder; schizophrenia; bipolar I disorder with psychotic features; major depression, recurrent, with psychotic features; panic disorder; reactive attachment disorder; conversion disorder; anorexia nervosa; erectile disorder (primary impotence); and pedophilia, exclusive type. I agree that judgments about biological design are sometimes difficult, but nosological categories tend to start from cases in which such judgments, although fallible, can be made with relative plausibility.

Kincaid's Analogy between "Cancer" and "Mental Disorder"

In arguing that psychiatry doesn't need an analysis of the concept of disorder, Kincaid's primary argument is by analogy to oncology that, he has argued elsewhere (Kincaid 2008), neither has nor needs a conceptual analysis of "cancer" and yet gets along fine as a perfectly respectable medical specialty without it: "there are no clear individually necessary and jointly sufficient conditions for being a cancer, but that does not mean oncology is based on a mistake and that its 'status as a medical discipline' is at stake."

Let's be charitable and put obvious disanalogies aside (e.g., for starters, no one is actually challenging oncology's status as a medical discipline based on "cancer" being incoherent, unlike psychiatry!). If one looks closely at Kincaid's analysis in support of this proposition, one finds that he is really arguing that various *theories* and *explanations* and *characterizations* of cancer do not apply in any simple or straightforward way across the hundreds of distinct medical categories that fall within the category "cancer." However, cancer itself does have a standard definition, namely, diseases in which, due to uncontrolled cell division, a tumor spreads to other tissue: "Cancer is a large group of diseases that can start in almost any organ or tissue of the body when abnormal cells grow uncontrollably, go beyond their usual boundaries to invade adjoining parts of the body and/or spread to other organs" (World Health Organization 2020); "A term for diseases in which abnormal cells divide without control and can invade nearby tissues" (National Cancer Institute 2018); "Cancer is the name given to a collection of related diseases. In all types of cancer, some of the body's cells begin to divide without stopping and spread into surrounding tissues" (National Cancer Institute 2015). Indeed, Kincaid himself seems to agree with this definition that unites the category of cancer: "Finally, I should note that there are over 100 different forms of cancer, and what they at most all have in common is uncontrolled cell division sufficient to cause a health problem" (2008, 373). That's nothing to sneeze at as a useful and theoretically interesting reference fixer.

Kincaid's immersion in fascinating details that vary from cancer to cancer or do not distinguish cancer from noncancer seems a case of missing the forest for the trees. For example, arguing against the importance of the normal/dysfunction distinction, Kincaid observes that "the notion of 'normal' functioning of cells and tissues plays little role in identifying cancer because most tumors cells are normal" (2008, 373). But, first, the point of identifying a disorder is to identify the dysfunction responsible for the symptoms, so the normal cells in a tumor are on a first pass not relevant to that task, whereas a breakdown in regulation of cell growth by other cells is a relevant dysfunction. Second, the "uncontrolled" in Kincaid's own characterization is an implicit marker for "pathological"; obviously, there are endless "controlled" (i.e., biologically designed) rapid or extensive cell divisions, from a fetus's growth into an adult to the formation of a scab in a wound, so, contra Kincaid, the definition must contain an implicit reference to a needed baseline of "normal."

However, fruitful as "uncontrolled cell division that spreads" may be as a current reference fixer, a conceptual stickler has to say that this standard "definition" can't be right as a conceptual analysis. Cancer was known and named in ancient times long before it was known that the body is composed of cells. Hippocrates (460–370 BC) used *carcinoma*, Greek for "crab," to describe the projections of tissue and blood vessels reminiscent of a crab's shape that occurred as a tumor spread; the Roman physician Celsus (28–50 BC) translated *carcinoma* into the Latin word for crab, "cancer"; and the Greek physician Galen (130–200 AD) described the growth of tumors using the term "oncos" (Greek for "swelling"), the root of our term "oncology." Since then, there have been many theories of cancer having nothing to do with uncontrolled cell replication. We could conceivably wake up tomorrow and find out that we were wrong about cell division dysfunction and that one of those other theories of cancer is correct, and that would be a discovery about cancer and not a mere semantic manipulation. Cancer was long thought to be one disorder occurring at different locations in the body but now is thought to be many disorders due to diverse dysfunction etiologies, but such issues are not part of what "cancer" means because those are issues about cancer that are being decided empirically.

So, we have here an essentialist theory of cancer masquerading as a meaning, in the way that "H_2O" might be said to be what we mean by "water" when of course it is a theory of water. Lots of people throughout history and even nowadays understand the meaning of "water" without having any idea about H_2O, and entire technical and scientific hydrological disciplines existed before the discovery that water is H_2O. Similarly, cancer was a medical domain of theory, research, and treatment before the cell theory.

"Cancer" does have a meaning that determines its reference, anchored in a certain history. That meaning is more abstract than various theories about cancer and various proposals for how to differentiate cancer from other disorders. Very roughly, one might describe the meaning this way: if one looks back to the kinds of lesions and tumors that caught the eye of physicians from at least ancient Egyptian and Greek times on, they shared the property of inexorable tissue expansion of a tumor; even the Egyptians, who cauterized tumorous breast lesions, already observed that there is no curative treatment that stops the swelling of these masses. Let's call that recognized base set "*those tumors.*" "Cancer" means "tissue that pathologically expands into other tissues due to the same kind of dysfunction as the ones underlying *those tumors.*" Of course, this is rough and subject to revision in various ways. However, medical science has since established to our satisfaction that the processes underlying *those tumors* crucially involve various forms of dysfunction in which there is pathologically unregulated cell replication, and so as a general essentialist characterization of a pathological natural kind, cancer is "defined" as pathologically unregulated cell division that threatens harm through invasion of tissues. That there are over 100 known forms of this category of pathology does not diminish the importance of this "definition." Indeed, this very definition requiring an invasive nature is cited and deployed when borderline conditions come up for debate among oncologists, as in the recent debates over the diagnostic status of ductal carcinoma in situ, with the possibility raised of there being unknown differentiators between potentially invasive (and thus cancerous) forms and noninvasive (thus not really cancer) forms.

The "uncontrolled cell division" essentialist characterization of cancer, on which the World Health Organization (2020), National Institutes of Health (2015), and Kincaid all agree, delineates a broad natural kind that is the target of a medical specialty. Nonetheless, Kincaid insists that disorders are not natural kinds (see my reply to Lemoine in this volume for further discussion of essences and natural kinds). In fact, many categories of disorder are not initially natural kinds, but nosology tends to get reassembled to preserve natural kinds of etiologies. Once breast cancer is understood to be due to several different sets of mutations or multiple sclerosis as several different pathways to autoimmune neurological dysfunction, those distinct dysfunctions are gradually seen as separate diseases falling under the locational category "breast cancer" or the broader descriptive category "multiple sclerosis," respectively. Disease categories do not generally spring full blown as natural kinds, but they are by nature in search of natural kinds. Thus, the seemingly incoherent locution that a category of disorder is in fact several disorders.

Whose Intuitions Is the HDA Trying to Explain?

Kincaid, like some other critics, raises the question of who is to be included in the target community of those whose judgments are to be explained by the HDA's conceptual analysis: "We should first ask who gets to vote in the game of definition and counterexample that is to define 'mental disorder.'" Well, the initial community of clinicians, nosologists, and other professionals is pretty obvious. In any event, Kincaid knows well that a scientific theory and its target domain and boundary conditions tend to evolve together to optimize explanatory power and evidential support. Thus, precisely specifying a preset target community is not necessary. However, the intuitions that are used in the HDA's analyses are remarkably widespread, as nosologists like Spitzer (1999) observe, and there is no deep problem about identifying a target community of the analysis. Actually, I think the notion of the target community is a bit more complicated and interactive than that, analogous to the target domain of a scientific theory. I am after one particular meaning of "disorder," and I often write as if the target community has only that one meaning, but that is of course an idealization and a methodological artifact. The "community" is in effect a construct of those dispersed throughout the professional and lay communities who share a certain widespread concept of disorder that is a salient one among the many in circulation and has certain properties that make it important in scientific research and lay debate. Critics in this book, like many others, raise the obvious objection that there are many different meanings for "disorder" depending on the context (see my reply to Murphy on multiple meanings). That is a great point in general, but it is not germane here because in this case, the context of the analysis of mental disorder as I approach it is specified, and the resulting target concept is relatively determinate. Although the HDA is a conceptual analysis, the analysis of mental disorder in the context of our time is also what might be thought of as a transcendental argument that tries to identify whether there is a widespread concept of medical disorder that makes it possible to assert certain conclusions about mental disorder that are widely believed in the psychiatric and lay communities. These transcendental considerations include, most importantly, the following: (1) psychiatry is (in part, or at its core) a branch of medicine; correspondingly, (2) at the conceptual level, mental disorders are disorders in the same sense in which physical disorders are disorders; (3) there is an in-principle distinction between mental disorder versus social deviance and socially disvalued traits; and (4) mental disorder is at least in part a factual scientific concept that allows scientific research to bear on whether or not a psychological condition is a disorder. If an analysis of a widespread understanding of the concept of mental disorder satisfies these criteria and thus explains how it is possible for someone to believe these theses, it has met the antipsychiatric challenge and justified the beliefs at the heart of modern psychiatry.

This agenda is part of the reason I have not pursued the "harm" component as thoroughly as the "dysfunction" component (for other reasons, see my reply to Cooper in this volume). The value component presents urgent and important challenges. However, differences over nuances about the value component of "disorder" do not present an existential challenge to psychiatry, whereas in light of antipsychiatry, the "dysfunction" component does present what amounts to an existential issue for the standard view of psychiatry as a nonoppressive medical discipline. Many critics argue that "dysfunction" itself in fact harbors value assumptions. I don't think that evolutionary dysfunction hides any ineliminable value assumptions, but one can see why in the end this does not really matter as long as a factual component that can be studied scientifically apart from value assumptions can be extricated from "dysfunction." In effect, "dysfunction" is a placeholder for the factual element in "disorder," whatever it may be, that explains how we can scientifically show that some negatively valued conditions are disorders and some are not. In effect, all value considerations simply can be relocated to the "harm" component. But, again, I think a sheerly factual component is adequately identified as evolutionary dysfunction.

Kincaid also asks, "Do the intuitions of those outside the psychiatric professions count?" This is a point on which Christopher Boorse and I diverge; he limits the relevant community to pathologists, whereas I include professionals and laypeople. Obviously, professionals know much more than do laypeople about disorders, but do they have a different concept from laypeople? The continuity of the recent debates about the validity of proposed *DSM-5* diagnostic criteria across professional and lay contexts suggests that there is a shared concept. Here, my essentialist perspective plus the aforementioned evidence of continuity of discussion inclines me to follow other essentialist writers and to see ordinary concepts as continuous with scientific concepts. Here is Hilary Putnam on this issue:

> Ordinary language philosophers…tend to compartmentalize the language; the presence of water in the physical theory ('Water is H_2O') is held to involve a different use (i.e., a different sense) from the 'ordinary use'.…This compartmentalization theory seems to me to be simply wrong. Our language is a cooperative venture; and it would be a foolish layman who would be unwilling to ever accept correction from an expert on what was or was not water, or gold, or a mosquito, or whatever.…Ordinary language and scientific language are different but interdependent. (Putnam 2015, 361–362)

And here is Keith Donellan, in what is in some ways a critique of Putnam's account, nonetheless agreeing with him and elaborating this point:

> The Kripke-Putnam theory offers an answer to an important puzzle about the relationship of vernacular kind terms and scientific discovery. We seem willing to tailor the application of

many of our vernacular terms for kinds to the results of science and if necessary to allow our usual means of determining the extension of these terms to be overridden. There is, for example, a product on the market composed half of sodium chloride and half of potassium chloride. It looks like and tastes like ordinary salt. In most ordinary circumstances—in talking about how much to put in the stew, for example—we would be happy to call this product "salt" even if we knew its chemical composition. But if pressed to say whether this product is "really" salt, I think we would, if we know some elementary chemistry and the chemical composition of the product, concede that it is only half salt. To take a couple of more examples, I would give up calling a stone purchased as a diamond a 'diamond' if assured by experts that it did not possess a certain crystalline structure of carbon and I am prepared to be corrected when what I take to be a wolf in a cage at the zoo turns out to be identified by zoologists as being of a quite distinct species. (Donnellan 2014, 180–181)

The judgments of disorder versus nondisorder and the considerations in defending one or the other judgment in a controversial instance manifest equally impressive continuity across lay and professional communities, justifying the assumption that one analysis is likely to explain the conceptual underpinnings of both professional and lay disorder judgments. As with many other essentialist categories subject to scientific exploration, disorder and nondisorder appear to retain the same meaning across lay and professional judgments.

Kincaid's Approach to Mental Disorder

Kincaid says, "The alternative approach I favor denies that we must have a clear conceptual analysis of disorder in order to understand the practice of psychopathology research. … Instead, I think that the ideal for the sciences of psychopathology is to establish the existence of objective, explanatory classifications." The "instead" here is mystifyingly general. Every science attempts to establish objective, explanatory classifications. So, we are left with the question, what makes it the case that a system of objective, explanatory classifications is a system of nosology, that is, a system of mental disorder classifications, versus some other kind of classification? Remarkably, search as one might, Kincaid never answers this question.

Despite eschewing any conceptual analysis of "mental disorder," in order to argue that the HDA fails, Kincaid is forced to offer his own account of the distinction between disorder and nondisorder. He acknowledges the usefulness of some of my analyses that distinguish specific disorders from superficially similar normal reactions, yet wants to deny that those contributions are tied to the HDA's account of the concept of disorder and so attempts to provide an alternative account of the usefulness of the distinctions I have made. He argues that rather than considering my analyses to identify harmful dysfunctions versus biological design, "the question is whether these conditions allow for objective, explanatory classifications, a question that makes no essential judgment about evolutionary considerations." The problem, of course, is that objective ways of classifying things are a dime a dozen, and most of them don't impact the disorder-nondisorder distinction. For example, when writing about cancer, Kincaid explains, "Oncology, like the rest of medicine, studies and treats conditions that it can objectively and reliably identify and conditions where it can predict and alter the course of development in ways that people perceive to improve their lives." Agreed, but as alluded to by the phrase "like the rest of medicine," this characterization is a non sequitur if one is asked to characterize oncology because it does not differentiate oncology from proctology or, we now see, from psychiatry, for which Kincaid gives a more or less identical account.

One expects to get such an account in the final section of Kincaid's paper, in which he "sketches an alternative pluralist view of psychopathology that makes the search for objective explanatory classifications of psychopathology paramount, a goal inspired by and consistent with Wakefield's insightful critique of psychiatric practice." It turns out that the sketch just repeats what he has already said, namely, that psychopathology is distinguished from normality by being objectively characterized, using any theoretical means available: "I would argue that finding malfunctions in evolutionary mechanisms or breakdown of roles in a complex system are just valuable means to the end of getting objective, explanatory classifications of behavior that psychiatry and related disciplines study and treat."

Kincaid's most detailed statement of his view is the following: "the ideal for the sciences of psychopathology is to establish the existence of objective, explanatory classifications. ... *Objective* classifications as I use the term are ones that put individuals into classes based on real differences in facts about those individuals. ... *Explanatory* classifications as I am using the term are those that ground regularities and causal relations."

However, both normal and disordered categories can be objective and explanatory, and distinctions between two normal properties or between two disorders can be as objective and explanatory as a distinction between a disorder and a normal-range condition. So, the fact that a classification is objective and explanatory does not remotely make it an adequate classification of normal versus disordered conditions. Kincaid, avoiding any mention of biological design, has nothing at all to say about how that specific distinction is to be made.

A natural question is, if we take this substantively vacuous route, how do we fend off the antipsychiatric critique that all we are doing is creating spurious medical disorder categories to justify intervention into socially undesirable psychological features? Kincaid's answer is that we can refute social constructivism without any reference to evolutionary theory of functions and dysfunctions simply by using objectively characterizable differences to distinguish between disorder and normality: "What we need to show is that the psychiatric-related disciplines can produce objective and explanatory categorizations of behavior, ideally ones that lead to successful treatments. ... For example, the Big Five personality classification system relies on reliable and psycho-metrically validated measures; scores on those measures predict differences in behavior. Here psychological phenomena are classified in objectively grounded ways that refute pure social constructivist stories."

This response reveals some serious confusions. The objective evidence for the Big Five personality traits might be used to refute social constructivism about personality traits, but it has no bearing on social constructivism about disorder. More generally, the point of the social constructivist attack on psychiatry is not that there is no objective difference whatever between the people psychiatry places in categories of disorder versus nondisorder—there could be lots of objective differences, such as those associated with social deviance—but rather that whatever differences there are do not actually imply medical disorder versus nondisorder. It's the medicalization that is claimed to be spurious, not necessarily the group itself that is being medicalized. Thus, contra Kincaid, to refute social constructivist antipsychiatric claims, one must have an understanding of what it is to be a disorder, and this is one reason why the conceptual analysis of disorder became so important in the wake of the antipsychiatric movement.

As part of his "objective differences" approach to the distinction between disorder and nondisorder, Kincaid suggests that evolutionary dysfunction is just one objective indicator that might be used and neurobiological typical functioning another: "psychiatric research should get on without the concept of a disorder. If we can find compelling evidence of malfunctioning evolutionarily selected psychological mechanisms, then it would have a role in those cases. I also find it plausible that some behavior that gets labeled pathological involves a breakdown in the normal operation of cognitive and neurobiological systems, the idea promoted by competitors to Wakefield's analysis of function." Kincaid here begs the question by not explaining what it means to have a "breakdown in the normal operation of cognitive and neurobiological systems" as contrasted with "malfunctioning evolutionarily selected psychological mechanisms." We are learning that neurobiological mechanisms operate in highly idiosyncratic ways so that a sheerly statistical notion of "normal" neurological functioning won't do (Paulus and Thompson 2019). Kincaid appears to accept a statistical definition of pathological neurobiological performance, but generally, "something has gone wrong" is not be the same as "statistically unusual"; gum disease afflicts the vast majority of humans around the world, yet is considered a disorder, whereas lactose tolerance is statistically unusual among the human race, yet no one thinks it is a disorder because it is believed to be an adaptation in some groups to the availability of milk that resulted from the domestication of animals. As far as I can tell, the only way to distinguish normal neurobiological functioning from a breakdown in such functioning in the sense relevant to disorder judgments is by whether neurobiological systems are performing as they were biologically designed to perform. Thus, once placed within an HDA framework, I see no tension whatever between the evolutionary and neurobiological levels of explanation of function and dysfunction and would argue that they are complementary (for this argument, see my reply to Gerrans in this volume).

Are There Naturally Selected Disorders?

Like many other critics (see my replies to Cooper and to Garson in this volume), Kincaid argues that some conditions we are inclined to label as disorders could be naturally selected, falsifying the HDA. He thus claims there are "reasons to doubt that evolutionarily based dysfunction accounts fit with the kind of (reasonable) intuitive judgments that Wakefield wants to make about which symptoms constitute disorders and which do not. The problem is that there are plausible evolutionary stories where a wide range of behaviors that we are inclined to call disorders turn out to be the products of evolutionarily selected mechanisms." Focusing on depression and anxiety, he offers three scenarios in which this might occur.

Before examining Kincaid's three scenarios, it is important to keep in mind that what we are inclined initially to say is not always what we are inclined to say once we discover some condition is biologically designed. For example, the long-time general inclination to consider fever a disorder was based on the view that fever is a dysfunction caused by the toxic effects of illness, but when it was established that fever is a biologically designed defensive reaction, this inclination changed and we were no longer inclined to call fever itself a disorder. (Only when we think the fever mechanism itself has gone out of control and beyond its biologically designed parameters do we then consider it a disorder.) So, in considering Kincaid's stories, we have to consider what we are inclined to say about the diagnostic status of the condition in question if we believe one of Kincaid's stories to be true. In fact, I will argue, his three stories are explanations for what we would take to be normal variation, not disorder.

Disorders as Disproportionate Responses

The first of Kincaid's three stories that are supposed to show that disorders can be biologically designed is: "Success under natural selection requires a trade-off between costly unnecessary responses to threats to reproduction and between costly failures to detect such threats. Where the threat to reproductive success is death, it is not hard to imagine that natural selection would err on the side of false positives. A one strike and you are out threat would seemingly produce traits that produce lots of false positives in reacting to such threats, given the extreme consequences of a false negative." That is, Kincaid is arguing that there are cases in which "psychological mechanisms producing false positives would be fitness improving." With all of this, one can agree: to avoid disaster, we do seem to be biologically designed to be a vigilant, anxious, sadness-prone species.

those with chronic or traumatic stress, can cause disorders. However, that is because they create internal dysfunctions that become independent of the toxic environment. The fact that an individual has a negative reaction to a problematic environment mismatched to her biological design is not in itself considered a mental disorder. To take an extreme case of design-environment mismatch, it is not a disorder to be unable to breathe underwater, even though this limitation can kill you. It is not a mental disorder to desire infidelity in an environment that heavily punishes such desires, or to desire to eat fat and sugar in an environment where the novel easy availability of these high-calorie treats is problematic for long-term health, or to have a bothersome fight-or-flight reaction to the many anxiety-provoking situations that occur daily in a mass society. I do understand that it is very tempting to add chronic individual-environment mismatches that cause chronic misery to harmful dysfunctions under the disorder category. However, aside from the fact that that is not how intuitions about disorder work (as the above examples illustrate), there is the problematic outcome that if one locates mismatches under mental disorder, then psychiatry engulfs control of social deviation in which individuals' natures are mismatched to social demands (e.g., Soviet dissidents' longing for freedom was mismatched to their social environment). As the *DSM-5* definition of mental disorder indicates, "Socially deviant behavior (e.g., political, religious, or sexual) and conflicts that are primarily between the individual and society are not mental disorders unless the deviance or conflict results from a dysfunction in the individual" (American Psychiatric Association 2013, 20). Adding mismatches to the disorder category undermines the integrity of the concept in a way that legitimizes antipsychiatric objections.

Kincaid presents me with the following question: "A few miles from where I live, there are over a million people cramped into wall-to-wall corrugated metal shacks without running water and sanitation. Most live on less than $2 a day. Probably 50% are unemployed. ... Wakefield argues that depressive symptoms in response to a job loss should not be counted as a disorder. However, what if the job loss is a repeated or a permanent part of life as it is for the residents of these townships and the response is permanent depressive symptoms? Should we deny that they have a depressive disorder? ... Such examples should be a chance for clarification of his views."

I believe that I have always been crystal clear on this point: being chronically depressed due to chronic losses is not a mental disorder but a terrible misfortune, just as being chronically anxious due to chronic real threat is not a disorder. In some attenuated sense, such chronic negative responses to real environmental situations may be considered a "mental health problem" but not a disorder. I say this not because this is what I think but because I believe this is how laypeople and professionals tend to judge disorder under such circumstances, I have done empirical research on clinical judgment of conduct disorder in relation to chronic environmental triggering situations that suggests reactions to chronic stressors are not seen as disorders (Wakefield, Pottick, and Kirk 2002). Moreover, Kincaid's suggestion that the individuals in the horrifyingly afflicted community he describes should be understood as having depressive disorders due to their chronic reactions to chronic deprivations is in its own way horrifying, because it implies that the place where things are "going wrong" in creating this disaster is in the individuals, and the likely conclusion is that what is needed is a massive medical intervention such as provision of antidepressants, whereas what he describes is clearly a social problem inflicted on presumptively normal individuals that requires first and foremost a social response. (Drawing this sort of distinction is not merely a theoretical exercise; for example, United Nations relief agencies often must decide after a disaster whether the priority for limited resources in dealing with stress reactions is psychiatric treatment or environmental intervention [World Health Organization 2015].) Of course, some individuals in such circumstances do develop mental disorders and do need medical treatment. However, the crucial implication of the nondisorder judgment for the majority is that if improved circumstances and jobs are provided to these individuals, it is likely the distress will recede because there is no dysfunction in sadness-generating mechanisms. No such implication follows from the disorder attribution.

These judgments about disorder, the HDA emphasizes, are surrogates for causal hypotheses and consequently are important to scientific research. Although the experience of sadness and at one level the mechanisms involved in generating those experiences may be quite similar in the individuals in the community Kincaid describes and in those with out-of-the-blue chronic melancholic depression (as magnetic resonance imaging studies of disordered and normal sadness suggest [Mayberg et al. 1999]), one would expect to see divergent causal pathways at a deeper level. I have argued similarly that *DSM*'s invalidly lumping adolescent delinquency with true conduct disorder led to confused research outcomes as well as misplaced social priorities (Kirk et al. 1999; Wakefield et al. 2002; Wakefield et al. 2006).

Disorders as Extremes on Dimensions

Kincaid's third story of purported biologically designed disorder is: "The general fact that evolution produces traits with a wide reaction norm, raising the prospect that extremes of human behavior that we call pathological are the distributional tails of normal traits." Kincaid elaborates: "A third evolutionary approach arguing that psychopathology is the standard functioning of naturally selected traits points out that biological traits can have a wide reaction norm. Seemingly normal traits in common environments can exhibit extreme deviations from the average, given subtle changes in the developmental environment. The claim thus would be that major depression is just the tail of the expression of normal, presumably adaptive, trait of sadness. This is the kind of view advocated by the psychometric tradition that wants to treat psychopathology as a continuous trait and replace talk of disorders and psychopathology with talk of abnormal behavior."

The psychometrician's idea, popular in nosology at the moment, is that one scales symptoms or traits on a severity dimension, and we just label the extreme as disorder. Regarding evolution, the idea here is that naturally selected mechanisms generally yield not singular categorical traits but dimensions of symptoms or traits with continuously distributed variations in severity for a variety of reasons (such as interaction with other mechanisms and genes in the individual and with the environment), and thus all the points along the dimension are naturally selected, yet the extreme ones are labeled disorders. (There are also interactions between the fetus and the prenatal environment that alter later outcomes; see Garson's paper in this volume and my response.) If indeed some of the more extreme of the outcomes of a selected mechanism are classified as disorders, the argument goes, we have here disorders that are naturally selected.

This story is based on a manifestly invalid form of reasoning. To see why, consider instances of heterozygous advantage in which one copy of a gene is advantageous and selected for, whereas two copies cause a genetic disease. This is known to occur in single-gene mediated physical disorders such as cystic fibrosis and sickle cell anemia, but it is looking like this sort of situation could be quite a widespread phenomenon among polygenic disorders and even among mental disorders. For example, it appears that the risk genes for autism show evidence of positive selection for various cognitive capacities, yet in certain combinations of these, risk genes yield a devastating disorder (Polimanti et al. 2017). Phenomena such as heterozygote advantage explain why the genes conferring risk for mental disorders are so common and have not been eliminated from the population.

The clearest model of this situation is sickle cell anemia. Consider two individuals with sickle cell trait—a combination of one sickle cell gene and one standard gene—who are considered normal in a malaria-endemic environment in which sickle cell trait protects against malaria. Consider further that this trait that has been *selected for* (and that the sickle cell trait is in fact somewhat more fit than two standard genes). Let's imagine that these two individuals have children. Normal genetic distributional mechanisms operating on their genes will yield a "continuous" distribution along the genetic dimension of number of sickle cell genes and along the phenotypic dimension of degree of red blood cell sickling. (Actually, of course, the genetic distribution is not literally continuous, but neither are any other genetic distributions; they only have a lot more discrete steps, so the principle is the same.) So, this is an instance satisfying Kincaid's premises—namely, a naturally selected gene and a normal mechanism distributing intensities of that gene. Yet, his conclusion does not follow; the various outcomes are not considered equally naturally selected in their own right, and in fact, the tail end of the distribution that is considered a clear disorder—sickle cell anemia—is considered anything but naturally selected in itself. (This is the same error made by De Block and Sholl in their chapter in this volume; for a different worked-out example concerning hyperemesis gravidarum, see my reply to them in this volume.) This situation with regard to sickle cell anemia is of course due to the phenomenon of heterozygote advantage.

The moral of the sickle cell anemia story is that from normal naturally selected mechanisms for distribution of genotypes and consequent phenotypes, some parts of the distribution may be the ones that are responsible for the overall mechanism's natural selection, whereas other parts—due to processes of, or analogous to, heterozygote advantage—may be individually nonselected disordered variants, like sickle cell disease. The two-standard-gene configuration has a positive natural selection history, and sickle cell trait—one standard gene and one sickle cell gene—also has a positive selection history in malarial environments in which sickle cell trait arose, so both can be considered biologically designed, whereas sickle cell anemia—two sickle cell genes—came about as a nonnaturally selected and severely disordered side effect of those positive selection processes. One can consider sickle cell anemia a population-level trade-off for the enhanced fitness of sickle cell trait, but disorders are judged at the individual organism level, and for those with sickle cell anemia, there is no fruitful trade-off for the failure of multiple bodily systems and frequent early death.

Although the situation is much more complex in mental disorders such as depression, the critical point is the same. Depression, I agree, is a naturally selected defensive response that appears in varying degrees. However, the extreme of depressive feelings, which we label major depressive disorder, is judged a disorder because the nature, length, and independence from context of the symptoms (described earlier) suggest not an extreme of a naturally selected reaction but a breakdown in that naturally selected reaction. As in the distinction between pathological depression versus normal sadness, the HDA predicts that we judge disorder at the extreme of a dimension only if we believe that the extreme involves a dysfunction, either by being so severe as to counteract or override whatever effect the trait was selected for or by otherwise causing a dysfunction as collateral damage. Given how we think about disorder, if one really believed the evolutionary scenario as Kincaid presents it, the conclusion would be not that there are naturally selected disorders at the extremes of naturally selected dimensions but Plomin's (2003, 2018) much more radical and implausible conclusion that there are in fact no disorders at all, only dimensions (for more on this, see my response to De Block and Sholl in this volume).

References

American Psychiatric Association. 2013. *Diagnostic and Statistical Manual of Mental Disorders*. 5th ed. American Psychiatric Association.

Baller, E. B., S.-M. Wei, P. D. Kohn, D. R. Rubinow, G. Alarcón, P. J. Schmidt, and K. F. Berman. 2013. Abnormalities of dorsolateral prefrontal function in women with premenstrual dysphoric disorder: A multimodal neuroimaging study. *American Journal of Psychiatry* 170: 305–314.

Donnellan, K. (2014). Kripke and Putnam on natural kind terms. In *Essays on Reference, Language, and Mind*, J. Almog and P. Leonardi (eds.),179–203. Oxford University Press.

Dubey, N., J. F. Hoffman, K. Schuebel, Q. Yuan, P. E. Martinez, L. K. Nieman, et al. 2017. The ESC/E(Z) complex, an effector of response to ovarian steroids, manifests an intrinsic difference in cells from women with premenstrual dysphoric disorder. *Molecular Psychiatry* 22(8): 1172–1184.

First, M. B., and J. C. Wakefield. 2010. Defining 'mental disorder' in *DSM-V*. *Psychological Medicine* 40(11): 1779–1782.

First, M. B., and J. C. Wakefield. 2013. Diagnostic criteria as dysfunction indicators: Bridging the chasm between the definition of mental disorder and diagnostic criteria for specific disorders. *Canadian Journal of Psychiatry* 58(12): 663–669.

Horwitz, A. V., and J. C. Wakefield. 2012. *All We Have to Fear: Psychiatry's Transformation of Natural Anxieties into Mental Disorders*. Oxford University Press.

Kincaid, H. 2008. Do we need theory to study disease? Lessons from cancer research and their implications for mental illness. *Perspectives in Biology and Medicine* 51(3): 367–378.

Kirk, S. A., J. C. Wakefield, D. Hseih, and K. Pottick. 1999. Social context and social workers' judgment of mental disorder. *Social Service Review* 73: 82–104.

Mayberg, H. S., M. Liotti, S. K. Brannan, S. McGinnis, R. K. Mahurin, P. A. Jerabek, et al. 1999. Reciprocal limbic-cortical function and negative mood: Converging PET findings in depression and normal sadness. *American Journal of Psychiatry* 156(5): 675–682.

National Cancer Institute. 2015. What is cancer? February 9. https://www.cancer.gov/about-cancer/understanding/what-is-cancer.

National Cancer Institute. 2018. NCI dictionary of cancer terms. April 3. https://www.cancer.gov/publications/dictionaries/cancer-terms/def/cancer.

Nesse, R. M. 2001. The smoke detector principle: Natural selection and the regulation of defensive responses. *Annals of the New York Academy of Science* 935: 75–85.

Paulus, M. P., and W. K. Thompson. 2019. The challenges and opportunities of small effects: The new normal in academic psychiatry. *JAMA Psychiatry* 76(4): 353–354.

Plomin, R. 2003. Genes and behavior: Cognitive abilities and disabilities in normal populations. In *Disorders of Brain and Mind*, M. Ron and T. Robbins (eds.), vol. 2, 3–29. Cambridge University Press.

Plomin, R. 2018. *Blueprint: How DNA Makes Us Who We Are*. MIT Press.

Polimanti, R., and J. Gelerner. 2017. Widespread signatures of positive selection in common risk alleles associated to autism spectrum disorder. *PLoS Genetics* 13(2): e1006618.

Putnam, H. 2015. Reply to Ian Hacking. In *The Philosophy of Hilary Putnam*, R. E. Auxier, D. R. Anderson, and L. E. Hahn (eds.), 358–364. Open Court.

Quine, W. V. O. 1960. *Word and Object*. MIT Press.

Rind, B., and R. Yuill. 2012. Hebephilia as mental disorder? A historical, cross-cultural, sociological, cross-species, non-clinical empirical, and evolutionary review. *Archives of Sexual Behavior* 41(4): 797–829.

Schmidt, P. J., L. K. Nieman, M. A. Danaceau, L. F. Adams, and D. R. Rubinow. 1998. Differential behavioral effects of gonadal steroids in women with and in those without premenstrual syndrome. *New England Journal of Medicine* 338: 209–216.

Spitzer, R. L. 1997. Brief comments from a psychiatric nosologist weary from his own attempts to define mental disorder: Why Ossorio's definition muddles and Wakefield's "harmful dysfunction" illuminates the issues. *Clinical Psychology: Science and Practice* 4(3): 259–261.

Spitzer, R. L. 1999. Harmful dysfunction and the *DSM* definition of mental disorder. *Journal of Abnormal Psychology* 108(3): 430–432.

Vargas-Cooper, N. 2012. The billion dollar battle over premenstrual disorder. *Salon.* https://www.salon.com/2012/02/26/the_billion_dollar_battle_over_premenstrual_disorder/.

Wakefield, J. C. 1992a. The concept of mental disorder: On the boundary between biological facts and social values. *American Psychologist* 47: 373–388.

Wakefield, J. C. 1992b. Disorder as harmful dysfunction: A conceptual critique of *DSM-III-R*'s definition of mental disorder. *Psychological Review* 99: 232–247.

Wakefield, J. C. 1993. Limits of operationalization: A critique of Spitzer and Endicott's (1978) proposed operational criteria of mental disorder. *Journal of Abnormal Psychology* 102: 160–172.

Wakefield, J. C. 1995. Dysfunction as a value-free concept: A reply to Sadler and Agich. *Philosophy, Psychiatry, and Psychology* 2: 233–46.

Wakefield, J. C. 1997a. Diagnosing *DSM-IV*, part 1: *DSM-IV* and the concept of mental disorder. *Behaviour Research and Therapy* 35: 633–650.

Wakefield, J. C. 1997b. Diagnosing *DSM-IV*, part 2: Eysenck (1986) and the essentialist fallacy. *Behaviour Research and Therapy* 35: 651–666.

Wakefield, J. C. 1997c. Normal inability versus pathological disability: Why Ossorio's (1985) definition of mental disorder is not sufficient. *Clinical Psychology: Science and Practice* 4: 249–258.

Wakefield, J. C. 1997d. When is development disordered? Developmental psychopathology and the harmful dysfunction analysis of mental disorder. *Development and Psychopathology* 9: 269–290.

Wakefield, J. C. 1998. The *DSM*'s theory-neutral nosology is scientifically progressive: Response to Follette and Houts. *Journal of Consulting and Clinical Psychology* 66: 846–852.

Wakefield, J. C. 1999a. Evolutionary versus prototype analyses of the concept of disorder. *Journal of Abnormal Psychology* 108: 374–399.

Wakefield, J. C. 1999b. Mental disorder as a black box essentialist concept. *Journal of Abnormal Psychology* 108: 465–472.

Wakefield, J. C. 2000a. Aristotle as sociobiologist: The "function of a human being" argument, black box essentialism, and the concept of mental disorder. *Philosophy, Psychiatry, and Psychology* 7: 17–44.

Wakefield, J. C. 2000b. Spandrels, vestigial organs, and such: Reply to Murphy and Woolfolk's "The harmful dysfunction analysis of mental disorder." *Philosophy, Psychiatry, and Psychology* 7: 253–269.

Wakefield, J. C. 2001. Evolutionary history versus current causal role in the definition of disorder: Reply to McNally. *Behaviour Research and Therapy* 39: 347–366.

Wakefield, J. C. 2006. What makes a mental disorder mental? *Philosophy, Psychiatry, and Psychology* 13: 123–131.

Wakefield, J. C. 2007. The concept of mental disorder: Diagnostic implications of the harmful dysfunction analysis. *World Psychiatry* 6: 149–156.

Wakefield, J. C. 2009. Mental disorder and moral responsibility: Disorders of personhood as harmful dysfunctions, with special reference to alcoholism. *Philosophy, Psychiatry, and Psychology* 16: 91–99.

Wakefield, J. C. 2011. Darwin, functional explanation, and the philosophy of psychiatry. In *Maladapting Minds: Philosophy, Psychiatry, and Evolutionary Theory*, P. R. Andriaens and A. De Block (eds.), 143–172. Oxford University Press.

Wakefield, J. C. 2014. The biostatistical theory versus the harmful dysfunction analysis, part 1: Is part-dysfunction a sufficient condition for medical disorder? *Journal of Medicine and Philosophy* 39: 648–682.

Wakefield, J. C. 2016a. The concepts of biological function and dysfunction: Toward a conceptual foundation for evolutionary psychopathology. In *Handbook of Evolutionary Psychology*, D. Buss (ed.), 2nd ed., vol. 2, 988–1006. Oxford University Press.

Wakefield, J. C. 2016b. Diagnostic issues and controversies in *DSM-5*: Return of the false positives problem. *Annual Review of Clinical Psychology* 12: 105–132.

Wakefield, J. C., and M. B. First. 2003. Clarifying the distinction between disorder and nondisorder: Confronting the overdiagnosis ("false positives") problem in *DSM-V*. In *Advancing DSM: Dilemmas in Psychiatric Diagnosis*, K. A. Phillips, M. B. First, and H. A. Pincus (eds.), 23–56. American Psychiatric Press.

Wakefield, J. C., and M. B. First. 2012. Placing symptoms in context: The role of contextual criteria in reducing false positives in *DSM* diagnosis. *Comprehensive Psychiatry* 53: 130–139.

Wakefield, J. C., K. J. Pottick, and S. A. Kirk. 2002. Should the *DSM-IV* diagnostic criteria for conduct disorder consider social context? *American Journal of Psychiatry* 159: 380–386.

World Health Organization. 2015. *mhGAP Humanitarian Intervention Guide (mhGAP-HIG): Clinical Management of Mental, Neurological and Substance Use Conditions in Humanitarian Emergencies.* WHO.

World Health Organization. 2020. Health topics: Cancer. https://www.who.int/health-topics/cancer #tab=tab_1.

II   The Demarcation Problem

9   Psychiatric Disorders and the Imperfect Community: A Nominalist HDA

Peter Zachar

I.   The Concept of Psychiatric Disorder: Why Wakefield Matters[1]

There has been extensive scholarly discussion about how to define psychiatric disorder (Gert and Culver 2004; Graham 2010; D. Murphy 2006; Wakefield 1992b). Developing an official definition of psychiatric disorder became important, in part, because of the disagreement in American psychiatry during the 1970s about whether homosexuality is a disorder. The *Diagnostic and Statistical Manual of Mental Disorders* (*DSM*) definition (developed by Robert Spitzer and first published in the *DSM-III* and revised in later editions) was proposed to support the exclusion of homosexuality from the class of psychiatric disorders (Bayer 1981; Zachar and Kendler 2012). It was not, however, offered to *justify* that exclusion. The primary justification for the exclusion was an empirical one, specifically, the discovery that gay male relationships are not more compulsive and short term in nature than are heterosexual relationships.

Prior to the 1970s, the conventional argument for the pathological nature of homosexuality was that such relationships lacked the depth and commitment of mature sexual relationships. Once this was shown to be false, it became evident that the mental health benefits of sexual relationships in general can accrue to homosexual relationships; that is, sex between two men or two women can have positive effects on their mental health. Being gay was not inherently distressful, nor did it necessitate social or occupational dysfunction. For these reasons, making distress or impairment definitional of a psychiatric disorder supported removing homosexuality from the classification system. In its original formulation, the *DSM* definition began as follows: in *DSM-III*, each of the mental disorders is conceptualized as a clinically significant behavioral or psychological syndrome or pattern that occurs in an individual and that is typically associated with either a painful symptom (distress) or impairment in one or more important areas of functioning (disability) (American Psychiatric Association 1980, 6).

Our working concept of psychiatric disorder, therefore, has significant cultural implications, and defining it is more than an intellectually entertaining puzzle.

Consider the following nominalist definition: *psychiatric disorder is a name for what psychiatrists treat.* A definition of this sort was once suggested by Lilienfeld and Marino (1995). In making this proposal, they were calling attention to the heterogeneity of psychiatric disorders. The definition implies that for the class of psychiatric disorders as a whole, there is no essence or set of necessary and sufficient properties that all of them share and that distinguish them from other medical disorders and from normality.

The problem with such an austere definition is that, as happened in the 1850s, a community of psychiatrists could label recurrent attempts to escape slavery a psychiatric disorder, and no one could reject that label by arguing that runaways do not "really" have a psychiatric disorder. According to the austere definition, if these psychiatrists decide to conceptualize recurrent escape attempts as a "compulsion" and to treat it, then it is a psychiatric disorder. Under the guidance of such a relativistic concept, any kind of political or cultural dissident could be labeled as disordered by a community of psychiatrists.

Szasz's (1961) opposition to psychiatry as a medical specialty is based on his claim that psychiatric disorders are disliked because they represent not legitimate diseases but social norm violations. Consider slavery again. In 1851, the American physician Samuel Cartwright proposed that slaves who evidenced a rebellious desire to run away had a psychiatric disorder that he named *drapetomania.* For those slaves who did succeed in absconding, Cartwright claimed that misery in the form of an even worse disorder called *dysaesthesia aesthiopis* (or rascality) would follow them because they were not constituted to cope with freedom. But all was not lost, he said: "With the advantages of proper medical advice, strictly followed, this troublesome practice that many negroes have of running away, can be almost entirely prevented" (Cartwright 1851/2004, 34).

According to the Szaszian view, the only difference between Cartwright's including drapetomania under the umbrella of psychiatric disorder and the modern psychiatric community's abhorrence of Cartwright's proposal is that the modern psychiatric community holds different values than did Cartwright. The concept of psychiatric disorder, says Szasz (1960/2004), is an abstract name for those problems in living that society considers deviant and deserving of remediation.

1.1 The Harmful Dysfunction Analysis
In light of the Szaszian critique, one of the purposes of a conceptual definition of psychiatric disorder is to help psychiatrists demarcate valid disorders from all other problems in living. With respect to this goal, the most philosophically influential analysis of "psychiatric disorder" is Wakefield's (1992a, 1992b, 2000, 2004) *harmful dysfunction* (HD) model. Wakefield combines the metaphysical essentialism of Kripke (1972) and early Putnam (1975) with the psychological essentialism of Medin and Ortony (1989) under the name *black-box essentialism.* According to this view, the nature of a psychiatric disorder should be subject to scientific authority just as the nature of gold is subject to scientific authority.

Humans noticed and started working with gold at least 4,000 years ago. At various points in history, there was occasional disagreement about the criteria of "real" gold, but people were generally consistent in what they took to be gold. In the twentieth century, scientists discovered that every atom of gold (defined as the metallic element between platinum and mercury on the periodic table) has seventy-nine protons in its nucleus. "The element having seventy-nine protons in the nucleus" was arguably the object of people's talk about gold from the very beginning, even though it was hidden from view—or *in the black box*. The concept of gold *indirectly referred* to the element having seventy-nine protons, but the empirical meaning of the term was not properly specified until scientists discovered atomic structures.

Ancient people also noticed and named behavioral aberrations such as melancholia and mania, although, unlike gold, the concept of "mental/psychiatric disorder" is a term of art that is linked to the medical profession. Within medicine and related professions, there is some intuitive consistency in the concept's use, but according to Wakefield, the meaning of "psychiatric disorder" can and should be clarified just as the meaning of gold was clarified. The harmful dysfunction model is proposed as such a clarification.

Wakefield agrees that psychiatric disorders represent norm violations as the Szaszians claim, but he also argued that "dysfunction" is an objectivist concept—referring to the failure of some biological or psychological mechanism to perform as it was designed to perform during evolution. In Wakefield's synthesis of objectivism and normativism,[2] the attribution of "psychiatric disorder" to a particular condition involves a judgment on the part of mental health professionals that there exists an objective psychological dysfunction that, in addition, is harmful to its bearer and deserving of treatment. Murphy (2006) dubbed this the two-stage picture.

An important aspect of Wakefield's model is the concept of *natural function*. In evolutionary theory, natural functions are adaptive capacities such as vision and temperature regulation whose contribution to a species' survival explains why the mechanism underlying those capacities were selected during evolution (Millikan 1984; Wright 1973). According to this approach, the eyes were designed through natural selection for seeing; if they cannot see (due to something like cataracts), then there is a dysfunction (i.e., a failure of their naturally selected function).

One must also understand that Wakefield's model, like many other evolutionary models in psychology, is an interactive and contextual, not a reductionist, model. For example, many natural psychological functions were selected because they are adaptive responses to social and psychological situations. According to Wakefield, the underlying biological mechanisms for intense sadness may be the same in a grief reaction and a depressive disorder, but a grief reaction is a normal selected response to bereavement, whereas a depressive disorder occurs in response to situations in which intense sadness would not have been selected.

The key problem with the harmful dysfunction model is that it offers limited empirical guidance in distinguishing disorders from nondisorders because identifying objective natural functions depends on conceptual analysis, not factual evidence. Samuel Cartwright's own argument for drapetomania was predicated on the *inability* of some slaves to accept the submissiveness that he speculated represented natural functioning for black Africans enslaved in the United States.

As argued by Richardson (2007), there is not enough information about the selection pressures that were operating during human evolution, particularly on the evolution of the brain, to support empirically based theories of natural function. Wakefield (2001) contends that careful reasoning can reveal what natural psychological functions exist, but one has to worry that reason unconstrained by evidence can be marshalled to defend many different conclusions.

For example, Horwitz and Wakefield (2012) use a conceptual analysis of what we should and should not be expected to do to identify what lies within our biologically designed, naturally selected range of behaviors. According to them, talking to family members without intense anxiety lies in this range, but handling snakes without intense anxiety does not. Only psychiatric symptoms that interfere with what we should naturally be expected to do are considered objective dysfunctions. In this analysis, the distinction between disordered and normal is being made not by discovering an objective dysfunction but by reasoning.

The HD analysis cannot, therefore, empirically do what it was proposed to do, *factually* demarcate valid psychiatric disorders from the larger class of problems-in-living. It is quite likely that no model could do so given all the different considerations that might be deemed relevant in considering something to be dysfunctional and harmful.

1.2 Essentialism versus Empiricism

Spitzer's definition of mental disorder was a listing of features, not an abstract concept such as *harmful dysfunction*. Wakefield's conceptual analysis—that something has "really" gone awry inside the person and that it is harmful to its bearer—is parsimonious and useful. It is also an important advance in our thinking following the challenges posed by the Szaszian critique. For good reasons, Wakefield's analysis has become the de facto definition of mental disorder in psychiatry.

In adopting Wakefield's concept, however, psychiatrists and psychologists have also, maybe unwittingly, adopted a de facto essentialism. This would not displease Wakefield. In a penetrating analysis of the work of the eminent psychologist and philosopher Paul Meehl, Wakefield (2004) argues that when Meehl gave up strict operationalism in favor of scientific realism and construct validity, he made a mistake in not also abandoning empiricism. As an empiricist, Meehl continued to advocate for treating scientific concepts as open. The notion of an open concept was promulgated by the philosopher Arthur Pap (1958) in his critique of the analytic-synthetic distinction. This neo-empiricist notion, says Wakefield, is a myth.

According to Meehl (1986), *DSM* depression is an open diagnostic concept because the cluster of signs and symptoms in the *DSM* are, at best, indirect measures of an underlying pathology and its associated etiology. Clearly, Meehl construes depression in a medical model framework as a disease entity that results from an underlying pathological process, and Wakefield makes a good point that the medical model's conventional notion of a disease entity coheres with essentialism (perhaps even an essentialism that is more reductionist than Wakefield would prefer).

But Meehl also said that a psychological disorder such as depression is different from an infectious disease. It is also different from gold. For instance, key features of depression such as low positive emotionality and cognitive distortion are *conceptual interpretations* of behavior. The notion of an open concept refers to how the meaning of an abstract, dispositional concept such as "depression" is distributed (Meehl 1978). It is distributed among more observable indicators (e.g., lack of positive emotionality) and other theoretical concepts by which depression is implicitly defined (e.g., psychiatric disorder, cognitive distortion, and object loss). The meaning of an open concept cannot be defined *only* by a set of measurements (or partial definitions). Furthermore, open concepts are potentially extendable so that a new measurement *may* also become part of our definition of the concept. An open concept refers to what it is that the different operationalizations of it have in common, but it is not reducible to any of those operationalizations.[3]

The network of concepts that indirectly define an open concept such as depression is called the concept's surplus meaning. Meehl's notion of construct validation is, in part, about clarifying those surplus meanings that are of interest to us (Cronbach and Meehl 1955). Such meanings and the generalizations they allow can evolve as new facts are discovered and related concepts are modified (including our causal hypotheses). The goal is to calibrate our understanding of the concept so that it is adequate to both facts and well-supported theories (Zachar 2012), but the extendable/open nature of these concepts challenges the essentialist goal of treating them as rigid designators.

For example, the discovery that most cases of depression are precipitated by stress in the previous six months may lead us modify the concept of depression one way, and the discovery that cases of depression that lack precipitants are more treatment resistant may lead us to modify the concept (and related concepts such as psychiatric disorder) in another way. Each of these decisions could lead to elucidating different causal trajectories for "depression." If we narrow the depression construct by eliminating cases with clear precipitants, we can tell ourselves that this (and its causal story) is what we were "really" referring to all along, but that is a post hoc, even Whiggish assertion.

From a neo-empiricist standpoint, essentialism is an excessive metaphysical elaboration that is needlessly grafted onto this complicated network of "observations" and allied concepts. Some developmental psychologists have argued that essentialism is a cognitive bias that emerges by the time we are five or six years old (Gelman 2003, 2004; Gelman and Wellman 1991). The bias is reinforced by the science curriculum in high school and college because using essentialist frameworks makes scientific concepts easier to understand. The essentialist framework thereafter becomes accepted as a scientific ideal—a model of what a real science is. As scientists gain experience in their own domains of expertise, however, they increasingly adopt nonessentialist thinking. For example, as one learns more about depression, the population of depressive symptom clusters is more likely to be seen in a nonessentialist way as: (a) the result of multiple causal trajectories, (b) with no necessary and sufficient set of causes that are identity determining, and (c) regularly overlapping with normality, anxiety disorders, obsessive-ness, and psychosis.

Doubtlessly, the essentialist bias makes Wakefield's concept attractive, whereas the relativism of Lilienfeld and Marino's nominalism leaves psychiatric classification too ungrounded. If philosophical empiricists do not want to cede the ground to the essentialism (or to Meehl's putative crypto-essentialism) but avoid extreme nominalism and relativism, a variation upon Wakefield's, Meehl's, and Lilienfeld and Mariono's analyses is needed. The variation I propose is called the imperfect community model.

II. The Imperfect Community Model

2.1 The Experience of Dysfunction

In early onset Alzheimer's disease, the experience of dysfunction includes getting lost while driving in familiar places or continually forgetting recent events. Such experiences are salient examples of a *decline-in-functioning* that is developmentally unexpected and not a part of the typical course of life (Zachar 2011; Zachar and Kendler 2010). They are intrusive and unwanted failures of capacities that used to be there. Declines-in-functioning should also occur across multiple contexts—they travel with the person.

There are three important differences between this minimalist notion of dysfunction-as-decline and Wakefield's more ontologically elaborate concept of objective natural dysfunction. First, its objectivity does not depend upon speculation about natural functions. Rather, declines-in-functioning are objective in two different senses: (a) they are often intersubjectively confirmable, and (b) denying that they have occurred, although common, is a distortion. Eventually, people who are open to the evidence are compelled to accept that an important change has occurred, no matter what they may prefer to be the case.

Second, this minimalist notion is also normative. Wakefield separates dysfunction from harm, but these concepts are tightly integrated in noncontroversial examples of disorder such as Alzheimer's disease. The affected person experiences declines that *should not* have happened. They are *unwanted* declines. They represent something being *broken.* They are capacity *failures.* One can understand the attractiveness of stipulating that dysfunctions are out there and those that are harmful are disorders, but that does not seem consistent with how we come to identify dysfunctions.

What does making dysfunction both objective and normative do to the two-stage picture? The second stage is the attribution of disorder. I join Wakefield in using the term "disorder" as a general concept that encompasses diseases (e.g., tuberculosis), injuries (e.g., broken bones), vulnerability conditions (e.g., hypertension), and numerous painful states such as tension headaches that can be associated with "the sick role." They actively or potentially interfere with functioning and are reasonable targets for treatment. To name something a disorder, practically speaking, is to say that it a potential target for treatment. As we will see shortly, however, what unites psychiatric disorders is not only a belief that they are deserving of treatment but also the kinds of symptoms that characterize them.

Third, if we examine the set of things currently called psychiatric disorders, it is clear that a decline-in-functioning is not an essence. It is neither necessary for the attribution of psychiatric disorder nor sufficient. Many cases of intellectual disability (and other neurodevelopmental disabilities) do not manifest as declines in functioning.

2.2 The Domain of Psychiatry

Berrios (1996) reports that at the beginning of the nineteenth century, the main categories of psychiatric disorder were melancholia, mania, phrenitis, delirium, paranoia, lethargy, carus, and dementia. All these conditions are unambiguous examples of declines-in-functioning, and those conditions causing the greatest degree of impairment would presently be called psychotic conditions. People who become psychotic represent a psychiatrically vulnerable population. If one examines these cases over time, in addition to the florid psychotic symptoms such as hallucinations and delusions, one sees panic, obsessiveness, hypochondriasis, mood instability, impulsivity, and lack of empathy—in fact, much of our extant psychiatric symptom space.

In their studies of folk conceptions of mental disorder, Haslam (2005) and his colleagues propose that behavior that is unexpected, hard to understand or explain, and owned by the person (as opposed to compelled by an outside agent) is seen as pathological in all societies (Giosan et al. 2001; Haslam et al. 2007). "Pathologizing" refers to a sense that something is not right with the person—an inference that is easiest to make if there is a change/decline from a previous level of functioning.

Social constructionists sometimes suggest that in other cultures, people who become psychotic are valued and given meaningful roles like that of the shaman (Silverman 1967). This is better considered a myth (Boyer 2011; Haslam et al. 2007). For example, my colleague Jim Phillips spends part of his year working in Ayacucho, Peru—a rural city in the Andean Mountains. He claims that psychosis in the Ayacucho looks much like psychosis in the United States and that no one is inclined to give it a positive spin.

Similar observations about Eskimos in Alaska and the Yorubas in rural Nigeria were offered independently by the anthropologist Jane Murphy (1976).

In the domain of psychiatric disorders, psychotic states are *exemplars* in Medin's (1989) sense of the term. The larger domain was assembled, initially, in reference to them. Historically, psychiatry as a field developed in the nineteenth century when the exemplary psychotic disorders managed by the doctors who worked in mental asylums (called alienists) were expanded upon by the addition of the functional disorders of the neurologists that occupied some of the same symptom space as psychosis. To the extent that these combined symptom clusters explain why the discipline of psychiatry first appeared, their inclusion in the domain cannot be simply relativized to the idiosyncratic preferences of small communities of psychiatrists.

This development is usually discussed with respect to how the psychological approach associated with Freud came to replace the organic model of the alienists, but for our purposes, the important thing was the expansion of the symptom domain to cover the kinds of problems encountered in both the inpatient settings of the alienists and the outpatient settings of the neurologists. The link between the two settings was the group of premorbid and residual symptoms that resided in the penumbra of the psychoses.

Particularly in the United States, there was a major expansion of psychiatry into the outpatient population after World War II—in the 1950s and thereafter. The establishment of the clinical and counseling psychology specialties in the Veterans Administration hospitals and on college campuses at this time was also important. It is crucial to point out that this expansion cannot be simply attributed to the activity of mental health professionals because people with psychiatric symptoms actively sought out both treatments and diagnoses. In many respects, the expansion in the number of diagnostic constructs in the *DSM-III* was a belated recognition of this new reality.

The result of this mélange of functional disorders is an imperfect community— meaning that there is no set of properties that all psychiatric disorders share and that distinguish them from nondisorders. The "conditions" that were added to the psychiatric domain overlapped with the psychosis cluster in a variety of ways. These include but are not limited to the following:

Decline-in-functioning and other statistically abnormal developmental trajectories

The presence of reality distortion

Suicidal ideation

Confusion and other cognitive difficulties

Intrusive thoughts

Difficult to control impulses and compulsions

Agitation, anger, and excitement

Excessive anxiety and fear

Emptiness and anhedonia

Somatic preoccupations

Seeming more amenable to the skill set of psychiatry than other medical specialties

Interestingly, anthropologist Jane Murphy also indicated that among both the Eskimos and the Yorubas, a greater number of people suffer from the kinds of symptoms that psychiatrists would call depression-anxiety. These symptoms are considered different from being "crazy." Although Eskimos and the Yorubas do not lump this cluster of symptoms under a single name like "depression" or "neurosis," both groups consider them problems that are under the purview of the shaman/healer.

The "imperfect" part of the community of psychiatric disorders has been eloquently described by Allen Frances (2013):

> Some mental disorders describe short-term states, others life-long personality; some reflect inner misery, others bad behavior; some represent problems rarely or never seen in normals, others are just slight accentuations of the everyday; some reflect too little self-control, others too much; some are intrinsic to the person, others are culturally determined; some begin early in infancy, others emerge only late in life; … some are clearly defined, others not; and there are complex permutations of all of these possible differences. (17)

Although imperfect, the notion of *a community* suggests that the collection is not simply random or arbitrary. The various symptoms and symptom clusters are included as members for reasons. The domain of psychiatry should not be limited primarily to psychosis but also include what was added in the merging of the disorders of the alienists and the neurologists, of inpatient and outpatient, and of decline, distress, and disability into the imperfect community of psychiatric disorders.

III. The Causal Network Approach

Rachel Cooper (2005) claims that the concept of psychiatric disorder refers to unwanted psychological-behavioral conditions just as the concept of weed refers to unwanted plants. Cooper also notes that although "weed" is a heterogeneous category, the same cannot be said for particular kinds of weeds. For example, a dandelion is a kind of weed. Dandelions also have shared underlying properties, and generalizations about them can be made. She suggests that the same can be said for psychiatric disorders such as major depressive disorder and schizophrenia.

Wakefield argues that particular disorders such as major depressive disorder and schizophrenia, if valid, are the expressions of underlying psychopathological structures that represent design failures. According to Wakefield (2004), talk about these disorders directly refers to their symptomatic manifestations but indirectly refers to their underlying mechanisms. The mechanisms represent what the disorders really are.

3.1   Latent Variables versus Causal Networks

In psychometrics, the hidden patterns that causally produce observable symptoms are called *latent variables*.[4] When depicted visually, latent variables are represented as circles with causal arrows pointing at squares, which represent observed variables (see figure 9.1).

In clinical psychology, latent variables are considered to represent the psychopathological reality behind the appearances. They are causally important, the same from case to case, and make disorders what they are (identity determining). As a result, they correspond to the philosopher's notion of real essences. Although this essentialist model still remains largely promissory, it continues to hold sway—and understandably so.

Essentialism, however, is not scientifically necessary. A group of psychologists associated with the psychological methods program at the University of Amsterdam, including Han van der Maas, Denny Borsboom, and Angélique Cramer, argues that latent variables do not have to be interpreted as referring to real essences. Consider the latent variable called *psychometric g*. This variable is a mathematical index of the positive correlations that exist between different measures of cognitive ability. It is often conceptualized as a psychological ability called "general intelligence," which refers to what it is that all cognitive abilities share. In the realist interpretation of latent variables, the positive correlations between the abilities exist because they are all the outcomes of a shared causal entity represented by *g*.

According to van der Maas et al. (2006), an alternative to a causally potent latent variable (or common cause) model is a model in which cognitive abilities are in direct causal relationships with each other. For example, being able to process information quickly might have positive effects on working memory. Cognitive abilities can enter into mutual interactions in a variety of ways. Some people may naturally have high abilities across the board, whereas others are gifted in one or two areas—such as

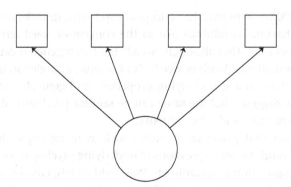

Figure 9.1
Visual representation of a latent variable model.

processing speed and attention capacity—but these skills permeate through the ability network and raise scores on tests of general intelligence. For example, in neuropsychology settings, temporary problems with focused attention just after a brain injury will depress scores on other cognitive abilities. An assessment of lasting deficits cannot occur until attention improves.

Van der Maas and his colleagues simulated data sets that were consistent with both the common cause scenario and the mutual interaction scenario and discovered that the latent variable model "fit" both of them. This means that psychometric g will mathematically appear if the positive correlations between the variables are the result of direct causal relationships rather than the result of an underlying common cause. Both scenarios can be analyzed to produce the shared correlations that are lumped together as psychometric g.

One implication of this research is that the psychological concept of general intelligence as the ability to perform well across multiple cognitive domains is an empirically supported phenomenon, but it need not be the result of an underlying causal entity called g. Another implication is that the relevant causal structure from which a latent variable emerges does not have to be a universal (or the same from case to case).

Likewise, in psychiatry and psychology, latent variables are interpreted realistically—meaning that the cluster of symptoms that constitute depression is considered correlated because they are manifestations of a shared underlying psychopathological process (Borsboom et al. 2003; Kendler et al. 2011). Furthermore, the more reliable the symptomatic criteria, the better they are supposed to be at estimating a person's *true score* on the underlying variable. In contrast, for causal networks, the symptoms hold together because they are in direct, possibly causal, relationships with each other (Borsboom 2008). For example, rather than both sleep problems and fatigue being manifestations of a single underlying cause called "depression," sleep problems (SP) likely directly influence the level of fatigue (F). In addition, such factors as depressed mood (DM) and loss of interest (LI) are central symptoms, meaning they enter into a high number of mutual relationships with other symptoms in the network. As a result of these connections, when central symptoms are activated, it is more likely that other symptoms will follow. A pathological state of depression would represent the emergence of feedback loops between symptoms that become self-sustaining (see figure 9.2).

Abandoning the realist interpretation of latent variables in favor of symptom networks, however, does not make depression a theoretical fiction. Depression is instead understood as the activation of a network within the larger symptom space of psychiatric disorders. According to Borsboom (2008), requiring five out of nine symptoms for a diagnosis does not indicate the presence of an underlying entity called depression. Instead, it indicates the extent to which the symptom network (named depression) has been entered.

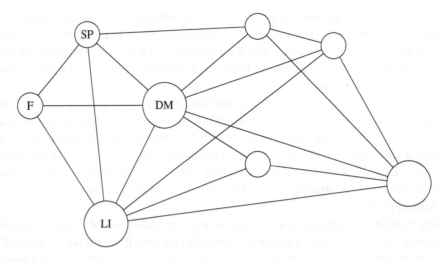

Figure 9.2
A causal network model for major depressive disorder.

3.2 Comorbidity

The network model also offers a new understanding of comorbidity. In traditional medicine, comorbidity is defined as the simultaneous occurrence of two causally independent diseases such as liver cancer and heart disease (Feinstein 1970). Presumably, the presence of one disease has consequences for the development and treatment of the second. The problem in psychiatry is that such co-occurrences tend not to be independent. *Psychiatric comorbidity* refers to complicated, multisymptomatic cases that tend to occur in vulnerable populations (Klein and Riso 1993; Neale and Kendler 1995; Zachar 2009).

According to one very influential latent variable model, the high rate of comorbidity between a depressive episode and generalized anxiety disorder (GAD) is explained with reference to a common vulnerability factor—the personality trait of neuroticism (Clark 2005; Kahn et al. 2005). In contrast, the causal network approach conceptualizes comorbidity in terms of the relationships between symptoms within the larger network of psychiatric symptomatology (Borsboom et al. 2011).

Using data from the National Comorbidity Survey Replication, Cramer et al. (2010) mapped reciprocal relationships between the symptoms in both the depression and GAD clusters. They discovered that some symptoms have connections to symptoms in both networks. They labeled these bridge symptoms.

In depression and GAD, the bridges connecting the two networks include sleep problems (SP), fatigue (F), concentration problems (CP), and irritability (I). For example, the central symptom of depressed mood (DM) has multiple relationships with other depression symptoms. It is also connected to several bridge symptoms and, through them, to symptoms in the GAD network. DM even does double duty as a bridge symptom by being directly connected to chronic anxiety (CA), which is itself a central symptom in the GAD network. In this model, comorbidity is the result of a spreading activation process. In more vulnerable persons, once activated, a symptom network stays activated via feedback loops (see figure 9.3).

In traditional medical classification, good diagnostic criteria are both sensitive and specific indicators of a disorder. For this reason, a symptom such as irritability is not an ideal criterion for depression because it is sensitive to depression but not specific to depression. Highly anxious people are also irritable. Within the network perspective, however, rather than being ignored because they are not specific to a single disorder, overlapping symptoms contribute to our understanding of how complicated cases might develop. When bridge symptoms are ignored, the gaps between clusters look larger (or more "real") than they are.

An important implication of the symptom network model is that diagnosticians should be attending not only to the diagnostic categories for which a patient meets criteria but also to the number of symptoms activated. If two separate individuals each meet four criteria for a major depressive episode, neither would be diagnosed. But if the first person meets criteria composed of symptoms that are also bridges to another network such as the anxiety disorders network, he might be experiencing considerably more social and occupational dysfunction than the second person who meets criteria for fewer bridge symptoms. Not all subthreshold conditions are the same. Consider

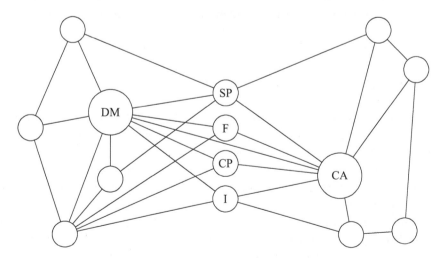

Figure 9.3
A causal network mode for the comorbidity of depression and generalized anxiety disorder.

this statement from the *DSM-5*: "the boundaries between many disorder 'categories' are more fluid over the life course than the *DSM-IV* recognized, and many symptoms assigned to a single disorder may occur, at varying levels of severity, in many other disorders" (American Psychiatric Association 2013, 5).

Given the empirically demonstrated patterns of comorbidity, it would not be unexpected for a person diagnosed with depression to experience anxiety-related symptoms that are not typically listed as falling under the depression concept. From an essentialist standpoint, these extra symptoms are accidental rather than essential properties of a patient's depression. From a symptom network perspective, these symptoms may be an integral part of the symptom cluster for that person.

It should be noted that the network model does not eliminate underlying causal structures. For example, a symptom such as a sleep disturbance can be understood with respect to a multiplicity of underlying mechanisms at many levels of analysis (genetic, physiological, anatomical, etc.). In addition, researchers could also investigate whether the causal relationship between sleep problems and concentration problems involves relations between two sets of underlying mechanisms, that is, the presence of direct causal relations between endophenotypes.

A symptom such as "sleep problem" is also a conceptual abstraction that summarizes a variety of symptoms. Particular kinds of sleep problems (early awakening, difficulty falling asleep, etc.) are themselves the result of underlying causal mechanisms. If the imperfect community is a swarm made up of points that represent a cluster of symptoms, for multifaceted symptoms such as "sleep problems," we can expect that a plurality of underlying nested mechanisms is present. In such a multilevel "bushy" network, some of the basic insights of essentialism such as the importance of underlying causal properties are preserved, but the conventional essentialist framework in which these properties are seen as identity-determining universals is abandoned.

IV. Identifying Disorders in the Imperfect Community

The disorders of psychiatry are the result of a gradual addition of variations on the symptom clusters of the alienists and, after psychodynamic theories made their mark, variations on the neurotic clusters as well. What we are left with is a large symptom space that can be organized in multiple ways. The *DSM* and the *International Classification of Diseases* (*ICD*) are two ways of organizing the symptom space, but because of the way the domain was built (by the addition of variants on variants), no single organization can model all of the overlapping relationships. It is important to establish standards of adequacy and work to improve the classification system, but that goal does not entail the discovery of a classification that is uniquely privileged in nature.

What does such a model do to resolve the problem of defining psychiatric disorders arbitrarily as "what psychiatrists decide to treat?" Let us consider depression. According to the essentialist model, valid depressive disorders are caused by dysfunctional mood-regulating mechanisms. From an empiricist standpoint, referring to objective dysfunctions hidden in the black box introduces an unnecessary metaphysical elaboration that distorts the actual basis for the distinction.

Jerry Wakefield has taught us that a careful conceptual analysis can help constrain what psychiatrists and other mental health professionals treat. However, rather than making the distinction using an inferred essentialist criterion such as objective dysfunction, it is more commonly made using a polythetic criterion set (i.e., a collection of conceptual elaborations). As more of these conceptual criteria are met, the more it makes sense to start thinking of a symptom cluster as disordered. Rather than being absolutely present or absent, disorders are a matter of degree.

Considerations that are relevant in making the depressive disorder attribution include (a) the extent to which the person has entered a psychiatric symptom network. The most important criterion is the presence of a decline in functioning, although it is not a necessary criterion. Sometimes symptoms are related to impaired functioning only, not to decline. Also, (b) those symptom networks that are locked in rather than transient and flexible are also more disorder-like. Additionally, (c) more severe symptoms and more complex symptom networks support the disorder attribution. For distressing psychological symptoms such as anhedonia, (d) if there are no compensatory factors that allow the person to continue to function (and flourish), then a disorder attribution is more warranted. It is also important not to limit assessment to a single slice of time because (e) a past history of symptoms and a family history of symptoms alter the base rates and make the disorder attribution more plausible. In these cases, the appearance of milder symptoms might signal a risk for more impaired functioning in the future. In addition, as Horwitz and Wakefield (2007) persuasively argue, the attribution of disorder to a cluster of depression symptoms is more warranted when the depressive symptoms appear out of the blue—for no apparent reason—or if there is a precipitant, the response is excessive and not in proportion to the trigger.

Acknowledgments

Andrea Solomon, Denny Borsboom, Bob Krueger, Ken Kendler, Katie Tabb, and Steve Lobello provided helpful commentary on an early version of this chapter.

Notes

1. Part of this chapter draws on material previously published in Zachar, P. (2014). *A Metaphysics of Psychopathology*. MIT Press. Reprinted with permission here.

2. Both Boorse and Fulford use the term "illness" to describe the confluence of fact (an underlying pathology) and value (being *bad* for its bearer). See Boorse, C. (1975). On the distinction

between disease and illness. *Philosophy and Public Affairs* 5, 49–46, and Fulford, K. W. M. (1989). *Moral Theory and Medical Practice.* Cambridge University Press.

3. Since this chapter was written in 2013, I have thought more about open concepts. See Zachar, P., E. T. Turkheimer, and K. S. Schaffner (2020). Defining and redefining phenotypes: operational definitions as open concepts. In *The Cambridge Handbook of Research Methods in Clinical Psychology,* A. G. C. Wright and M. N. Hallquist (eds.), 5–17. Cambridge University Press.

4. For neo-empiricists, signs and symptoms index a latent variable, and the latent variable is an index of a causal trajectory. A latent variable cannot be eliminated in favor of what indexes it or what it indexes.

References

American Psychiatric Association. 1980. *Diagnostic and Statistical Manual of Mental Disorders.* 3rd ed. American Psychiatric Association.

American Psychiatric Association. 2013. *Diagnostic and Statistical Manual of Mental Disorders.* 5th ed. American Psychiatric Publishing.

Bayer, R. 1981. *Homosexuality and American Psychiatry: The Politics of Diagnosis.* Basic Books.

Berrios, G. E. 1996. *The History of Mental Symptoms.* Cambridge University Press.

Borsboom, D. 2008. Psychometric perspectives on diagnostic systems. *Journal of Clinical Psychology* 64(9): 1089–1108.

Borsboom, D., A. O. J. Cramer, V. D. Schmittmann, S. Epskamp, and W. Lourens. 2011. The small world of psychopathology. *PLoS ONE* 6(11): e27407.

Borsboom, D. G., G. J. Mellenbergh, and J. van Heerden. 2003. The theoretical status of latent variables. *Psychological Review* 110(2): 203–219.

Boyer, P. 2011. Intuitive expectations and the detection of mental disorder: A cognitive background to folk-psychiatries. *Philosophical Psychology* 24(1): 95–118.

Cartwright, S. A. 1851/2004. Diseases and physical peculiarities of the negro race. In *Health, Disease, and Illness,* A. L. Caplan, J. J. McCartney, and D. A. Sisti (eds.), 28–39. Georgetown University Press.

Clark, L. A. 2005. Temperament as a unifying basis for personality and psychopathology. *Journal of Abnormal Psychology* 114(4): 505–521.

Cooper, R. 2005. *Classifying Madness: A Philosophical Examination of the Diagnostic and Statistical Manual of Mental Disorders.* Springer.

Cramer, A. O. J., L. Waldrop, H. L. J. van der Mass, and D. Borsboom. 2010. Comorbidity: A network perspective. *Behavioral and Brain Sciences* 33(2–3): 137–150.

Cronbach, L. J., and P. E. Meehl. 1955. Construct validity in psychological tests. *Psychological Bulletin* 52(4): 281–302.

Feinstein, A. R. 1970. The pre-therapeutic classification of co-morbidity in chronic disease. *Journal of Chronic Diseases* 23(7): 455–468.

Frances, A. 2013. *Saving Normal*. William Morrow.

Gelman, S. A. 2003. *The Essential Child*. Oxford University Press.

Gelman, S. A. 2004. Psychological essentialism in children. *Trends in Cognitive Science* 8(9): 404–409.

Gelman, S. A., and H. M. Wellman 1991. Insides and essences: Early understandings of the non-obvious. *Cognition* 38: 213–244.

Gert, B., and C. M. Culver. 2004. Defining mental disorder. In *The Philosophy of Psychiatry: A Companion*, J. Radden (ed.), 415–425. Oxford University Press.

Giosan, C., V. Glovsky, and N. Haslam. 2001. The lay concept of 'mental disorder': A cross-cultural study. *Transcultural Psychology* 38(3): 317–322.

Graham, G. 2010. *The Disordered Mind*. Routledge.

Haslam, N. 2005. Dimensions of folk psychiatry. *Review of General Psychology* 9(1): 35–47.

Haslam, N., L. Ban, and L. Kaufmann. 2007. Lay conceptions of mental disorder: The folk psychiatry model. *Australian Psychologist* 42(2): 129–137.

Horwitz, A. V., and J. C. Wakefield. 2007. *The Loss of Sadness: How Psychiatry Transformed Normal Sorrow into Depressive Disorder*. Oxford University Press.

Horwitz, A. V., and J. C. Wakefield. 2012. *All We Have to Fear: Psychiatry's Transformation of Natural Anxieties into Mental Disorders*. Oxford University Press.

Kahn, A. A., K. C. Jacobson, C. O. Gardner, C. A. Prescott, and K. S. Kendler. 2005. Personality and comorbidity of common psychiatric disorders. *British Journal of Psychiatry* 186: 190–196.

Kendler, K. S., P. Zachar, and C. Craver. 2011. What kinds of things are psychiatric disorders. *Psychological Medicine* 41(6): 1143–1150.

Klein, D. N., and L. P. Riso. 1993. Psychiatric disorders: Problems of comorbidity. In *Basic Issues in Psychopathology*, C. G. Costello (ed.), 19–66. Guilford.

Kripke, S. 1972. *Naming and Necessity*. Reigel.

Lilienfeld, S. O., and L. Marino. 1995. Mental disorder as a Roschian concept: A critique of Wakefield's 'harmful dysfunction' analysis. *Journal of Abnormal Psychology* 104(3): 411–420.

Medin, D. L. 1989. Concepts and conceptual structure. *American Psychologist* 44(12): 1469–1481.

Medin, D. L., and A. Ortony. 1989. Psychological essentialism. In *Similarity and Analogical Reasoning*, S. Vosniadou and A. Ortony (eds.), 179–195. Cambridge University Press.

Meehl, P. E. 1978. Theoretical risks and tabular asterisks: Sir Karl, Sir Ronald, and the slow progress of soft psychology. *Journal of Consulting and Clinical Psychology* 46(4): 806–834.

Meehl, P. E. 1986. Diagnostic taxa as open concepts: Metatheoretical and statistical questions about reliability and construct validity in the grand strategy of nosological revision. In *Contemporary Directions in Psychopathology: Toward the DSM-IV*, T. Millon and G. L. Klerman (eds.), 215–231. Guilford.

Millikan, R. G. 1984. *Language, Thought, and Other Biological Categories*. MIT Press.

Murphy, D. 2006. *Psychiatry in the Scientific Image*. MIT Press.

Murphy, J. M. 1976. Psychiatric labeling in cross-cultural perspective. *Science* 191(4231): 1019–1028.

Neale, M. C., and K. S. Kendler. 1995. Models of comorbidity for multifactorial disorders. *American Journal of Human Genetics* 57(4): 935–953.

Pap, A. 1958. *Semantics and Necessary Truth*. Yale University Press.

Putnam, H. 1975. *Mind, Language and Reality: Philosophical Papers*. Vol. 2. Cambridge University Press.

Richardson, R. C. 2007. *Evolutionary Psychology as Maladapted Psychology*. MIT Press.

Silverman, J. 1967. Shamans and acute schizophrenia. *American Anthropologist* 69(1): 21–31.

Szasz, T. 1960/2004. The myth of mental illness. In *Health, Disease, and Illness*, C. A. L. Caplan, J. J. McCartney, and D. A. Sisti (eds.), 43–50. Georgetown University Press.

Szasz, T. S. 1961. *The Myth of Mental Illness*. Harper & Row.

van der Maas, H. L. J., C. V. Dolan, R. P. Grasman, J. M. Witchers, H. M. Huizenga, and M. E. Raijmakers. 2006. A dynamical model of general intelligence: The positive manifold of intelligence by mutualism. *Psychological Review* 113(4): 842–861.

Wakefield, J. C. 1992a. The concept of mental disorder: On the boundary between biological facts and social values. *American Psychologist* 47(3): 373–388.

Wakefield, J. C. 1992b. Disorder as harmful dysfunction: A conceptual critique of *DSM-III-R*'s definition of mental disorder. *Psychological Review* 99(2): 232–247.

Wakefield, J. C. 2000. Aristotle as sociobiologist: The 'function of a human being' argument, black box essentialism, and the concept of mental disorder. *Philosophy, Psychiatry, and Psychology* 7(1): 17–44.

Wakefield, J. C. 2001. Spandrels, vestigial organs, and such. *Philosophy, Psychiatry, and Psychology* 7(4): 253–269.

Wakefield, J. C. 2004. The myth of open concepts: Meehl's analysis of construct meaning versus black box essentialism. *Applied & Preventive Psychology* 11: 77–82.

Wright L. 1973. Function. *Philosophical Review* 82(2): 139–168.

Zachar, P. 2009. Psychiatric comorbidity: More than a Kuhnian anomaly. *Philosophy, Psychiatry, and Psychology* 16(1): 13–22.

Zachar, P. 2011. The clinical nature of personality disorders: Answering the neo-Szazian critique. *Philosophy, Psychiatry, and Psychology* 18(3): 191–202.

Zachar, P. 2012. Progress and the calibration of scientific constructs: The role of comparative validity. In *Philosophical Issues in Psychiatry II: Nosology-Definition of Illness, History, Validity, and Prospects*, K. S. Kendler and J. Parnas (eds.), 21–34. Oxford University Press.

Zachar, P., and K. S. Kendler. 2010. Philosophical issues in the classification of psychopathology. In *Contemporary Directions in Psychopathology*, T. Millon, R. F. Krueger, and E. Simonsen (eds.), 126–148. Guilford.

Zachar, P., and K. S. Kendler. 2012. The removal of Pluto from the class of planets and homosexuality from the class of psychiatric disorders: A comparison. *Philosophy, Ethics, and Humanities in Medicine* 7: 4.

10   Can a Nonessentialist Neo-Empiricist Analysis of Mental Disorder Replace the Harmful Dysfunction Analysis? Reply to Peter Zachar

Jerome Wakefield

I have watched with amazement the extensive and diverse contributions Peter Zachar has made to philosophy of psychiatry over time. He has done it in the way that I think is most productive yet rarely pursued, by being immersed in and publishing in both philosophy and psychiatry at once, with close ties to colleagues in both fields. I thank him for his contribution to this volume and his illuminating description of various positions including my harmful dysfunction analysis (HDA) of medical, including mental, disorder. The HDA claims that "disorder" refers to "harmful dysfunction," where dysfunction is the failure of some feature to perform a natural function for which it is biologically designed by evolutionary processes and harm is judged in accordance with social values (First and Wakefield 2010, 2013; Spitzer 1997, 1999; Wakefield 1992a, 1992b, 1993, 1995, 1997a, 1997b, 1997c, 1997d, 1998, 1999a, 1999b, 2000a, 2000b, 2001, 2006, 2007, 2009, 2011, 2014, 2016a, 2016b; Wakefield and First 2003, 2012). I especially appreciate Zachar's recognition that "Wakefield's model, like many other evolutionary models in psychology, is an interactive and contextual, not a reductionist, model." Indeed, I have been arguing for years and continue to argue (Wakefield 2017) that mental disorders can occur at the intentional-system level without there being any disorder describable at a purely neurobiological level and that context is critical to evaluating whether a disorder exists (Wakefield and First 2012), points often missed by critics and defenders alike.

However, as with Harold Kincaid's Quinianism (see Kincaid in this volume and my reply), my reply to Zachar is made more challenging by the fact that he and I have deep differences on broader philosophical issues. Specifically, our differences regarding Zachar's neo-empiricism versus my essentialist realism go well beyond the present topic of the concept of mental disorder and cannot be fully aired in this interchange. I will comment briefly on a few of the broader philosophical issues Zachar raises in his paper and then focus on his substantive views of the concept of mental disorder and especially on points of divergence between us.

One point of apparent convergence is important to mention at the outset. Judging by his comments early in his paper, Zachar and I agree that a requirement of any successful account of mental disorder—and thus of any account of medical disorder that encompasses mental disorder—is that it respond to the Szaszian type of antipsychiatric attack on psychiatry's legitimacy as a medical discipline. We also agree that, whatever else one thinks of the HDA, it does offer such a response. In the course of his paper, in a quest for a nonessentialist account of disorder, Zachar offers several characterizations of mental disorder, and I will apply this test of adequacy when evaluating his various suggestions.

Essentialism versus Neo-Empiricism

I am going to focus mostly on assessing Zachar's positive suggestions for how to understand disorder from a neo-empiricist perspective. However, before proceeding to those issues, in this first section, I briefly present some background and address some of the comments Zachar makes about the inadequacies of the HDA.

My modest form of essentialism (see my reply to Lemoine in this volume for discussion of modest essentialism) allows for multiple meanings of terms depending on context and on an ontological marker that indicates the type of thing being defined from among the many possible essences identifiable based on any base set. Generally, essentialist definitions take the form "something belongs to this category if it has the same nature as X," where X is some base set of observably identifiable instances. The concept then generalizes not along the lines of the observable characteristics of the base set but along the lines of the underlying nature of the base set. In principle, modest essentialism allows that meanings can include neo-empiricist-type observational meanings that don't refer to any underlying essence. Thus, in some contexts, "depression" can refer to a certain phenomenology and set of experiences that can be normal or disordered, and in others—including typical *Diagnostic and Statistical Manual of Mental Disorders* (*DSM*) diagnostic contexts—it can refer specifically to a disorder, in which case it has an essentialist loading that requires some inferred dysfunction. If it is eventually established that there are several quite different types of dysfunction that lead to the same symptom syndrome, then there is the option of concluding that depressive disorder as conceptualized fails to be construct valid and is in fact several disorders. "Essentialist" meanings encompass virtually any meaning that refers directly or indirectly to nonobservational properties that explain and unify the members of the category and thus goes beyond neo-empiricist constraints that limit concepts to sets of observational properties. While allowing that terms are sometimes used in neo-empiricist ways, modest essentialism holds that most scientific concepts—and certainly psychiatric concepts such as "mental disorder"—have salient primary essentialist meanings. This is particularly so if one is trying to identify the senses of "function" and "dysfunction" that underlie medical diagnosis.

Zachar uses the standard example of "gold"—eventually identified as the element having atomic number 79—to illustrate an essentialist concept, but this may be misleading in one respect. "Gold" has an essence that is an actual structural underpinning. Obviously, there is no such substantial real essence shared among disorders such as infections, injuries, poisonings, allergies, and so on. The nature of disorders is endlessly variable, so what unites disorders is not any real-essence commonality but rather the "essential" (nonobservational) property that they are failures of natural functions, and natural functions do have an essential (although not structural) commonality, namely, they are naturally selected effects. Unlike gold, neither natural functions nor their failures share a specific material essence. Their essences are more analogous to the modest quasi-essentialist account of artifact categories such as "chair"; chairs have no material substrate or even physical similarities in common (think of bean bag chairs and tree-stump chairs), but they are chairs roughly because they share the fact that they were designed (or retained, if a natural object) to be a place for someone to sit, which is not an immediately observable property of chairs but nevertheless determines their category. This is quite different from the situation with "gold."

One must distinguish the concept of medical disorder in general from the concepts of specific disorders. Specific disorders are individuated by the specific dysfunction(s) that cause the symptoms and that constitute the essence of the disorder. Zachar says, "Ancient people also noticed and named behavioral aberrations such as melancholia and mania." The use here of "behavioral aberrations" to suggest no reference to inferred explanatory properties beyond behavior is tendentious. Ancient people noticed and named lots of behavioral aberrations (e.g., hubris, impiety, erotic love, grief), and they, like us, considered melancholia and mania and other mental disorders to be more than mere "behavioral aberrations." They even recognized that the very same set of symptoms could represent distinct disorders or even disorder versus nondisorder (e.g., melancholia versus grief or despair over romantic rejection). They already used medical concepts as etiologically inferential theoretical concepts, with disorders sometimes named after the theory popular at the time of the unobservable etiology of the symptom syndrome (e.g., hysteria, melancholia, malaria). Given that a dysfunction might have a unique pathophysiology, this is somewhat closer to the "gold" situation.

Trying to portray the HDA's essentialism as discordant with *DSM*'s prominent definition of disorder, Zachar claims that "Spitzer's definition of mental disorder [in *DSM-III*] was a listing of features, not an abstract concept such as *harmful dysfunction*." In his paper, Zachar reproduces the first few sentences of the definition, and they do indeed focus on the observable harms of distress and impairment of role functioning, and remarkably he then ends the quote, tendentiously leaving out the very next sentence that directly falsifies his claim: "In addition, there is an inference that there is a behavioral, psychological, or biological dysfunction" (American Psychiatric Association 1980, 6).

Zachar cites the epistemological difficulties in knowing what was naturally selected as an objection to the HDA. The HDA is a conceptual analysis aimed at understanding what we mean by "mental disorder" and has little to do with epistemological issues in identifying mental disorders, other than setting the conditions for something being a mental disorder and thus setting the overall conceptual ground rules for epistemological inquiry. Nonetheless, Zachar objects, "The key problem with the harmful dysfunction model is that it offers limited empirical guidance in distinguishing disorders from nondisorders because identifying objective natural functions depends on conceptual analysis, not factual evidence." A conceptual analysis gives you the conditions under which a concept applies to an object. Finding out whether the conditions actually apply to a given object is an empirical matter that requires factual claims and cannot be determined by the concept alone.

Zachar argues that the guidance offered by the HDA is not effective because evolutionary function and dysfunction are so difficult to establish: "As argued by Richardson (2007), there is not enough information about the selection pressures that were operating during human evolution, particularly on the evolution of the brain, to support empirically based theories of natural function. Wakefield (2001) contends that careful reasoning can reveal what natural psychological functions exist, but one has to worry that reason unconstrained by evidence can be marshalled to defend many different conclusions."

Of course, I strongly agree with the last point, and that is why so much of my work is critical of psychiatric diagnosis. However, one has to do more than worry. One has to critically evaluate claims and fight the tendency of societies to interpret their local values as an expression of human nature so as to make social deviance into disorder amenable to interventions using medical power. This is the sort of direct answer to Szaszian antipsychiatry that, we shall see, Zachar's view fails to muster because, lacking an adequate understanding what it is that society means by "disorder," he cannot argue persuasively about what society is getting wrong.

Zachar, we saw, cites Richardson's (2007) critique of evolutionary psychology as showing the flaws in an evolutionary approach to psychology, and there are many good such critiques. I am not a partisan of any particular evolutionary psychological views, other than what I take to be plausible hypotheses about natural selection of psychological features that underlie typical psychopathological categories. Mostly, these critiques, like Richardson's, deal with issues that do not bear on the broad assumptions about function and dysfunction underlying most major *DSM* or *International Classification of Diseases (ICD)* categories of mental or physical disorder. It is pretty obvious or at least plausible for most of them that something is going wrong relative to biological design. Of course, all such judgments about function and dysfunction are fallible, and we not only can be wrong but often have been wrong about what seems obvious. Nonetheless, looking at Richardson's book, I could not find even one example in his many critiques of evolutionary psychological hypotheses that would cast doubt on a diagnostic judgment among *DSM*'s categories of disorder.

In any event, what seems epistemically challenging now may not be in the future. For example, there are scientific methods now that did not exist a few decades ago for examining the patterns of genetic loci near a target locus and determining whether it is likely that the target locus was the result of positive selection pressures or not (e.g., Ding et al. 2002; Lind et al. 2019; Polimanti and Gelernter 2017), offering a degree of ability to enter into evolutionary inquiry sans time machine that was unimagined even a few years ago. In philosophy of science, our epistemic position with regard to specific factual questions can change radically and relatively quickly, and this makes it additionally important to keep epistemic and conceptual/ontological issues separate. When the positivists wrote, it was impossible to observe the back of the moon; until very recently, the existence of exoplanets was not empirically establishable; and just a few decades ago, before ultrasound, it was impossible to know the sex of a baby before birth, yet no one thought that these epistemological challenges—all overcome in time—somehow undermined the standard meanings of these concepts or demanded a redefinition pegged to what one could at the time establish.

A problem with Zachar's critique of the HDA's conceptual account of "medical disorder" is that, in the examples he offers, he consistently seems to confuse the speculative theorizing on the basis of known facts with conceptual analysis, which is a wholly different thing. For example: "Horwitz and Wakefield (2012) use a conceptual analysis of what we should and should not be expected to do to identify what lies within our biologically designed, naturally selected range of behaviors. According to them, talking to family members without intense anxiety lies in this range, but handling snakes without intense anxiety does not.... In this analysis, the distinction between disordered and normal is being made not by discovering an objective dysfunction but by reasoning."

Zachar bewilderingly assumes that the described reasoning must be conceptual analysis, but reasoning is not the same as conceptual analysis. To the contrary, speculative reasoning about theoretical matters based on whatever facts and theoretical assumptions one has at hand occurs in science all the time, and that is not conceptual analysis. It is not the result of a conceptual analysis of "disorder" or "anxiety" that Horwitz and I suggested that intense anxiety about speaking with family members might be a sign that the functioning of social anxiety mechanisms has gone awry; it is a result of pondering what we know about anxiety, how we are biologically designed, how reliant we are on family intimacy and support, and what makes sense in light of what we know about human nature. Given how little evidence we have, admittedly we were forced to judge this issue on flimsy grounds, but we argued that, contra the *DSM*, this is a much more likely indicator of pathology than, say, public speaking anxiety. This sort of "reasoning" is not at all the same as "conceptual analysis."

Zachar says, "The HD analysis cannot, therefore, empirically do what it was proposed to do, *factually* demarcate valid psychiatric disorders from the larger class of problems-in-living." To the contrary, the HDA specifies the kinds of facts (and values) that demarcate disorders from problems-in-living, which is what it is supposed to do. It is science's, not the HDA's, responsibility to ascertain when the facts apply and thus which conditions actually are disorders.

Zachar treats us to a brief history of the notion of "open concepts." He explains that "open concepts are potentially extendable so that a new measurement *may* also become part of our definition of the concept. An open concept refers to what it is that the different operationalizations of it have in common, but it is not reducible to any of those operationalizations." So, it changes but it is the same. I am not sure this makes sense, but if it does, it can't be right. I (Wakefield 2004) have dealt with this notion elsewhere, showing why it is confused and problematic and why essentialism is a better way to address the problems that open concepts are supposed to address. One problem is that neo-empiricism, even when supplemented by open concepts, yields theory incommensurability, which implies that we can't constructively disagree because, having different beliefs, we don't have the same concepts and so there is no common language in which to conduct the dispute and no common agreed construct about which to have our disagreement. This is the sort of problem that caused philosophers of science to largely abandon neo-empiricism. In the course of his discussion, Zachar illustrates my point. He says, "The discovery that most cases of depression are precipitated by stress in the previous six months may lead us modify the concept of depression one way, and the discovery that cases of depression that lack precipitants are more treatment resistant may lead us to modify the concept (and related concepts such as psychiatric disorder) in another way." He is saying that every change in belief, because it alters how you might empirically test for the construct, alters the meaning of the concept and is thus a change of the concept. Consequently, you never actually discover anything about a construct because the discovery makes it a different construct. But, one can discover something about depression without changing the meaning of "depression," and two people can have different beliefs about the very same entity, depression. Essentialism explained how this is possible and was a breath of fresh air that resolved all these self-inflicted problems of neo-empiricism.

Zachar's "Decline-of-Functioning" Account of Disorder

Zachar expends considerable energy defending a "decline-of-functioning" analysis of disorder. A similar idea was suggested by Lilienfeld and Marino (1995) and rebutted (Wakefield 1999a) by obvious counterexamples to sufficiency (declines that are not disorders) and necessity (disorders that are not declines). Zachar evades such easy rebuttal by asserting that the "decline" criterion is neither necessary nor sufficient, just a strong indicator. When examples don't fit the criterion, he brings in qualifiers in an unsystematic and ad hoc way to fix the problem, such as that the declines must be "unwanted" or that they "represent something being *broken*." However, he ignores what if any inferential theoretical assumptions, for example, about biological design, might lie behind such qualifiers as "broken." Later (see below), he even redescribes the criterion as "decline-in-functioning and other statistically abnormal developmental trajectories," which is a wholly different and much broader notion—many developmental deviations involve no decline at all (see below)—that raises the new problem that a statistical deviation account of disorder opens the door wide to Szaszian antipsychiatric objections. Zachar emphasizes that the "decline-in-functioning" criterion has the virtue of being an objective fact just like dysfunction ("declines-in-functioning are objective…they are often intersubjectively confirmable")—but, like the overemphasis on achieving reliability in *DSM-III* at the expense of validity, the fact that one's criterion is objective is irrelevant if it is not identifying what you are trying to identify.

Of course, in certain contexts, decline in functioning offers persuasive evidence of disorder. However, decline in functioning is common, and it is taken to be a disorder when and only when the decline is taken to indicate harmful dysfunction. There are many forms of decline in function that occur occasionally and are seen as biologically designed parts of life and thus not considered disorders, such as sleep that leaves one unconscious, semi-paralyzed, and periodically hallucinating for about one-third of one's entire life span; the decline in various areas of physical functioning experienced by women in advanced stages of pregnancy; and the decline in capability due to muscular fatigue after vigorous exercise. Then, there are conditions that are considered disorders and involve no decline in functioning but only a failure to proceed to new biologically designed developmental milestones, such as neurological disorders in which children fail to develop the capacity to sit, walk, or speak or psychiatric disorders such as intellectual disability, classic autism, and schizoid personality disorder. Similarly, the "lifelong generalized" subtype of erectile disorder or orgasmic disorder (which has one specifier, "never experienced an orgasm under any situation") involves no decline but rather failure to develop biologically designed functioning. Again, lead poisoning need not cause a decline in functioning or even a statistical deviation from the normal range of development but may be a disorder nonetheless by simply preventing full development of potential capacities. And so on. Adding a qualifier like "unexplained" or "unexpectable" to "decline in functioning" won't help because many well-explained and expectable declines in functioning (e.g., when someone breaks an arm or contracts pneumonia) are considered disorders. The very same decline in strength, say, might be a nondisorder with nothing broken in one instance (e.g., due to stopping one's exercising) and represent something broken because due to a dysfunction in another (e.g., an early stage of a neurological disorder). Zachar says that decline in functioning is not an essence, and of course he is right; it is a descriptive term, and this is why, as he himself observes, it is neither necessary nor sufficient for disorder. It is the type of explanation of the decline that makes a decline of functioning a disorder or nondisorder, and the theoretical notion of dysfunction is necessary to make sense of the distinctions we routinely make between declines that are pathologies and declines that are normal.

Perhaps most troubling is that Zachar embraces the decline-of-functioning criterion despite the fact that it cannot address the Szaszian challenge. Social deviance and oppressed conditions often involve declines or decrements in functioning as socially defined, and without a theory of natural functions, it is the social perspective that will be relied on for such judgments. Decline of functioning encompasses socially disapproved changes in functioning, opening the door to the pathologization of social deviance. If a teenage student attends a new high school and experiences a steep decline in grades for one reason or another, if someone enters a life of criminality, if a couple begins to have major conflicts that decrease their well-being, or if someone experiences boredom or burnout at their job, these declines in social functioning seem to be candidates for mental disorder according to Zachar's "decline" criterion. This is the Szaszian nightmare realized. The HDA blocks such categorizations because decline in functioning is considered indicative of disorder when and only when it is due to a dysfunction, and such social failings are not necessarily indicative of evolutionary dysfunctions.

A bit later in his paper, Zachar expands on the decline-in-functioning account, listing a series of features that to some extent suggest disorder but presumably are not meant as either necessary or sufficient criteria by themselves or even in combination: "decline-in-functioning and other statistically abnormal developmental trajectories; the presence of reality distortion; suicidal ideation; confusion and other cognitive difficulties; intrusive thoughts; difficult to control impulses and compulsions; agitation, anger, and excitement; excessive anxiety and fear; emptiness and anhedonia; somatic preoccupations; seeming more amenable to the skill set of psychiatry than other medical specialties." This list fails to characterize many disorders, and many conditions that are characterized by these features singly or in combination are not considered disorders, so the list is not explanatorily compelling. My hypothesis is that, singly or in combination, the features on this list will be considered indicative of disorder when and only when they are believed to support an inference to dysfunction. But, because dysfunction is a theoretical concept rooted in an essentialist inference about biological design, neo-empiricist Zachar is unable to test my hypothesis against actual judgments because his philosophical blinders preclude any such theory from being considered. That's too bad, because such tests are easy to do! One might get started by asking questions such as: When is suicidal ideation considered indicative of disorder and when is it not (e.g., Masada)? When is reality distortion considered suggestive of disorder and when is it not (e.g., "love is blind")? When are problematic conditions more amenable to the skill set of psychiatry than other medical specialties considered disorders and when are they not (e.g., see the extensive list of nondisorder Z Code conditions in *DSM-5*)? There is no need to allow an esoteric and outmoded philosophical doctrine that was an overreaction to the metaphysical excesses of the nineteenth century to stop one from testing the explanatory power of a reasonable alternative conceptual hypothesis.

Moreover, once again, Zachar's amplified list fails to satisfy the sine qua non requirement of an analysis of "disorder" of rebutting Szaszian antipsychiatry. All sorts of socially deviant or socially disapproved nondisorders, from interpersonal conflict to criminality, can possess one or more of Zachar's conditions. Thus, a Szaszian would point out that Zachar's list confirms that psychiatric criteria for disorder go way beyond the bounds of true medical conditions and serve as a means of social control. If Zachar's long list of not-really-necessary and not-really-sufficient features is all there is to the concept of mental disorder, then it is compellingly arguable that the antipsychiatrists are correct and psychiatry has no legitimate foundation as a medical discipline.

At the end of his paper, after explaining the network approach (see below), Zachar takes a last shot at listing "considerations that are relevant in making the depressive disorder attribution." He says these include "(a) ... decline in functioning ... (b) ... locked in rather than transient and flexible ... (c) more severe symptoms and more complex symptom networks ... (d) no compensatory factors that allow the person to continue to function (and flourish)." Perusing this list, it seems to me that one could easily satisfy three or possibly all four criteria in a normal reaction to losing a spouse on whom one relied for one's social network, or in losing a job on which one depended, or if one became involved in criminal activity, or if one were involved in a long legal suit. Zachar's list potentially confuses lengthy normal distress and decreased role functioning with mental disorder, offering no answer to the antipsychiatrist.

"Imperfect Community": Zachar on the History and Heterogeneity of Psychiatric Disorders

To block the notion that one can provide an essentialist or any necessary-and-sufficient conceptual analysis of "disorder," Zachar throughout his paper emphasizes the heterogeneity of psychiatric disorders. In support of his position, Zachar presents a brief history of psychiatry that makes it seem as though all sorts of random accretions of psychological conditions to the disorder category took place discontinuously over time: "The disorders of psychiatry are the result of a gradual addition of variations on the symptom clusters of the alienists ... but because of the way the domain was built (by the addition of variants on variants), no single organization can model all of the overlapping relationships." Zachar adopts the dubious Roschian notion that psychosis is the prototype of mental disorder (I have shown elsewhere that this approach just does not work; conduct disorder, dyslexia, and erectile dysfunction are not disorders because of any family resemblance to psychosis [Wakefield 1999a]) and argues that via similarities to similarities, all sorts of conditions got into the category. Zachar seems here to adopt Frances and Widiger's (2012) view that "historically, conditions have become mental disorders by accretion and practical necessity, not because they met some independent set of abstract and operationalized definitional criteria. Indeed, the concept of mental disorder is so amorphous, protean, and heterogeneous that it inherently defies definition—creating a hole at the center of psychiatric classification" (111). This is a bizarrely skeptical view given that Frances vigorously argued that many conditions added as disorders to *DSM-5* are not in fact disorders, and he sometimes anchors his arguments about disorder in evolutionary theoretical considerations consistent with the HDA's essentialist perspective—but, I digress.

Zachar's historical sketch provides an extraordinarily tendentious picture. He fails to examine how specific added conditions were considered prior to the supposed change, does not consider whether the change was one of terminology or refinement of categories rather than a real change of view of disorder versus nondisorder, and ignores the possible theoretical rationale for each supposed accretion that emerged in the inevitable professional disputes over such nosological adjustments. In my own historical work, I have found enormous continuity in what is considered a disorder and in the rationale for disorder versus nondisorder judgments, but with much recategorization and elaboration in response to shifting theories, frequent refinement of single categories into multiple subcategories, changing of emphasis, and terminological shifts reflecting larger theoretical programs, all of which potentially confuse the picture and make it seem like new disorder categories are appearing out of nowhere when in fact disorder versus nondisorder judgments are surprisingly stable (Horwitz and Wakefield 2007; Wakefield 2001). Zachar's description of the history of psychiatry as semirandom accretions is about as illuminating as someone arguing that the chemical substance "water" is in reality just a random collection of things, as evidenced by the history; first people labeled clear liquids in lakes and rivers "water," then people expanded the category to include the totally different materials of ice and steam that happen often to occur near water or transform into water, and then astronomers expanded the category to include, for example, stuff detected by spectrometers floating in the Horsehead Nebula that isn't anything like any of the other instances and is not near any liquid water; the chemical substance water is certainly a "very imperfect community" with variations upon variations and so no unifying criterion!

This brings me to a central thesis of Zachar's, that "mental disorder" is what he calls an "imperfect community," a term derived from Nelson Goodman denoting the phenomenon of a class of objects in which any two bear some features in common but the entire class has no one feature in common. The "imperfect community" view of concepts has strong affinities to Wittgensteinian family-resemblance and Roschian prototype-similarity views of concepts. Let me make clear that I believe that concepts can be defined in myriad ways, ranging from empiricist to Roschian to essentialist. However, the evidence is that an essentialist account best represents the structure of the concept of mental disorder, at least at one crucial level—the level needed to rebut Szaszian antipsychiatry.

Zachar goes the Roschian route and claims that whether someone has a disorder is a matter of degree depending on how many of a set of criteria he presents are possessed by the condition: "As more of these conceptual criteria are met, the more it makes sense to start thinking of a symptom cluster as disordered. Rather than being absolutely present or absent, disorders are a matter of degree." This mini-argument is wholly invalid. The second sentence—the conclusion that disorder is a matter of degree—does not follow from the first sentence's premise, that as more criteria are met, it makes more sense to conclude that there is a disorder. In theory, as more *DSM* criteria are met, the strength of the evidence that there is a disorder increases, but either there is or there isn't a disorder—leaving aside the inevitable boundary fuzziness and unclear cases that afflict most concepts. However, a condition can satisfy just one of Zachar's criteria and be a crystal-clear disorder or satisfy many criteria and be a crystal-clear nondisorder. On average, the more criteria that are met, the more secure is an inference to the existence of dysfunction and thus the more likely that there is a disorder, but the degree of strength of the evidence for inferring a disorder is not the same as there being a degree of disorder (First and Wakefield 2013; Wakefield 1999a, 2012).

Zachar argues that the fact that there are so many varieties of disorders supports his conception of an "imperfect community" of conditions, that is, conditions not answering to a single conceptual analysis of "disorder." Other than his questionable history of psychiatry, Zachar supports this position by observing that "the 'imperfect' part of the community of psychiatric disorders has been eloquently described by Allen Frances," the chair of the *DSM-IV* Task Force. Zachar then quotes the following passage describing the multiplicity of types of things that are disorders as evidence in support of his "imperfect community" position:

> Some mental disorders describe short-term states, others life-long personality; some reflect inner misery, others bad behavior; some represent problems rarely or never seen in normals, others are just slight accentuations of the everyday; some reflect too little self-control, others too much; some are intrinsic to the person, others are culturally determined; some begin early in infancy, others emerge only late in life.... Some are clearly defined, others not; and there are complex permutations of all of these possible differences. (Frances and Widiger 2012, 111)

This is a surprising argument for Zachar to use because as a philosopher, Zachar knows full well that Frances and Widiger's argument is patently fallacious. The fact that various pairs of mental disorders have some opposite properties shows *nothing whatsoever* about the univocal analyzability of "disorder." Does Zachar think that the fact that there are red spheres and blue spheres shows the unanalyzability of "sphere," or the fact that there are large numbers and small numbers shows that numbers form an "imperfect community" with no defining features? There is simply nothing to this argument.

Instead of citing irrelevant contrary properties, we might take Wittgenstein's advice to *look and see* whether the entities with these properties share some further unifying features. In any of the categories mentioned, the vast majority of conditions are not considered disorders, so what determines which of the conditions with that property are disorders and which are not? To approach an answer, one might scrutinize actual examples of psychopathology instantiating each pair of the cited contrary categories: short term versus long term (e.g., brief psychotic reaction versus borderline personality disorder), inner misery versus behavior (e.g., generalized anxiety disorder versus pyromania), accentuation of the common versus distinctive rarity (e.g., dysthymia versus fugue states), too little control versus too much control (e.g., intermittent explosive disorder versus sexual sadism disorder), innate versus culturally shaped (e.g., intellectual disability versus reading disorder), and emerges early versus emerges late (e.g., autism spectrum disorder versus Alzheimer's disease). One finds that the inference that there is a harmful dysfunction is common to all of these disordered conditions whatever their other properties and distinguishes them from the vast number of conditions that have the same contrary properties but are not considered disorders.

The vague and stretchable criteria Zachar proposes in his lists noted earlier of considerations for entering his "imperfect community" of psychiatric disorders can serve to rationalize just about any judgment one wants to make. Zachar's analysis thus leaves us right back where we started when it seemed like an analysis of disorder would be an important and useful endeavor: without a principled difference between disorder and nondisorder. With no clear conceptual firewall, every agreed abuse or mistake of psychiatry from drapetomania and sluggish schizophrenia to Victorian surgery for female clitoral orgasm and even the repathologization of homosexuality could find a place within this spongy set of guidelines. Zachar tries so hard to avoid constraining psychiatry by the supposed bogeyman of essentialism that his criteria would leave us with a psychiatry unclear about its own foundational concepts and unconstrained in labeling whatever clinicians want to treat as a disorder, posing a threat to our civil liberties and offering a legitimate target of antipsychiatry.

Zachar on the Causal Network Approach to Intelligence

I now turn to an examination of the pivotal section of Zachar's chapter in which he attempts to show that "essentialism … is not scientifically necessary" for an account of disorder. The HDA implies that "disorder" is inherently an explanatory-sketch concept that applies only if there is an explanation of a condition in terms of a dysfunction. Zachar argues that no such explanatory loading is implied by disorder attributions. To support his claim that "from a neo-empiricist standpoint, essentialism is an excessive metaphysical elaboration that is needlessly grafted onto this complicated network of 'observations,'" Zachar elaborates the currently much-discussed "causal network approach" to psychopathology. This view, he explains, holds that "latent variables do not have to be interpreted as referring to real essences," thus illustrating that a theory of psychopathology need not be essentialist. The network approach, an offshoot of some traditional behaviorist ways of thinking about psychopathology, has recently been elaborated and championed by Denny Borsboom and his colleagues, and I rely on Borsboom's (2017) recent summary in examining this approach. Although there is much of interest that one might say about the network approach and its implications in general, I limit my remarks to aspects that bear on evaluating Zachar's attempt to leverage it into an antiessentialist argument.

Zachar initially uses the example of network theorists' rethinking of the construct of general intelligence (often referred to as *g*) to explain the network approach. According to this approach, general intelligence, as manifested in high performance across a range of intellectual tests, may not be a general factor or cause underlying all cognitive abilities (e.g., rapid neuronal conduction) but rather simply the expression of how networks of cognitive abilities interact. Zachar explains,

> An alternative to a causally potent latent variable (or common cause) model is a model in which cognitive abilities are in direct causal relationships with each other. For example, being able to process information quickly might have positive effects on working memory. Cognitive abilities can enter into mutual interactions in a variety of ways. Some people may naturally have high abilities across the board, whereas others are gifted in one or two areas—such as processing speed and attention capacity—but these skills permeate through the ability network and raise scores on tests of general intelligence.

Without getting too deeply into issues regarding the network analysis of intelligence, I offer a few comments before turning to Borsboom's approach to psychopathology. At one level, intelligence is just a descriptive concept—close to a neo-empiricist understanding—referring to an individual's performance on intellectual tests of various kinds. However, like all scientists, psychologists generally construe their concepts in an essentialist manner that goes beyond sheer description and refers to the deeper nature of the initial phenomenon because that is how one reaches perspicuous explanation, prediction, and interventive possibilities. Thus, the question "what is intelligence" has many potential levels of meaning depending on semantic or ontological markers that are part of the meaning of a specific usage. (See my reply to Murphy in this volume for further discussion of the multiple levels of concepts.) Zachar's claim is that, in formulating a theory of intelligence, one can possibly trade the classic theory that there is a latent as-yet-unknown inferred essential explanatory variable that directly explains the performance of all of the individual domains for a network theory that hypotheses that only certain domains have intrinsically high performance but they interact with other domains in distinctive patterns so as to confer high test performance on those other domains as well. If so, then no further across-domain underlying essence of intelligence is explanatorily required.

    This network characterization is perfectly sensible as a possible alternative theory of what constitutes intelligence at a certain level. However, the possibility of such a theory does not accomplish Zachar's goal of discounting the need for essentialism. The problem is that Zachar's description of high intelligence in terms of network interactions begs the question of the nature of intelligence by already referring to the presence of either "high abilities across the board" or being "gifted in one or two ways [that] ... permeate through the ability network." The network theory thus assumes that there is some variable of ability or giftedness that applies not generically but to specific psychological modules, and that such intrinsically high-performance modules along with certain forms of modular interaction yield generally high modular test performances. None of this relieves us of the question of the essence of intelligence; it just pushes it back a step and relocates the question in the essence of specific modules' ability or giftedness.

    One might of course shift more and more of the explanation to specific interactive patterns rather than intrinsic characteristics of key modules. However, if one identifies specific patterns of modular interaction with intelligence, first, one can then say that intelligence does have an essence—namely, those distinctive patterns of modular interaction—and second, one will want to know for each such pattern what is the essential set of conditions that bring it about. Conceivably, intelligence theory might then split into several essentialist theories of the different patterns of interaction that manifest as high intelligence, in the way that there are essentialist chemical theories of each of the two types of mineral that fall under the concept "jade" or in the way that theorists suggest that *DSM* categories of "major depression" or "schizophrenia" in fact encompass multiple disorders with distinct essential etiologies. In sum, the network account of intelligence does not somehow allow the scientist to escape the scientific necessity of identifying what constitutes the essence of high intelligence.

    However, for our purposes, perhaps the most critical point about Zachar's use of the intelligence example as an exemplar of the network account is the obvious one that high intelligence is a prototypical normal-range quality, not a form of psychopathology. This reflects the fact that the applicability of network analysis is independent of whether one is dealing with normal or pathological conditions. Consequently, whatever it is that characterizes psychopathology as opposed to normal-range features must be some property over and above whether the phenomenon can be characterized using network analysis. Consequently, even if network analyses in themselves did not require an essentialist approach, the key question would remain unanswered: must one cite some essentialist (i.e., nonobservational explanatory) properties to distinguish those networks that are disorders from those that are not? To answer this question, I examine Borsboom's account of how network theory is applied to psychopathology.

Borsboom on the Causal Network Approach to Psychopathology

The HDA implies that whatever makes a network pathological involves factors such as etiology and history that go beyond a description of the network itself in observational terms. For example, a network analysis that indicated a statistically average intellectually functioning human brain might indicate normality or, if it was the brain of a genius who suffered lead poisoning as a youth or brain trauma as an adult, it might be the result of pathology. A network analysis that revealed that an individual's intellectual functioning is high but emotional functioning is very low might be a schizoid pathology or someone from an emotionally suppressive culture. The distinction between normality and pathology seems to require information that goes beyond the network's manifest performance.

A persuasive piece of evidence that the network approach is not, as Zachar claims, an inherently nonessentialist approach opposed to the HDA is that Borsboom's presentation implicitly presupposes the HDA's rather than Zachar's view. Consider this abstract of Borsboom's (2017) recent paper setting forth the theoretical foundations of the network approach to psychopathology:

> In recent years, the network approach to psychopathology has been advanced as an alternative way of conceptualizing mental disorders. In this approach, mental disorders arise from direct interactions between symptoms.... At the heart of the theory lies the notion that symptoms of psychopathology are causally connected through myriads of biological, psychological and societal mechanisms. If these causal relations are sufficiently strong, symptoms can generate a level of feedback that renders them self-sustaining. In this case, the network can get stuck in a disorder state. The network theory holds that this is a general feature of mental disorders, which can therefore be understood as alternative stable states of strongly connected symptom networks. This idea naturally leads to a comprehensive model of psychopathology. (5)

What is striking about this statement is that Borsboom directly addresses the problem that Zachar insists on ignoring, namely, precisely how pathological networks differ from nonpathological networks. He proposes that a general feature of mental disorders is that exceedingly strong causal relations between symptoms can trigger a sustained pathological feedback loop that becomes stable and inflexible at the severe level ("If these causal relations [between symptoms] are sufficiently strong, symptoms can generate a level of feedback that renders them self-sustaining. In this case, the network can get stuck in a disorder state"). Borsboom is clearly implying that in the formation of such a self-sustaining loop, something has gone wrong and that getting stuck in such a symptom feedback loop is a failure of how these symptom links were biologically designed to occur (see below). It is the unnatural intensity and stuckness in the self-sustaining inflexible symptom pattern that constitutes the dysfunction that, according to Borsboom, is at the core of every mental disorder, a view consistent with the HDA.

I claim that the process of a normal linkage between experiences getting stuck in an intense self-sustaining symptom cycle is best understood as a harmful dysfunction, and Borsboom seems to agree. Later in his paper, he observes that most symptom linkages involved in pathology start out as normal associations due to various normal biological, psychological, and social processes. The switch to a disordered self-sustaining feedback loop, he notes, "thus may involve harmful dysfunctions in these processes" (11):

> As may be clear from the examples given in this paper, connections between symptoms are often prosaic. If you do not sleep, you get tired; if you see things that are not there, you get anxious; if you use too much drugs, you get into legal trouble, etc. It is, in my view, likely that these symptom-symptom connections are rooted in very ordinary biological, psychological and societal processes (and thus may involve harmful dysfunctions in these processes). This is surprising, because it means that disorders are not ill-understood ephemeral entities, the nature of which will have to be uncovered by future psychological, neuroscientific or genetic research (which appears a widespread conviction, if not the received view, among researchers). Rather, the fact that we have the set of basic symptoms, and also understand many of the relations between them, means that we already have a quite reasonable working model of what disorders are and how they work. (11)

In other words—and even according to Borsboom's own understanding—the network approach's postulation of how things go wrong does require some understanding of the difference between normality and pathology of the sort provided by the HDA, contrary to Zachar's interpretation. There must be some such differentiating standard because some tight and inflexible linkages between reactions are part of biologically designed functioning and entirely normal, so such reactions can indicate pathology only when they are dysfunctions. Indeed, the above passage indicates that it is not network links per se, which are omnipresent and prosaic, but, consistent with the HDA, deviations from the natural levels of linkage tightness and feedback looping that suggest pathology. Deeper processes sustaining such a dysfunction is its essence.

Before leaving the network perspective, it is worth observing in passing that it harbors some facile assumptions. Network theory's standard hypothesis, we have seen, is that pathology often emerges from known linkages between phenomena, and it consists of the development of excessively powerful linkages between those phenomena with circular feedback loops forming between symptoms that keep the network going. However, none of these generalizations are as obvious or generalizable as network theorists suggest. Consider Borsboom's example of the insomnia-fatigue link in depression. First, fatigue can be caused by insomnia, but it can also be phenomenologically and functionally different from insomnia-induced tiredness, involving not sleepiness per se but low energy levels (ask those who have experienced both), and fatigue independent of insomnia can be an important vegetative symptom of depression. As much as one might enjoy heaping ridicule on *DSM* for not recognizing such a commonsensical connection as that between lack of sleep and fatigue, the reality is that fatigue appears as a symptom because sometimes depression does include an independent fatigue symptom. (However, Zachar's using the link between insomnia and fatigue as an objection to essentialism because the symptoms are not independently explained by the hypothesized dysfunction is a straw-person argument in the extreme because there is nothing in essentialism that is violated by such a link among observable phenomena.) Second, when severe fatigue does result from insomnia during a depression, this does not imply that the link between insomnia and fatigue has been pathologically strengthened; pathological levels of insomnia can naturally produce correspondingly high levels of fatigue. Finally, the notion that when depressive insomnia causes severe fatigue, a pathological feedback loop occurs in which the fatigue sustains the insomnia, is questionable because in most instances when sleep returns to normal, insomnia-induced fatigue correspondingly recedes rather than triggering renewed insomnia.

Nonetheless, network theory is smarter than symptom lists in several ways. Network theory correctly emphasizes that not just the list of symptoms but the dynamics of the causal network of symptoms—whether the system of symptoms itself comprises the dysfunction as network theory holds or are the effects of some underlying dysfunction—matters enormously to diagnosis and treatment. Mapping symptom causal relations can yield additional insight that is lost in the literal-minded symptom-list approach. Indeed, such analysis can lead, for example, to the insight that more or less the same set of depressive symptoms in fact is generated by insomnia and is a sleep disorder rather than a depressive disorder. As well, I heartily agree with several broader theses defended recently by Borsboom, Cramer, and Kalis (2019), including the irreducibility of some mental disorders to brain disorders and the need to take into account intentional content and not just brain-level descriptions in understanding symptom-symptom linkages.

Returning to the issue of essentialism, the network theory of disorder that Zachar presents as his trump card in demonstrating the possibility of a neo-empiricist account of disorder in fact demonstrates the opposite. Like all serious theories of disorder, network theory distinguishes between the natural functioning of the organism consistent with how it is biologically designed and the ways in which that functioning can go wrong—that is, dysfunctions. These implicit assumptions allude to a theoretical distinction that goes beyond anything in the symptom network itself. There is thus nothing in network theory that supports Zachar's attempt to escape the fact that the distinction between normality and disorder implies a distinction of (inferred) types of causes, which in turn requires an essentialist analysis that goes beyond the conceptual straightjacket of neo-empiricism. The failure of Zachar's earnest series of attempts, from decline in functioning to imperfect community to network theory, to vindicate his neo-empiricist approach both in terms of defending against the antipsychiatric challenge and in terms of simply explaining common intuitions about disorder makes the point manifest that "disorder" is an inherently essentialist concept.

References

American Psychiatric Association. 1980. *Diagnostic and Statistical Manual of Mental Disorders.* 3rd ed. American Psychiatric Association.

Borsboom, D. 2017. A network theory of mental disorders. *World Psychiatry* 16(1): 5–13.

Borsboom, D., A. O. J. Cramer, and A. Kalis. 2019. Brain disorders? Not really: Why network structures block reductionism in psychopathology research. *Behavioral and Brain Sciences* 42(e2): 1–63.

Ding, Y. C., H. C. Chi, D. L. Grady, A. Morishima, J. R. Kidd, K. K. Kidd, et al. 2002. Evidence of positive selection acting at the human dopamine receptor D4 gene locus. *Proceedings of the National Academy of Sciences* 99(1): 309–314.

First, M. B., and J. C. Wakefield. 2010. Defining 'mental disorder' in *DSM-V*. *Psychological Medicine* 40(11): 1779–1782.

First, M. B., and J. C. Wakefield. 2013. Diagnostic criteria as dysfunction indicators: Bridging the chasm between the definition of mental disorder and diagnostic criteria for specific disorders. *Canadian Journal of Psychiatry* 58(12): 663–669.

Frances, A. J., and T. Widiger. 2012. Psychiatric diagnosis: Lessons from the *DSM-IV* past and cautions for the *DSM-5* future. *Annual Review of Clinical Psychology* 8: 109–130.

Horwitz, A. V., and J. C. Wakefield. 2007. *The Loss of Sadness: How Psychiatry Transformed Normal Sorrow into Depressive Disorder.* Oxford University Press.

Lilienfeld, S. O., and L. Marino. 1995. Mental disorder as a Roschian concept: A critique of Wakefield's 'harmful dysfunction' analysis. *Journal of Abnormal Psychology* 104(3): 411–420.

Lind, A. L., Y. Y. Y. Lai, Y. Mostovoy, A. K. Holloway, A. Iannucci, A. C. Y. Mak, et al. 2019. Genome of the Komodo dragon reveals adaptations in the cardiovascular and chemosensory systems of monitor lizards. *Nature Ecology & Evolution* 3(8): 1241–1252.

Polimanti, R., and J. Gelernter. 2017. Widespread signatures of positive selection in common risk alleles associated to autism spectrum disorder. *PLoS Genetics* 13(2): e1006618.

Richardson, R. C. 2007. *Evolutionary Psychology as Maladapted Psychology.* MIT Press.

Spitzer, R. L. 1997. Brief comments from a psychiatric nosologist weary from his own attempts to define mental disorder: Why Ossorio's definition muddles and Wakefield's "harmful dysfunction" illuminates the issues. *Clinical Psychology: Science and Practice* 4(3): 259–261.

Spitzer, R. L. 1999. Harmful dysfunction and the *DSM* definition of mental disorder. *Journal of Abnormal Psychology* 108(3): 430–432.

Wakefield, J. C. 1992a. The concept of mental disorder: On the boundary between biological facts and social values. *American Psychologist* 47: 373–388.

Wakefield, J. C. 1992b. Disorder as harmful dysfunction: A conceptual critique of *DSM-III-R*'s definition of mental disorder. *Psychological Review* 99: 232–247.

Wakefield, J. C. 1993. Limits of operationalization: A critique of Spitzer and Endicott's (1978) proposed operational criteria of mental disorder. *Journal of Abnormal Psychology* 102: 160–172.

Wakefield, J. C. 1995. Dysfunction as a value-free concept: A reply to Sadler and Agich. *Philosophy, Psychiatry, and Psychology* 2: 233–46.

Wakefield, J. C. 1997a. Diagnosing *DSM-IV*, part 1: *DSM-IV* and the concept of mental disorder. *Behaviour Research and Therapy* 35: 633–650.

Wakefield, J. C. 1997b. Diagnosing *DSM-IV*, part 2: Eysenck (1986) and the essentialist fallacy. *Behaviour Research and Therapy*: 35: 651–666.

Wakefield, J. C. 1997c. Normal inability versus pathological disability: Why Ossorio's (1985) definition of mental disorder is not sufficient. *Clinical Psychology: Science and Practice* 4: 249–258.

Wakefield, J. C. 1997d. When is development disordered? Developmental psychopathology and the harmful dysfunction analysis of mental disorder. *Development and Psychopathology* 9: 269–290.

Wakefield, J. C. 1998. The *DSM*'s theory-neutral nosology is scientifically progressive: Response to Follette and Houts. *Journal of Consulting and Clinical Psychology* 66: 846–852.

Wakefield, J. C. 1999a. Evolutionary versus prototype analyses of the concept of disorder. *Journal of Abnormal Psychology* 108: 374–399.

Wakefield, J. C. 1999b. Mental disorder as a black box essentialist concept. *Journal of Abnormal Psychology* 108: 465–472.

Wakefield, J. C. 2000a. Aristotle as sociobiologist: The "function of a human being" argument, black box essentialism, and the concept of mental disorder. *Philosophy, Psychiatry, and Psychology* 7: 17–44.

Wakefield, J. C. 2000b. Spandrels, vestigial organs, and such: Reply to Murphy and Woolfolk's "The harmful dysfunction analysis of mental disorder." *Philosophy, Psychiatry, and Psychology* 7: 253–269.

Wakefield, J. C. 2001. Evolutionary history versus current causal role in the definition of disorder: Reply to McNally. *Behaviour Research and Therapy* 39: 347–366.

Wakefield, J. C. 2004. The myth of open concepts: Meehl's analysis of construct meaning versus black box essentialism. *Applied & Preventive Psychology* 11: 77–82.

Wakefield, J. C. 2006. What makes a mental disorder mental? *Philosophy, Psychiatry, and Psychology* 13: 123–131.

Wakefield, J. C. 2007. The concept of mental disorder: Diagnostic implications of the harmful dysfunction analysis. *World Psychiatry* 6: 149–156.

Wakefield, J. C. 2009. Mental disorder and moral responsibility: Disorders of personhood as harmful dysfunctions, with special reference to alcoholism. *Philosophy, Psychiatry, and Psychology* 16: 91–99.

Wakefield, J. C. 2011. Darwin, functional explanation, and the philosophy of psychiatry. In *Maladapting Minds: Philosophy, Psychiatry, and Evolutionary Theory*, P. R. Andriaens and A. De Block (eds.), 143–172. Oxford University Press.

Wakefield, J. C. 2012. Are you as smart as a 4th grader? Why the prototype-similarity approach to diagnosis is a step backward for a scientific psychiatry. *World Psychiatry* 11: 27–28.

Wakefield, J. C. 2014. The biostatistical theory versus the harmful dysfunction analysis, part 1: Is part-dysfunction a sufficient condition for medical disorder? *Journal of Medicine and Philosophy* 39: 648–682.

Wakefield, J. C. 2016a. The concepts of biological function and dysfunction: Toward a conceptual foundation for evolutionary psychopathology. In *Handbook of Evolutionary Psychology*, D. Buss (ed.), 2nd ed., vol. 2, 988–1006. Oxford University Press.

Wakefield, J. C. 2016b. Diagnostic issues and controversies in *DSM-5*: Return of the false positives problem. *Annual Review of Clinical Psychology* 12: 105–132.

Wakefield, J. C. 2017. Addiction and the concept of disorder, part 2: Is every mental disorder a brain disorder? *Neuroethics* 10(1): 55–67. https://doi.org/10.1007/s12152-016-9301-8.

Wakefield, J. C., and M. B. First. 2003. Clarifying the distinction between disorder and nondisorder: Confronting the overdiagnosis ("false positives") problem in *DSM-V*. In *Advancing DSM: Dilemmas in Psychiatric Diagnosis*, K. A. Phillips, M. B. First, and H. A. Pincus (eds.), 23–56. American Psychiatric Press.

Wakefield, J. C., and M. B. First. 2012. Placing symptoms in context: The role of contextual criteria in reducing false positives in *DSM* diagnosis. *Comprehensive Psychiatry* 53: 130–139.

III   The Dysfunction Component

11 Is the Dysfunction Component of the "Harmful Dysfunction Analysis" Stipulative?

Maël Lemoine

Introduction

The harmful dysfunction analysis (HDA) goes like this: for a condition to be a disorder, it is necessary and jointly sufficient to be harmful, according to a value judgment, and to be dysfunctional, according to a value-free appraisal. This is a simple, original, and powerful way to combine the "naturalist" and "normative" aspects of the concept of disease, and it is indeed a highly faithful account of what both laymen and psychiatrists mean by "disorder." However, in their "Conceptual Analysis versus Scientific Understanding," Murphy and Woolfolk have contested this point: "Wakefield's final position... demonstrates that his overall project represents a counterproductive attempt to stipulate conceptually the character and domain of scientific inquiry into psychopathology" (Murphy and Woolfolk 2001, 271). What he stipulates is, according to them, some sort of "folk psychology" consisting of our commonsense intuitions about mental disorders. I disagree. I think that there is indeed something stipulative in Wakefield's position about the concept of mental disorder but also something descriptive. Yet what is stipulative is not the general framework for the concept of mental disorder (what I will call the HAA: harmful abnormality analysis): it is rather the evolutionary concept of dysfunction and, most of all, the way in which Wakefield has tried to conflate two good ideas into one. As Bolton puts it, "Definition of mental disorder in evolutionary terms, whatever other virtues it may have, does not capture the usage of the term mental disorder in the diagnostic manuals" (Bolton 2008, xxv). I would like to add that it also fails to capture the lay public's usage of this term. Ultimately, I think that Wakefield's arguments hide an incompatibility (at some point) between two purposes: on one hand, to give an account of what is usually meant by "mental disorder"; on the other hand, to give a satisfactory scientific account of the concept of dysfunction. The key problem here is in "stipulation": while a descriptive account must not stipulate, a scientific account has to.

I. What Kind of Definition Does the HDA Aim at?

The HDA provides a definition of disorder. What kind of definition is it? Hempel's classic presentation of definitions contrasts the nominal, *stipulative* definition of an expression or concept, which cannot be true or false but has to be syntactically determined, univocal, and consistent (Hempel 1952, 12–14, 17–18, 18–19), with real definitions, which consist of true or false claims (7–8), whenever they conform (or not) to the given meaning of an expression or concept (*meaning analysis*) or to given facts (*empirical analysis*: 8). *Rational construction* or *logical analysis*—that is, *explication*—draws from both of them. On one hand, explication consists of a synthesis of choices between available senses of the word in question and new elements, to the effect that the term is given a much more precise meaning that was not originally contained in natural language. On the other hand, the synthesis is guided by an empirical purpose: generally, to provide some useful predictive and explanatory features (10–12). Explication differs from stipulation in that we stipulate each time we need to introduce a new concept in science (e.g., "tachyon" or "prion") and explicate a term each time we arrange and stabilize its existing meanings (e.g., the definitions of "probability$_1$" and "probability$_2$" in Carnap [1962]).

To illustrate, let me take a simple definition of disease:

(1) *disease* = state of an organism with a lesion.

It would be a *stipulative* definition if I took every existing usage of the term as unavailable or not relevant: "I (for myself) call 'disease' the state of an organism with a lesion" (the existence of so-called diseases with no lesions, or lesions without so-called diseases, does not speak against it in any way). It would be a *meaning analysis* if I intended to capture its usual meaning (or meanings) among physicians, laymen, or both: "we use the term and the concept of disease whenever speaking of the state of an organism with a lesion" (what I compare my definition to is the common usage of the term). It would be an *empirical analysis* if my definition formulated laws of nature of the kind: "every state of disease is associated with an organic lesion" (what I have in mind are actual cases, experiments, statistics, etc.). In the end, it would be an *explication* if it was a less vague and more empirically powerful concept than the one captured in the common meaning of the term (as was the case at the beginning of the nineteenth century for the definition of disease).

The HDA explicitly rules out stipulation. Speaking of Spitzer's analysis as well as of his own, Wakefield remarks that "such analyses do not stipulate how we should use mental disorder" (Wakefield 1999d, 1011). He is also clear about rejecting empirical claims. In his view, a definition of mental disorder initially requires "conceptual validity" (Wakefield 1992b, 232; 1993, 170), that is, a correct discrimination between disordered and nondisordered conditions. Only after that can operational criteria be sought and the issue of reliability addressed (Wakefield 1992b, 233; 1993, 163; 1997a, 634).[1]

Wakefield's suggestion of a "conceptual analysis," though, does not explicitly distinguish between meaning analysis and explication. "In a conceptual analysis, proposed accounts of a concept are tested against relatively uncontroversial and widely shared judgments about what does and does not fall under the concept. To the degree that the analysis explains these uncontroversial judgments, it is considered confirmed, and a sufficiently confirmed analysis may then be used as a guide in thinking about more controversial cases" (Wakefield 1992b, 233; Wakefield 1999a, 376). Those "widely shared judgments" about what is disordered and what is not are supposed to be "largely shared by professional and the lay public" (Wakefield 1992a, 374). Any hypothetical definition must be assessed according to those judgments, and counterintuitive consequences are supposed to rule it out (example in Wakefield 1993, 166). This approach seems to be inclining in favor of meaning analysis. Yet "formulating theories to explain a distinction we already make" (Wakefield 1999d, 1011) involves not only an analysis of the distinction but explication as well.

In my view, the distinction between meaning analysis and explication implicitly follows from the distinction between the three steps of the HDA (Wakefield 1999a, 375):

1. *disorder* means dysfunction;
2. *function* and *dysfunction* are "straightforward scientific, causal terms"; and
3. the only available scientific account of such a dysfunction is evolutionary.

Only the first two steps claim to be analytically determined from "a widely shared, intuitive medical and lay concept." The last one alone is supposed to be explicative and is expected to one day provide a means to "distinguish natural functions from other effects in a manner more precise than that afforded by commonsense intuitions."

In any case, the dysfunction clause in the definition of disorder is on no account supposed to be stipulative, whether it is analytic or explicative. Therefore, my questions are as follows:

1. Is it *description* or stipulation to define mental disorders as dysfunctional states and to define dysfunction as a scientific concept?
2. Is it *explication* or stipulation to define dysfunction (in mental disorders) as an evolutionary concept?

II. Is the Definition of "Mental Disorder" as Dysfunction Descriptive or Stipulative?

After a quick glance at the problem, it seems that defining a condition as a mental disorder may represent an instance of stipulation when considering the requirement that the condition must be judged harmful according to values; in contrast, the requirement of a genuine, value-free type of dysfunction prevents the definition of such a condition from being stipulative. Therefore, the harmful dysfunction (HD) definition of mental disorder would avoid stipulation thanks to the concept of dysfunction. However, this statement requires the following qualifications: (1) a value-free concept of dysfunction does not necessarily provide a value-free definition of disorder, (2) some concepts of disorder are stipulative precisely because there are uncertainties about the existence of the dysfunction that supposedly defines them, and (3) defining mental disorders as dysfunctional states is not trivial and requires taking sides in theoretical controversies. My conclusion will be that the HDA does not avoid stipulation by introducing the concept of dysfunction in the definition of mental disorders.

2.1 A Stipulation Is a "Value-Free" Definition, Not the Definition of a "Value-Free" Concept

Stipulating often implies a commitment to some theory or, at least, some specified views on a subject. Here, we may neglect the possible, but improbable, cases of a stipulation made randomly and/or a stipulation made erroneously. For instance:

(2) *"mental disorder* = some kind of small, brown banana from the Caribbean"

is likely a random stipulation, and

(3) *"mental disorder* = the mental image of an untidy room"

is likely an erroneous stipulation. Putting aside such cases, stipulation always comes from some particular theoretical background. Therefore, a good strategy for providing a descriptive account of the meaning of "mental disorder" would be to provide a "value-free" definition. This is, I think, the purpose of the HDA.

First, we must consider that a value-free definition of a concept is not the same as a definition of a value-free concept. On one hand, we can stipulate (for normative motives) that some concepts are not normative. A definition could be biased in that way if, for instance, we wanted to say that

(4) *"depression* = a flaw in chemistry, not in character"

to avoid being judgmental about depressed people. On the other hand, there may be nonstipulative definitions of normative concepts. For instance, one could claim that

(5) *"dysfunction* = whatever prevents one from doing what is expected by a majority of people in a given culture"

is an analytic definition of a normative concept. Fulford, Cooper, and others have tried to provide such analytic definitions of disease, mental disorder, or dysfunction as normative concepts (see, e.g., Fulford 2001; Cooper 2002; Nordenfelt 2007). Although it might be contested that they are indeed value concepts, there is no contradiction between merely describing the usage of a given phrase and assuming it is value laden.

The HD definition of mental disorder may well be in the same situation as that in (4). Whether it is or not, it is clear that one does not avoid stipulation by defining mental disorder through a value-free concept of dysfunction.

2.2 The Value-Ladenness of Some Concepts of Mental Disorder Also Comes from the Dysfunction Component of Mental Disorder

A value-free concept of dysfunction appears to permeate through to the concept of disorder itself. In other words, we cannot consider whatever state we like to be a mental disorder. By using a dysfunctional condition for the definition of mental disorder, *stipulative* definitions of various disorders would be dismissed. However, this inference requires further scrutiny.

First, I do not think that the reference to dysfunction in the definition of a given disorder implies stipulation in the sense of a commitment in favor of a given theory. Of course, given our present imperfect state of knowledge, many hypotheses are in competition, so the question is: how can the dysfunction component avoid stipulating any of them? According to Wakefield, the HD approach is "theory-neutral" but "inferential" (Wakefield 1993, 171). "Theory-neutral" means that "criteria...are framed in terms that are independent of any particular theory of the nature and genesis of mental disorder, such as psychoanalytic, cognitive, behavioral and biological theories" (Wakefield 1992a, 385; 1992b, 232). For instance,

(6) "*depression* = sadistic drives turned toward the self"

is not a theory-neutral definition of depression. Theory-neutral means that observational terms are not laden with any particular, *well-known* theory, not that they are not laden with any theory at all (Wakefield 1999c, 966: "avoid definitionally ruling out any of the major competing theories of etiology"). But the definition of a mental disorder cannot be atheoretical in the sense of being "non-inferential" in the sense that "criteria...are framed in terms that are entirely observational and do not depend for their application on inferences about internal, historical, evolutionary, or other unobservable features" (Wakefield 1993, 171). Definition (6) fails to be theory-neutral but is inferential, because it refers to so-called theoretical entities, that is, nonobserved processes (the "drives"). The concept of dysfunction the HDA refers to is inferential, because it has to refer to an unobserved dysfunction that explains what is observed: "diagnosing disorder is inherently theoretical in the sense that it goes beyond sheer symptoms to hypothesize the existence of a dysfunction, without necessarily specifying the exact nature of the dysfunction or its etiology" (Wakefield 1999c, 966). How can it be at the same time theory-neutral and inferential? Is not an inference to etiology theoretical per se? Indeed, it is; but Wakefield propounds the "black-box" (Wakefield 1997b, 658; 1999b, 471–472; 2001, 359–362) view of dysfunction, according to which it is permissible to speak of a dysfunction before knowing what it consists of exactly. A definition can thus be inferential, because it assumes the existence of a dysfunction, and theory-neutral, because it does not "explain the behavior in any substantial or full way" (Wakefield 1999c, 986). Thanks to this black-box view, the concept of dysfunction can avoid theoretical stipulation.

Second, the concept of dysfunctional states is expected to stand against normative views of what is desirable and what is not. This means that it can oppose normative aspects of the choices made by authors of the diagnostic manuals. It is important not to conflate this kind of impartiality with reliability. There could be "reliable"—that is, shared and highly reproducible—clinical judgments based on precise, operational, and yet normative criteria (Wakefield 1992b, 233). For instance,

(7) *"antipsychiatric behavior* = denial, either in acts or in words, of the facts of psychiatric science, as assessed by the results of the tests of the Scientific Antipsychiatric Scale."

Third, the necessity to assess dysfunction in a suspected case of mental disorder also addresses the clinical level. It limits the operative role of the values of the clinician in clinical judgments. For instance,

(8) *"antipsychiatric behavior* = excessive denial of the facts of psychiatric science according to the feeling of the clinician"

and

(9) *"mental distress* = whatever state a subject may be in, which requires help from a mental practitioner (according to the practitioner)"

can be applied to a given situation without referring to anything other than the clinician's value judgment. Definition (9) may be reliable depending on the homogeneity of the clinical community (see Bolton 2008, 14–15), but it is value-laden nevertheless.

In helping to guard against both arbitrary categories and false-positive cases (Wakefield et al. 2010), the dysfunction component presents a further problem in the determination of what should properly be called a mental disorder. With Horwitz, Wakefield has emphasized the importance of the assessment of context in *The Loss of Sadness* (Horwitz and Wakefield 2007). The problem here is linked to the dysfunction component, not to the harm component. The difficulty lies in appraising whether there is indeed a dysfunction involved in some state (e.g., sadness) or whether the state is best understood as a normal response to a life event. This does not suggest that the general framework of the HD definition of mental disorder is stipulation, but it suggests that the dysfunction component is in part responsible for some stipulations about both definition and application of categories. This is, so to speak, the side effect of the black-box view.

2.3 The Concept of Mental Disorder Does Not Necessarily Imply a Concept of Dysfunction

Until now, it has not been proven that the HD definition of mental disorders is a stipulation but only that the presence of the dysfunction component does not immunize either the general definition of mental disorders or specific definitions of mental disorders against stipulation. I would not assert here that Wakefield stipulates a dysfunction concept of mental disorders, but I would not consider defining mental disorder as dysfunction a trivial point to make either. Derek Bolton has rightly emphasized this:

> What we know as mental disorder—or at least, as mental health problems—can involve factors other than *dysfunction*. Among the most important and readily understood key ideas in an evolutionary theoretic framework that point in this direction are (1) design/environment mismatches, (2) highly evolved design features of human beings, (3) defensive strategies, and (4) strategies that involve disruption of function. (Bolton 2000, 146)

For the purposes of this chapter, the point to be made is just to emphasize the incompatibility between the dysfunction thesis and an analytic purpose. With Bolton, I think that Wakefield is correct in saying that the folk and scientific core concept of mental disorder requires a scientific component. But I do not think that it is merely *description* to assume that this scientific component is dysfunction.

So a description of the general framework of the concept of mental disorder ought to be some sort of deflationary or downgraded version of the harmful-dysfunction analysis (I propose "HAA" for harmful abnormality analysis). By "abnormality" here, I mean a much broader concept than that of dysfunction and one that is not restricted to the statistical concept of abnormality. In a nutshell, "abnormality" addresses the notion of the objective basis of the concept of mental disorder, whether it is a dysfunction, a mismatch, a strategy, and so on. Abnormalities are observed facts; they are not supposed to be spotted after value judgments and *they* are expected to limit arbitrary disease entities and false-positive cases. The preceding sums up an analytic or descriptive approach to the HAA. The HAA is the only uncontroversially descriptive general framework for the concept of mental disorder: every further specification is stipulation and constitutes a theoretical move.

III. Is the Definition of "Dysfunction" as an Evolutionary Concept Explication or Stipulation?

Is the evolutionary concept of dysfunction some kind of elucidation of what we usually mean by dysfunction (as "probability$_1$" and "probability$_2$" are for the general concept of probability), or is it a brand-new scientific concept (as "prion," "tachyon," "money supply," or "energy")? Obviously, stipulation would be a legitimate approach in the field of philosophy of psychiatry as well as in science, but perhaps equally obviously, Wakefield means it to be an explication of the common term and not a stipulation of a new, specific concept of dysfunction. I would like to make a few points, though, in favor of a stipulative interpretation of the HDA: (1) there are other scientific definitions of dysfunction than the evolutionary definition contained within the HDA, and were the evolutionary approach to provide the best scientific account available, it could as well be stipulation; (2) even a theory-neutral concept of dysfunction can imply stipulation; (3) the obviousness of the concept of dysfunction does not mean that its definition is explicative; and finally, (4) Boorse's naturalist account of dysfunction seems to fit an explicative purpose best.

3.1 The Best Scientific Account of Dysfunction May Be Stipulation All the Same

Some of us are inclined to consider abnormalities, as previously defined, to be statistical entities. Others view abnormalities in terms of biological defects, and yet another approach describes them as information-processing failures, social conflicts, and so on. Some of these positions equate abnormality with dysfunction, yet they do not all necessarily mean the same thing by "dysfunction" (for this line of arguments against the HDA, see, e.g., Murphy and Woolfolk 2001; Schramme 2010). Wakefield considers the question to be as follows: is a definition of abnormality as a biological dysfunction in the evolutionary sense the best one available or even the "most viable one" (Wakefield 1992b, 237)? He has made a strong case against several kinds of alternative definitions—for example, statistical definitions (Wakefield 1992a, 377–378; 1999a, 388–390, etc.), "disadvantage" definitions (Wakefield 1992a, 378), and "current causal role" definitions (Wakefield 2001), among others. He has also made a strong case for his definition of dysfunction against many different critiques. The more successful he is in defending his definition against his critics, the more his definition appears to be the best one available. This is not my point here, though. My point is more to question the implicit argument that states a scientific (i.e., evolutionary-based) definition of dysfunction would be the best one available, therefore making it impartial and nonstipulative.

As a matter of fact, impartiality has nothing to do with explication (as opposed to stipulation). Wakefield's account of abnormality as a dysfunction could well be the best one available, yet fails to elucidate the common meaning of "mental disorder." At the end of the nineteenth century, for instance,

(10) *"Diabetes mellitus* = pancreatic condition"

was indeed impartial in that it was the best definition available, based on the discoveries of Oscar Minkowski. Yet in no way would this have been an explication, for no one had yet thought of this as the definition of diabetes mellitus. What if, for instance, the evolutionary account of dysfunction was the best one on scientific grounds, yet was definitely not what scientists themselves usually meant by dysfunction? On the other hand, Wakefield's definition of dysfunction could also draw from no arbitrarily determined goals, yet be stipulation, precisely because a lot of effects we want to call functions might be value-laden (aside from any harm done by the condition). For instance,

(11) *"old age* = universal dysfunction of the telomerase in animals"

might happen to be impartial, yet we could oppose the claim that aging is the result of a dysfunction (see Wakefield 1999b, 468). Hence, an impartial definition of dysfunction is not a sufficient condition for an explicative definition of dysfunction.

3.2 A Theory-Neutral Definition of Dysfunction Is Not Necessarily Explication

The fact that all the major theories of mental disorder (see, e.g., Bolton 2008, 15 sqq.) are *compatible* with a definition of disorder as a dysfunction in the evolutionary sense does not imply that disorder analytically means dysfunction in the evolutionary sense. For instance,

(12) *"light* = visible manifestation of the divine radiance known as uncreated light or Tabor's Light"

does not, in my view, rule out any claim from the corpuscular or wave theory of light and thus does not take sides. It is undoubtedly stipulative, though. Therefore, the theory-neutrality of the HDA does not make it immune to stipulation (not of course because it would be theological or nonscientific but rather because it is a new hypothesis and works on a different level of analysis with regard to the question of mental disorders).

3.3 A Self-Explicatory Concept of Dysfunction Is Not Necessarily Explicative

According to Wakefield, the evolutionary concept of dysfunction is not only the best available theory-neutral concept we possess but also the clearest: "natural selection is the only known means by which an effect can explain a naturally occurring mechanism that provides it" (Wakefield 1992a, 383; 1999b, 465). In other words, the evolutionary concept of dysfunction is explicative rather than stipulative in that it replaces an obscure and vague concept of dysfunction by an obvious or self-explicatory one.

Elsewhere, I have given a cursory account of what I mean by "self-explicatory" in biomedical science more generally (see Lemoine 2011). Let us assume here simply that scientific explanations can never be satisfactory except in a special kind of predicament where the scientist is bound to acknowledge that this particular explication takes everything important into account. In a scientific explanation, necessity comes free with some beliefs that make this predicament possible. For instance,

(13) *"Recessive genetic disease* = any disease that must affect 25% of the offspring of heterozygous parents as to this trait"

is an obvious definition, given the laws of Mendelian genetics. (In other senses, of course, it is not obvious at all, because it is not operational. First, no "must affect" can be observed; second, "25%" is probabilistic here.) On the other hand,

(14) *"mental disorder* = state of a person endowed with statistically rare (less than 2.5%) representations of some significant item of her environment"

and

(15) *"dysfunctional* = belonging to the first 2.5 percentiles of a Gaussian distribution of mean performances to a task"

are not obvious in the sense of self-explanatory, because they rest upon an arbitrary, obscurely determined threshold of normality or functionality.

I think that the evolutionary concept of dysfunction is indeed obvious and self-explanatory. But the fact that a concept is obvious within one particular predicament, say, the theory of evolution, does not prove that it is the only predicament possible in which an obvious concept of dysfunction is possible. Therefore, even if we could think of no other self-explanatory account of dysfunction, one cannot assume that this is the only one possible. Yet this would be a necessary condition for us to assume that this definition is explication.

3.4 Boorse's Account of Dysfunction Is Better Than Wakefield's as a Naturalist Explication of the Concept of Dysfunction

The challenge for a naturalist account of mental disorder is to elucidate it by shielding entirely the dysfunction component from values "partitioned off in the harmful part of the analysis" (Bolton 2008, 121, 231–233 on Gert and Culver's appraisal of the HDA). By assuming that *harm* and *dysfunction* are to be thought of as entirely separate things, the HDA stays at equal distance from two opposed lines of thought. One is the idea that dysfunctions are precisely the kind of mechanisms associated with the states we disvalue or those that an organism seems to disvalue itself. Valued or disvalued states do not change, but as we discover biological mechanisms and their links to valued and disvalued states, we change our views on their being functional or dysfunctional. In the end, we are expected to know what is functional and dysfunctional because we want to know what is linked to harmful states and how. The other line of thought is that what we conceive of as "harmful" is what we understand as dysfunctional in at least one respect. On this view, it would be precisely because we do not know every function and dysfunction, that the concept of harm is value-laden, and that the definition of mental disorder is too. Once function and dysfunction were properly understood, the concept of harm would be as value-free as the concept of function, and so would be the concept of mental disorder.

It is easy to understand how an ultimate evolutionary theory of what is dysfunctional could be contrasted with what we consider to be harmful or not. But it is not easy to understand how we can consider dysfunctional states and harmful states to be different things in an imperfect state of knowledge. In the case of *mental* conditions, "this ignorance is part of the reason for the high degree of confusion and controversy concerning which conditions are really mental disorders" (Wakefield 1992a, 383). Confusion and controversy do not imply that dysfunction is a value-laden concept, given that there are scientific controversies (at least let us suppose that). However, it is clear that if we do not know of everything in a given mechanism (e.g., walking), everybody will agree with the idea that we can say it is malfunctioning all the same. How do we do that, if we must not use the concept of harm? An explicative, naturalist concept of dysfunction has to explain this fact. Wakefield is correct, I think, in saying that "evolutionary design and human values do also often diverge" (Wakefield 2001, 352) and even in saying that "natural function is a scientific concept that cannot be reduced to values" (Wakefield 1992a, 376). But is it true that an evolutionary or "etiologic" account of *dysfunction* elucidates this independence of the concept of dysfunction best?

The general theoretical framework of Wakefield's analysis of dysfunction is "Hempel's challenge" on function (Wakefield 2001, 359): How can we discriminate among the natural effects of a biological mechanism so as to determine which one(s) is (are) its function(s) (Wakefield 1992a, 382)? A function, as Wakefield puts it, conforms to the "explanation criterion" (385). It is this special kind of effect that can explain the presence of its cause (Wakefield sometimes also talks of functions as the cause of natural effects). What is *dysfunction*, then? According to Wakefield, "dysfunction is the failure of a mechanism to perform its natural function" (383; Wakefield 1999b, 465: "failure of biologically designed functions"). Here, dysfunction is obviously an underlying cause, not its effects. We understand underlying dysfunction due to the absence of natural effects (what Wakefield calls "circumstantial evidence": Wakefield 1999b, 465; 1999c, 988).

In a strictly naturalist view, I can think of two ways to know that functional effects are absent. One is by comparing the effects of a mechanism in an individual to the effects of the same mechanism in the proper subgroup of the relevant species. This is a statistical definition of function, which we owe to Boorse (1977) and not to Wakefield. The other approach—and I presume it to be Wakefield's—is to *appraise* those observed effects that replace the natural ones. Some effects obviously run contrary to what could possibly be the natural function of a biological organism. This does not mean that every effect that cannot possibly explain the existence of a mechanism that is causing it is a dysfunction. For instance, the sound of the heart cannot explain the cardiac mechanism, but it is not a dysfunction. Rather, it means that a dysfunction is a failure of a mechanism to perform its natural function because this effect is somehow at odds with the presumed natural function of the mechanism.

I think that the only naturalist way to distinguish between nonnatural and harmful effects of a mechanism in an imperfect state of knowledge is to adopt Boorse's biostatistical views on dysfunction. Significantly, when considering the possibility of harmless dysfunctions, Wakefield appears to turn to this competing conception of dysfunction. For instance, he gives the imaginary example of "a dysfunction that slow[s] the aging process and lengthen[s] life" (Wakefield 1992a, 384; 2001, 352), but the question is how could this be imagined as a dysfunction except by comparison? The same goes for albinism, fused toes, *dextrocardia situs inversus*, and having one kidney. This is not a proof, but it is a sign. I am not saying that Boorse's views on function are compatible with Wakefield's examples on harmless dysfunction. I am suggesting that Wakefield's examples of harmless dysfunction are only compatible with Boorse's views on function.

This leaves us with a challenge to the HDA. If it cannot give any example of a harmless condition, which would be thought of as dysfunctional without any comparison to a biological reference class, it has either to consider every dysfunctional state to be harmful in one way or to adopt Boorse's view on dysfunction, at least as a temporary stage, in providing a naturalist account of dysfunction. The latter is the least damaging to the HDA. But it means that the HDA works best to clarify what we currently mean by "dysfunction," therefore, that any other view on it is stipulative.

Conclusion

My first point was that the HD definition of mental disorder may rightly introduce the concept of dysfunction as the best way to define it, but this is not really a description of the common usage of the term. My second point was that in defining dysfunction as an evolutionary concept, Wakefield propounds a sound scientific hypothesis, but one that works poorly in elucidating the common meaning of the term. My conclusion is that there is a fundamental choice to make between a descriptive or explicative "conceptual analysis" and a stipulative, scientific contribution.

Because the HAA I suggested here as the most faithful description of the meaning of the term is probably not a very useful definition, I suggest that the HDA should be resolute in proclaiming stipulation instead and entering the scientific arena of competition between theories (compare with Wakefield 1999c, 965). In doing so, maybe Wakefield should abandon any belief that there exists an independent, precise content of the notion of mental disorder as belonging to folk psychology, as Murphy and Woolfolk have suggested. Or maybe he would have to acknowledge that there is not much to gain in a descriptive definition of mental disorder. In view of this, it would be possible to adopt a fully fledged naturalist conception of mental disorder as well as of dysfunction: here, I mean "naturalism" as the rejection of *any* legitimate independence of the folk concept of disease from science. I think that what prevents Wakefield from doing so is the strong strategic argument from plausibility: for instance, "Freud was sophisticated enough to realize that, to offer a persuasive theory of etiology, one must define a disorder in such a way that it can be identified by those who do not initially share one's theory" (1999c, 968). Besides, how could we consider mental disorder independently of commonsense views of it being harmful, if this is not possible even for a concept such as "dysfunction"? (This is a point one could reject in favor of Wakefield's position and against Murphy and Woolfolk.) In defense of naturalism, though, I think that this strong strategic constraint of folk plausibility on our conceptual definitions of mental disorder can be understood *extensively*, not necessarily *intensively*. I mean that as long as roughly the same patients are considered to be affected by mental disorders, the intensional content of the definition does not matter to the lay public, and the requirement of "conceptual validity" is respected. Besides, current boundaries are both fuzzy and plastic, and they do not constitute such a stringent constraint on theoretical plausibility They are plastic because, thanks to science, the lay public has been convinced to view some conditions as disorders. This comes precisely from the fact that any mental disorder is stipulated; "because the actual identity of the essence is often unknown at the time that the term is defined, the definition uses a stipulated base set of known initial instances of the natural kind to establish the reference of the term" (Wakefield 1997b, 657). Moreover, "treatable conditions" in Bolton's sense (Bolton 2000, 149 sqq.; 2008, 191) are a broader class within which scientists might feel rather free to delineate classes without directly intervening in social conflicts about mental health. And this is the class philosophers actually have to address if they want to step in.

Note

1. "In making criteria more reliable, *DSM-III-R* has sacrificed some aspects of validity" (Wakefield 1992b, 241). See also Wakefield (1993, 161): "I suggest an alternative approach to diagnosis in which operational criteria for specific disorders are based on nonoperational functional definitions of mental disorder and of specific disorders." At last, Wakefield says, "A reference to dysfunction that is not translated into operationalized criteria leaves it entirely open to clinicians to make a global judgment of whether a dysfunction exists. This introduces a highly unreliable element into the criteria" (Wakefield, 1997a, 646). This last quotation addresses the "dysfunction" component of the harmful dysfunction analysis. This is the one I will focus on, leaving aside interesting questions about the stipulative or descriptive nature of the "harm" component.

References

Bolton, D. 2000. Alternatives to disorder. *Philosophy, Psychiatry, and Psychology* 7(2): 141–153.

Bolton, D. 2008. *What Is Mental Disorder? An Essay in Philosophy, Science, and Values. International Perspectives in Philosophy and Psychiatry.* Oxford University Press.

Boorse, C. 1977. Health as a theoretical concept. *Philosophy of Science* 44(4): 542–573.

Carnap, R. 1962. *Logical Foundations of Probability.* 2nd ed. University of Chicago Press.

Cooper, R. 2002. *Disease. Studies in History and Philosophy of Science Part C: Studies in History and Philosophy of Biological and Biomedical Sciences* 33(2): 263–282.

Fulford, K. W. 2001. 'What is (mental) disease?': An open letter to Christopher Boorse. *Journal of Medical Ethics* 27(2): 80–85.

Hempel, C. G. 1952. *Fundamentals of Concept Formation in Empirical Science.* University of Chicago Press.

Horwitz, A. V., and J. C. Wakefield. 2007. *The Loss of Sadness: How Psychiatry Transformed Normal Sorrow into Depressive Disorder.* Oxford University Press.

Lemoine, M. 2011. *La désunité de la médecine. Essai sur les valeurs explicatives de la science*. Hermann.

Murphy, D., and R. L. Woolfolk. 2001. Conceptual analysis versus scientific understanding: An assessment of Wakefield's folk psychiatry. *Philosophy, Psychiatry, and Psychology* 7(4): 271–293.

Nordenfelt, L. 2007. *Rationality and Compulsion: Applying Action Theory to Psychiatry. International perspectives in philosophy and psychiatry*. Oxford University Press.

Schramme, T. 2010. Can we define mental disorder by using the criterion of mental dysfunction? *Theoretical Medicine and Bioethics* 31(1): 35–47.

Wakefield, J. C. 1992a. The concept of mental disorder: On the boundary between biological facts and social values. *American Psychologist* 47(3): 373–388.

Wakefield, J. C. 1992b. Disorder as harmful dysfunction: A conceptual critique of *DSM-III-R*'s definition of mental disorder. *Psychological Review* 99(2): 232–247.

Wakefield, J. C. 1993. Limits of operationalization: A critique of Spitzer and Endicott's (1978) proposed operational criteria for mental disorder. *Journal of Abnormal Psychology* 102(1): 160–172.

Wakefield, J. C. 1997a. Diagnosing *DSM-IV*, Part I: *DSM-IV* and the concept of disorder. *Behaviour Research and Therapy* 35(7): 633–649.

Wakefield, J. C. 1997b. Diagnosing *DSM-IV*, Part 2: Eysenck (1986) and the essentialist fallacy. *Behaviour Research and Therapy* 35(7): 651–665.

Wakefield, J. C. 1999a. Evolutionary versus prototype analyses of the concept of disorder. *Journal of Abnormal Psychology* 108: 374–399.

Wakefield, J. C. 1999b. Disorder as a black box essentialist concept. *Journal of Abnormal Psychology* 108: 465–472.

Wakefield, J. C. 1999c. Philosophy of science and the progressiveness of the *DSM*'s theory-neutral nosology: Response to Follette and Houts, Part 1. *Behaviour Research and Therapy* 37(10): 963–999.

Wakefield, J. C. 1999d. The concept of disorder as a foundation for the *DSM*'s theory-neutral nosology: Response to Follette and Houts, Part 2. *Behaviour Research and Therapy* 37(10): 1001–1027.

Wakefield, J. C. 2001. Evolutionary history versus current causal role in the definition of disorder: Reply to McNally. *Behaviour Research and Therapy* 39(3): 347–366.

Wakefield, J. C., M. F. Schmitz, and J. C. Baer. 2010. Does the *DSM-IV* clinical significance criterion for major depression reduce false positives? Evidence from the National Comorbidity Survey replication. *American Journal of Psychiatry* 167(3): 298–304.

12 Is the Harmful Dysfunction Analysis Descriptive or Stipulative, and Is the HDA or BST the Better Naturalist Account of Dysfunction? Reply to Maël Lemoine

Jerome Wakefield

I thank Maël Lemoine for his provocative and nuanced critique of my harmful dysfunction analysis (HDA) of the concept of medical, including mental, disorder. The HDA claims that "disorder" refers to "harmful dysfunction," where dysfunction is the failure of some feature to perform a natural function for which it is biologically designed by evolutionary processes and harm is judged in accordance with social values (First and Wakefield 2010, 2013; Spitzer 1997, 1999; Wakefield 1992a, 1992b, 1993, 1995, 1997a, 1997b, 1997c, 1997d, 1998, 1999a, 1999b, 2000a, 2000b, 2001, 2006, 2007, 2009, 2011, 2014, 2016a, 2016b; Wakefield and First 2003 2012). There are more points of contention raised by his wide-ranging paper than I can address here, and some are best pursued in future personal interactions in which I look forward to extending the enjoyable interchange that started when we met at a conference in honor of Christopher Boorse some time ago. In this reply, I focus on the most important questions raised by his paper's main line of argument challenging the HDA. Some of these are questions I have not dealt with before, and I thank Lemoine for prodding me to address them.

A brief word about terminology and abbreviations: there is a general "selected effects" account of functions that is applied across domains (e.g., biology, artifacts) and is commonly abbreviated as "SE" functions. But, here I am concerned only with biological functions and with the theory of natural selection, and when the SE account is so restricted, I will label it the "evolutionary" or "NSE" (i.e., naturally selected effects) approach to functions. Cummins puts forward the very broad view that functions are simply the causal roles played by various mechanisms, commonly labeled "CR" functions (see my response to Murphy for a detailed analysis of CR functions). Boorse employs a form of CR functions that he terms the "general goal contribution" (GGC) account, which restricts relevant causal roles to the ones that contribute to goals, and he applies the GGC across domains. When applied to biology, Boorse claims that the goals of organisms are survival and reproduction, so the GGC view becomes the view that a biological function is the causal contribution made by a mechanism to survival and reproduction, which he labels the "S&R" view of biological functions.

First, it is important to clarify that a central point raised by Lemoine as a criticism is in fact one on which he and I entirely agree. Lemoine argues that when I call the HDA a descriptive conceptual analysis, I "conflate two good ideas into one" because the HDA's evolutionary analysis of "dysfunction" is in fact not a descriptive conceptual analysis but something different, which he calls a "stipulation" (I will come back to the stipulation issue later): "there is indeed something stipulative in Wakefield's position...but also something descriptive. Yet what is stipulative is not the general framework for the concept of mental disorder...: it is rather the evolutionary concept of dysfunction." Lemoine further claims that the descriptive versus stipulative distinction reveals a tension within the HDA: "Wakefield's arguments hide an incompatibility (at some point) between two purposes: on one hand, to give an account of what is usually meant by 'mental disorder'; on the other hand, to give a satisfactory scientific account of the concept of dysfunction...: while a descriptive account must not stipulate, a scientific account has to."

Now, if we momentarily put aside the question of whether the proposed nonconceptual-analytic part of the HDA should be interpreted specifically as a "stipulation," *Lemoine's account is precisely the position I have always put forward*! "Harmful dysfunction" is a conceptual analysis prior to the evolutionary interpretation of "dysfunction," and the evolutionary interpretation of "function" is an essentialist theoretical move that is not conceptual-analytic or sheerly descriptive but a theoretical identification. Thus, if I can be excused a lengthy self-quote to make this point clear, near the beginning of my main article defending the evolutionary part of my account (1999a), which Lemoine cites in his references, I said,

> One technically must distinguish the analysis of disorder as harmful dysfunction from the evolutionary theory of dysfunction, which together comprise the HD view. The HD analysis cannot directly define disorder in evolutionary terms because the analysis aims to capture a widely shared, intuitive medical and lay concept that existed long before evolutionary theory and is shared by many who are ignorant of or who reject evolutionary theory. Simply put, you do not have to understand or accept evolution to possess the concept of disorder. It is a momentous scientific discovery, not a matter of definition, that natural selection is the essential process that explains functions and dysfunctions. So, harmful dysfunction is the meaning of disorder, and evolution is the most incisive theory of the nature of functions and dysfunctions.
>
> The HD analysis may be thought of as arriving at the evolutionary account in three steps. First,...a disorder exists only when an internal mechanism is dysfunctional, specifically in the sense that it is incapable of performing one of its natural functions (at this stage of the analysis, natural function is used in an intuitive sense that has existed for millennia, not in a technical evolutionary sense)....Second,...natural function[s]...like the intentionally designed functions of artifacts, must somehow be part of the explanation of why the underlying mechanisms exist and are structured as they are. (By analogy with artifacts, such functions are often said to be what the mechanism is "designed" to do.)....Disorders, then, are failures of mechanisms to perform their natural functions....

Strictly speaking, these two steps complete the conceptual analysis of disorder. However, the analysis inevitably leads to the question, What kind of underlying process could possibly be responsible for such seeming design in natural systems without any designer?...Evolutionary theory provides the only plausible scientific account that presently exists of how the natural functions of a mechanism can explain the existence and structure of the mechanism....This third, theoretical argument leads to the conclusion that disorders are failures of mechanisms to perform functions for which they were naturally selected. (1999a, 374–375)

So, I have been quite explicit about this, and Lemoine is simply agreeing with me about the dual nature of my argument for the HDA. As Lemoine observes, I link the conceptual analysis and evolutionary theory via a "black-box essentialist" analysis of "function" (Wakefield 1999b, 2000a); a natural function is, conceptually, whatever is due to the same essential process that brings about a base set of obvious examples of apparent biologically designed features, such as eyes seeing, hands grasping, thirst causing us to drink needed water, fear causing us to flee danger, and so on. It is an empirical discovery that that essential process is natural selection, implying that a dysfunction (in the sense relevant to medical disorder) is failure of a mechanism to be capable of having its naturally selected effect. Note that there is no comparable unified and direct essentialist account of dysfunctions, only the indirect one that they are failures of natural functions, because such failures occur for myriad diverse reasons.

In fairness to Lemoine, in some of my writings, when it seemed not to matter, I have been sloppy about distinguishing the conceptual-analytic and scientific-theoretical aspects, misleadingly compressing my description to characterize the entire HDA as a conceptual analysis. However, in my more careful theoretical writings, I have clearly drawn the distinction that Lemoine accuses me of ignoring and have even critiqued (e.g., Wakefield 2000a) both Neander (1991a) and Millikan (1989) for making the error, in different ways, of interpreting the link between "function" and natural selection as a conceptual one, and this should have made my position clear.

The Conceptual Analysis (Strictly Speaking) of "Medical Disorder"

Given the agreed division of the HDA into a conceptual-analytic and scientific-theoretical component, Lemoine's discussion raises two important questions: (1) Exactly how far can conceptual analysis take us before we must turn to scientific theory? (2) What degrees of freedom to "stipulate" do we have in moving via the black-box essentialist structure from the conceptual analysis to a theory of functions and dysfunctions? Lemoine answers both questions in ways I will dispute.

Lemoine agrees with what he interprets as the conceptual-analytic part of the HDA. He says that other than the evolutionary interpretation of dysfunction, the HDA "is probably the best account of the concept of mental disorder" and "is indeed a highly faithful account of what both laymen and psychiatrists mean by 'disorder.'" He also seems to accept or at least acknowledges the advantages of my black-box essential-ist account of function and dysfunction as allowing a theory-free conceptual analy-sis: "Thanks to this black-box view, the concept of dysfunction can avoid theoretical stipulation."

For the HDA's conceptual-analytic part prior to the evolutionary interpretation of function and dysfunction, Lemoine coins the term "harmful abnormality." The use of the vague term "abnormality" is specifically aimed at stepping back from a more specific notion of "dysfunction." Lemoine does not offer any actual counterexamples to support his rejection of "dysfunction" in favor of the broader notion of "abnor-mality" but rather relies on an assertion by Derek Bolton: "What we know as mental disorder—or at least, as mental health problems—can involve factors other than *dys-function*. Among the most important and readily understood key ideas in an evolu-tionary theoretic framework that point in this direction are (1) design/environment mismatches, (2) highly evolved design features of human beings, (3) defensive strate-gies, and (4) strategies that involve disruption of function" (Bolton 2000, 146). Citing Bolton's assertion, Lemoine concludes that the conditions that fall under the intuitive concept of disorder are of many kinds that go well beyond dysfunction.

Lemoine's conclusion is mistaken and based on lack of attention to actual intuitive examples (see, e.g., Wakefield 1999a). For example, defensive strategies (e.g., cough-ing in response to dust in the air), functions that are designed to disrupt subsidiary functions (e.g., impairment of a man's ability to urinate when sexually aroused), and design/environment mismatches (e.g., problems with desiring high-fat and high-sugar foods in modern environments in which they are all too readily available) are not generally judged to be disorders. Additionally, if organism-environment mismatches are classified as disorders, that immediately makes every problematic social deviation into a mental disorder, which is one of the main outcomes that the analysis of mental disorder is meant to prevent.

In fact, Bolton hedges his claim by specifying that his list consists of conditions that "we know as mental disorder—*or at least, as mental health problems*" (emphasis added). Elsewhere in the same article, Bolton cites my arguments and notes that my analy-sis leads to the conclusion that not all such potentially treatable problematic mental health conditions are literally disorders: "there may be a broader class of behaviors relevant to 'mental health' than the class of disorders defined by Wakefield.... Wake-field acknowledges that *disorder* and *treatable conditions* do not coincide" (145). Note that the scope of Bolton's term "mental health problems" goes well beyond failures of health in the medical sense and encompasses almost any negative psychological state. For example, a very extensive list of Z coded mental conditions that are not disorders but are frequent targets of clinical intervention is included in the *Diagnostic and Statis-tical Manual of Mental Disorders (DSM-5)* (American Psychiatric Association 2013) and the *International Classification of Diseases (ICD-11)* (World Health Organization 2018).

Writers sympathetic with the HDA (e.g., Cosmides and Tooby 1999), including me (Wakefield 2015), have argued that there are many problems that the medical professions ought to be mandated to treat but that are not mental disorders, ranging from substance abuse without addiction to marital conflict. Consequently, Lemoine's use of the broad category of abnormality instead of dysfunction in his rendition of the HDA conceptual component is unsupported.

Having rejected dysfunction as a conceptual requirement for disorder, Lemoine elaborates his broader analysis:

> So a description of the general framework of the concept of mental disorder ought to be some sort of deflationary or downgraded version of the harmful-dysfunction analysis (I propose "HAA" for harmful abnormality analysis). By "abnormality" here, I mean a much broader concept than that of dysfunction and one that is not restricted to the statistical concept of abnormality. In a nutshell, "abnormality" addresses the notion of the objective basis of the concept of mental disorder, whether it is a dysfunction, a mismatch, a strategy, and so on. Abnormalities are observed facts; they are not supposed to be spotted after value judgments and *they* are expected to limit arbitrary disease entities and false-positive cases. The preceding sums up an analytic or descriptive approach to the HAA. The HAA is the only uncontroversially descriptive general framework for the concept of mental disorder: every further specification is stipulation and constitutes a theoretical move.

Lemoine does not explain how such an extraordinarily broad notion that allows any problematic objective internal state to be a dysfunction can possibly serve to "limit arbitrary disease entities and false-positive cases." In any event, as we have seen, there are ample reasons why this analysis cannot be correct. Beyond the earlier examples of nondisordered defenses, mismatches, and so on, "abnormality" in the sense that Lemoine defines it encompasses a vast terrain of problematic nondisorders (e.g., ignorance, lack of talent, negative personality traits, social deviance), defeating the point of an analysis of disorder. (For further explanation of why such a view fails, see my reply to De Vreese in this volume.)

The history of medicine from Hippocrates to our own time indicates that the concept of a medical disorder involves more than problematic states caused by internal conditions, for there are many normal problematic states caused by internal conditions. It involves a presupposition that, as Robert Spitzer used to put it, *something has gone wrong*, which, I have argued (and Spitzer eventually agreed [Spitzer 1997, 1999]), involves the presupposition that there is a failure of some internal mechanism to perform as it was biologically designed to perform. Biological design, which is apparent to laypersons and scientists alike, has been the central puzzle of biology from Aristotle to Darwin, and it is anchoring in the objective feature of biological design that allows disorder to transcend values and gives it a distinctive social status. (For further comments on the historical centrality of biological design to biology, see my reply to Murphy in this volume.) Thus, conceptual analysis can take us further than Lemoine allows. The purely conceptual-analytic meaning of "disorder" is "harmful dysfunction" in which "dysfunction" is not evolutionarily interpreted but understood in intuitive biological-design natural-function terms.

Bolton (2000), in the same article cited by Lemoine, seems to understand better than Lemoine the logic and appeal of natural function as part of the foundation for the prescientific concept of disorder:

> Wakefield (1999a) clarifies his position as being that "harmful dysfunction is the meaning of disorder, and evolution is the best theory of the nature of functions and dysfunctions." ...
>
> This is an important and helpful line of thought. The suggestion is that we have first an analysis of a folk concept of disorder, or its reasonably close cognates, appealing essentially to what is natural—or of our nature. This we may plausibly suppose not only captures the principles of common usage of terms related to disorder, but is also at work among physicians, including mental health professionals in the clinic. (145)

So, the answer to the first question raised by Lemoine's critique—namely, what the conceptual analysis of "disorder" can yield—is that "disorder" means "harmful dysfunction" where "dysfunction" means "failure of a natural function" (or "failure of a biologically designed function") in a preevolutionary sense, and "natural function" is understood in terms of a black-box essentialist descriptive naturalist definition. Note that this answer to the first question imposes limits on the answer to the second question regarding the potential scope for stipulation in specifying a theory of dysfunction, a point to which I will later return.

Modest Black-Box Essentialism

Before addressing stipulation, I need to clarify my understanding of essentialism—a term to which some critics seem allergic—because the question of stipulation will be considered within the context of the black-box essentialist analysis of "function." I construe an essentialist view of natural kind concepts in a minimalist way that avoids the metaphysical doctrinal loading of Kripke's (1980) account and the strawman formulations of critics (e.g., Kendler, Zachar, and Craver 2011). On most issues, I adopt Putnam's nonmetaphysical and more scientific and pragmatic account that, simply stated, is that "to be water, or gold, or some other natural kind, is to have *the same nature* as 'this,' where the 'this' can be any one of the [majority of the] paradigms we point to, *and the 'sameness of nature' is a scientific or protoscientific concept, not a metaphysical one*" (Putnam 2015c, 359). (Putnam more frequently calls the paradigm cases "stereotypes" and I call them the "base set.") In particular, the "nature" or "essence" of the category is a nonobservable feature that is explanatorily and theoretically potent, in that it plays a major role in formulating theories that explain the important features of the base set, including the salient observable features that made us pick out the base set to define a broader category in the first place. I also accept a flexible version of Kripke's notion of "baptism," in which one identifies an initial set of instances as the basis for reference fixation of the overall category. This construct seems necessary to make good on Putnam's reliance on a reference-fixing sample of "stereotypical" category members.

The essence is not explicitly identified in the category's definition but is rather referenced via the indirect description, "whatever is the same in nature as the base set." This allows the category to be defined without any explicit reference to, and often without any knowledge of, the specific hypothesized essential property that determines its members and explains their salient properties. The basic point is that new category members are added based not on their superficial similarity to the members of the base set but on the basis of the judgment that they share the relevant underlying nature with the base set. The base set may be defined descriptively in terms of observable features, but that description does not define the entire category: "The stereotype, that gold is yellow, precious, etc., is *not* analytic; it may well turn out to be wrong; but nevertheless the shared stereotype plays a role in stabilizing the use of 'gold'" (Putnam 2015a, 77). The kind can always transcend the stereotypical observable properties (e.g., the base set of tigers are large striped felines, but there are still dwarf albino tigers). Despite this definitional structure, essentialistic categories, like most categories, generally have fuzzy boundaries in virtue of the fuzziness of the various component concepts.

Admittedly, the term "essence" has a disturbing resonance with bygone metaphysical doctrines. However, it is generally used today as a philosophical term of art shorn of such doctrines. As noted above, it refers to hidden explanatorily potent structures, as in gold being the element with atomic number 79 or water being the chemical H_2O. Moreover, the "hidden structure" characterization cannot be taken too literally. We can of course use terms in all sorts of ways for varying purposes, including positivist observable-property meanings. However, especially in science, the conceptual and theoretical undertow pulls us toward structures beyond observable properties because they generally support a more perspicuous theory and deeper understanding. "Hidden structure" is best understood as simply a term of art covering almost any not-directly-observable property that determines category membership. So, on this modest interpretation, if the intentions of designers determine artifact category membership or the history of an interbreeding population in addition to its genetics partly determines a species, these can still be essentialist concepts.

Essentialism in this modest form has a number of benefits, from correcting positivist accounts of concept meanings in terms of superficially observable or operationalizable properties, to offering a path to reject positivist-meaning holism and thus an escape from Kuhnian incommensurability. The descriptive elements in the identification of the base set preserve a link to observables but in a nonpositivist way that, reflecting scientific reality, allows category reference to go beyond any reductionistic tie to the observable. Consequently, the common scientific occurrence of being surprised by the novel way things with certain observable properties are theoretically categorized is explained by modest essentialism.

There is a problem for essentialism known as the *"qua"* problem (Devitt and Streleny 1987) that might be mistaken for indeterminacy or an opportunity for stipulation but is quite different and reveals the importance of an additional element of natural kind definitions. The *qua* problem arises from the fact that the very same baptized base set has many different levels and types of hidden explanatory structures that, if identified as the sought-after "nature" of the base set, determine various distinct categories: "Any sample of a natural kind is likely to be a sample of many natural kinds; for example, the sample is not only an echidna, but also a monotreme, a mammal, a vertebrate, and so on…a term refers to all objects having the same underlying nature as the objects in the sample. But which underlying nature? The samples share many" (Devitt and Streleny 1987, 73).

Putnam proposes that the relevant essence of a kind in a given context is determined by an additional often-implicit element of the definition, a "semantic marker"—or what I call an "ontological marker"—that specifies what kind of thing is being defined. · I agree with Putnam that many terms are used with a multiplicity of varying ontological markers indicating varying related kinds. Putnam embraces the resulting diversity and observes that for the same term and base set, the category reference can vary but remain determinate in each context based on the interests of those doing the defining ("in one context, 'water' may mean *chemically pure water,* while in another it may mean the stuff in Lake Michigan"), and he labels such judgments "interest-relative and context-sensitive" (Putnam 2015a, 80). These divergences occur in science as well as ordinary language: "'Is it part of the essence of dogs that they are descended from wolves?' The answer seems to be 'yes' from an evolutionary biologist's point of view and 'no' from a molecular biologist's point of view" (Putnam 2015b, 333).

It is important to keep in mind here that multiplicity is not the same as indeterminacy. Despite the plurality of ontological markers, there is not a stipulative free-for-all because in each context there is an anchoring in specific aspects of reality: "I believe that given the interests that structure the various natural sciences, some classifications are objectively more natural than others. This does not mean that all the natural sciences must use the same classification: a molecular biologist may legitimately classify organisms differently than an evolutionary biologist" (Putnam 2015c, 359).

Several critics raise the question of whether the concepts with which I deal are ordinary folk concepts or experts' scientific concepts. In the case of "medical disorder," I see no decisive *conceptual* separation between ordinary and professional technical concepts, although there are of course vast differences in ordinary and expert beliefs. This view is consistent with the essentialist view that science is often filling in the black boxes in vernacular essentialist concepts, but the concept itself generally stays the same and only the identification of the indirectly-referred-to essence is at stake: "Our language is a cooperative venture; and it would be a foolish layman who would be unwilling to ever accept correction from an expert on what was or was not water, or gold, or a mosquito, or whatever. ... Ordinary language and scientific language are different but *interdependent*" (Putnam 2015c, 361–362; see also Putnam 2015b, 333).

With this elaboration of a modest essentialism in hand, I turn to the question of whether or in what senses identifying the essence of natural functions allows for stipulated choice between the HDA and the biostatistical theory (BST).

Do the HDA and BST Offer Competing Theories of "Function"?

Because the HDA's evolutionary account of function and dysfunction is not a conceptual analysis, Lemoine leaps to the conclusion that it is no longer linked tightly to an analysis of meaning and that the evolutionary component of the HDA is in fact a sheer stipulation and should be explicitly pursued as such: "it is suggested that the 'conceptual analysis' approach be replaced by a full-fledged naturalist approach of mental disorder that is openly stipulative." To fill the proposed space open to stipulation, Lemoine thinks he can simply choose Boorse's (1987) "biostatistical theory" of disorder over the HDA as a better stipulation.

From the fact that the evolutionary account of function is not a conceptual analysis, it does not follow that it is a stipulation. According to the HDA's black-box essentialist analysis of "natural function," the evolutionary account of "natural function" is an explanatory scientific theory of the nature or essence of natural functions. Such theories are not stipulations in any usual sense of the word. They are scientific discoveries that are embraced on the basis of evidential support, explanatory power, and the scientific goals and methodological canons of a given scientific discipline. For example, the identity of the essence of water as the chemical structure H_2O is not a conceptual analysis, but neither is it a stipulation. Rather, it is a scientific discovery about the nature of water. It is embraced on the basis of a judgment that it is evidentially the best supported theory. Similarly, it is a matter of the scientific evidence and not stipulation whether evolution versus, say, creationism better specifies the essential nature of the process that explains biological design. In sum, the HDA's evolutionary component is best construed not as a stipulation or choice of how to think about functions but as a scientific theory of the nature of natural functions yielding biological design.

However, even if Lemoine accepts the black-box essentialist framework for formulating a theory of natural functions (in a later section, I will consider these issues apart from any essentialist assumptions), he could claim that the HDA and the BST are competing essentialist theories of this domain. If the BST is a viable alternative theory of natural functions, perhaps it could legitimately be "stipulated" or selected as the best available theory consistent with the constraints of scientific methodology and the goals of theory formation. Scientific domains are, after all, filled with rival theoretical formulations that compete for evidential vindication.

From a black-box essentialist perspective, the statistical-contribution-to-S&R and evolutionary theories in principle can be construed as essentialist scientific theories that attempt to explain adaptation, natural functions, and biological design, and they can be compared in terms of explanatory power and evidential support. Lemoine does not attempt such a comparison. However, on Lemoine's behalf, we might consider the following scenario. If Boorse's S&R theory of biological function and the HDA's evolutionary theory are construed as rival scientific theories of the same target domain of natural functions, but no clear deciding evidence exists, then one might imagine a "stipulation" of one or the other theory for certain purposes. Analogously, for example, at a point when there was genuine scientific uncertainty about whether the phlogiston theory or the oxidation theory of fire would prove to be true, in a discussion of fire, various theorists might simply have stipulated one theory or the other for the sake of that discussion.

However, to have such a situation in which stipulation might enter into theory selection, both theories would in fact have to be attempting to explain roughly the same domain of phenomena, and both would have to do a reasonably good job. That domain, which we saw in the discussion above, is the nature or essence of whatever explains the presence of biological design. The BST simply identities S&R-productive organismic features. Contrary to the "stipulation" scenario, it is a confusion to think that the HDA's evolutionary account and the BST's S&R account are plausibly construed as rival accounts of "natural function." They are in fact attempts to explain different things. In keeping with the analysis presented earlier, the target of the evolutionary account is to explain biological design. Whereas the BST account is explaining how the organism's nature causes it to have capacities for survival and reproduction, which, as it happens, are the two most salient domains of biological design. These are different explanatory problems of how biological design works.

What, then, even in very rough schematic form, would a black-box essentialist definition of "natural function" look like, and how is it different from a BST-type explanation? Let me approach this question via a well-known example of Aristotle's, that acorns have the remarkable ability under suitable circumstances to grow into oak trees, which in turn produce such acorns. That, one intuitively judges, can't be a mechanistic accident; this is such an unlikely and remarkable process that acorns in some sense must be "designed" to grow into oak trees. Aristotle understood that in explaining such a puzzling phenomenon, there are two different causal explanations required: efficient and final causes. Aristotle had no idea of the details of either explanation but understood that both types of explanation must be involved. The efficient cause of the acorn's turning into an oak tree is a standard causal explanation of how it works, addressing the puzzle of how an acorn can possibly produce an oak tree. The explanation will be couched in terms of the nature of the acorn's internal structures and parts, its interaction with the soil's nutrients, its positioning relative to sunlight, and so on. This explanation will be complex, and it will involve many initial conditions given that, according to some estimates, perhaps only 1 in 10,000 acorns actually grows into an oak tree even under standard conditions. The efficient causal explanation of how the parts of an acorn contribute to its ability to become an oak tree is the type of explanation provided by Cummins's causal role (CR) functions. And, because the acorn turning into an oak tree that in turn produces acorns is the act of reproduction of the oak tree that produced the acorn, the efficient causal explanation provides the Boorsean S&R biological functions of the parts of the acorn—that is, their contributions to the oak tree's S&R. A full efficient causal account will allow us to understand how this biologically designed acorn-to-oak-tree process works.

What is lacking here? How the acorn's nature explains its capacity to grow into an oak tree is one major scientific mystery, but it is not the only scientific mystery. Aristotle saw that a second scientific mystery—and perhaps the more profound one—is to explain what in nature shapes organisms to have parts with the specific causal powers that enable them to produce such design-like effects and contribute in such unlikely ways to S&R. This is a second-level explanatory mystery, and the inferred cause by which the end shapes the means is what Aristotle referred to as the "final cause." The problem Darwin addresses is analogous to this Aristotelian puzzle of final causation, which is the second-order causal puzzle of what causes organisms to have efficient causal properties that are instances of and produce biological design—for example, why things like acorns have an unlikely, coordinated, and remarkably complex system of causal powers such that they yield things like oak trees, where the entire process appears biologically designed. The final cause is not about how an acorn's structure gives it the power to become an oak tree but about how an acorn comes to have the kind of structure that enables it to become an oak tree when that very structure must in some way have been shaped by the very fact that they have that oak tree outcome. The challenge of natural functions, then, is the explanation of biological design, and natural functions are in the first instance the category of effects that are design-like. The mystery that Aristotle labeled "final causation" is what explains why the efficient causation by the acorn's parts has effects that are design-like. Functions as causal contributions to S&R offer an efficient-causal analysis of the most salient acknowledged domains of biological design. Functions as *naturally selected* contributions to S&R offer a final-causation analysis of biological design itself and explain why there are so many substantial S&R functions.

So, in a black-box essentialist vein, one might say: for an effect of an organism's feature to be a natural function of that feature is for it to be due to the right effect-sensitive causal process (i.e., a process in which the effect somehow causally shapes the feature's mechanisms that lead to it and where, in this case, the effect is part of the organism's biological design; I here alter Cummins and Roth's [2009] terminology of "function-sensitivity" that explains standard examples of biological design such as eyes seeing, hands grasping, and acorns growing into oak trees). The hypothesized process that explains why organisms have so many S&R functions that are structured in an apparently biologically designed way to produce biologically designed outcomes could have been some mystical inherent final-causation principle in the universe, or God's handiwork, or many other processes that have been proposed through the ages, but it turned out (based on the best scientific theory we have at present) to be natural selection. But, of course, that discovery of the essence of natural functions and biological design does not enter into the definition of the category in a black-box essentialist definition.

Consequently, whereas S&R functions are standard causal properties, natural functions presuppose second-order causal properties—that is, natural functions presuppose that there is a distinctive effect-sensitive causal explanation of the organism's features having certain distinctive kinds of the standard effects they have. This distinctive type of second-order causal explanation is precisely what evolutionary theory and natural selection provide. So, a first approximation to a black-box essentialist definition of "natural function" might look something like this: "*A natural function N of an organismic feature X is an S&R-function of X, the presence of which is at least partly explained by the same (presumptively) effect-sensitive natural process that explains the base set of instances of biological design, such as the presence of the eyes' S&R function of enabling sight, the hands' S&R function of enabling grasping, fear's S&R function of taking us away from danger, thirst's S&R function of causing us to seek out and drink water needed to survive, and an acorn's capacity to grow into an oak tree.*"

If this is correct, then there is no opportunity for the sort of stipulation Lemoine suggests, at least not within an essentialist framework for theorizing about the relevant function concept. This is because the BST and HDA are not rivals in explanatory competition. Rather, evolutionary theory and the BST's S&R functions address two different questions. The BST's S&R notion of function, basically a restriction of causal-role functions to those that contribute to the S&R of the organism, attempts to describe how the processes that constitute biological design work but has no capacity to explain what the concept of natural function addresses, namely, why such an ample number of S&R functions constituting biological design exist in the first place. So, one cannot choose to stipulate the BST as the account of "natural function" because it simply does not address that issue.

I provisionally conclude that S&R functions are not rivals to the etiological account of natural functions but rather address a different first-order domain of causal relations. If so, there is no room for stipulation of one theory over another because they are not competitors. Only evolutionary theory attempts to identify the essence referenced in the definition of natural function.

Boorse on the Explanatory Power of the BST

Naturally selected effect (NSE) function theorists hold that "function statements are intrinsically explanatory: to ascribe a function to a device is to offer an explanation of its presence" (Price 1995, 153). They thus object to the S&R account of "function" because, they claim, it offers no such explanations. However, Boorse (2002) disputes the claim that S&R functions "cannot accommodate functional explanation" (63) and have "insufficient explanatory power" (78) to match that of the NSE account aimed at explaining a feature's presence. Thus, the conclusion arrived at earlier that the NSE and S&R accounts are not rival explanatory accounts of "natural function" must remain provisional until Boorse's arguments that the two approaches provide similar explanatory power are considered.

Boorse first says, "In the first place, however, there was never any basis for assuming function statements to be inherently explanatory of anything, any more than statements about organisms, cells, … or most other objects of biology" (2002, 78). This is clearly not true specifically for natural functions, for which a 2,300-year tradition concerning final causation provides such a basis. We saw that in the case of natural functions, there is explanatory content both in the presumed effect sensitivity that explains a feature's nature or presence or maintenance and in the reference to an inferred natural process that explains why so many of such features yield apparent biological design. Boorse here simply begs the question.

Boorse proceeds: "In the second place, even if function statements have to be inherently explanatory, a satisfactory kind of non-etiological functional explanation is available: Cummins's functional analysis (1975), undeniably prominent in biological fields like physiology" (2002, 78). The attribution of a CR function does imply a causal role in producing the organisms' capacities and thus is explanatory in that way. However, as we saw, such CR functions are presupposed and built upon by the concept of natural function, which involves second-order causal attributions of the process that causes CR functions to come about in a way that yields biological design and is presumptively effect-sensitive. Citing the fact that CR functions have some causal explanatory power is thus a non sequitur with regard to the question of the specific forms of causal power attributed to natural functions.

Boorse further argues, "In the third place, that there are unselected biological functions is part of the current 'consensus'. … To attribute such functions is not to offer any etiological explanation. … Once one recognizes unevolved functions, their prevalence or rarity is, of course, an empirical question" (2002, 78). That is, the acknowledgment of CR functions (which I do acknowledge; see my response to Murphy in this volume) implies that not all things labeled "functions" are etiologically defined, and thus the general claim that functions must be etiological is defeated. However, this argument depends on interpreting the term "function" as univocal in meaning and as referring to S&R functions, where some functions as conceptual accidents just happen to have natural-function properties as well. This interpretation ignores the obvious possibility that S&R and NSE functions are two distinguishable senses of "function" with somewhat different meanings. Taking the latter approach, the "current consensus" is best understood as a consensus that biology uses "function" in two distinct senses (or perhaps in a primary NSE sense and a secondary derived synecdochical S&R or CR sense; see my reply to Murphy in this volume). If so, throwing all the uses together into one bin and pointing to the CR sense as evidence that functions need not be explanatory is a confused non sequitur that makes no more sense than, say, rejecting the assertion that "water is a liquid" on the grounds that the substance concept, "water," covers ice and steam as well as liquid water. Clearly, there is an alternative sense of "water" that refers strictly to the liquid (thus the waiter really has made a mistake if in response to a request for a glass of water, he delivers a glass of ice, although in a chemistry class, maybe that would be fine). In citing features of CR functions to dispute claims about natural functions, Boorse is similarly confusing matters by running together broader and narrower meanings of "function." This is further problematic in that it potentially obscures the precise senses of "function" and "dysfunction" that form the basis for medical judgments of health and disorder.

As a further point, Boorse says of S&R functions, "What the analysis does not do is to write even the existence of such an [evolutionary] explanation, let alone its details, into the meaning of the function statement itself. But there is no reason why it should....There is no reason why all the premises of a full evolutionary explanation, including background theory and initial conditions, must be part of a function statement's meaning" (2002, 80). I agree with Boorse (contra some etiological theorists) that it would be inappropriate for "a full evolutionary explanation" to be written into the concept of natural function. The concept "natural function" existed long before those evolutionary details were known, and surely its meaning makes no reference to those details. However, Boorse is incorrect in claiming that the analysis of "natural function" should not include reference to the existence of some effect-sensitive type of explanation. The concept of natural function rests on an inference to the existence of some such process that explains the bewildering existence of so many apparently adaptive S&R features that contribute to the quintessential biologically designed outcomes of survival and reproduction. The existence of effect-sensitive feature shaping is built into the meaning of the concept via the specification of the kind of shared "nature" that defines the category using base-set instances that exemplify biological design.

Boorse mounts another argument in defense of the explanatory power of S&R functions when he considers common function attributions, such as "the function of the giraffe's long neck is to reach up into the trees for food." Such a statement seems to be a way of explaining why the giraffe has a long neck, yet the S&R function attribution seems to offer no such explanations. Boorse (2002) argues that the explanation is indirect, arrived at by uniting the function attribution with what we know about the link between S&R functions and natural selection: "What I believe, with nearly all other current writers on biology, is the following: a disposition D of a trait type T causally to contribute to the goal of individual fitness can, via evolutionary theory, explain the prevalence of present tokens of T by D's manifestation in past tokens. Since such contribution is a GGC function, that immediately solves…the 'Explanation Problem' of 'understanding how ascribing a function to a biological trait can help explain the trait's existence'" (79); "However one explains the origin of traits like…long necks via their fitness benefits, any such evolutionary explanation is in terms of these organs' GGC functions—namely, their causal contributions to goals of the organism, survival and reproduction. So the GGC account has no defect of missing explanatory power" (80).

Boorse's argument here is, again, a non sequitur. He is of course correct that, generally speaking, certain S&R functions influenced natural selection and thus over evolutionary history explain biological design via natural selection. So, he is correct that if you conjoin the S&R function of a feature with evolutionary theory, then maybe you will get an explanation of the presence of the feature (but, as noted earlier, not always, because lots of current S&R functions are not the S&R effects that actually shaped the selection of a feature). However, first, S&R functions in themselves have no *conceptual* implications that involve any effect-sensitive process let alone natural selection as a directly or indirectly referenced process or outcome. This is why Aristotle felt the need to add the final cause to the efficient cause. If the goal is a conceptual analysis of "function," Boorse has now left that domain and is linking "function" to etiology via a scientific discovery, thus failing to place the claim of an effect-sensitive causal process within the meaning of "natural function." Second, this supposed solution depends on the details of Darwin's discoveries and thus cannot possibly explain how it was that for the 2,100 or so years between Aristotle and Darwin, there was a teleological notion of "natural function" and a continuing deep mystery of biological design, the unknown solution of which was implicitly referenced in the meaning of "natural function."

Boorse notes that in some contexts such as evolutionary biology, "one can *agree* to mean by 'the function of X' *the evolutionary function of X*. If so, one's function statements will have essential etiological explanatory force—they will be 'equivalent to' or 'tantamount to' an evolutionary explanation" (2002, 80). This seeming concession evades the issue. Of course, one can always stipulate a meaning of a term. However, this dispute is about the conceptual analysis of an existing meaning, not the possibility of stipulating a deviant meaning. Moreover, "function" had explanatory force before we understood evolutionary theory and so we would like to understand that meaning, which was not determined by an evolutionary context.

I conclude that Boorse's attempted rebuttal fails to counter the explanatory-power objection, and so the earlier conclusion can stand. The HDA and the BST are not explanatory rivals, and so there is no option to choose or stipulate between them. This conclusion does, however, pose an interesting question. If the BST and HDA are not theoretical rivals in the way most observers have assumed, then what precisely is their relationship? I will return to this question in my conclusions.

Essence Indeterminacy and the Limits of Stipulation

The idea that one might stipulate an essence is not an idiosyncratic notion of Lemoine's but the topic of an active philosophical literature. Before proceeding to the remainder of Lemoine's argument, I briefly consider the implications of that literature for Lemoine's claim.

When I argued for the evolutionary theory of function and dysfunction, I gave no thought to possible stipulated choices because I thought of the essence of "natural function" as being firmly fixed by Darwin's theory, which provides the only respectable scientific explanation of biological design. However, the philosophical literature raises the possibility that in linking a vernacular essentialist concept to a scientific theory of the relevant essence, the process can be more complicated than simply discovering *the* essence. As Wilson (1982) puts it, "The 'natural kind' doctrine makes the uniqueness of this [essential] property seem more likely than is reasonably plausible" (579).

Keith Donnellan (1983/2014) offers perhaps the most influential example of a possible indeterminacy and stipulation in essence identification. He argues that, when there are multiple ways of dividing things up to form essences, different background senses of what is important can yield different judgments about how best to translate vernacular concepts into the terms of a new theory. Donnellan constructs his argument in the context of an imagined Putnam-style "Twin Earth" situation, but to simplify matters—and for those unfamiliar with the Twin Earth scenario—I paraphrase Donnellan's thought experiment without his parallel-worlds apparatus.

Each atom of a given element has the same characteristic number of positively charged protons in its nucleus, which is the element's "atomic number" and largely determines its chemical properties. For this reason, the periodic table of elements is organized by periodicities in atomic number that determine similar patterns of chemical reactions. In addition to protons, the nucleus can also contain varying numbers of neutrally charged particles, "neutrons," where each number of neutrons determines an "isotope" of the element. Neutrons are about as massive as protons, so the "atomic weight" of the same element's isotopes varies (electrons are of negligible weight in this context). Although chemical reactions are generally similar across the isotopes of an element, there can be significant nonchemical differences. For example, some isotopes of an element can be radioactive and others not, and some isotopes can be unstable and break down into another element, whereas others are stable.

Given the possible differences among isotopes of an element, Donnellan argues that, despite the overwhelming importance of elements' atomic numbers for chemical reactions, in principle, for those with interests different from ours, "it might be a close question as to whether isotope number or atomic number has more importance" (197). Thus, he claims, it was a *choice* whether the periodic table was organized so that atomic numbers or atomic weights are the essences of elements.

Interestingly, this thought experiment comes close to describing an actual historical occurrence. When the elements' atomic weights were calculated for Mendeleev's original periodic table of elements, the average of available samples was used and so the atomic weights represented an amalgam of the weights of isotopes readily available on earth. This led to some anomalies in the grouping of elements in terms of chemical properties. In a momentous scientific advance, Henry Moseley figured out in 1913 that the anomalies were eliminated if atomic number rather than atomic weight was used as the organizing principle, yielding the modern periodic table.

Of more relevance to the translation of vernacular terms, Donnellan extends his argument to the chemical substance, water. Scientists have given the names "protium," "deuterium," and "tritium" to the three isotopes of hydrogen in which the nucleus, along with hydrogen's one proton, have zero, one, and two neutrons, respectively. Since all three can combine chemically with oxygen, there are three types of H_2O or "water": protium, deuterium, and tritium water (deuterium water is known as "heavy water"). Donnellan argues his analysis "can, obviously, be extended to the vernacular term 'water.' ... In my story, because isotopes are taken more seriously for one or another practical or historical reason, we can suppose that [we] will identify water with protium oxide and exclude what we call 'heavy water'—deuterium or tritium oxide" (Donnellan 1983/2014, 198). That this might have been an option makes some sense because earth's water is almost entirely protium water (99.98%), with a little deuterium "heavy water" thrown in (tritium is unstable and rare). Moreover, although protium and deuterium water have the same basic pattern of chemical reactions, there are some differences in the rate of some chemical reactions that can make a difference to the health of an organism. A glass of heavy water is harmless, but about 50% replacement of protium water with heavy water can be lethal. Also, heavy water plays a unique role in certain types of nuclear reactors. These practical nonchemical differences led Donnellan to argue that despite the importance of atomic numbers in explaining chemical reactions, in principle, scientists might judge that isotope number has more importance in identifying the essence of water. Thus, he claims, it was to some degree a *choice* to identify water (as understood in the vernacular) with the substance H_2O (including all hydrogen-isotope variations) rather than identifying water exclusively with protium water and leaving deuterium and tritium H_2O outside of the "water" category altogether.

Donnellan concludes his analysis with the following thoughts:

What do I conclude from my story? I do not draw the conclusion that Putnam has failed to describe how natural kind terms in the vernacular function. The story does not show that. But ... there is a certain slackness in the machinery which Putnam does not, I feel, prepare us for. ... The slackness comes from how ordinary language terms for kinds are mapped onto the same classifications. In my story I have envisaged only a small wobble; how much latitude there might be in theory I do not know. ... The "slackness" I have talked about seems to allow that from the very same linguistic base we may, after the very same scientific discoveries, move in different directions. (1983/2014, 199–200)

Donnellan's argument leaves the door ajar for possible stipulation in essence identification. However, his conclusion does not support Lemoine's exuberant claims. The indeterminacy Donnellan identifies merely indicates "a certain slackness...from how ordinary language terms for kinds are mapped onto" new scientific classifications and represents a "small wobble" from the standard determinate essentialist story (although he leaves open how large a wobble is possible). Rather than freely selecting from among alternative competing theories of water, there is one overwhelmingly supported chemical theory of water, but the discovery of isotopes, unanticipated by the vernacular concept's pretheoretical background assumptions, led to ambiguities in precisely how to map water onto chemical theory. If Donnellan is correct, then some rectification of chemical theory and the vernacular concept of water is required. Whether the rectification allows for stipulation in accordance with external interests as Donnellan suggests or is decided for chemists by the canons of scientific theory formation as Putnam holds remains disputed, as we shall see. Either way, the ambiguity is limited by the fact that it occurs within a theory that overall is understood to identify the nature of water. Although Donnellan argues that it is open to stipulation whether water is all of H_2O or just protium H_2O, he accepts that science has discovered, not stipulated, that the water is H_2O in some form that includes protium.

Joseph LaPorte (2004) systematically expands the Donnellan type of argument to additional areas of science and makes the case that essence indeterminacy often dominates over scientific discovery in identification of essences of vernacular kinds. Going beyond the standard element and substance-type examples, LaPorte argues, for example, that biologists, consistent with the discoveries they have made but contrary to their actual decisions, might have chosen to classify whales as fish and guinea pigs as rodents, yielding different essences of vernacular kinds. LaPorte distinguishes such classificatory decisions from changes in the meaning of a term, which everyone agrees can occur. Rather, there are areas of inherent boundary fuzziness in the vernacular concept yielding a choice of how to form categories. A theory of essence can be stipulated to resolve those ambiguous fuzzy cases one way or another, thus "precisifying" the concept rather than changing the term's meaning.

Alexander Bird (2010) lucidly summarizes LaPorte's position as follows:

> Concentrating on theoretical identities such as 'water is H2O', LaPorte argues that there is considerable vagueness in the use of kind terms, especially vernacular kind terms....For a kind term 'K', some things will be determinately K and other things will be determinately not K. But there will be a boundary of things for which there is no determinate fact of the matter whether they are K or not....According to LaPorte, when a natural kind identity is established as being determinately true, that is because scientists have made a *decision* to adopt the identity as true. In so doing, it will now be determined of items that were previously in the boundary (neither K nor not-K) whether they are K or not. For example, we now regard heavy water (deuterium oxide [D_2O]) as a subspecies of water; but scientists could have decided to exclude deuterium

oxide from the extension of 'water'. So 'water is H2O' is true in virtue of a decision. That truth…is not the discovery of some previously hidden essence. Rather, it is an empirically motivated *stipulation*. (2010, 125)

Bird objects to LaPorte's view that "there is rather less room for conceptual choice and stipulation than LaPorte supposes" (125), for two reasons. First, the fuzzy boundary area is limited, so there is limited freedom for stipulative precisification: "Vagueness between red and orange leaves it determinate nonetheless that a ripe tomato is red. … The concept water may have open texture so that it is not determinate whether D_2O is water. But that is consistent with its being determinate that all water is H_2O" (Bird 2010, 135).

Second, science is more determinate than it seems because it eschews the kinds of practical concerns cited by LaPorte and others (e.g., Zachar 2002) as grounds for essence indeterminacy. Here Bird follows Putnam in holding that scientists have methodological standards for determining essences that are distinct from general interests. Bird argues that any choice other than identifying water with H_2O would violate the scientific canon that requires chemists to determine substances based strictly on chemical theoretical properties: "it will be chemical facts that determine the identity of substances. The chemical facts class D_2O with other kinds of H_2O" (2010, 127). Bird argues that, because the differences between D_2O and protium water primarily "come from outside chemistry," they "are not pertinent to the science whose job it is to investigate the nature of and to classify water" (2010, 127–128).

Bird's point seems fundamental. It is difficult to imagine how science could progress otherwise. The introduction into chemical theory of considerations of human concerns or practical uses would introduce myriad issues distant from what is needed to identify the classification that offers the deepest and most perspicuous understanding of how the world works. Such an approach would hobble the kind of scientific theory development that is chemistry's task. Practical concerns should be and are reflected in other available concepts and terminology but not in chemical theory per se. Thus, the nature of science's own standards for successful theory sets a limit on the scope for stipulation in essence identification.

Whatever one thinks of Bird's or Putnam's responses, the examples presented by Donnellan and LaPorte at least raise the possibility—if not in the discussed examples, then perhaps elsewhere—of the need for rectification of some degree of indeterminacy and stipulation in essence identification due to theoretical anomalies relative to vernacular background assumptions. However, the scope of indeterminacy suggested by these arguments is quite limited and does not alter the big picture of scientific accounts of essence. Even for Donnellan and LaPorte, water is a form of H_2O. None of the surveyed arguments open Lemoine's stipulationist spigot to radically different theories. There is nothing in this fascinating literature that would cast doubt on the overwhelming scientific primacy of the evolutionary explanation of the nature of natural functions. However, even if the evolutionary account is inevitably the theory of the essence of natural functions, these debates suggest that there could there be a degree of indeterminacy and possible stipulation in the precise specification of the evolutionary essence of function. If so, this remains unexplored territory.

So, where does this leave Lemoine's first core claim that, because the HDA's evolutionary theory of function and dysfunction is not a conceptual analysis, one can choose to stipulate Boorse's biostatistical theory (BST) of function rather than the HDA's evolutionary account of function, as one pleases? The literature suggests that even if in rare cases stipulation is an option, its scope is quite limited and intratheoretic, concerned with nuanced indeterminacies in how the terms of a dominant essentialist theory are precisely mapped onto pretheoretical concepts and not a matter of freely selecting among theories. There can be little question that evolutionary theory is the dominant theory that explains the essential nature of natural functions and biological design. We have seen that the BST cannot be considered an alternative theory of the essence of "natural function" in the relevant sense because it does not correspond to the right kind of explanatory essence. The BST, being a variant of Cummins's CR-function approach, is by its nature not explanatory at the same level, Boorse's claims to the contrary notwithstanding. So, there is no competition and no support for Lemoine's proposed stipulative choice of the BST over the HDA as an account of "function" or his suggestion of a stipulative free-for-all. If there is any minimal domain of detail of terminological mapping open to stipulation, it is insufficient to support Lemoine's ambitious claims and poses no threat to the HDA's evolutionary component.

Is the BST a Better Naturalist Account of Dysfunction Than the HDA?

In the final section of his paper, Lemoine pivots from his focus on the HDA's account of dysfunction as a mere stipulation to a straightforward argument that the BST's statistical account is superior to the HDA's evolutionary component as a naturalistic account of dysfunction: *"Boorse's account of dysfunction is better than Wakefield's as a naturalist explication of the concept of dysfunction."* For those who, like Lemoine, have naturalist aspirations, this question of whether the evolutionary or statistical approach provides the best naturalist account of dysfunction is a crucial issue.

Lemoine argues that although the concept of evolutionary dysfunction is in principle not dependent on the concept of harm ("It is easy to understand how an ultimate evolutionary theory of what is dysfunctional could be contrasted with what we consider to be harmful or not"), we are unable, due to our relative ignorance of psychological and physiological causal mechanisms, to make dysfunction claims that do not rely on harm as a heuristic for dysfunction ("it is not easy to understand how we can consider dysfunctional states and harmful states to be different things in an imperfect state of knowledge"). (This criticism was also posed by De Block and Sholl in their chapter and addressed in my reply in this volume.) Lemoine then asks whether the HDA has any strictly naturalist approach to identifying dysfunction without reliance on harm. He answers that, once divorced of the harm criterion, and given our ignorance of mechanisms and evolutionary history, the evolutionary account must rely on the BST's statistical approach to get off the ground, so the BST is the superior naturalist account.

Lemoine can think of only two possible harm-independent naturalist ways to recognize that a mechanism is failing to perform its natural function. The first way is by a statistical comparison of the mechanism's performance to the performances of analogous mechanisms in promoting survival and reproduction (S&R) in some reference class of other individuals; this is the naturalist statistical criterion proposed by Boorse. The second way is by directly appraising the degree to which the actual performance replaces and runs contrary to the presumed natural function of the underlying mechanism; this naturalist failure-of-function criterion is the one proposed by me. However, Lemoine argues that the failure-of-function criterion presumes knowledge of the proper natural functioning of the underlying mechanism, but "in an imperfect state of knowledge" (as Lemoine describes our situation of ignorance about most internal mechanisms and their functions), we do not have such knowledge, and so the HDA's distinctive failure-of-function approach cannot be used. Thus, the only way to appraise failure of function is to use Boorse's statistical comparison method to establish what is normal functioning: "I think that the only naturalist way to distinguish between non-natural and harmful effects of a mechanism in an imperfect state of knowledge is to adopt Boorse's biostatistical views on dysfunction."

Lemoine's analysis seems to run together conceptual and epistemological issues. Both the BST and the HDA aim to address the conceptual question of the nature of normal function and dysfunction. Lemoine's argument concerns the epistemological question of how we identify a dysfunction in circumstances of ignorance. However, Lemoine might reply that if the BST's conceptual analysis better illuminates the epistemology of dysfunction identification as we know it, then to this extent, it is a better account of the concept we actually use. So, I will take Lemoine's epistemological analysis as an indirect conceptual claim based on the claimed superiority of the BST in explaining dysfunction identification. I will return to the epistemological issue at the end of my analysis.

The HDA versus the BST on Setting the Mean and Range of Normal Functioning

Lemoine's argument that the evolutionary view ultimately must depend on statistics is based on his intuition that there is no other way to decide what is a normal function versus dysfunction. However, his argument needs elaboration and evaluation. Fortunately, the view that the evolutionary view ultimately rests on the statistical view has also been defended by Boorse himself, who claims that there are "reasons to think that no evolutionary approach can analyze biomedical normality without appealing to statistics, as I do" (2002, 101). So, to understand how one might defend Lemoine's claim, I examine Boorse's arguments for the same point.

Boorse's primary argument is that a purely evolutionary account, unlike a statistical account, cannot "determine the mean and endpoints of normal function.... Even theoretically, it seems impossible... to avoid statistics" (2002, 101). He first considers the mean, asking, "How can evolution alone locate the mean of, say, normal human visual acuity?" (2002, 101). He pursues this question by analyzing a discussion of Neander's (1991b) on why penguins have poor vision when on land, Neander's answer being that their vision is primarily designed for seeing underwater in order to catch fish, and poor vision on land is a by-product of the way penguins' eyes were biologically designed in response to selective pressure for water vision. In response, Boorse says, "Neander confuses two questions: what the normal level of penguin vision is, and how one explains its origin. Penguin land myopia is normal because it is typical of penguins, not because it is somehow endorsed by evolution as a byproduct of something else, underwater visual acuity" (101–102).

However, it is Boorse who confuses two questions: what is the current statistically typical level of penguin visual acuity on land, and what is the biologically designed normal level of acuity? To that extent, the BST represents a confusion of the concepts of statistical normality and functional normality. That penguins statistically see with modest visual acuity on land can have several explanations, only one of which is that their eyes are biologically designed to see with that acuity on land. Alternative hypotheses tend to be improbable, and given the reach of biological design, we generally rely on what is statistically typical as the defeasible default hypothesis to tell us what is likely normal. However, various alternatives lurk in the background and reveal that the typical need not be the normal. For example, one alternative hypothesis— analogous to there being almost universal gum disease and tooth decay—is that penguins are subject to an almost universal eye infection that limits visual acuity on land. Another is that environmental conditions have changed in a way that creates vision-obscuring atmospheric distortions or allergens in the penguin habitats that has reduced penguins' previously much sharper terrestrial vision. A third is that penguins now suffer from a critical-period developmental dysfunction due to lack of some expectable stimulation that triggers development of greater land-based visual acuity, in the way that early close-focus visual experiences may cause near-sightedness in humans.

Boorse asks, "If it is as easy as Neander thinks for whole species to be diseased, why are penguins not diseased for not seeing well both on land and in the sea?... Why was that genetic deficiency not itself a pandemic penguin disease?" (2002, 101). The answer is that there was no "genetic deficiency." The level of visual acuity on land results from or is a by-product of the way penguins' visual system is biologically designed through natural selection and can be explained by the pattern of selective pressures exerted on the penguin population. The answer to Boorse's first question is that the mean of normality on a dimension is determined by the mean of the range for which it was naturally selected.

Boorse's second question concerns the range of normal function: "How can a purely evolutionary concept set boundaries to the normal range? If we seek to capture the biomedical idea of normality, it must be possible to have even pathologically myopic penguins.... So how does penguins' evolutionary history determine a lower limit of normal penguin myopia? Pending such an explanation, I conclude that ... even an etiological theory requires a concept of statistical normality to match basic logical features of biomedical concepts" (2002, 102).

Again, the answer at a theoretical level is obvious. Although there will be a fuzzy boundary zone as there is for most legitimate conceptual distinctions (day/night, red/ orange, child/adult), the setting of the normal range is basically a matter of judging the range over which positive selective pressures played a significant role in shaping the capacity in question through an effect-sensitive causal process. Boorse's "in theory" challenge is thus answered, although Lemoine's question about how this works in a state of ignorance still needs to be addressed (see below).

There is an irony in Boorse's critique of the evolutionary account for not specifying the range of normality. Boorse fails to consider how well the statistical view does in comparison, and it seems assumed that a statistical view must automatically resolve statistical-like questions about range. However, in fact, Boorse's statistical view has no answer to the question of how to set the range of normality of a function, declaring the boundary between normal function and dysfunction to be wholly arbitrary: "the lower limit of normal functional ability—the line between normal and pathological—is arbitrary" (1987, 371); "the term 'normal functional ability' had been defined dispositionally, as the readiness of an internal part to perform all its normal functions on typical occasions with at least typical efficiency. 'Typical efficiency' of a part-function, in turn, is efficiency above some arbitrarily chosen minimum in its species distribution" (1997, 8); "the BST is consistent with disease prevalence of 35%, 20%, 5%, 1%, or, I suppose, even 0%, and with prevalence varying from disease to disease. What it is inconsistent with is prevalences ≥50%" (2014, 714). According to the BST, the prevalence of dysfunction for any function can be decided arbitrarily anywhere from 0% to 49%, and there is no further conceptual reason or justification for favoring any given level, only pragmatic reasons extraneous to the concept of dysfunction itself.

These limitations of the BST mean that accepting Boorse's—and Lemoine's— position would be disastrous for achieving one of the primary goals that motivated the search for a definition of disorder in the first place: to limit false-positive diagnoses in which social deviance is mislabeled mental disorder and thus to respond to antipsychiatric claims that psychiatric diagnosis is misused for social control purposes by creating overly inclusive categories. Boorse's view provides a conceptual warrant for arbitrarily pathologizing up to half the population on every single functional variable without any conceptual recourse, a breathtakingly ill-considered approach.

The Pandemic Disease Objection to a Statistical Criterion for Dysfunction

The above discussion of the range of normality indicates a bewildering feature of the BST's statistical approach to dysfunction. The BST's statistical subtypicality account of dysfunction implies that a dysfunction cannot be typical; that is, it cannot occur in more than half of the population. Critics have rightfully taken this claim to be demonstrably false and argued that there is nothing contradictory or even puzzling about statistically common disorders: "There is nothing incoherent in the idea of typical dysfunction, as our concepts of epidemics and pandemics attest" (Neander 2012, 2). If correct, this objection implies that, although most dysfunctions are subtypical, there must be some criterion beyond statistics that forms a backbone for the concepts of function and dysfunction and overrides the statistical approach.

Lemoine ignores this problem, whereas Boorse, to his credit, squarely confronts this problem, admitting that, contrary to the BST, the concept of medical disorder clearly allows for dysfunctions occurring in a majority of a species: "Any account of normality must concede that medicine recognizes a tiny number of diseases that are typical or even universal, either in the whole species (atherosclerosis) or in an age group (osteoarthritis or prostatic cancer in men of a certain age)" (2002, 102–103).

The problem is larger than Boorse suggests. First, the list of such pandemic conditions could easily be expanded beyond Boorse's "tiny" number. For example, tooth decay and gum disease afflict about 90% of humanity and apparently have for a long time, judging from jawbone and tooth remains, and Boorse elsewhere notes that, on his view, if children generally suffer bruised knees, that pandemic condition would not be a disorder. (I note in passing that if Boorse were correct that any dysfunction is a disorder, then the problem would be much larger because there are many pandemic dysfunctions, such as mutations in skin DNA due to sunlight exposure or some number of dysfunctional sperm, that would then constitute pandemic disorders, but since he is plainly incorrect—a pathologist would label a sperm without a tail as a dysfunctional sperm but not thereby necessarily label the individual as medically disordered because there is no harm—I leave this problem aside.) Boorse uses the example of prostate cancer, but the disorder of benign prostatic hyperplasia, which can obstruct urine flow to the point of retention and can lead to kidney damage, is a better example, with about half of men in their fifties and about 90% of men in their eighties suffering from this condition. Second, given that Boorse claims that the BST is a conceptual analysis, an additional problem is the endless number of *possible* pandemic diseases one can easily imagine developing or being discovered. For example, one can easily imagine humanity generally suffering from a dramatic increase in antibiotic-resistant infections coincident with the worldwide spread of infectious disorders due to global warming or the discovery of formerly unrecognized almost universal parasites. Though counterfactual, such examples of what is clearly possible represent legitimate counterexamples to the BST.

So, how does Boorse address this issue? Rather than conceding that the existence of medically acknowledged pandemic disorders requires abandonment or modification of a statistical view of disorder, he says that "the question is how we should explain this fact" (2002, 102–103). He notes that he has changed his mind more than once on the explanation and offers his then-latest view: "I currently favor the view that medicine is wrong to recognize any universal diseases, since it lacks any coherent concept of pathology that can make them pathological. On this view, what is pathological is only age excessive atherosclerosis, premature prostate cancer, and so on … I will embrace the conclusion of my analysis. If nearly all human left legs have been broken throughout human history … , then that is their normal condition" (2002, 103). Thus, in the face of seemingly conclusive counterexamples, Boorse offers no explanation but rather simply insists on his view and rejects the judgments of the medical field. Nothing Lemoine says extricates him from this problem with the statistical view. The most plausible "explanation" of the facts is simply that Boorse's analysis is incorrect. As to Boorse's claim that there is no coherent view that explains the conceptual possibility of pandemics, of course he is wrong there too, for the HDA's evolutionary account readily explains such judgments.

Reference Classes and the Myth of a Statistical Theory of Dysfunction

I now come to the foundation of the statistical approach to distinguishing normal function from dysfunction endorsed by Lemoine, namely, the process by which the typical and subtypical are statistically identified. To understand why Lemoine's faith that evolutionary judgments must rest on the BST's statistical judgments is misguided, one needs to examine the conceptual bedrock underlying the statistical judgments themselves. So, in this section, I examine Boorse's notions of normality and dysfunction and the BST's critical notion of "reference classes" that underlies the identification of the statistically typical and subtypical.

Boorse defines normal function and dysfunction in strictly statistical terms of typical versus atypical levels of contribution to survival and reproduction (S&R): "normal function of a part or process is a statistically typical contribution by it to their individual survival and reproduction" (1977, 555); "medically normal function of any token item (for example, a single human heart) is analyzable as an output within a statistically typical range of contributions to survival and reproduction by tokens of that type in an age group of a sex of a species" (2002, 72); "what is pathological in medicine is statistically subnormal … function" (2002, 94).

A basic challenge for the BST's statistical conception of dysfunction is that statistical typicality and deviance measures vary depending on the "reference class" that forms the background for the measure. For example, relative to sighted people, a blind person has eyes that make a subtypical contribution to S&R, but relative to other blind people, a blind person's eyes may make a typical contribution to S&R. So, for a statistical account of dysfunction as subtypical S&R contribution to make sense, an account must be provided of the reference classes on which the statistical claims are based. The reference class cannot simply be the entire human race because, for example, then children who normally have less capability than adults could be labeled as dysfunctional and women (who comprise slightly less than half the world population) could be classified as having a dysfunction due to their lack of various male organs and processes. Thus, some more refined reference class must be defined to distinguish normal function from dysfunction. Boorse is well aware that his account of normal function and dysfunction requires the specification of such reference classes: "I make normal function in physiology or medicine a statistical concept, involving generalization over a reference-class. I defined medical normality as 'the readiness of each internal part to perform all its normal functions on typical occasions with at least typical efficiency'—that is, at an efficiency level not far below the reference-class mean" (2002, 90).

The problem for the BST is how to identify such reference classes in a way that yields results consonant with medical intuitions without invoking evolutionary theory. For example, benign prostate hyperplasia (BPH) is considered a disorder, according to the HDA, based on the judgment that in BPH, the biologically designed functioning of the urinary and prostate system is harmfully failing. This evolutionary judgment, Lemoine would claim, is based on the statistical abnormality of the features of urinary and prostate functioning in BPH. However, relative to what reference class is BPH statistically subtypical functioning? One cannot use all human beings as the reference class because half are women without prostate glands, and that lack is not a dysfunction. Nor can one use all males because children do not yet have fully functioning prostates and would skew the results. At the other extreme, if one uses just those males who present for urinary flow problems, then what is truly a dysfunction would be classified as statistically typical and thus normal. So, one has to choose the group that is "just right." If that class is all male adults, then BPH is statistically infrequent. If it is limited to the age-sex class of males over fifty years old, then more than half have some degree of BPH and (counterintuitively) it would not be a disorder in that age-sex cohort, according to the statistical approach. So, the identification of reference classes is crucial for the statistical view.

"For medical purposes," Boorse defines a reference class as "a natural class of organisms of uniform functional design: specifically, an age group of a sex of a species" (Boorse 1977, 555; Boorse 2002, 90). Note that the use of the term "functional" in "uniform functional design" is not circular or begging the question of how to establish normal function versus dysfunction because all that "functional" means for Boorse is the causal contributions made by various parts under various circumstances to S&R. Thus, "design" with its evolutionary connotation is a bit misleadingly teleological, and elsewhere Boorse uses "functional organization" in explaining what he means: "Once one knows that functions are causal contributions to goals of the organism, one can classify the functional organization of different individuals—that is, the ways their parts contribute to their survival and reproduction—as similar or dissimilar" (2002, 91). In theory, the levels of such contributions under varying circumstances can be established independently of and without any reference to normality versus dysfunction, which are identified at a later stage of the analysis by the levels of contribution to S&R in the reference class that are typical and subtypical, respectively.

Boorse's above definition of reference classes contains two criteria. He first specifies that the class must be of "uniform functional design" and then elaborates that it is, "specifically, an age group of a sex of a species." This raises the question of the relationship between the two criteria, and which is primary. The "uniform functional design" criterion is clearly intended as the rationale for the specific sex and age dimensions of the reference classes; otherwise, the specification of age and sex appears arbitrary. However, in "specifically" indicating age and sex subgroups, Boorse appears to be claiming that these are the only dimensions that yield reference classes of uniform functional design, or at least the ones he is selecting as relevant to medical judgments. (He at times has suggested that perhaps race would be another such dimension, but I set that issue aside here.) However, it is not obvious that limiting reference classes to sex and age dimensions follows from the "similar functional organization" criterion. Consequently, given the potential divergence between the two criteria, in evaluating Boorse's approach to reference classes, it seems charitable to consider separately each of the two possible approaches he suggests, one that specifies that reference classes are limited to age and sex categories, and the other that relies on the general characterization of "uniform functional organization."

I start by evaluating the specification of age and sex categories as the unique reference classes. The idea that age and sex divisions are legitimate reference class divisions may seem innocent enough given that these groupings (e.g., male versus female, child versus adult) have evolutionarily shaped differences. However, using age and sex reference classes independently of evolutionary judgments allows diagnostic absurdities that are inconsistent with medical thinking and thus falsify the statistical view.

First, if reference classes are limited to age and sex categories, then all those naturally selected features that result from such processes as niche selection or balancing selection are in danger of being considered dysfunctions by virtue of their comparison to typical functioning in species-level age and sex categories. Yet, these processes produce specific adaptive features in response to specific environmental contexts—for example, lactose tolerance in cultures with the availability of milk, sickle cell trait in environments with endemic malaria, blood alterations in high altitudes—that are considered normal functioning and not disorders. Age and sex reference classes cannot take account of more fine-grained normality based on such niche natural selection.

Another domain of falsifications concerns the BST's prediction of allowable age-dependent medical diagnoses. If the BST were correct, then whether a kind of condition could be considered a disorder in a given age cohort would depend on the statistics of the condition at that age, and the answer can vary from age to age. One could delay coming to the physician for a year and find that one's condition, which has stayed entirely constant, was a disorder the year before but is no longer so because it afflicts the majority at your older age. Aside from Boorse's examples mentioned earlier of children with bruised knees and prostate cancer or atherosclerosis in the elderly not being disorders, it is possible that, before the advent of vaccination, children of a certain age who contracted measles and elderly who contracted pneumonia were not disordered by the statistical criterion. None of these predictions comport with medical thinking.

Moreover, for many developmental stages, from puberty and menopause to children learning to walk or speak, there is enormous normal variation in the age at which the changes occur and physicians do not consider such variations in themselves to be disorders. However, the BST, using age to define reference classes, potentially pathologizes almost half of the normal-variation population. For example, the age of onset of puberty in females and thus the capacity for childbearing, which has direct S&R implications, varies greatly, and there is an age at which puberty has occurred in the majority of females and thus has become species typical, so the BST using age cohorts for reference classes allows all those who are still not pubescent because they fall in the later part of the onset curve to be classified as disordered. (Thus, age-cohort reference classes undermine any advantage Boorse might claim for the statistical account's ability to yield means for typical functioning.)

Needless to say, this is simply not how medical diagnosis works. Medicine considers such differences in age of reaching developmental milestones up to a point to be normal variation and generally does not change a diagnosis in response to the changing statistics at the patient's age. Given that Boorse presents the BST as a conceptual analysis of medical thinking, these radical divergences from medical thinking are legitimate counterexamples that falsify the BST.

The age-and-sex account of reference classes is thus both too refined and too unrefined. It is falsified both by the existence of normal naturally selected categories (e.g., lactose tolerance) that require more refined reference classes and by the pathologization of normal variation (e.g., age of puberty) that occurs with the use of overly refined age cohorts as reference classes. These falsifications are avoided by the evolutionary natural-function approach.

This suggests that the more charitable interpretation of Boorse's view may be to abandon the age-and-sex approach to reference classes and give priority to the more abstract "uniform functional organization" characterization of reference classes, to which I now turn. Despite Boorse's equating of the two approaches, they diverge because functional organization in Boorse's sense of a part's contribution to S&R can vary enormously within sex and age categories, yielding "similar functional organization" reference classes that do not correspond to age and sex categories. For example, twenty-five-year-old women who are blind do not have the same functional organization as normally sighted women of the same age, given that their eyes and their senses of hearing and touch perform such different roles in their survival and reproduction, nor does the pancreas play the same functional role in those with and without diabetes. This problem is not limited to disorders that confer distinct functional organizations but also applies to myriad normal variations. For example, physical appearance plays a different functional organizational role in those who are attractive versus those who are homely, and anxiety plays a different functional role in those high and low on normal-range neuroticism. So, given Boorse's definition of "uniform functional design" as similar contributions of the parts to S&R, reference class distinctions can go well beyond sex and age differences.

The implications of this proliferation of potential reference classes for the statistical view of normal function versus dysfunction are devastating. For example, consider again the distinction between blind and normally sighted twenty-five-year-old females. If they were included in the same reference class of twenty-five-year-old females, then the former women could be judged as having a vision dysfunction because of a lesser contribution to S&R by their eyes relative to others' eyes in that reference class. (It is not clear what one would say about females born without eyes, but I leave that sort of complication aside.) However, as noted, it would seem that the two groups of women do not have similar functional organizations by Boorse's criterion because of the radically different roles that their eyes and other senses play in promoting S&R. Thus, according to the uniform-functional-organization criterion, the blind women would (or could) be placed in a distinct reference class of blind female adults and not the same reference class with sighted female adults. This creates a major problem for the statistical view, because within the reference class of blind female adults, a given blind woman's eyes may well make a typical (low) level of S&R contribution and so she would not be judged to be subtypical and would not be considered to have a vision dysfunction—even though in fact she is blind and has an obvious dysfunction and medical disorder. There are endless variations in functional design—indeed, almost any significant genetic variation may define a distinct functional design (in the sense of a distinct pattern of the parts' contribution to S&R)—implying that reference classes will proliferate, dividing along myriad lines ranging from darkly pigmented skin versus less pigmented skin to pygmy versus Watusi height and morning people versus night people, and so on.

The problem this poses for the statistical view is that if reference classes can be so fine-grained, then the entire system for recognizing dysfunctions as subtypical functional contribution collapses because dysfunction, from kidney failure to schizo-phrenia, generally implies a different functional organization than those with nor-mal functioning. That is, the uniform-functional-organization criterion for reference classes threatens to create separate baselines of "normal" functioning for every signifi-cant human variation, including every significant genetic normal variation but also every significant dysfunction, thus effectively erasing the distinction between medical disorder and health and undermining the very point of the statistical analysis.

Note that it would be circular for Boorse to try to escape this problem by saying that the blind and the sighted are of uniform design and belong in the same reference class but only seem different because one group has a dysfunction that interferes with that design, because at this stage of the analysis, there is not yet a concept of dysfunction available; the whole point of independently defining the reference classes is to then identify normal function versus dysfunction. Thus, Neander argues that Boorse's defi-nition of reference classes "involves an intolerable circularity" (Neander 1983, 94): "For instance, those with adult onset diabetes might be said to have a 'uniform functional design', if we consider just the actual causal roles of traits. But we would not want to count those with adult-onset diabetes as a distinct reference class or else it will follow that their condition would then count as normal. How to discount this reference class, however, but for the fact that the peculiarities in functioning of those in the class are dysfunctions? One can speak of what is normal in the sense of typical for adult-onset diabetes, but what is normal in the sense of typical for those with adult-onset diabetes involves malfunction" (Neander 2012, 1).

If it seems remotely possible that diabetics and nondiabetics might be seen as having similar functional organizations, then consider more extreme cases such as the class of individuals with the lack of both sight and hearing, such as Helen Keller, or the class of individuals born without multiple limbs (e.g., due to their mothers taking thalido-mide). There seems to be no way, without prior reference to natural functions and dys-function, to argue that such individuals have the same functional organization as the functionally normal individuals without those infirmities and thus no noncircular way to distinguish the dysfunctions from the normal functions using the statistical approach. The only sense in which those without sight and hearing are similar in functional orga-nization to those with intact senses is if one equates their functional organization with their evolutionary biological design and observes that the deviations are not part of bio-logical design. That, however, would be to admit that the statistical view cannot succeed without reference to evolutionary presuppositions.

Boorse attempts to answer the reference-class circularity objection by explaining that he doesn't need to know what a dysfunction is prior to judging uniformity of functional design and forming reference classes: "The circularity charge rests on a con-fusion. Once one knows that functions are causal contributions to goals of the organ-ism, one can classify the functional organization of different individuals—that is, the ways their parts contribute to their survival and reproduction—as similar or dissimilar" (2002, 91).

This answer does not resolve the problem. It is true, as noted above, that there is no circularity in the reference to "functional design" because Boorse defines that as the pattern of S&R contributions, which does not presuppose anything about normality versus dysfunction. The problem lies with "uniform." It begs the question for Boorse to assume without any explanatory account that, say, the blind will be judged similarly enough functionally organized to be placed in a common reference group with the sighted so that the they come out statistically dysfunctional relative to the others in their reference group. Some severe pathologies are likely to be judged organizationally different from normality no matter where the "similarity" boundary is located, and then they will be placed in their own reference classes in which they are statistically typical, misclassifying them as normally functioning.

The statistical view using the uniform-functional-organization criterion for reference class formulation, like the age-and-sex account of reference classes considered earlier, fails to explain the distinction between dysfunction and normal function in a way that is noncircular, properly reflects medical judgments, and does not rely on prior evolutionary considerations of biological design. I conclude that the statistical account of dysfunction on which Lemoine rests his case against the HDA has no coherent foundation without reference to the HDA's evolutionary considerations.

Conclusion

Lemoine is surely correct that statistical comparisons are important to intuitive function judgments. When we look around and intuitively judge what for our species are normal functions versus dysfunctions, we often depend to some extent on statistical observations and comparisons. Eyes seeing, hands grasping, fear taking us away from danger, and so on impress us as biologically designed partly because they are obvious, common features of our species. Generally speaking, naturally selected functions become species typical, so species typicality is a powerful guide in assessing normal function. Statistical commonality is thus a useful epistemological adjunct to basic intuitions about candidates for biological design and normal function, especially when evolutionary history is unknown.

However, one has to distinguish epistemological from conceptual claims. Epistemologically, of course, initial judgments about what is a natural function often do rely on some statistical observation based on species typicality. However, conceptually the issue is whether the feature is biologically designed, that is, whether natural selective pressures led to the feature. Any evidential pathway, statistical or otherwise, that you can take to gain such understanding can lead to legitimate function judgments. Indeed, modern genetic analysis techniques are giving us new ways to establish what was and was not naturally selected (e.g., Ding et al. 2002; Lind et al. 2019; Polimanti and Gelernter 2017) without the need for a time machine. It is true that such methods involve such statistical methods as cross-species and intraspecies comparisons of mutation rates around target loci, but such tests of genetic stability are used to establish the likelihood of positive natural selection that may then be used in inferences about normality and dysfunction; they are not used to directly infer normality and dysfunction from statistics alone without reference to natural selection. Such methods are at this time largely limited to single-loci analyses, but it is an open and growing area of research. Consequently, Lemoine's single-minded focus on the epistemological situation of our being in a perpetual state of gross ignorance about natural selection is scientifically out of date and excessively pessimistic. Additionally, regarding Lemoine's claim that the purely statistical view of normal function and dysfunction is presupposed by the HDA's evolutionary approach and thus a better naturalist account of dysfunction, the analysis reveals that, due to challenges in identifying reference classes, the statistical approach cannot get off the ground on its own steam without an implicit appeal to biological design. Thus, the statistical approach implicitly depends on the evolutionary approach.

In his attempt to find an alternative to an evolutionary account of natural functions, Lemoine fails to critically examine the coherence and evidential plausibility of the statistical approach before embracing it. Close examination reveals that the statistical account is not viable as an exclusive stand-alone statistical foundation for medical judgments for a variety of reasons. Biological design literally overrides statistics in judging dysfunction in ways that provide persuasive counterexamples to the statistical subtypicality account's necessity and sufficiency for dysfunction. Regarding necessity, statistically typical and pandemic conditions (e.g., tooth decay and gum disease, atherosclerosis) can be medically classified as dysfunctions, and regarding sufficiency, many conditions that are subtypical (e.g., high neuroticism, homeliness) or are present in a minority (sickle cell trait, lactose tolerance) are medically classified as normal variations. The absurdity of the age dependency of dysfunction accepted by Boorse (e.g., knee bruises and prostate cancer are not dysfunctions at certain ages), the conceptual allowability according to the BST of arbitrarily pathologizing almost half of the population on any functional variable without any further conceptual justification, and most of all the inability of the proposed reference classes to adequately separate dysfunction from normal function all provide compelling objections and counterexamples to anything like the BST's statistical theory. Contrary to what initially might seem like common sense, one cannot simply go out and do statistical analysis to decide the normal versus dysfunctional status of a feature without some further guidance. Given that Lemoine embraces the BST precisely because it is by far the most sophisticated statistical theory around, the most reasonable conclusion is that the statistical approach to dysfunction must be rejected and that the idea that a purely statistical approach can escape theoretical loading while adequately identifying dysfunction is a myth.

Finally, let me return to a question raised earlier: if Lemoine is wrong in arguing that the evolutionary account of dysfunction rests on the statistical account, then what is the correct relationship between the naturalistic components of the BST and the HDA? Boorse has often been criticized for his selection of survival and reproduction as the effects that determine a function as an implicit value judgment. One might also argue that in selecting these criteria, he is trying to mimic evolutionary theory without acknowledging its role. In my view, the explanation of Boorse's choice is more benign. Boorse has correctly observed the fact that long before evolutionary theory and reaching back to antiquity, survival and reproduction are the two domains that were routinely used to justify function attributions.

What Boorse fails to observe is that there is a deeper rationale for why the two specific areas of survival and reproduction are linked to function judgments. The reason is that they are the areas that most distinctively manifest the mystery of biological design, from eyes seeing to acorns growing into oak trees. That is, while eschewing the theoretical explanatory implications of "natural function" linking it to biological design, Boorse has nonetheless picked as his criterion for the overall function category the causation of precisely those outcomes that form the most plausible base set of biologically designed phenomena for the definition of "natural function."

Thus, the relationship between the S&R concept of function and the etiological concept of function is simply that some S&R functions—where the choice is guided by intuitions about biological design—form the base set for defining natural etiological functions. This would make natural functions and S&R functions complementary parts of one account rather than competitor analyses, like the relationship between the base-set description "clear thirst-quenching liquid in lakes and rivers" and the category of (substance) "water" as anything with the same chemical essence as the base-set examples. According to this integration of the views, the S&R view would descriptively pick out some presumptive instances of a natural kind of "natural functions" and thus would indeed be an epistemologically accessible subset of the larger essentialistically defined category of such functions, where the larger category defined in terms of the base set can encompass instances that do not fit that initial base-set descriptive criterion.

Interestingly, this possibility is hinted at in a passing prescient remark of Lemoine's. Near the end of his paper, he mentions that one possibility is for the HDA to "adopt Boorse's view on dysfunction, at least as a temporary stage, in providing a naturalist account of dysfunction." If one interprets that "temporary stage" as the formulation of the base set of apparently biologically designed effects that forms the foundation for the fuller black-box essentialist definition of "natural function," then the two views can be integrated, with Boorse's view capturing the more readily observable base set of species-typical intuitively biologically designed features that requires further explanation in terms of some explanatory nature that forms the essence of natural functions.

References

American Psychiatric Association. 2013. *Diagnostic and Statistical Manual of Mental Disorders*. 5th ed. American Psychiatric Association.

Bird, A. 2010. Discovering the essences of natural kinds. In *The Semantics and Metaphysics of Natural Kinds*, S. Beebee, N. Sabbarton-Leary, and F. Longworth (eds.), 125–136. Routledge.

Bolton, D. 2000. Alternatives to disorder. *Philosophy, Psychiatry, and Psychology* 7(2): 141–153.

Boorse, C. 1987. Concepts of health. In *Health Care Ethics: An Introduction*, D. Van DeVeer and T. Regan (eds.), 359–393. Temple University Press.

Boorse, C. 1997. A rebuttal on health. In *What Is Disease?* J. M. Humber and R. F. Almeder (eds.), 1–134. Humana Press.

Boorse, C. 2002. A rebuttal on functions. In *Functions*, A. Ariew, R. Cummins, and M. Perlman (eds.), 63–112. Oxford University Press.

Boorse, C. 2014. A second rebuttal on health. *Journal of Medicine and Philosophy* 39: 683–724.

Cosmides, L., and J. Tooby. 1999. Toward an evolutionary taxonomy of treatable conditions. *Journal of Abnormal Psychology* 108(3): 453–464.

Cummins, R. 1975. Functional analysis. *Journal of Philosophy* 72: 741–765.

Cummins, R., and M. Roth. 2009. Traits have not evolved to function the way they do because of a past advantage. In *Contemporary Debates in Philosophy of Biology*, F. Ayala and R. Arp (eds.), 72–86. Blackwell.

Ding, Y. C., H. C. Chi, D. L. Grady, A. Morishima, J. R. Kidd, K. K. Kidd, et al. 2002. Evidence of positive selection acting at the human dopamine receptor D4 gene locus. *Proceedings of the National Academy of Sciences of the United States of America* 99(1): 309–314.

Donnellan, K. 1983/2014. Kripke and Putnam on natural kind terms. In *Essays on Reference, Language, and Mind*, J. Almog and P. Leonardi (eds.), 179–203. Oxford University Press.

First, M. B., and J. C. Wakefield. 2010. Defining 'mental disorder' in *DSM-V*. *Psychological Medicine* 40(11): 1779–1782.

First, M. B., and J. C. Wakefield. 2013. Diagnostic criteria as dysfunction indicators: Bridging the chasm between the definition of mental disorder and diagnostic criteria for specific disorders. *Canadian Journal of Psychiatry* 58(12): 663–669.

Kendler, K. S., P. Zachar, and C. Craver. 2011. What kinds of things are psychiatric disorders? *Psychological Medicine* 41(6): 1143–1150.

Kripke, S. A. 1980. *Naming and Necessity*. Harvard University Press.

LaPorte, J. 2004. *Natural Kinds and Conceptual Change*. Cambridge University Press.

Lind, A. L., Y. Y. Y. Lai, Y. Mostovoy, A. K. Holloway, A. Iannucci, A. C. Y. Mak, et al. 2019. Genome of the Komodo dragon reveals adaptations in the cardiovascular and chemosensory systems of monitor lizards. *Nature Ecology & Evolution* 3(8): 1241–1252.

Millikan, R. G. 1989. In defense of proper functions. *Philosophy of Science* 56: 288–302.

Neander, K. 1991a. Functions as selected effects: The conceptual analysis defense. *Philosophy of Science* 58: 168–184.

Neander, K. 1991b. The teleological notion of function. *Australasian Journal of Philosophy* 69: 454–468.

Neander, K. 2012. Biological function: Statistical theories of function. *Routledge Encyclopedia of Philosophy*. https://www.rep.routledge.com/articles/thematic/biological-function/v-1.

Polimanti, R., and J. Gelernter. 2017. Widespread signatures of positive selection in common risk alleles associated to autism spectrum disorder. *PLoS Genetics* 13(2): e1006618.

Price, C. 1995. Functional explanations and natural norms. *Ratio* 7: 143–160.

Putnam, H. 2015a. Intellectual autobiography of Hilary Putnam. In *The Philosophy of Hilary Putnam*, R. E. Auxier, D. R. Anderson, and L. E. Hahn (eds.), 3–110. Open Court.

Putnam, H. 2015b. Reply to Alan Berger. In *The Philosophy of Hilary Putnam*, R. E. Auxier, D. R. Anderson, and L. E. Hahn (eds.), 332–336. Open Court.

Putnam, H. 2015c. Reply to Ian Hacking. In *The Philosophy of Hilary Putnam*, R. E. Auxier, D. R. Anderson, and L. E. Hahn (eds.), 358–364. Open Court.

Spitzer, R. L. 1997. Brief comments from a psychiatric nosologist weary from his own attempts to define mental disorder: Why Ossorio's definition muddles and Wakefield's "harmful dysfunction" illuminates the issues. *Clinical Psychology: Science and Practice* 4(3): 259–261.

Spitzer, R. L. 1999. Harmful dysfunction and the *DSM* definition of mental disorder. *Journal of Abnormal Psychology* 108(3): 430–432.

Wakefield, J. C. 1992a. The concept of mental disorder: On the boundary between biological facts and social values. *American Psychologist* 47: 373–388.

Wakefield, J. C. 1992b. Disorder as harmful dysfunction: A conceptual critique of *DSM-III-R*'s definition of mental disorder. *Psychological Review* 99: 232–247.

Wakefield, J. C. 1993. Limits of operationalization: A critique of Spitzer and Endicott's (1978) proposed operational criteria of mental disorder. *Journal of Abnormal Psychology* 102: 160–172.

Wakefield, J. C. 1995. Dysfunction as a value-free concept: A reply to Sadler and Agich. *Philosophy, Psychiatry, and Psychology* 2: 233–46.

Wakefield, J. C. 1997a. Diagnosing *DSM-IV*, part 1: *DSM-IV* and the concept of mental disorder. *Behaviour Research and Therapy* 35: 633–650.

Wakefield, J. C. 1997b. Diagnosing *DSM-IV*, part 2: Eysenck (1986) and the essentialist fallacy. *Behaviour Research and Therapy*: 35: 651–666.

Wakefield, J. C. 1997c. Normal inability versus pathological disability: Why Ossorio's (1985) definition of mental disorder is not sufficient. *Clinical Psychology: Science and Practice* 4: 249–258.

Wakefield, J. C. 1997d. When is development disordered? Developmental psychopathology and the harmful dysfunction analysis of mental disorder. *Development and Psychopathology* 9: 269–290.

Wakefield, J. C. 1998. The *DSM*'s theory-neutral nosology is scientifically progressive: Response to Follette and Houts. *Journal of Consulting and Clinical Psychology* 66: 846–852.

Wakefield, J. C. 1999a. Evolutionary versus prototype analyses of the concept of disorder. *Journal of Abnormal Psychology* 108: 374–399.

Wakefield, J. C. 1999b. Mental disorder as a black box essentialist concept. *Journal of Abnormal Psychology* 108: 465–472.

Wakefield, J. C. 2000a. Aristotle as sociobiologist: The "function of a human being" argument, black box essentialism, and the concept of mental disorder. *Philosophy, Psychiatry, and Psychology* 7: 17–44.

Wakefield, J. C. 2000b. Spandrels, vestigial organs, and such: Reply to Murphy and Woolfolk's "The harmful dysfunction analysis of mental disorder." *Philosophy, Psychiatry, and Psychology* 7: 253–269.

Wakefield, J. C. 2001. Evolutionary history versus current causal role in the definition of disorder: Reply to McNally. *Behaviour Research and Therapy* 39: 347–366.

Wakefield, J. C. 2006. What makes a mental disorder mental? *Philosophy, Psychiatry, and Psychology* 13: 123–131.

Wakefield, J. C. 2007. The concept of mental disorder: Diagnostic implications of the harmful dysfunction analysis. *World Psychiatry* 6: 149–156.

Wakefield, J. C. 2009. Mental disorder and moral responsibility: Disorders of personhood as harmful dysfunctions, with special reference to alcoholism. *Philosophy, Psychiatry, and Psychology* 16: 91–99.

Wakefield, J. C. 2011. Darwin, functional explanation, and the philosophy of psychiatry. In *Maladapting Minds: Philosophy, Psychiatry, and Evolutionary Theory*, P. R. Andriaens and A. De Block (eds.), 143–172. Oxford University Press.

Wakefield, J. C. 2012. Are you as smart as a 4th grader? Why the prototype-similarity approach to diagnosis is a step backward for a scientific psychiatry. *World Psychiatry* 11: 27–28.

Wakefield, J. C. 2014. The biostatistical theory versus the harmful dysfunction analysis, part 1: Is part-dysfunction a sufficient condition for medical disorder? *Journal of Medicine and Philosophy* 39: 648–682.

Wakefield, J. C. 2016a. The concepts of biological function and dysfunction: Toward a conceptual foundation for evolutionary psychopathology. In *Handbook of Evolutionary Psychology*, D. Buss (ed.), 2nd ed., vol. 2, 988–1006. Oxford University Press.

Wakefield, J. C. 2016b. Diagnostic issues and controversies in *DSM-5*: Return of the false positives problem. *Annual Review of Clinical Psychology* 12: 105–132.

Wakefield, J. C., and M. B. First. 2003. Clarifying the distinction between disorder and nondisorder: Confronting the overdiagnosis ("false positives") problem in *DSM-V*. In *Advancing DSM: Dilemmas in Psychiatric Diagnosis*, K. A. Phillips, M. B. First, and H. A. Pincus (eds.), 23–56. American Psychiatric Press.

Wakefield, J. C., and M. B. First. 2012. Placing symptoms in context: The role of contextual criteria in reducing false positives in *DSM* diagnosis. *Comprehensive Psychiatry* 53: 130–139.

Wilson, M. 1982. Predicate meets property. *The Philosophical Review* 91(4): 549–589.

World Health Organization. 2018. *International Statistical Classification of Diseases and Related Health Problems.* 11th rev. https://icd.who.int/browse11/l-m/en.

Zachar, P. 2002. The practical kinds model as a pragmatist theory of classification: Comment. *Philosophy, Psychiatry, and Psychology* 9(3): 219–227.

13 Function and Dysfunction

Dominic Murphy

Introduction

Few ideas in the philosophy of psychiatry have been discussed as widely as Jerry Wakefield's harmful dysfunction analysis (HDA) of mental disorder in the twenty years or so since its original promulgation (Wakefield 1992a, 1992b, 1993). This is unsurprising, since it is a tour de force of simple, elegant analysis. And it does seem to get the basic picture right; there is something compelling about the idea that the attribution of mental illness rests on both a value judgment and a belief that something is wrong with the inner systems of a sufferer. On closer inspection, though, I think that the HDA turns out to be unconvincing when it comes to the details. The HDA's account of function is not the right one for the job. The philosophical literature on functions has uncovered many nuances that Wakefield misses, and the evolutionary analysis of functions makes a number of commitments that do not seem to be part of the general tendency to attribute mental illness that Wakefield relies on as evidence for his account. It also seems that medicine and other branches of experimental biology rely on a different account of function than the evolutionary one. I shall lay out Wakefield's analysis and, in doing so, point to some of its attractions. I will take a while to describe the HDA as I understand it. This is partly because I think that some criticisms of the HDA are unfounded and I want to dissociate myself from them, but more important because some of those criticisms would, if correct, tell against a broader naturalistic family of analyses of which the HDA is a member. I think that once the HDA is laid out and its attractions manifest, we can see that there are further options for naturalistic analyses.

Although I will be critical of Wakefield's HDA in what follows, I do wish to be constructive and exploratory, as well. Wakefield has for the most part been clear and concise in advancing his theory and bitten some bullets in defending it. This lets us see what is at stake, and one important result is that Wakefield has opened up ways to develop a family of views that are not simply normative. In what follows, then, I will suggest ways in which the details of the HDA might be changed but remain in keeping with its basic philosophical orientation.

I. The Components of Wakefield's View

1.1 The HDA as a Two-Stage View

I class Wakefield's HDA as a two-stage account of mental disorder, in the tradition of Boorse (1975, 1976). Two-stage theorists hold that there are two individually necessary and jointly sufficient conditions for disorder. First, there is a biological dysfunction. Wakefield's innovation was to see this as specifically a failure by a bodily system to perform the naturally selected function that explained the system's replication in past generations: "the failure of a mechanism in the person to perform a natural function for which the mechanism was designed by natural selection" (Wakefield 1993, 165).

Second, the dysfunction must result in harm to the individual. "Harm" is generally recognized to be a normative notion, and Wakefield thinks we follow a simple rule when judging that someone is harmed. It is judged by prevailing social norms: "defined by social values and meanings" (1993, 373). The fact that this is a simple rule does not mean that it is a simple matter to tell where and how it applies. Whether somebody is harmed may be difficult to assess, and although judgments can be uncontroversial (a terminal disease or a serious injury is obviously harmful), they often won't be. But although assessing harm is often difficult or controversial, the rule is simple: harm is assessed relative to the prevailing norms of the society, not the views of the individual concerned, who may not feel as though they are badly off at all.

In sum, we have the two components of the HDA (Wakefield 2006, 157), which state that for a condition to count as a mental disorder: (1) it is negative or harmful according to cultural values, and (2) it is caused by a dysfunction (i.e., by a failure of some psychological mechanism to perform a natural function for which it was evolutionarily designed).

The mix is part normative and part objective. Clause (1) tells us that what counts as harmful will differ across times and cultures, but clause (2) tells us that dysfunction will not. Our psychology, like our physiology more generally, is made up of numerous mechanisms that combine to cause normal behavior. Each of these has the job that it was selected for, and if it does not work as selected, it is dysfunctional. On some occasions, that dysfunction causes some phenomenon—physiological, mental, behavioral—that is judged to be harmful by the wider group that the person with the dysfunction belongs to. At other times, the dysfunction might not be a source of harm. In theory, a dysfunction could make you better off. For example, if your liver metabolism departed from its historically adaptive range in a way that enabled you to drink all you want without suffering ill effects, people might not think that you were harmed, at least in the circles I move in. I think it is clear that a view of this type—a two-stage view—has many attractions, which perhaps come out if we compare it to its main rivals. Doing so will also raise some important issues that will detain us later. I will go over these attractions and questions now.

1.2   The HDA and Normative Views

Two-stage views sit between purely normative views and those that deny that our disease concepts employ any human norms at all. On one hand, a purely normative view would argue that an attribution of mental illness is solely a value judgment: it merely reflects the way we evaluate people with respect to prevailing social norms. A view like this faces the great problem that we distinguish many forms of departures from normality. Sometimes we judge people to be ill or mentally disordered, but we can also judge them to be deviant in a host of other ways. They might be criminal, or eccentric, or immoral, or indeed they might depart from normal forms of behavior in ways that we prize, in which case we call them geniuses. What, on the purely normative view of mental disorder, makes the difference in these cases? Why do we call some behavior eccentric or criminal and other behavior disordered? One big advantage of a two-stage account of mental disorder is the answer it gives to this question. We call people disordered or diseased when we think that there is something wrong "under the hood." Some part of them is not working the way that a normal component of human being naturally works, and it is responsible for the salient features of their behavior. I take it that this is the basic intuition Wakefield is working with. We respond to the mentally ill as if there is something wrong under the hood—that is the dysfunction, and we take the salient harm to be evidence for it.

Another way of asserting the purely normative view is to insist that calling something a dysfunction expresses a stance toward it, perhaps based on what we take to be the best interests or purposes of the owner of the system. I think Wakefield is quite correct to push back against claims of this kind (e.g., in Wakefield 2009, 92–93): it is one thing to identify a system as relevant for its owner but another to assert that its function is just normative. If you are training someone to be an athlete or an opera singer, it might pay to enhance their lung capacity. In that sense, their respiratory system is a site of our joint interests, but the function of that system is still perfectly objective. What a sophisticated proponent of the purely normative view should do is argue that disease concepts have a different structure altogether. Cooper (2007) and Murphy (2006) have drawn an analogy between the concept of mental disorder and that of weed. Weeds are not a natural kind. We can perhaps say that a weed is a fast-growing species that negatively impacts on economically valuable crops, usually through competition for nutrients, sunlight, and space. What fixes the extension of "weed" (and similar concepts like "vermin" or "precious metal") is a set of contingent human interests that can change over time. Suppose that determining that a condition is a disorder is like determining that a plant is a weed. The judgment is determined by normative considerations that we have already made. But nonetheless, there is real, explanatory mind-independent knowledge to be had about each sort of "weed."

A skeptic about the objectivity of mental disorder could exploit this point. She could admit that there are correlations between psychologically salient behavior and the performance of underlying systems. Such a skeptic might also argue that although there is perfectly objective knowledge to be had about those systems, they only count as disordered because of our prior decision to insist that they are disordered—anything that produced that behavior would be called dysfunctional, because it is productive of mental illness. Such a skeptical view would also combine a claim about judgments of disorder with a claim about the objective nature of underlying systems. It could even agree that commonsense attributions of mental illness involve detection of systems that strike us as broken "under the hood." It would, however, deny that there is any sense to calling such systems dysfunctional. So a two-stage theory like the HDA needs a way to show that a system is dysfunctional that meets this skeptical challenge.

The last point raised by a purely normative analysis of the concept of mental disorder is that of relativity. If being mentally ill is just a matter of how it strikes the other members of one's society, then it seems that whether you are mentally ill depends on where and when you live. The history of psychiatry—indeed, of the sciences of the mind in general—is full of episodes in which some disfavored group has been condemned as pathological in the light of considerations that strike us as fraudulent. Homosexuals, notoriously, were diagnosed as mentally ill until the revision of the *Diagnostic and Statistical Manual of Mental Disorders (DSM)* in the 1970s. The HDA lets us say that such judgments are incorrect unless they involve the detection of some underlying disorder, whereas a purely normative view seems to have no resources to avoid relativism.

So far in this section, I have contrasted the HDA with views that insist on the purely normative character of the concept of mental disorders. The other option would be a completely nonnormative view, insisting that judgments of harm are just as objective as those of dysfunction. A two-stage view incorporates values judgments and, in so doing, fits both medical practice and ordinary thought better, because it does seem undeniable that we argue about whether something is a disease based on whether we think it makes a life go less well, and the relevant considerations are indeed a matter of socially constituted meanings.

The story so far is this: the HDA is one of a family of two-stage analyses of the concept of disorder that combine normative evaluations of harm with criteria of dysfunction that aim to be objective and scientifically grounded. In the second part of the chapter, I will discuss whether, as Wakefield contends, the analysis of function that this account needs is an evolutionary one. But first, I will mention one last issue in the characterization of the HDA. Whose concept is being analyzed?

1.3 Whose Concept?

Conceptual analysis in philosophy is often undertaken with the aim of regimenting nontheoretical talk. We might pick out a term that plays a role in commonsense description of the world and try to define it. Many philosophers of science, though, are interested in how terms work in theoretical contexts; concepts exist in unfolding scientific projects, and we want to understand how they work. When we do this, we often uncover differences or ambiguities in scientific practice. Philosophers of biology, for example, have largely come to agree that there is no unified concept of the gene throughout biology (Griffiths and Stotz 2013). Rather, different areas of biology, or even the same scientist at different times, will use the gene concept to pick out different aspects of the underlying genetic and developmental processes. I think *function* is scientifically polysemous in just this way and will argue for that claim in the next section. Right now, I want to ask what sort of project Wakefield is engaged in.

Wakefield typically argues that his project involves the analysis of *mental disorder* in scientific and clinical contexts. However, Wakefield is also happy to argue that some diagnoses are in error because they ignore the lessons of common sense.

Horwitz and Wakefield (2007), for example, argue that the *DSM-IV* fails to respect common sense or previous psychiatric consensus about depression, and as a result is diagnosing many people as depressed when they are just normally miserable. Since classical antiquity, Western thought has recognized a condition of melancholy, as people slip into depression without any observable, proportionate cause. This is to be distinguished from ordinary understandable sadness that people suffer when they are visited by life's misfortunes. The tradition sees pathology only in the former case, insisting that "pathological depression is an exaggerated form of a normal human emotional response" (Horwitz and Wakefield 2007, 71). They conclude that the concept of depression defined by the contemporary diagnostic syndrome represents a major conceptual break with both past psychiatry and commonsense thought about human nature. This has led to needless alarmism about an epidemic of depression and caused misfortune for many individuals diagnosed in error.

It is correct that the *DSM* concept of depression, on the face of it, lumps together different psychological and behavioral types in the same category because of observable similarities, and it is quite true that observable similarities may nonetheless reflect diverse etiologies. The response (Kendler et al. 2008; Zisook and Kendler 2007) is to argue that the populations are too similar on the relevant measures to justify treating them as different. This argument was made with great force in the run-up to the *DSM-5*, when various parties debated whether it was appropriate (as in *DSM-IV*) to exempt the bereaved from a diagnosis of depression or to, in effect, treat grieving as form of depression.

Wakefield has weighed in on the statistical issues involved in this debate (Wakefield et al. 2007), but it is the conceptual argument I want to focus on here. If we are trying to capture a scientific concept, on what grounds can we argue that it should be criticized for departing from traditional conceptions? A chemist who was told that traditional usage did not regard objects as made of atoms would be unmoved. So, one possibility is that Wakefield is just being inconsistent, appealing to scientific practice in some cases and traditional or commonsense views in others. A more charitable reading would be that Wakefield thinks that the underlying logic of psychiatric practice accords with the HDA but that sometimes psychiatrists depart from the logic of their own projects. Nonetheless, this does raise the question of how revisionist the HDA might turn out to be. It is unusual for scientific developments to vindicate traditional modes of thought, such as the venerable distinction between melancholy and depression, but Wakefield's view, as has been pointed out (Kingma 2013; Murphy and Woolfolk 2000a, 2000b), looks to be very revisionist for independent reasons, connected to the HDA's requirement that dysfunction is necessarily a property of evolved systems.

1.4 Revisionism

Many critics have argued that the existence of evolutionary by-products is a problem for Wakefield's account (Kingma [2013, 375–379] has an excellent review). Wakefield himself notes that acalculia, dyslexia, and amusia are disorders that do not involve selected effects but side effects of other systems (2011, 169). On the face of it, the HDA would have to rule these conditions out, but Wakefield has a reply. He argues that in dyslexia, the problem must arise because of a dysfunction in some other system that does have a selection history.

Now, as Kingma (2013, 376) notes, it is quite possible for a linked trait to be abnormal for independent reasons that have nothing to do with a dysfunction in the system it is linked to. Wakefield (2011, 170) argues that students of reading disorders assume that there is a dysfunction involved in the condition, which they do not do for cases of ordinary illiteracy. This is correct, but it only meets the objection if those researchers are committed to an evolutionary account of function, which is the very point at issue. The fact that they take for granted the existence of a dysfunction (or some other proximate cause of the condition) does not show that they take for granted the existence of an evolutionary dysfunction. Wakefield thinks that he can rule this out because there is no viable concept of dysfunction other than an evolutionary one, but that is not correct, as the next section will show.

Kingma argues that Wakefield's position is potentially very revisionist indeed: if a large number of disorders turn out not to be linked to selected effects but to be the product of other processes, such as developmental or genetic linkage, then he will have to say that they are not really disorders. Wakefield seems to think that this is not a live possibility and that one can always postulate the existence of a selected function that is linked to the condition. As Kingma (2013) and Nordenfeldt (2003) argue, this seems grossly ad hoc: one can indeed always postulate such a dysfunction, however remote the causal chain may be, but this just makes the HDA immune to counterexample by stipulation. Whenever the apparent cause of a disorder seems to be something other than a dysfunctional selected system, Wakefield can just insist that there must be one somewhere.

Suppose the view is revisionist, and we have to revise our thinking about mental disorder. Is that so bad? Well, psychiatric concepts, like some others, are impure: although they involve scientific criteria, they also speak to urgent practical needs. Part of the appeal of the HDA is its impurity, since it incorporates both scientific assessment and normative, cultural assessment. If it turned out that a lot of what we consider to be mental disorders are not disorders at all, we would still worry about the people who fall under those diagnoses, and we would still want concepts that differentiate them from others. And those concepts would need to direct our attention to the causes of the conditions, because we would want to be able to intervene in order to improve their lot. Certainly, some human traits have come to be seen as normal rather than disordered, and others have gone the other way. But widespread revisionism seems unattractive, and if it can be avoided, I take that to be a point in favor of an analysis.

1.5   Some Desiderata

I have argued that Wakefield's HDA is an instance of a two-stage view that combines a normative component and a naturalistic understanding of function. The question now before us is whether his evolutionary understanding of function is the correct one. I extract three desiderata from the discussion so far that can serve as constraints on the account of function we need. First, it should be able to make precise the idea that attributions of mental illness rely on something being objectively wrong under the hood of a human being. Second, it should capture relevant scientific practice. Third, it should not be too revisionist but make sense of the idea that some conditions may have causes that cannot be shown to depend on failures of selected effects. In the next section, I will argue that there are accounts of function available that do a better job of meeting these constraints than the evolutionary account that Wakefield prefers. Therefore, there are two-stage analyses of the concept of mental illness that are superior to the HDA while still retaining its benefits.

II.   The Concept of Function[1]

As I said in the last section, the HDA is based around the fundamental intuition that our ascriptions of mental disorder reflect the view that something is wrong under the hood of a human being. It assumes that what is wrong is a dysfunction in a system whose normal function can be objectively discovered. Wakefield claims (2011, 144) that Darwin discovered the nature of biological function, just as atomic chemistry discovered the nature of water. Therefore, the Darwinian understanding is what people have always referred to when talking of natural functions. Hence, the HDA (or any two-stage theory) must appeal to a Darwinian notion of function to make sense of attributions of dysfunction in medicine, psychiatry, and ordinary unscientific talk, for "function" identifies a set of beneficial capacities of living things, and Darwin has told us what those are. When there is a failure of natural order, it is of the order imposed by natural selection.

If it were correct that a Darwinian account of function was the only scientifically respectable adumbration of that concept, then Wakefield's position would be unimpeachable. But it is not correct. In contemporary philosophy of biology, analyses of function derive from two important papers. Wright (1973) argued that ascriptions of function to a structure are causal-historical, where function depends on a prior selection process. Wright is sometimes taken to have adopted an evolutionary account of function that relies on the notion of natural selection, but he did not. It was Millikan (1984) and Neander (1991) who developed Wright's account into an explicitly evolutionary one. Wakefield's understanding of function is squarely in this tradition.

Cummins (1975) was the other key paper. Cummins's concept of function was not historical but dispositional. He understood the function of an entity to be the contribution it makes to "an adequate analysis" of the capacity of the overall system that includes it. According to Cummins, a component may have a function even if the component was not "designed," and therefore, parts with no selection history can be ascribed a function. Wakefield argues that Cummins's account was introduced to capture functional explanation in the philosophy of mind and is not relevant to biology (2011, 149). However, philosophers of biology (including Cummins himself) have elaborated the analysis, just as Millikan and Neander did with Wright's historical account, and they have done so in order to capture the important role that nonhistorical concepts of function play in many areas of biology. In doing so, they have shown how this concept of function fits into the mechanistic explanations that are common in biomedicine. In this section, I will introduce the selectionist analysis of function that Wakefield prefers, then the alternative causal-mechanical analysis, and argue that the latter better fits medical practice, is epistemically less committed, and is at least as good a fit for common sense.

2.1 The Selectionist View

Evolutionary views of function involve causal-historical explanations of traits that I will call *selectionist*. The heart is a standard example. Millikan (1984) said that *the heart is a pump because it is the heart's pumping that contributes to the successful reproduction of organisms with hearts*: if x is a member of a biological category, it is not because of "the actual constitution, powers, or dispositions" of x, but because of the "proper function" of x (Millikan 1984, 17). X's proper function depends on the history of x's lineage, which explains x's being supposed to do whatever it does. Neander (1991, 180) agrees that a biological part is only identifiable in terms of its proper function.

The point is quite subtle because the relevant history consists of correlations obtained between ancestors of x having a certain character and their having been able to perform x's function. So the structure of a heart explains why it pumps, but it does not count as a heart (or a pump) in virtue of having that structure.

The selectionist account of function seems to offer two big benefits. First, it promises to give a definite specification of the function of an organic system and hence a clear criterion for calling it dysfunctional. Second, it seems to offer a scientifically unproblematic way to say what a system ought to be like. If you are worried about the accusation that function talk is normative, you can embrace natural selection. Teleological notions are commonly associated with the pre-Darwinian view that the biological realm provides evidence of conscious design by a supernatural creator. The point about selectionist concepts of function is that they assuage this metaphysical concern by showing how norms are part of nature. I am not going to suggest that there is something wrong with the Darwinian picture of natural order. But I will suggest that selectionist concepts of function and dysfunction are a poor bet for psychiatry. I will now introduce a rival account of function, but before developing it philosophically, I will try to motivate it: the point is not just to argue that there is a philosophical option that Wakefield has not considered but to argue that this unconsidered option fits the relevant sciences better. So I will start with the science.

2.2 Why We Need Other Concepts of Function

Wakefield argues that selectionist accounts of function solve the "essential explanatory puzzle posed by function attributions within biology" (2011, 149), namely, how can there be apparently designed systems in a world devoid of purpose. However, this metaphysical question, despite its importance, is not the only context within which functional talk appears in the sciences. As Amundson and Lauder (1998, 227) put it, "Philosophers' special interests in purposive concepts can lead to the neglect of many crucial but non-purposive concepts in the science of biology." Amundson and Lauder maintain that a selectionist analysis of function fits evolutionary biology, but they argue that a different concept of function is used in comparative and functional anatomy. They contend that this alternative concept of function is well captured by a Cummins-style account, which they call a causal-role analysis. In contrast to Millikan and Neander, they point out that it is entirely possible to identify anatomical units by anatomical considerations, regardless of proper function. They also argue for the ineliminability of a causal-role analysis of function, on the grounds that an anatomical unit can have a function even in the absence of a selectionist history: the fact that a biological system has a selective history does not imply that all of its components have a distinct selective history that makes them what they are. Their functions, in the sense of their causal contribution to the overall system, are independently identifiable on morphological and physiological grounds, regardless of history.

The biomedical sciences routinely try to work out what a system contributes to the overall functioning of the organism. In doing so, they typically do not try to establish that a biological component has a selectionist function. For example, take Hubel and Wiesel's famous program of mapping the receptive fields of cells in the visual cortex and then establishing further visual information-processing channels in the brain. That program, and the research on the neurobiology of vision inspired by it, depended on a set of engineering assumptions about the way the brain is organized to process information. It did not test assumptions about the selective advantage and history of the components of the visual brain. Hubel and Wiesel never sought to show that the cats whose visual system they interfered with produced fewer descendants than other cats.

It may be that the facts uncovered in physiology are evidence for evolutionary relationships, and of course, all biological systems have an evolutionary history, but when we determine what normal function is, in medicine, we do not even try to establish what that history is: selectionist, or broader historical, considerations do not arise. It is the mechanistic relations between parts of the system that matter.

Schaffner (1993) argued that although medicine might use teleological talk in its attempts to develop mechanistic explanations, that talk is just heuristic. It focuses our attention on entities that are useful to the organism. Schaffner suggested that as we learn more about the role a structure plays in the overall functioning of an organism, the need for evolutionary functional ascriptions drops out. It is replaced by the vocabulary of mechanistic explanation: the causal relationship of parts that jointly produce phenomena of explanatory interest. Functional explanations that draw on evolutionary considerations are, he claimed, "necessary, but empirically weak to the point of becoming almost metaphysical" (Schaffner 1993, 389–390).

Normal biomedical ascription of function to a system makes no claims about selective history. It requires only that we can identify the role played by a system in the overall economy of the organism. How is dysfunction determined? By the use of a biomedical concept of normality that is an idealized description of a component of a biological system in an unperturbed state. It does not rest on the failure of a biological part to replicate as its ancestors did, or to reduce overall fitness, but by its failure to be close enough to the causal contribution of the analogous part in the idealized overall system.

Wachbroit (1994, 588) argues persuasively that when medicine or physiology says that an organ is "normal," the relevant conception of normality "is similar to the role pure states or ideal entities play in physical theories." Such an idealization represents actual organs or systems in unperturbed states (see also Ereshefsky 2009). To understand a real case, we add information to develop a model that resembles actual hearts (Wachbroit 1994, 589). For instance, Gross (1921) was able to establish post mortem that anastomotic communication between main arteries increases over a typical life span, thereby establishing that we need to model younger and older hearts differently. The point of such idealizations is not to represent the statistically average heart but to describe hearts in a way that allows departures from the ideal to be recognized and to serve as template from which more realistic models can be built.[2] In general, physiological theories are families of such idealizations, and bodily systems are understood as functional parts of larger systems, typed unhistorically.

Insofar as psychiatry is a branch of medicine, the concept of function it needs resembles those of physiology and biomedicine. Evolutionary considerations are just beside the point. Wakefield argues that the selective account of function is one that should be embraced by the philosophy of medicine because it is the working assumption of medical scientists. That is just not so: most parts of medicine and biology, including the areas closes to psychiatry, use a mechanistic, ahistorical account of function. The concepts of psychiatry should be continuous with those of medicine and physiology more generally. The life sciences ask all sorts of questions, but the questions that medicine asks are not those that a selectionist account of function can answer. Most biomedical research is based on establishing the components, as well as the functional relations between components, in biological systems. It is not aimed at uncovering evolutionary relationships. Health and fitness are different concepts, with different functional analyses. As Gluckman et al. (2009, 4–8) argue in their textbook on evolutionary medicine, for example, medicine is about health, and evolutionary biology is about fitness, and the latter does not provide a definition of disease.

At the end of section II, I suggested that there were three constraints on a satisfactory account of function from the point of view of a two-stage analysis of mental disorders such as the HDA. The second of these was that it should capture biomedical practice. The selectionist account of function does not do this as well as the rival, ahistorical account, which from now on I will call the *systemic capacity* account. That leaves two other constraints: whether the account can provide an objective articulation of the intuition that there is something inner—under the hood—that is wrong with the mentally ill and whether it will deal with cases of disorders that do not seem to depend on failures of selected effects. I think that the systemic capacity account does well on both counts, and I will now try to show why. I have argued for the ubiquity of an alternative analysis of function in "experimental biology" (Weber 2005b) and medicine but not provided many details. In the last part of the chapter, I will sketch the account I prefer and argue for its virtues.

2.3 The Systemic Capacity Account

Cummins (1975) introduced his account of function in the context of explaining how the overall capacity of system—its ability to do something—depends on the subcapacities that interact to produce it. A components function in a system is whatever it does that contributes to the overall capacity of the system that contains it. As it stands, this view does not tell us why the entity with the component's function is there in the first place, which is what the historical account was designed to do. However, as Cummins (2002) points out, a selectionist account of function does not say why the entity is there in the first place either. Selection accounts for the spread of a trait, not its origin. In order to outcompete its variant, a system must exist, and the selectionist story does not tell us why it exists.

The bigger problem with Cummins's analysis is that, notoriously, attributions of function on this account are interest relative: if you are interested in the heart's contribution to the circulation of the blood, you can analyze it one way, and if you are interested in its contribution to the sum total of the noises the body makes, you can treat it as a "lub-dup" generator. In both cases, it counts as a part of the overall system you wish to decompose. Cummins thought that the overall system depended on the interests of the investigator. In that sense, he was not really trying to articulate a naturalistic concept of function that captures biological practice but to understand the logic of functional analysis. This is, however, a problem for such a view with respect to the first of my three constraints: we want an objective characterization of dysfunction rather than a mere acknowledgment that we decompose a system into its contributory parts. If that were all that the account gave us, it would threaten the objectivity that is appealing about two-stage views a like the HDA. It would be possible to argue like the skeptic I imagined in section 2.2. The skeptic contends that our analysis of what biological systems do is driven by a prior judgment that they are disordered. It is not independent of that judgment *but is a scientific analysis of what we have decided to call a disorder on evaluative grounds.* To rebut the skeptical point, we need a way of characterizing biological systems that sees them as mind-independent components of nature, not just reflections of human concerns.

As Amundson and Lauder note (1998, 237), even within unambiguously scientific contexts, it is possible to cook up "whimsical Cummins functions" such as Neander's (1991) example of the function of geological plate movements in tectonic systems. What the whimsical examples trade on is the absence in Cummins's account of any commitment to the overall goal of the system; there is nothing that the tectonic system is for, so attributing functions to its parts looks weird. However, Amundson and Lauder argue that these examples do "not apply to the real world of scientific practise." They argue that in fields like comparative anatomy, one finds anatomical, rather than purposive or functional, characterizations of living systems with causal relations among their parts that a Cummins-style account is needed to deal with.

I have some sympathy with the idea that the whimsical objections to Cummins's analysis are scientifically irrelevant. Nonetheless, it would be good to have some principled way of identifying natural systems. Recent attempts to do this attempt to identify some metaphysical relation that holds natural systems together.

Weber (2005a) argues for *coherence*. A coherent system is one that displays a complex network of capacities with contributory relations among them, so that capacities contribute to other capacities that contribute to other capacities. In his example (193), ion channels in nerve membranes "regulate ion permeability because this capacity is part of an account of the nervous system's capacity to process information. Therefore, it is a function of nervous membranes to fire action potentials. Furthermore, the nervous system's capacity to process information is part of an analytic account of the organism's capacity to locate food and sexual partners" and so on. Organisms are webs of integrated explanatory relations, and respecting these webs provides a constraint on individuating systems that makes them not just choices of an investigator but genuine parts of nature.

A related account tied to a fuller account of explanation is Craver's (2007) development of Cummins-style functional analysis into mechanistic explanation. Craver begins his book by discussing the mechanism by which neurotransmitters are released

(4–6). This involves finding answers to questions such as the following: why does depolarization of an axon terminal lead to neurotransmitter release, and why are neurotransmitters released in quanta? Answers identify anatomical entities, such as specific types of calcium and various intracellular molecules, and show how they interact with each other to give rise to the explanandum. This picture applies to mental disorders just as it does to the activities of the normal mind: they depend on the interaction of biological systems that manifest a given phenomenon. An explanation with these features is mechanistic: it appeals not to natural laws but to the interaction of natural systems.

In recent years, philosophers have stressed the way in which explanation in many sciences, above all the biological and cognitive, depends on finding the parts within a system whose interactive structures and activities explain the phenomena produced by the system. Philosophers disagree over exactly how to characterize mechanisms, but it is agreed that mechanisms comprise (1) component parts that (2) do things. Strife arises over how to see the activities of the parts. Are they also primitive constituents of a mechanism or just activities of the constituent components (for full references and a review, see Tabery 2004). A mechanistic explanation shows how these parts and what they do give rise to the phenomenon we want to explain.

I take it that the affinity with a Cummins-style account of function is clear. Craver (2007, 161) asks, "How must Cummins-style functional analysis be restricted to provide a normatively adequate of mechanistic explanation" (i.e., one that displays the properties that good explanations have)? His answer, which is in the spirit of Weber's story, is that relations between subcomponents of a system must be constitutive. A mechanism has parts that hang together and jointly compose a system, and the causal relations among them must be genuine ones, rather than mere correlations. I will not go over Craver's full account, which is thorough and elaborate. The point is that philosophers of biology have worked to develop a Cummins-style analysis into a genuine causal-explanatory account that fits into a wider picture of how organisms fit together and how mechanistic explanation reveals the explanatory relations among parts of biological systems. Wakefield's claim (2011, 149) that the Cummins picture *"does not attempt to elucidate how functional relations are explanatory"* of causal relations in biology is true of the original account. But it overlooks the extensive work done in recent years by philosophers of biology who have developed it into a causal-explanatory account.

2.4 The Scoreboard

At the end of section II, I listed three constraints on an account of function suitable for a two-stage theory of mental disorder like the HDA. It is time to take stock. I have already shown that when it comes to capturing biological practice, the systemic capacity view is superior, because it accords with the understanding of function used in the parts of biology and medicine that are most relevant to psychiatry, rather than evolutionary biology. What about the other two constraints that the account of function should meet? One of them was the extent to which an account of function can provide an objective understanding of what we mean when we attribute a dysfunction. I have argued, although not shown in detail, that a systemic capacity account can comport with an objective understanding of natural systems. Exactly what ordinary attribution of dysfunction means is unclear. However, there is no reason to suppose that it must be articulated in an evolutionary fashion—certainly we don't check whether someone has low biological fitness before we call them disordered. Perhaps we should say here that no view has a clear advantage. My own hunch is that there is no one view that is the best candidate for the scientific articulation of every kind of selection talk, including the ways in which we attribute dysfunction. But there is no reason to think that the systemic capacity view cannot serve as well as the selectionist view when it comes to the relevant contexts. There is no reason to think that comparative anatomy or neurophysiology is less objective than evolutionary biology, not that they are lesser candidates than evolutionary biology for the role of capturing the sorts of judgment Wakefield is interested in.

Last, I suggested that a view might want to escape the apparent revisionism that lurks in Wakefield's commitment to the necessary existence of an evolutionary dysfunction. Here the systemic capacity view wins easily. The systemic capacity view can ask what in the individual is contributing to the salient behavior without worrying about history. Wakefield stipulates that there must be some evolved system somewhere that has departed from its historical design and is connected to the current problem. In contrast, the systemic capacity view just asks *what the underlying system is that is misbehaving*. This is what I mean by calling it less epistemically committed. It has one less bet to make. We both agree that researchers in dyslexia, say, are looking for dysfunctions. Wakefield assumes that they must be concerned with the history of the systems they scrutinize. The systemic capacity view just says that they must be concerned with what the systems are like. Even if a system has no selective history, it can still fail to exhibit its normal capacity and be treated as dysfunction. The systemic capacity view can deal with these cases, and the selectionist view cannot.

So the systemic capacity view is a winner on at least two counts out of three, and one is at best a stalemate. I suggest that this means that the "dysfunction" part of the HDA needs to be rethought and brought into line with contemporary biology and philosophy of biology. The HDA remains a very elegant and attractive analysis, but its concept of function will not do.

Notes

1. Parts of this section draw on Roe and Murphy (2011).

2. Notice that some degree of idealization is required by a selectionist account too; one indisputable result of Darwin's work is the demonstration that variation is ubiquitous in nature. Any determination of the normal range of function of a biological system requires some idealization to cope with that variation.

References

Amundson, R., and G. Lauder. 1998. Function without purpose. In *The Philosophy of Biology*, D. L. Hull and M. Ruse (eds.), 227–257. Oxford University Press.

Boorse, C. 1975. On the distinction between disease and illness. *Philosophy and Public Affairs* 5: 49–68.

Boorse, C. 1976. What a theory of mental health should be. *Journal for the Theory of Social Behavior* 6: 61–84.

Cooper, R. 2007. *Psychiatry and the Philosophy of Science*. Acumen.

Craver, C. F. 2007. *Explaining the Brain: Mechanisms and the Mosaic Unity of Neuroscience*. Oxford University Press.

Cummins, R. 1975. Functional analysis. *Journal of Philosophy* 72: 741–764.

Cummins, R. 2002. Neo-teleology. In *Functions: New Essays in the Philosophy of Psychology and Biology*, R. Cummins, A. Ariew, and M. Perlman (eds.), 157–173. Oxford University Press.

Ereshefsky, M. 2009. Defining "health" and "disease." *Studies in the History and Philosophy of Biology and Biomedical Sciences* 40(3): 221–227.

Gluckman, P., A. Beedle, and M. Hanson. 2009. *Principles of Evolutionary Medicine*. Oxford University Press.

Griffiths, P., and K. Stotz. 2013. *Genetics and Philosophy: An Introduction*. Cambridge University Press.

Gross, L. 1921. *The Blood Supply to the Heart in Its Anatomical and Clinical Aspects*. New York: Hoeber

Horwitz, A., and J. C. Wakefield. 2007. *The Loss of Sadness: How Psychiatry Transformed Normal Sorrow into Depressive Disorder*. Oxford University Press.

Kendler, K. S., J. Myers, and S. Zisook. 2008. Does bereavement-related major depression differ from major depression associated with other stressful life events? *American Journal of Psychiatry* 165(11): 1449–1455.

Kingma, E. 2013. Naturalist accounts of mental disorder. In *The Oxford Handbook of Philosophy and Psychiatry*, K. W. M. Fulford, M. Davies, R. G. T. Gipps, G. Graham, J. Z. Sadler, G. Stanghellini, and T. Thornton (eds.), 363–384. Oxford University Press.

Millikan, R. G. 1984. *Language, Thought and Other Biological Categories*. MIT Press.

Murphy, D. 2006. *Psychiatry in the Scientific Image*. MIT Press.

Murphy, D., and R. L. Woolfolk. 2000a. The harmful dysfunction analysis of mental disorder. *Philosophy, Psychiatry, and Psychology* 7(4): 241–252.

Murphy, D., and R. L. Woolfolk. 2000b. Conceptual analysis and scientific understanding. *Philosophy, Psychiatry, & Psychology* 7(4): 271–293.

Neander, K. 1991. Functions as selected effects: The conceptual analyst's defense. *Philosophy of Science* 58(2): 168–184.

Nordenfeldt, L. 2003. On the evolutionary concept of health: Health as natural function. In *Dimensions of Health and Health Promotion*, L. Nordenfeldt and P.-E. Liss (eds.), 37–53. Rodopi.

Roe, K., and D. Murphy. 2011. Function, dysfunction, adaptation? In *Maladapted Minds*, P. Adriaens and A. Block (eds.), 216–237. Oxford University Press.

Schaffner, K. F. 1993. *Discovery and Explanation in Biology and Medicine*. University of Chicago Press.

Tabery, J. 2004. Synthesizing activities and interactions in the concept of a "mechanism." *Philosophy of Science* 71: 1–15.

Wachbroit, R. 1994. Normality as a biological concept. *Philosophy of Science* 61: 579–591.

Wakefield, J. C. 1992a. The concept of mental disorder: On the boundary between biological facts and social values. *American Psychologist* 47(3): 373–388.

Wakefield, J. C. 1992b. Disorder as harmful dysfunction: A conceptual critique of *DSM-III-R*'s definition of mental disorder. *Psychological Review* 99(2): 232–247.

Wakefield, J. C. 1993. Limits of operationalization: A critique of Spitzer and Endicott's (1978) proposed operational criteria for mental disorder. *Journal of Abnormal Psychology* 102(1): 160–172.

Wakefield, J. C. 1999. Disorder as a black box essentialist concept. *Journal of Abnormal Psychology* 108: 465–472.

Wakefield, J. C. 2006. Personality disorder as harmful dysfunction: *DSM*'s cultural deviance requirement reconsidered. *Journal of Personality Disorders* 20: 157–169.

Wakefield, J. C. 2009. Mental disorder and moral responsibility: Disorders of personhood as harmful dysfunctions, with special reference to alcoholism. *Philosophy, Psychiatry, and Psychology* 16: 91–99.

Wakefield, J. C. 2011. Functional explanation: Aristotle, Lucretius, Darwin. In *Maladapted Minds*, P. Adriaens and A. Block (eds.), 143–172. Oxford University Press.

Wakefield, J. C., M. F. Schmitz, M. B. First, and A. V. Horwitz. 2007. Extending the bereavement exclusion for major depression to other losses: Evidence from the National Comorbidity Survey. *Archives of General Psychiatry* 64: 433–440.

Weber, M. 2005a. Holism, coherence and the dispositional concept of functions. *Annals of the History and Philosophy of Biology* 10: 189–201.

Weber, M. 2005b. *Philosophy of Experimental Biology*. Cambridge University Press.

Wright, L. 1973. Functions. *Philosophical Review* 82(2): 139–168.

Zisook, S., and K. S. Kendler. 2007. Is bereavement-related depression different than non-bereavement-related depression? *Psychological Medicine* 37(6): 779–794.

14 Can Causal Role Functions Yield Objective Judgments of Medical Dysfunction and Replace the Harmful Dysfunction Analysis's Evolutionary Component? Reply to Dominic Murphy

Jerome Wakefield

I thank Dominic Murphy for his contribution to this volume and for his philosophically sophisticated writings over the years, including his illuminating *Psychiatry in the Scientific Image* (2006). In his present chapter, Murphy challenges the evolutionary component of my harmful dysfunction analysis (HDA) of medical, including mental, disorder. The HDA claims that "disorder" refers to "harmful dysfunction," where dysfunction is the failure of some feature to perform a natural function for which it is biologically designed by evolutionary processes and harm is judged in accordance with social values (First and Wakefield 2010, 2013; Spitzer 1997, 1999; Wakefield 1992a, 1992b, 1993, 1995, 1997a, 1997b, 1997c, 1997d, 1998, 1999a, 1999b, 1999c, 2000a, 2000b, 2001, 2006, 2007, 2009, 2011a, 2014, 2016a, 2016b; Wakefield and First 2003, 2012).

Murphy has long been a critic of my claim that the sense of "dysfunction" that is most relevant to understanding psychiatric attributions of disorder and nondisorder is failure of natural (or biologically designed) function, which cashes out in evolutionary terms. He frames his argument as a contest between the HDA's "selected effects" (SE) approach to "function" and Robert Cummins's "systemic capacity" or "functional analysis" or "causal role" (CR) understanding of "function" that Murphy embraces. My blurry recollection is that this dispute has been going on ever since our first (and I think only) face-to-face meeting many years ago when he was a graduate student and I a guest speaker in Stephen Stich's seminar at Rutgers. I have addressed this issue elsewhere (e.g., Wakefield 2000b, 2001), but I am happy to have this opportunity to tackle this central disagreement between us from the fresh perspective of his chapter, especially knowing that many others in our field share Murphy's preference for the causal role approach.

Murphy finds the CR function approach so persuasive that he suggests that my choice of an evolutionary approach must be due either to my missing nuances or not considering other options in the function literature. In fact, it was immersion in the function literature that persuaded me to reject Cummins's CR-function account and construct my own "black-box essentialist" evolutionary version of the nature of natural or biological function concepts. A central impetus for my formulating the HDA was my rejection of Boorse's (1976) critique of Larry Wright's (1973) seminal work on the etio-logical approach to function when applied to the specific case of biological functions. I concluded that Boorse's critique was flawed and left untouched a correct core idea in Wright's analysis when applied specifically to biological or natural functions and that this core idea is essential to the foundations of medicine. Another formative influence was a graduate seminar I sat in on at Berkeley with Charles Taylor—if memory serves, with Mark Bedau and Robert Wachbroit also attending, both of whom later published on functions—in which issues concerning function raised by Taylor's book *The Explanation of Behavior* (1964) were discussed. An additional provocation was the contro-versy about the evolutionary and function-related issues in regard to female orgasmic dysfunction raised by Don Symonds's (1979) book *The Evolution of Human Sexuality* (later examined in depth by Elizabeth Lloyd [2005]) as well as by research on orgasmic dysfunction that I was pursuing at the time with my colleague, Nadine Payn (Payn and Wakefield 1982) (for comments on my early papers on sexuality, see Demazeux's chapter in this volume).

So, if I have gotten "dysfunction" in its diagnostic sense wrong—and I don't think I have—it is not because I have missed or failed to consider various options regarding how to construe biological functions. It is because I think there are powerful arguments that other views are inadequate to provide a foundation for psychiatric and medical diagnosis. However, Murphy's pushing me on this point has usefully prodded me to address this topic in greater depth and thoroughness than I have before.

Murphy tends to emphasize a sharp divide between folk concepts and scientific concepts, and this has been the basis for another criticism by him, that in my criticisms of false-positive psychiatric diagnostic criteria, I give priority to folk psychology over science. Although I remain unclear about the precise basis for this claim, I am happy to see that in the present chapter, he adopts an alternative interpretation: "A more chari-table reading would be that Wakefield thinks that the underlying logic of psychiatric practice accords with the HDA but that sometimes psychiatrists depart from the logic of their own projects." That is correct; my critiques of psychiatric overdiagnosis are based on inconsistencies between psychiatry's classification of certain conditions as disorders and what I take to be psychiatry's own HDA concept of disorder. There is in my view no in-principle tension between common sense and science and certainly no dominance of folk theories over science. On my view, the intuitive concept of disorder and the sci-entific concept are basically the same with science's essentialist theory added, so there is no in-principle conflict at that level. And, common sense succumbs to science on the facts that determine whether specific conditions satisfy the conceptual and essentialist criteria and thus warrant disorder attribution. In any event, Murphy's more nuanced view of my position allows me to put aside this previous misunderstanding and focus on what is now the central issue between us, the nature of function and dysfunction in the medically relevant sense that pertains to disorder attributions.

The Ubiquity of CR Functions and the Reality of SE Functions

It is important to be crystal clear at the outset that I completely accept with Murphy that non-SE functional language is of course an integral part of biology's vocabulary. It is extremely common in biology to distinguish structure from function (which is a parallel task to distinguishing anatomy from physiology), with "function" most often simply meaning causal action. Indeed, an about-to-be-issued new journal in physiology sponsored by the American Physiological Association will be titled *Function* and almost certainly won't be limited to biologically designed causal roles. Throughout the contemporary biological sciences, and historically from William Harvey to Bock and von Wahlert (1965; see below) and on to Murphy's example of Hubel and Wiesel, "function" has been used by researchers to specify the "causal action" or "causal role" of a feature within a larger system being studied.

It is true, as SE theorists have often pointed out, that the language of function as causal action is often weaker in syntactic structure than the characteristic SE-function assertion such as "the natural (or biological) function of X is to Y" and may be more like "X functions to Y," "X functions as a Y," "X functionally interacts with Y," "the functional effect of X is Y," "X divides into functional units of type Y," and so on. For example, if one examines Hubel and Wiesel's (1959, 1962) classic work on the workings of the visual perceptual system of the cat cited by Murphy as an example of CR functions, it is true that they are primarily trying to understand the details of causal interactions and are not explicitly concerned with background assumptions about the biological design of the visual system, although such assumptions guide the kinds of hypotheses they formulate. Consequently, they almost never use "function" in the strong sense of "the function of" of an anatomical feature. Rather, consistent with their focus on causal role, their uses of "function" generally occur in adjectival and adverbial forms such as "functional architecture," "functionally different," "functional cell types," "functionally separated," "functional description," "functional subdivisions," "functionally disrupt," "functional role," "functional connexions," and "functional units." Only once do they step back and look at the big picture of the meaning of their detailed causal-action discoveries for overall biological roles in perceptual discrimination, and there they use "function" in a noun form that is at least ambiguous between CR and SE function: "Our findings in the striate cortex would suggest two further possible functions...to determine the form, size and orientation of the most effective stimuli, and secondly,...perception of movement" (1959, 588). So, Murphy's example supports his point that "function" and its cognates are used in CR-type ways. One need not go back to Hubel and Wiesel to nail down this point; surveying recent biological literature quickly proves the point. Indeed, I would argue that most theoretical terms have several or many meanings and can be used fluidly with different "semantic markers" (in Putnam's terminology; see my reply to Lemoine in this volume) in a multiplicity of ways.

Locutional nuances are not always a reliable indicator of meaning, and even the strong locution, "the function of X," is ambiguous and can be used in a CR-function context as a variant of "the functioning of X" even though it generally refers to SE functions. "Function" sometimes is used this CR way when describing pathological causal actions, as in the article title, "Retinoid X Receptors: X-ploring Their (Patho) physiological Functions" (Szanto et al. 2004). Similarly, in an editorial commenting on Engle et al.'s (2019) discovery that glycan carbohydrate antigen CA19–9, a known biomarker for pancreatic cancer, actually plays a pathogenic causal role in the disease, Halbrook and Crawford (2019) say that the Engle et al. study "ascribes a critical function to the most commonly used biomarker of the disease" (1132), that "there has been little understanding of CA19–9 function in pancreatic pathophysiology" (1132), and "the discovery of a new function of CA19–9 is exciting" (1133). Sometimes, CR and SE uses of "function" appear side by side. Thus, the same article that refers to "erectile dysfunction" with a clear implication of objective failure of natural function also refers to the effects of genetic variation on "sexual function" in the CR sense that encompasses causation of disorder: "Because the variants associated with erectile dysfunction are not associated with differences in BMI, our findings suggest a mechanism that is specific to sexual function" (Jorgenson et al. 2018, 11018), and the same article uses "function" to report the identification of the biologically designed SE-function role of a gene: "Finally, through in silico and in vitro functional investigations, we linked our risk locus to gene function. As evolutionary conservation is a strong marker of functional genomic sequences, we focused our follow-up analyses on … the only SNP located in an evolutionarily conserved region" (Jorgenson et al. 2018, 11019).

Although the focus on CR analysis often without explicit reference to biological design is ubiquitous in biological research, the depth of this separation can easily be overstated. Design considerations are almost always at least implicitly or potentially in the CR-analytic background in studies of normal functioning. Papers in functional anatomy almost always assume that salient anatomical structures have adaptive biological roles (even if the study examines a pathogenic causal role), and CR-type analyses are generally guided by implicit biological-design hunches. Analysis of functional mechanics is generally accompanied or followed by hypotheses about design function that guide further research. For example, consider these excerpts from article abstracts:

In 1678, Stefano Lorenzini first described a network of organs of unknown function in the torpedo ray-the ampullae of Lorenzini (AoL). An individual ampulla consists of a pore on the skin that is open to the environment, a canal containing a jelly and leading to an alveolus with a series of electrosensing cells. The role of the AoL remained a mystery for almost 300 years until research demonstrated that skates, sharks, and rays detect very weak electric fields produced by a potential prey. The AoL jelly likely contributes to this electrosensing function, yet the exact details of this contribution remain unclear.…We hope that the observed high proton conductivity of the AoL jelly may contribute to future studies of the AoL function. (Josberger et al. 2016, 1)

We report on the discovery of a remarkable defensive specialization in stonefishes that was identified during a phylogenetic study of scorpionfishes. ...The lachrymal saber, involves modifications to the circumorbitals, maxilla, *adductor mandibulae*, and associated tendons. At its core, the lachrymal saber is an elongation of an anterior spine...that stonefishes are capable of rotating from the standard ventral position to a locked lateral position....that we hypothesize reduces predation on stonefishes. (Smith, Everman, and Richardson 2018, 94)

Upon continued submersion in water, the glabrous skin on human hands and feet forms wrinkles. The formation of these wrinkles is known to be an active process, controlled by the autonomic nervous system. Such an active control suggests that these wrinkles may have an important function, but this function has not been clear. In this study, we show that submerged objects are handled more quickly with wrinkled fingers than with unwrinkled fingers, whereas wrinkles make no difference to manipulating dry objects. These findings support the hypothesis that water-induced finger wrinkles...may be an adaptation for handling objects in wet conditions. (Kareklas, Nettle, and Smulders 2013, 1)

These cases illustrate that analysis of how an organism CR-functions is almost always in service of understanding in the long run how the organism SE-functions. So, I agree with Murphy that reference to CR functions (in some broad sense) is a regular and perhaps predominant occurrence in biological science, because mostly researchers focus on how things work, which is both a practical concern and a foundation for attributing SE functions. I also assume that CR functions exist alongside SE functions and the investigation of CR functions generally takes place within the broader assumption of biological design, which waits in the background for occasional but pivotal illumination. I proceed on this basis to examine whether there are grounds for Murphy's position that medical and psychiatric diagnosis of disorder can be based on CR functions alone.

One Doubt about CR Functions

Before proceeding, I want to express one possible doubt about CR functions. This is not a doubt about the existence of CR functions as causal roles, because such causal roles obviously do exist. Rather, it is a doubt about whether CR functions really are a second, *independent* and scientifically interesting sense of "function" beyond SE functions that adds to the ontology of science. Such usage of "function" might be understandable instead as a common synecdochical usage that simply captures the causal-role aspect of SE functions and is parasitic on the primary SE usage. Consider an analogy: "reason," which inherently refers to a psychological cause of action, is commonly used for nonpsychological causation as well. There are no literal reasons (i.e., belief-desire pairs) that cause headaches or earthquakes or hearts to beat, yet "reason" is used in phrases such as "the reason for earthquakes" (Reason 2019), "28 Reasons for a Sudden or Throbbing Headache and Nausea" (Steinberg and Buoy Medical Review Team 2019), and the "reason for the motion and beat of the heart" (Harvey 1628/1993, as quoted in Ribatti 2009). This can be construed as a parasitic usage that expresses the causal power of reasons without there actually being any reasons. Or, one could on the basis of such usage assert that "reason" is polysemous. Similar options may be available in regard to the use of "function" as causal action.

The reason one might choose to understand CR-function talk as a derivative synecdochical form is out of concern about the ontological superfluousness of adding CR functions to the furniture of science. In his original article introducing CR functions, Cummins (1975) challenges the SE notion by asking, "We know why evolutionary biologists are interested in effects contributing to an organism's capacity to maintain its species, but *why call them functions*?" (756, emphasis added). He argues that one can just describe all of the biological facts without the additional label. Let's agree with the implied "semantic Occam's razor" that one does not want to needlessly introduce terminology into science that does not represent a substantive value-added ontological commitment. If so, then Cummins seems to have a problem if his question, "*why call them functions*?" is directed at his own proposed "CR function" terminology.

"Causal roles" are, after all, nothing more than abstract descriptions of causes within complex systems, an ontology that is already succinctly describable using standard causal language. Every causal analysis, whether explaining systemic capacities or describing billiard ball causation, involves abstracting from the many concrete features of the causal process and selecting causal sequences that are of interest. So, if the label denotes nothing substantive other than causation, *why call them "functions"*? (I will address this question in the case of SE functions below.) For example, in a science news article about the remarkable discovery that a long-known biomarker for pancreatic cancer actually has a causal role in causing the cancer, one author is quoted as explaining, "We serendipitously noted that the mice developed inflammation of the pancreas...and further studies then showed they had accelerated pancreatic tumor progression. CA19–9, in other words, was actively causing pancreatitis, leading to pancreatic cancer," and an independent expert who wrote an editorial about the discovery is quoted as saying, "This is a whole different paradigm. ...What used to be a marker is now [taking] a functional role in pancreatic disease" (Blanco 2019). What is notable is that there would be no content or implication lost if "functional role" in the second quote were replaced by "cause" or "causal role" from the first quote because they are both expressing the same idea. This seems true of CR-function mentions in general.

There thus seems to be no ontological profit in introducing CR function as a scientific concept, which as we shall see is decidedly not true of SE functions due to their distinctive feature of what Cummins calls "effect-sensitivity." Cummins seems to implicitly recognize this oddity about CR functions when he states that he is open to not calling them "functions": "It is, of course, perfectly possible to acknowledge that what we are calling functional analysis is both a useful and ubiquitous form of explanation in science and engineering, while denying that the analyzing capacities appealed to in such explanations are functions" (Cummins and Roth 2009, 75). However, CR functions would have more of a claim on ontological relevance if the concept of medical disorder could be adequately anchored in CR functions, and it is to that question that I now turn.

The Problem of the Objectivity of Biological Dysfunction

In a medical context, the idea that function and dysfunction and thus health and disorder are entirely relative to the interests or concerns of the observer is a nonstarter. There may be vast value-based disagreements about what to do about various functions and dysfunctions, and our ignorance of functions and dysfunctions of body and mind remains vast as well. However, the objectivity of the fact that, for example, the heart's function is to pump blood and that its failure to do so is a dysfunction is part of the scientific foundation on which medicine rests.

Cummins's view of the nature of functions and dysfunctions denies any such objectivity. Cummins (2002) begins one of his papers on functions with the following striking statement: "There are two subpopulations of functional explanation roaming the earth: teleological explanation, and functional analysis. The two are in competition" (2002, 157). Murphy follows Cummins in accepting as a starting point what is now often referred to as the consensus view (Godfrey-Smith 1993), that there are two forms of functional explanation and thus two kinds of function statements of the form, "The function of X is to Y," comparing it to the situation of the term "gene" in biology: "Different areas of biology, or even the same scientist at different times, will use the gene concept to pick out different aspects of the underlying genetic and developmental processes. I think *function* is scientifically polysemous in just this way" (Murphy, this volume). That is, "function" is used in both the CR and SE senses.

One might well ask: if there really are two different (legitimate) meanings of "function" and corresponding forms of functional explanation, then why are they in competition? Murphy's own analogy to the polysemous use of "gene" suggests a more pluralistic stance. If there really are two senses of "function," then the problem would seem to be which sense applies in which contexts. It would make no more sense to say that they are in competition than it would to say that "there are two different subpopulations of water roaming the earth, liquid water and substance water, and the two are in competition." In a restaurant, when I ask for water, I presumably mean the liquid, but in a chemistry lab or when studying molecules floating in the Horsehead Nebula, I probably mean the substance. If someone proposed that because these two related ideas are expressed using the very same word, we must decide on one meaning or the other for all contexts, that would not be taken seriously.

Nonetheless, Murphy follows Cummins in arguing that the CR view of functions is better than the SE view. Given that the major objection to CR functions has been that they are incapable of supporting objective dysfunction attributions and thus cannot be a basis for diagnosis, this is a risky position for Murphy to take. Indeed, Murphy acknowledges that this is a major problem with Cummins's view:

> The bigger problem with Cummins's analysis is that, notoriously, attributions of function on this account are interest relative: if you are interested in the heart's contribution to the circulation of the blood, you can analyze it one way, and if you are interested in its contribution to the sum total of the noises the body makes, you can treat it as a "lub-dup" generator. In both cases, it counts as a part of the overall system you wish to decompose. Cummins thought that the overall system depended on the interests of the investigator. In that sense, he was not really trying to articulate a naturalistic concept of function that captures biological practice but to understand the logic of functional analysis. This is, however, a problem for such a view.... We want an objective characterization of dysfunction rather than a mere acknowledgment that we decompose a system into its contributory parts. If that were all that the account gave us, it would threaten the objectivity that is appealing about... the HDA.... We need a way of characterizing biological systems that sees them as mind-independent components of nature, not just reflections of human concerns.

This problem defines the major task of Murphy's paper, which is to show that CR functions can provide an objective naturalist account suitable to medical diagnosis. Murphy proposes three tests that he will use to determine which of the two views of function is best suited to the foundations of medical diagnosis: "First, it should be able to make precise the idea that attributions of mental illness rely on something being objectively wrong under the hood of a human being. Second, it should capture relevant scientific practice. Third, it should not be too revisionist but make sense of the idea that some conditions may have causes that cannot be shown to depend on failures of selected effects."

Immediately below, I consider the second and third tests, which I think are based on misunderstandings and misguided assumptions. Then, for the remainder of this reply, I focus on addressing the first and conceptually most fundamental test: can CR functions explain the idea central to psychiatric diagnosis of "something being objectively wrong under the hood of a human being," as Murphy puts it? This is the essence of the idea of mental disorder, and if a view of function cannot explain this, then it is not the view of function that is relevant to medical and psychiatric diagnosis. Murphy's other two tests become irrelevant if the first test fails to support the CR approach as a viable alternative.

Is the HDA Too Revisionist?

Murphy proposes that an analysis of function and dysfunction for medical purposes "should not be too revisionist but make sense of the idea that some conditions may have causes that cannot be shown to depend on failures of selected effects." That is, Murphy accuses the HDA of being too revisionist because, he claims, there are many disorders that are not failures of selected effects, so the HDA would misclassify them as nondisorders. This claim begs the central question at issue unless Murphy can demonstrate that there are such conditions, which he attempts to do. It is a surprising claim given that the HDA attempts to explain actual disorder and nondisorder judgments and so should follow these judgments rather closely.

I am going to answer the charge of revisionism, but I note in passing that the charge is questionable as a claimed deep flaw in the HDA, depending on the kind of revisionism. Revisionism of specific disorder judgments is perfectly acceptable scientifically. Behaviorists, social constructivists, family systems theorists, and antipsychiatrists all had accounts that if true would have radically altered and virtually eliminated our usual disorder judgments. The reason for rejecting those views was not that they were revisionist—that is hardly scientifically problematic, and it was generally agreed that if these theories were correct, then there would be few or no mental disorders—but that they were false theories. If the HDA is correct about the concept of disorder, then it is up to advances in scientific knowledge to tell us which conditions satisfy that concept, and I would let the chips fall where they may.

To support his "too revisionist" claim about the HDA, Murphy compares the HDA and CR views on their potential for revisionism and claims that the "systemic capacity view wins easily." This is because the HDA's evolutionary requirement sets a much higher bar for disorder attribution than the CR view. The HDA "stipulates that there must be some evolved system somewhere that has departed from its historical design and is connected to the current problem," but the CR view "just asks what the underlying system is that is misbehaving." Murphy thus concludes that the CR view is less revisionist because it is "less epistemically committed" and it "has one less bet to make."

Murphy argues that because the HDA classifies much fewer conditions as disordered, it forces us to revise many of our judgments about disorder. This is a patently invalid argument unless one has already independently established that the conditions excluded from the disorder category by the HDA are in fact legitimate disorders. In fact, the real problem—and the real threat of massive unjustified revisionism—is just the opposite and lies with the looseness of the CR view. Because the CR view holds that what is a dysfunction (or what underlying system is misbehaving, as Murphy would have it) depends on researcher or clinician interests, CR diagnostic practice is subject to arbitrary expansion to reflect diagnosticians' preferences. Murphy's view that lack of sufficiently all-encompassing diagnosis is of central concern reveals a failure to appreciate that the goal is not to maximize diagnosable conditions such that all systemic "misbehavior" qualifies as a psychiatric disorder (which was exactly the criticism of the antipsychiatrists that psychiatry has labored to answer) but to get diagnosis right as medically legitimate. Recent debates over *Diagnostic and Statistical Manual of Mental*

Disorders (*DSM-5*) as well as ongoing critiques of psychiatry as in the current "neuro-diversity" movement underscore that overdiagnosis remains a major issue. The HDA's higher diagnostic threshold (or, actually, the fact that it has a threshold at all, because the interest-relative CR approach has none other than the diagnosticians' preferences) protects against false positives and the use of diagnosis for social control and locates psychiatric disorder within a legitimate medical domain. The CR-function approach is deeply and catastrophically revisionist because, as antipsychiatrists would quickly note, whether a system is "misbehaving" is in the eye of the beholder and not a matter of science.

Unlike the CR's free-for-all, the HDA's account of the concept of disorder is *appropriately* potentially revisionist in light of what we may discover about the scientific facts. It is important to recognize that revisionism at the level of specific disorder judgments is not intrinsically problematic, as long as one is observing the meaning of "mental disorder." Some scientific theories of the conditions generally labeled as mental disorders are truly massively revisionist at the level of specific judgments because they imply that those conditions generally do not satisfy the requirements to be a medical disorder. For example, certain forms of classic behaviorism and of extreme social constructivism imply that there are few actual dysfunctions underlying the conditions generally labeled mental disorders and so, consistent with the HDA, they claim that few conditions are genuine mental disorders. The HDA more modestly suggests that, in light of the facts, some revision of our bloated nosology is needed, including depathologization of certain types of what is now classified as attention-deficit/hyperactivity disorder (ADHD) (see my reply to De Vreese in this volume), depressive disorder (Horwitz and Wakefield 2007), autism spectrum disorder (Wakefield, Wasserman, and Conrad 2020), anxiety disorder (Horwitz and Wakefield 2012), and others (Wakefield 2016b). The ability to identify such justified revisions correcting diagnostic overreach allows psychiatry to respond to criticisms that specific categories go beyond the domain of medicine proper and have become a tool of social control, thus constructively addressing the legitimate concerns of the antipsychiatrists. The CR approach offers psychiatry no such response to antipsychiatric concerns.

Remarkably, the only example of the HDA's supposedly being "too revisionist" that Murphy offers is the tired (and unrepresentative; see my comments below on Kingma) "dyslexia"-type examples that I have addressed at length elsewhere (e.g., Wakefield 1999a; see also my reply to De Block and Sholl in this volume for further discussion of dyslexia). It is worth commenting on a couple of faulty assertions in Murphy's discussion. First, echoing other critics, Murphy suggests that in my portraying dyslexia in HDA terms as a social harm (inability to learn to read) caused by an inferred (but as yet not clearly established) brain dysfunction, the dyslexia example shows that I simply make up dysfunctions in an ad hoc manner so that my position is unfalsifiable: "Wakefield seems to think that…one can always postulate the existence of a selected function that is linked to the condition. ... This seems grossly ad hoc; ... this just makes the HDA immune to counterexample by stipulation ... Wakefield can just insist that there must be one somewhere."

This common objection reveals a misunderstanding of the HDA. The HDA is a conceptual analysis that explains when we are justified in our attributions of disorder; it is not a substantive theory of any particular condition's status as a disorder or nondisorder. Dyslexia is considered a disorder because it is believed to be due to a dysfunction, and one can excavate from the literature the reasoning that supports this hypothesis in the minds of clinicians and researchers. The HDA makes no claim that dyslexia actually is caused by a dysfunction; that is a matter of scientific evidence, not conceptual analysis, and nothing about the HDA's validity depends on whether there is or is not such a dysfunction. The HDA asserts that people attribute disorder when they believe there is a dysfunction; it says nothing about whether people are right in any given case. The relevant evidence consists of whether the way that reading disorder specialists and others think about and justify diagnosis of dyslexia is consistent with the HDA's conceptual-analytic claim. This evidence is publicly available and cannot be made up in an ad hoc manner. The question for the CR view is whether specialists believe that diagnosis of dyslexia is justified whenever a child does not learn to read given that we have an interest in children reading and thus failure to learn to read constitutes the "misbehaving" of some system in the child and warrants being labeled a disorder. When I reject that view and claim that dyslexia presupposes a dysfunction in the stronger HDA sense, I am reporting what a close examination of dyslexia diagnosis and research clearly reveals, namely, that dyslexia is commonly distinguished from all other manner of nondysfunction "misbehaving" (e.g., lack of education, emotional distraction, lack of motivation, low general intelligence, etc.) that causes lack of ability to read, any of which could be classified as CR dysfunctions, and moreover that, in the course of diagnosis, symptoms suggestive of neurological dysfunction (such as, in former days, letter reversal, although this particular symptom is now questioned) are accorded special significance as confirming the diagnosis. One can dispute my reading of the evidence, but there is nothing ad hoc or unfalsifiable about this approach to testing the HDA's explanatory power.

Moreover, there is a false background assumption underlying Murphy's dyslexia argument for the HDA's revisionism. Like some other critics (e.g., see Garson in this volume), Murphy presumes that we would continue to consider a condition such as dyslexia a disorder even if we discovered it is not due to a dysfunction, as if the attribution of disorder to a condition is atheoretical and remains fixed no matter how we explain it. The history of psychiatry shows this is false. When problematic psychological conditions come to be understood either as naturally selected or as just something other than failures of natural functions, they also come to be understood as nondisorders (see my replies to Garson, to De Vreese, and to Cooper in this volume).

In response to my claim that clinicians and researchers limit disorder attributions to what they believe to be dysfunctions, Murphy actually agrees but retorts, "This is correct, but it only meets the objection if those researchers are committed to an evolutionary account of function, which is the very point at issue. The fact that they take for granted the existence of a dysfunction…does not show that they take for granted the existence of an evolutionary dysfunction." This objection again confuses substantive essentialist theorizing with conceptual analysis. Obviously, most clinicians and researchers and laypeople are not explicitly thinking about evolution in judging there is a disorder, any more than people are thinking about the chemical formula H_2O when they ask for a glass of water in a restaurant. The concept of disorder was around long before Darwin and is understood by evangelical Christians who reject evolutionary theory, so someone need not have evolution in mind or even know about or believe in evolution to understand the concept of disorder. As I have explained elsewhere (Wakefield 1999a, 1999b; see also my reply to Lemoine in this volume), "disorder" means "harmful dysfunction" where dysfunction is understood intuitively in terms of failure of natural function, that is, failure of how we are biologically designed, which is a notion that has been at the center of biology and available to common sense ever since the discipline began. However, since Darwin, we know that the best theoretical explanation of natural functions and biological design is evolution by natural selection. The HDA proposes that evolutionary dysfunction is the best *theoretical explanation* of what clinicians and laypeople are aiming at when they identify disorders in the medical sense (see my reply to Forest in this volume for further comments on this point). So, in assuming there is a breakdown of some sort in the way the organism is designed to function, clinicians are in effect assuming there is an evolutionary dysfunction, just as in asking for water in a restaurant, one is in effect asking for H_2O even if one does not know anything about chemical theory. Note that the objectivity of dysfunction—Murphy's first test of an account of dysfunction, which is evaluated in detail below—is a salient aspect of disorder judgments that requires explanation, and evolutionary dysfunction explains this feature, whereas CR dysfunction cannot explain it unless, of course, Murphy can make good on his claim that objectivity can be teased out of the CR view, a claim that I evaluate below.

Reply to Kingma's Genetic Linkage Argument for the HDA Being Strongly Revisionist

There remains one central "revisionist" argument deployed by Murphy, which he largely outsources by citing a handbook chapter by Elsilijn Kingma (2013), in which she critiques the HDA as unacceptably revisionist. Kingma's and Murphy's argument is essentially that genetic linkage causes phenotypic effects that are not due to natural selection, so if those effects are valued but go wrong, then there are disorders that are not failures of natural functions to which the HDA denies disorder status, making it highly revisionist relative to current diagnostic practices. Murphy puts the linkage-based revisionism argument as follows: "Now, as Kingma notes, it is quite possible for a linked trait to be abnormal for independent reasons that have nothing to do with a dysfunction in the system it is linked to. … Kingma argues that Wakefield's position is potentially very revisionist indeed: if a large number of disorders turn out not to be linked to selected effects, but the product of other processes, such as developmental or genetic linkage, then he will have to say that they are not really disorders." This linkage criticism is closely related to a criticism earlier leveled by Murphy himself (Murphy and Woolfolk 2000) to which I replied (Wakefield 2000b). However, given this new more elaborated version, once more unto the breach.

Kingma cites several genetic linkage phenomena in addition to standard genetic linkage due to close positioning on a chromosome. The complexities of, for example, heterozygous advantage, developmental linkage, and antagonistic pleiotropy pose interesting challenges for any theory of health and disorder. These phenomena are so unanticipated that they might have required what I have called "conceptual rectification" with the intuitive concept of natural function, in the way that isotopes required rectification with the intuitive structural concept of substance (see my reply to Lemoine in this volume). However, Kingma acknowledges that the HDA can handle cases of heterozygous advantage (e.g., sickle cell trait versus sickle cell anemia) simply by distinguishing between the positively selected nondisordered trait and the negatively selected disorder, and a similar resolution can work when both effects are within one individual, as in antagonistic pleiotropy. So, I focus on Kingma's primary example of standard genetic linkage, which refers to the fact that a trait not at all selected for—thus either neutral or even deleterious with regard to fitness—may nonetheless be selected at higher than neutral statistical rates due to its proximity on the chromosome to a trait that is naturally selected. This is due to the mechanics of reproduction in which close-together genes tend to be kept together. Such linkage is not sensitive to the nature of the phenotypic results of the gene but is just a matter of the happenstance of where the gene falls on the chromosome, so it is unlikely to display apparent manifestations of biological design. Note that in trying to show that there are disorders without dysfunctions, Kingma has in mind examples in which there are no HDA-type dysfunctions to muddy the waters, so failure of the nonselected trait is neither due to nor causes any HDA-type dysfunction of any selected trait.

Kingma illustrates the possibility of nonselected traits due to linkage with the example of blue eyes, which is known to be linked to a skin coloration gene: "For example, the presence of blue eyes is not explained by an effect of blue eyes, but by the increased ability of lighter skin to absorb ultraviolet B radiation (which helps with vitamin D production). This can happen because the trait 'blue eyes' is linked to the trait 'light skin'" (392). Most people with the light-skin gene that causes lower production of melanin have the usual brown eyes, but in some people, the closely linked gene that regulates eye color has a genetic "switch" in an "off" position that blocks melanin production in the stroma of the iris and thus yields blue eyes. Kingma assumes that blue eyes are selectively neutral but are maintained or increased in the population because of the blue-eye gene's linkage to the pale-skin gene, which has been selected for in northern populations. (In actuality, there is some evidence that the blue eyes trait has been sexually selected and this explains the spread of blue eyes, but I leave this complexity aside here.)

Now, to Kingma's argument that "such linked traits pose a serious problem for Wakefield's account of disorder" (392). The problem is claimed to arise, first, because linked traits that are not themselves naturally selected have no natural function: "traits that are not selected for their own effect, but are selected because of their linkage to other successful traits, do not have a function on Wakefield's account" (392). Second, despite lacking a natural function, such nonselected linked traits may be socially exploited in various ways: "It is overwhelmingly likely that we have an abundance of traits that fulfill important roles for us and in our culture, particularly in the mental realm, but whose effects may not be what drove their selection" (395). Third, it is in principle possible for a linked trait to be interfered with without causing a problem for the naturally selected gene to which it is linked, and thus without causing any collateral evolutionary dysfunction: "it is not just possible, but in fact overwhelmingly likely, that all manner of things…could affect one out of a pair of genetically or developmentally linked traits without affecting the other" (393). So, for example, "even though the selection of blue eyes is explained by the effects of fair skin, it is entirely possible for something to happen to the blueness of my eyes without my skin being affected" (393). This potential for something to happen to a linked nonselected trait without affecting any selected trait applies to the aforementioned linked traits that we value and socially exploit. However, because these valued linked traits do not have a natural function, if they fail, the failure cannot be a dysfunction on the evolutionary account: "These traits therefore lack functions and, by consequence, the ability to dysfunction" (395). (I note in passing that all these premises would also apply to Boorse's view that Kingma embraces as superior because Boorse limits functions to the recent contributions of a part to survival and reproduction, and most nonselected linked traits will make no such contribution and thus lack Boorse-type functions.)

I agree with Kingma's premises but disagree with the conclusion that Kingma claims to follow from these premises that the HDA is highly revisionist. Kingma does not explicitly take the final steps to her conclusion, but the only route to get there is by adding something like the following suppressed premise: *the concept of disorder is such that any failure of a valued human trait qualifies as a disorder*. She indicates that the nonselected conditions that she thinks are truly disorders but revisionistically not classified as such by the HDA are "traits that fulfill important roles for us and in our culture." The suppressed premise of her argument is more general because there is nothing special about valued linked traits versus other valued nonselected traits that distinguish them in the argument. Moreover, linkage was unknown to those using the concept of disorder throughout medical history and so cannot play any distinctive conceptual role in the concept of disorder. Rather, linkage is just a vehicle for Kingma to make the correct point that some traits we value have no HDA-type natural function. Her suppressed premise that such conditions are disorders allows the argument to proceed to its suppressed conclusion, as follows: *Therefore, when valued linked traits fail, even though such failures are not dysfunctions, the failures fall under our concept of disorder and are in fact considered disorders. However, the HDA does not classify such failures of valued nonselected traits as disorders. Thus, the HDA is revisionist.*

The only example provided by Kingma is, like Murphy, a speculation that dyslexia might result from the failure of linked genes rather than from a dysfunction of selected brain mechanisms. Generalizing from the dyslexia example, Kingma further argues that such linked traits and their failures must be very common even among traits we (often mistakenly, according to Kingma) take to be biologically designed. This leads her to her unrestrained mincing-no-words conclusion: "Wakefield's account of disorder, it turns out, is very strongly revisionist" (394) (also, "highly," "so very," "terribly," and "so terribly" revisionist and "more revisionist than he realizes" [396, 394, 395]). I will examine each of the three aspects of this argument: the concept of disorder as failure of valued traits, the dyslexia example, and the argument for the frequency of nonselected traits constituting mental modules that we consider selected.

An argument that the HDA is revisionist is by nature comparative and relative to some accepted nonarbitrary baseline. Kingma's argument is built on her key assumption, never explicitly defended, that our baseline concept of medical disorder encompasses all failures of socially valued traits. Kingma relies on this inflated account of disorder to argue for the HDA's supposed revisionism in not properly classifying every socially disvalued trait as a disorder. This claim has no plausibility on its face because there are endless positive traits, the absence of which are not considered disorders. There is nothing special about genetic linkage here. With regard to any traits, socially undesirable normal variation—scoring low, for example, on dimensions of intelligence, height, mathematical or musical ability, verbal skill, social skill, emotional resilience, physical strength, physical attractiveness, and so on—is not considered a disorder as long as it is within a range that is not considered to indicate dysfunction. For those aware of the history of psychiatry, the claim that socially disvalued traits are disorders is not merely false but worrisome because it would be the basis for social control by psychiatry and invites antipsychiatric objections.

Consider, for example, the illustrations in the following passage in which Kingma claims that there are naturally selected disorders (see my supplementary response to Cooper for fuller discussion of this claim):

The first possible problem for Wakefield is that of "selected disorders." These are selected effects or strategies that have very negative effects in our present society. Possible examples include forms of antisocial behavior: rape, a violent disposition, or dependent or attention-seeking behavior. All of these may have been beneficial in selective terms: serial rape can be a good strategy for increasing one's reproductive output, for example, and violence, dependence, or attention-seeking may all increase one's access to resources that in turn increase fitness. But if it is true that these conditions have been selected, then they are not a disorder according to Wakefield—and this countervenes our current way of thinking about these conditions. (2013, 391)

Her examples, based on the criterion that conditions that "have very negative effects in our present society" are disorders, indicate that it is Kingma who "countervenes our current way of thinking about these conditions." There is no category in *DSM-5* or *International Classification of Diseases* (*ICD-11*) in which these undesirable conditions are generally labeled disorders. They are only labeled disorders in extraordinary, extreme cases in which there is a plausible argument that there is a dysfunction of the system that gives rise to them. For example, aggression and violence per se, even when they involve mass killing, are not necessarily considered a disorder (e.g., Knoll and Pies 2019). Engaging in multiple rapes is a crime, not a disorder (Wakefield 2011b). *DSM-5* did consider a rape-related paraphilic category of coercive sexuality in which the coerciveness itself becomes the primary arousing factor and rejected it partly because it could easily be confused with the nondisorder of serial criminal rape. Regarding antisocial behavior more generally, although universally considered undesirable, it is not in itself considered disordered (e.g., antisocial delinquent behavior and even gang behavior among youth is generally not pathologized). Moreover, as I have explained elsewhere in this volume (see my responses to Cooper and Garson), when researchers conclude that antisocial personality is a naturally selected strategy or the result of social conditions and not an HDA-type dysfunction, they tend to revise their belief that it is a disorder and come to understand it as an undesirable nondisordered normal variant. In *DSM-5*, regarding categories that address antisocial behavior (e.g., intermittent explosive disorder, antisocial personality disorder), *DSM-5* takes pains in the diagnostic criteria to try to separate dysfunctions of aggressive tendencies from the wider issue of antisocial behavior in general that Kingma seems willing to pathologize. Neither attention seeking nor dependence per se are generally considered disorders, despite being looked down upon in our society.

Kingma later presents what she sees as her "most damaging" revisionist objection. She argues that "most if not all of our physical, and the vast majority of our mental traits, fall within the domain of health and disorder...they are either disordered, and if not, they are healthy." She claims that "an evolutionary account of disorder can never bear this out" (395) because only selected traits can have functions and can dysfunction. She concludes that "Wakefield's account of disorder places a substantial portion of our physiological and mental traits out of the realm of health and disorder altogether" in "a clear violation of one core conceptual element of the health and disorder dichotomy" (396).

First, Kingma's argument that the HDA does not dichotomize health versus disorder is based on an elementary misunderstanding. Like Christopher Boorse, whose view Kingma in her chapter embraces as superior to the HDA, I define health for the purposes of these analyses as lack of disorder. Thus, any selectively neutral trait, whether it is positive or negative in terms of its social valuation, is part of normal variation and thus part of health along with every selected variant. The issue here is not dichotomizing health and disorder but where socially disvalued nondysfunction conditions fall in the dichotomy. Kingma's point in emphasizing the dichotomy is to locate all socially negative traits on the "disorder" side of the dichotomy rather than allowing for normal (nondisordered) variation that is socially disvalued and yet perfectly healthy. Her view fails to comport with standard medical concepts. Nor does it follow that socially disvalued normal variation cannot be treated. I (Wakefield 2015) have argued that if limitations to an individual's opportunity are primarily due to socially negative valuation of parts of normal variation, it is a matter of justice that the individual should be offered treatment, even though the condition is not a disorder.

So, who is the revisionist here? The issue here is not whether undesirable nonselected effects of linked traits may occur but whether such conditions are (or would be) considered *disorders*. Kingma's inclusion of socially undesirable traits within disorder has no foundation in the history or current practice of diagnosis and no coherent relationship to psychiatric diagnosis as it is codified in *DSM-5* or *ICD-11* or as it is generally practiced by mental health professionals. Kingma's expansive view eliminates the divide between immoral, illegal, ignorant, and other undesirable behavior, on one hand, and mental disorder, on the other, undermining psychiatry's distinctive validity and making it the agent of social control that antipsychiatry accused it of being.

Kingma and Murphy both use dyslexia (reading disorder) as their primary—indeed, only—example of the HDA's potential revisionism. They both think that to defend the HDA, I must claim that dyslexia is in fact caused by an evolutionary dysfunction and that this is uncertain: "Wakefield's response seems terribly ad hoc. Of course it may be the case that our ability to read is produced by a mechanism that was selected for a particular effect, and that dyslexia indicates a breakdown of that mechanism. But it is just as plausible that that mechanism is itself a by-product of the selection of a different, linked trait, and therefore lacking in function. Or that both the normal ability to learn to read and dyslexia are on a spectrum of normal variation in non-selected effects produced by a functioning underlying mechanism. ... Wakefield, therefore, seems to be making a risky bet" (393).

However, there is nothing to bet on here. The HDA is an explanation of how we think about disorder, not a substantive theory of any particular disorder. Classically, based on various arguments regarding similar symptoms occurring in brain trauma, brain studies that indicated anomalies, and such recently questioned beliefs as that dyslexia involves such neurologically suggestive symptoms as letter and word reversal, it was generally concluded that dyslexia is due to a brain dysfunction. This is still the majority view by researchers and clinicians. However, reading the literature on dyslexia, in fact there is much disagreement and debate, and the arguments reveal how people think about disorder versus nondisorder. There are some researchers who think dyslexia is a disorder, and they justify this belief with the claim that it is due to a malfunction of certain brain mechanisms. There are others who think that dyslexia is not a failure of brain mechanisms but some form of normal variation—perhaps along the lines of some of the linkage options offered by Kingma—and they deny that it is a disorder. It is clear from the literature that if dyslexia were to be proven to be due to variations in the effects of neutral linkages and thus was a form of normal variation and not something going wrong with the brain, then there would be a move to depathologize it. Indeed, the neurodiversity movement and many dyslexia support organizations already argue for Kingma's third option, that dyslexia is just the lower end of normal variation in the ability to learn to read and there is no dysfunction, but they conclude that, in virtue of this, there is no disorder. The HDA attempts to explain such differences in views of disorder by the differences in belief about dysfunction, and the literature on dyslexia tends to bear out the HDA's predictions. That literature sharply diverges from Kingma's views; all discussants agree that difficulty learning to read is a serious negative condition that warrants intervention in our society, yet there is a sharp and vigorous divide over whether it is a disorder based on differing views of whether there is a brain dysfunction. My discussions of dyslexia in regard to the HDA were never aimed at betting on one outcome or another but on explaining that those who believe that dyslexia is a disorder base that judgment on their belief that it is due to a dysfunction. For this account of the conceptual distinction, no hypothesis, ad hoc or otherwise, is necessary about the actual cause of dyslexia. (For various approaches to dyslexia, see, for example, the following: Armstrong 2015; Ap 2016; Artigas-Pallarés 2009; "Dyslexia Has a Language Barrier" 2004; "Dyslexia Is Not a Disease" n.d.; Habib 2000; Lilienfeld 2010; Protopapas and Parrila 2018, 2019; Schneps 2015; Treiman 2014; Ziegler et al. 2003).

Now, where does Kingma get her frequency estimation that the HDA is "very strongly" revisionist? Without evidence, based on the spurious accusation that postulates an ad hoc bet about dyslexia that can go wrong, Kingma generalizes the accusation to all disorders, for each purported disorder could be caused by failure of a linked trait rather than a failure of a selected effect: "Wakefield can bet against the odds in one case, dyslexia, and either win or lose. But if very many of our mental capacities are like reading—that is, effects of traits that do not themselves explain why those traits were selected, and that are therefore not functions—Wakefield's position starts to look more precarious" (394).

However, dyslexia is atypical precisely because the harm is not a failure of an apparently selected trait and so there is an unusual degree of inference involved in deciding whether or not there is a dysfunction. In contrast, most mental disorders in *DSM* and *ICD* are generally identified as disorders because they are occurring in what are pretty clearly biologically designed systems with complex regulatory features that are not plausibly due to linkage, and the failures that are labeled disorders compromise what appear to be the designed functions of the module. It is thus actually "overwhelmingly likely" that linkage is not the explanation for the vast majority of mental modules. Page through the chapters and categories of *DSM* and what you find are failures of the systems that are most plausibly biologically designed, such as human thought, perception, sadness, joy, grief, fear, psychological development, sleep, sex, eating, excretory function, and other categories of function, all of which are most plausibly the result of selection. This includes the vast majority of currently recognized physical and mental disorders.

Perhaps recognizing the flaw in the sheer "probability" argument for linkage, Kingma attempts to finesse the problem of the evidence for design by casting doubt on whether we are able to tell whether a system is likely biologically designed. She uses the example of reading: "It seems almost impossible that our ability to learn to read would not be designed: it is unique to humans, complicated, widespread, and incredibly useful, so how could it be a fluke? But it is a mistake to think that something is either selected, or a fluke" (395). Quite right, but what this example shows is that there are many sorts of processes that can lead to signs of design, which include biological selection, social construction, individual learning, and artifact-creation. After all, despite the design-like characteristics of our ability to read, no one in the diagnostic community has ever held that reading is a naturally selected trait.

Ignoring the fact that we theorize about mental modules based on evidence of likely design, Kingma tries to portray it as a matter of sheer probability whether a module is designed or not: "Here is one reason to suppose that more rather than fewer of our mental capacities will be like reading.... If a selected effect account is to bear out that mental modules have functions...those effects should...have been the drivers of the selection of those very modules. In other words, every single mental module or capacity must have been 'visible to natural selection' via its own effect rather than through any of the other possibilities discussed.... Given the developmental complexity of our mind, that seems extremely unlikely.... Wakefield's account of disorder, it turns out, is very strongly revisionist" (394).

I would say that, given the developmental complexity of our minds, selection was critical to getting all the pieces to work and interact correctly. Moreover, it is precisely due to the plausibility of biological design that we select modules, so there is nothing at all surprising or improbable about each module having been subject to selective pressures. It is not a matter of probability whether mental modules happen to fall within the selected for versus nonselected linked category. Mental modules are identified based on their apparent biologically designed and adaptive nature. Geneticists and evolutionary biologists affirm that natural selection is the only known process that reliably or frequently gives rise to apparent biological design. The nonselected effects of linkage that happen without reference to the content of the produced traits have no causal properties that are likely to produce such features.

Having argued that one can easily be mistaken about design, Kingma concludes, "Therefore the fact that our traits seem beautifully adapted to what they do should not tempt us into thinking that they were selected for what they do" (395). This overstated conclusion does not follow from anything she has said. Should we throw out Darwin and dismiss Aristotle's foolish notion that the acorn turning into an oak tree required a special form of design-like explanation? Should we perhaps resist the temptation of thinking that the artifacts in our homes have been designed? Taking seriously the evidence of design and adaptation has been the basis for the greatest breakthroughs in the history of biology. Just as in every other area of science, the fact that we can be mistaken does not obviate the general reliability and usefulness of our intuitions for generating initial hypotheses that allow us through testing to bootstrap to the truth.

Kingma ends up rejecting my view because "our concepts of health and disorder are not value-free" (397). This is of course my position as well, but Kingma never mentions the evaluative "harm" component of the HDA. Kingma prefers Boorse's (1975) view—which is genuinely nonevaluative—but never considers that Boorse's view is highly revisionist; its statistical criterion allows arbitrary classification of the bottom 50% of the population on any functional variable as disordered, and it classifies as a medical disorder any biological dysfunction no matter how harmless, of which each of us has millions (e.g., genetic mutations) (Wakefield 2014). Kingma prefers the "forward-looking model created by Boorse, not the backward-looking one by Wakefield" (397). Just as contemporary essentialist semantics builds causal history into the meaning of proper names and natural kind terms without thereby rendering the activities based on their meanings in any sense backward-looking, invoking history as part of the meaning of medical disorder has little to do with how forward-looking medical practice is. What is not forward-looking is to open the door wide to bogus diagnostic practices that support social control efforts and undermine the legitimacy of medicine, thus reawakening dormant antipsychiatric concerns that with decades of painstaking effort have been put to rest.

Does the HDA Cohere with Relevant Scientific Practice?

Regarding Murphy's proposed test that the concept of function "should capture relevant scientific practice," the most "relevant scientific practice" in this case is scientific practice that concerns the nature and treatment of disorders. Murphy says, "Insofar as psychiatry is a branch of medicine, the concept of function it needs resembles those of physiology and biomedicine. Evolutionary considerations are just beside the point." However, the concepts of function and dysfunction underlying medical diagnosis cannot be judged by adjacent disciplines that do not have the unique burdens and aims of medical diagnosis. Even if some other areas of science use "function" differently (which is not at all as clear as Murphy suggests), the real question is how medical diagnostic clinicians and researchers use the concept. Murphy here ignores his own point that "function" is polysemous, which suggests that it may have somewhat different meanings in different subdisciplines.

But what about the integration of different medical and nonmedical parts of biomedicine? As my analyses below will make clear, whether or not other areas of biology sometimes use CR functions, they also assuredly use evolutionary dysfunctions, so there will be no problem with an interface. In any event, a proper interface between psychiatry or medicine and the other biological sciences requires not that "function" is used in precisely the same way across disciplines but only that the various uses of function intermesh in a coherent and scientifically useful way even if they are somewhat different. And they do intermesh because, as Tinbergen (1963) famously observed, proximate causal explanation in terms of how things work and distal evolutionary explanations are complementary integral parts of an overall understanding of the biological design of organisms. Of course, most research on disorder is about how things work, not evolutionary functions, but, as we saw above, that research takes place within a framework set by the concept of biological design.

Murphy asserts that "the questions that medicine asks are not those that a selectionist account of function can answer." A glance at recent disputes about disorder status reveals that evolutionary considerations often do address basic questions of disorder versus nondisorder. For example, is lactose tolerance a disorder, given that it exists in a minority of the world's population and involves loss of an efficiency advantage after weaning? The answer, presented, for example, in the Gluckman (2009) reference that Murphy cites, is that because lactose tolerance has been naturally selected in environments where the domestication of animals made milk available during famines, it is not a disorder. Is ADHD partially caused by the DRD4 7-repeat allele a genetic disorder? Studies of sedentary versus nomadic populations suggest that this gene was naturally selected for interest in novelty and activity and that children who have this gene and display symptoms of ADHD are not suffering from a disorder but rather a normal variation that is mismatched to the demands of our current social environment (Eisenberg et al. 2008), and this information changed people's minds about the pathological status of this subset of ADHD diagnoses (see the discussion of ADHD in my reply to De Vreese in this volume). More generally, such considerations remain implicit because manifest (albeit fallible) indicators of design and dysfunction are taken as sufficient for judgment in most cases.

Murphy further argues, "Normal biomedical ascription of function to a system makes no claims about selective history. It requires only that we can identify the role played by a system in the overall economy of the organism. How is dysfunction determined? By the use of a biomedical concept of normality that is an idealized description of a component of a biological system in an unperturbed state. It does not rest on the failure of a biological part to replicate as its ancestors did, or to reduce overall fitness, but by its failure to be close enough to the causal contribution of the analogous part in the idealized overall system." Again, ascriptions of function and dysfunction generally operate at a more manifest level with the biological-design evolutionary underpinnings implicit, just as normal ascription that a liquid is water makes no explicit reference to chemical theory. In any event, Murphy's description of the situation begs the crucial objectivity question. It sounds objective—sort of like classic physics—to judge that a condition would exist in an "unperturbed" or "idealized" system. However, within a CR-function account of the kind that Murphy embraces, the notions of "unperturbed" and "idealized" are interest-relative terms that confer no objectivity, so the "overall economy of the organism" can be described in any way the investigator prefers with functions and dysfunctions distributed according to the investigator's interests. Such an account is not related to the medical target of health in the usual sense, unless, again, objectivity can be teased out of the CR view.

In sum, Murphy's claim that the CR view is superior to the HDA on the two tests of diagnostic revision and disciplinary integration fails. But can he make good on his further claim that the CR view passes the crucial test of yielding an objective measure of function and dysfunction corresponding with the way health and disorder judgments are actually made in medicine. I now turn in the rest of this reply to the question of whether the CR view can provide that kind of objective account of functions and dysfunctions.

Cummins on Interest Relativity and the Function of the Sound of the Heart

The interest relativity of CR functions implies that function judgments can occur in contexts in which they go against standard usage and intuition. Cummins unhesitatingly bites the bullet in such cases and insists that such attributions are entirely legitimate and the intuitions can be ignored. He maintains this position even in such classic cases of intuitive nonfunction as the sounds made by the heart: "Evolutionary biologists probably will not say that a function of the heart is to make sounds. But an ethnologist studying medical diagnosis probably wouldn't blink an eye. This relativity to a containing system and target capacity is just what the systematic account would predict, if it were in the business of predicting intuitions" (Cummins and Roth 2009, 83).

There are several problems with this facile claim if taken seriously. First, where is the evidence from the medical diagnostic literature that those studying medical diagnosis actually say the sorts of things that Cummins claims? There are endless sources that describe the functions of the heart, and not one of them that I have accessed, including the ones concerned with medical diagnosis, says that they include making a sound. The sound and pulse of the heart have played crucial roles in medical diagnosis since ancient times, so if Cummins's claim is true, there ought to be plenty of sources to illustrate its truth. If in fact the sources blink and refrain from such talk and Cummins's claim is unsupported, that reveals something about "function."

Second, according to Cummins's view, it should be a clear dysfunction if one's nose is shaped in such a way that it does not hold up one's glasses (Wang 2017; "Why Asian Fit?" 2019) or if one's blood vessels are hard to find and roll out of the way when a medical person is trying to take blood (as do mine in my left arm). Yet, no one describes these normal-variation situations as dysfunctions.

Third, even if medical diagnosticians were to apply "function" to heart sounds, they likely would not mean that the sounds have a natural or biological function, which is the sense relevant to medicine and relevant to the HDA. "Function" also applies to instrumental means in intentional action, including artifact construction. Medical diagnosis is an intentional human activity, and this creates the possibility of legitimate intentional-function attributions such as "the function of (listening to) heart sounds during a heart examination is to...." The HDA does not block such instrumental function attributions, but it does imply that the failure of an intentional function would not yield judgments of dysfunction and disorder relevant to medical diagnosis. So, the test of the HDA here is whether ethnodiagnostic researchers, when they come across individuals in a diagnostic context whose heart sound is muted or difficult to access for idiosyncratic anatomical reasons and thus the use of heart sounds diagnostically is disrupted, would judge the individual to have a biological dysfunction and thereby a medical disorder. This test would presumably not be passed by the claimed function attributions to heart sounds.

To all the arguments presented above, Cummins answers that they are based on intuitions we have about function attributions, but CR functions violate prior intuitions and so intuitions can be ignored. He compares this to what often happens in proposing breakthrough counterintuitive theories in the sciences: "We agree that the account does not square with intuitions about functions, in many cases.... But how seriously should we take this? Scientific treatments of motion have increasingly diverged from intuition since the seventeenth century.... Biology should be no more constrained by intuitions concerning functions than physics should be constrained by intuitions about motion. Physics is, in large part, counterintuitive, and so, it would be no knock against biology if it turns out it makes counterintuitive function attributions" (Cummins and Roth 2009, 82–83). Murphy follows Cummins in arguing that revisionism that overthrows common beliefs and intuitions should be no obstacle in science: "If we are trying to capture a scientific concept, on what grounds can we argue that it should be criticized for departing from traditional conceptions? A chemist who was told that traditional usage did not regard objects as made of atoms would be unmoved."

Cummins and Murphy here suggest that the reason we should not get too exercised by the counterintuitive conclusion that "the function of heart sounds is to alert the physician to medical problems" is because we should be ready to adjust to profound scientific insights that turn our view of the world upside down. However, such semantic deployment of "function" is scientifically trivial, based on no remarkable scientific discovery. In contrast, the discovery that biological functions are naturally selected effects is one of the most momentous and counterintuitive scientific discoveries in human history, comparable to Murphy's example of solid objects being made of atoms, and it did overthrow much prescientific understanding, supporting a distinctive term for naturally selected effects. The Darwinian image of "function" *is* the "scientific image" in the biomedical sciences.

Why Call SE Functions "Functions"?

We are now in the position to answer Cummins's "why call them functions?" argument and the answer is simple: functions are effects that are the products of biological design, and the best scientific theory we have of the intuitive concept of biological design is evolutionary theory. Even Cummins recognizes that there is something special along these lines about naturally selected effects:

> According to the selectionist, appeals to function to explain the spread of a trait are legitimate because there is a function-sensitive natural process that spreads traits: natural selection. … We have no problem with natural selection. So, if selectionists see functional explanation as simply a standard application of natural selection, then we can have no objections to selectionist accounts of functional explanation, so understood. (Cummins and Roth 2009, 77)

There are two crucial points. First, natural selection is a *function-sensitive* or, better, an *effect-sensitive* causal process because the *effects of traits* must be cited in explaining why the traits are present and how they are structured. This is a highly unusual situation. Such effect-sensitive processes are neither quite prototypically mechanistic nor quite prototypically teleological. Cummins's term "neo-teleology" is as good as any for labeling this sort of effect-sensitive causal process. Second, effect-sensitivity is not an explanatory desideratum or goal in itself. Rather, it is a necessary element in explaining biological design, and it is biological design that is the ultimate target domain of classic function explanations. As Aristotle already observed, oak trees can be explained mechanically in terms of the CR functions by which an acorn gives rise to an oak tree, but that misses something explanatorily crucial and distinctive, namely, how could it be that something could have those causal properties yielding species reproduction in a mechanical universe? It must be that acorns are the way they are *because* they give rise to oak trees. But, again, how can that be in a mechanical universe? Similarly, for William Harvey, the function of the heart is to pump the blood, and "this is the only reason for the motion and beat of the heart" (Harvey 1628/1993, as quoted in Ribatti 2009, 2), that is, the function of pumping somehow explains why the heart beats, and how this can be so is a mystery in addition to and transcending the mystery of the CR mechanics of the heart pumping the blood. What all this means is that adding the term "natural function" or, equivalently, "biological function" to the ontology of biological theory has real theoretical content that, while providing an initial minimal explanation sketch, identifies a fundamental and profoundly challenging explanatory target.

As Cummins and Roth (2009) point out, contra Aristotle, mechanics turned out not to be effect-sensitive or have use for a notion of natural function. There was no theoretically interesting sense in which objects were moving as they did because they were seeking to get to their natural place, nor was there any sort of feedback as to how they were doing in reaching that goal that then influenced their subsequent motion. Thus, the teleological effect-sensitivity aspect of ancient mechanics dropped away. Efficient-mechanical causation was deemed sufficient to explain motion and became the primary model for scientific explanation.

In biology, things went differently. The greatest puzzle about biological entities from ancient times was how, in a mechanical universe, organisms can possibly be so well adapted to the environment in a design-like manner and perform the seeming miracles of surviving and reproducing. Note that the process of reproduction takes the puzzle beyond sheer adaptation in the sense of a match between the needs of the organism for survival and the environment, as well as makes it a broader puzzle of biological design. Of course, as Murphy repeatedly points out, biological, anatomical, and biomedical investigations throughout history tried to figure out how things work (or how they function, where function is understood in CR-like terms as causal action) and do not generally refer explicitly to biological design, let alone natural selection (although selection-like theories of adaptation go back to ancient times).

Nonetheless, it is difficult to overstate the centrality of the issue of the design-like nature of organisms in the history of biology and the importance of Darwin's explanation for it in terms of natural selection. This point seems underappreciated by Murphy and Cummins, so allow me a brief historical anecdote. In 1880, the eminent German electrophysiologist and discoverer of the nerve action potential, Emil Du Bois-Reymond (1818–1896), delivered a famous lecture to the Berlin Academy of Sciences on the occasion of Leibniz's birthday, published two years later in *Popular Science Monthly* (Du Bois-Reymond 1882), in which he listed what he considered to be the seven most fundamental unsolved scientific puzzles. These basic mysteries, which he labeled the "seven world enigmas" (or "seven world problems"), ranged from "the origin of motion" and "the origin of life" to "the origin of sense perception [i.e., conscious experience]" and "the question of free will." The paper became a pivotal and enduring statement about the possibilities of scientific progress (e.g., the mathematician David Hilbert was still disputing its claims in a 1930 talk on BBC radio). In his talk,

Du Bois-Reymond identified a subset of the enigmas that he claimed were "transcendent," meaning that they could *never* be solved by science, such as the origin of motion and the origin of consciousness (of these, he famously said *"ignoramus et ignorabimus,"* "we do not know and we will not know"), versus those that seemed in principle scientifically resolvable.

Among Du Bois-Reymond's seven enigmas, the fourth was "the apparently teleological arrangement of nature," by which he meant the fact, observed since Aristotle, that the remarkable adaptiveness of organisms' features appeared "inconsistent with the mechanical view of nature" that Du Bois-Reymond himself strongly championed. This particular enigma, however, Du Bois-Reymond did not classify as "transcendent" and beyond science's reach despite the common attribution of the teleology of biology to God. The reason he considered it scientifically resolvable was the recent theory of Charles Darwin: "This difficulty is, however, not absolutely transcendent, for Mr. Darwin has pointed out in his doctrine of natural selection a possible way of overcoming it, and of explaining the inner suitableness of organic creation to its purposes and its adaptation to inorganic conditions…by a kind of mechanism in connection with natural necessity." Du Bois-Reymond not only classified the adaptiveness of biological features as one of the seven most fundamental mysteries in all the sciences but also acknowledged that for a nontheist, it appeared resolvable only because of the theory of natural selection, concluding, "Thus the fourth difficulty is no longer transcendent when it is earnestly, thoughtfully met."

It is this fundamental millennia-long scientific challenge of explaining the design-likeness of organisms that warranted adding "biological function" as an *ontological* rather than sheerly verbal-convenience category to the vocabulary of science and searching for this category's explanatory essence. That essence turned out to be natural selection.

Can SE Functions Be Understood as Fixed-Interest CR Functions?

Cummins tries to make it seem like effect-sensitivity of causal explanation—which is another way of referring to design-likeness in which somehow the causal role of a feature is shaped by the effects that it causes—is just another relativistic context or interest like any other: "You can make an instrumental norm look like a Norm by privileging a particular goal-state, but this is still just instrumental normativity—hence, relativized normativity—thinly disguised. … If you want to account for ('capture') the function attributions—including malfunction and failure of function attributions—of evolutionary biologists talking about natural selection, you can probably get a pretty good fit by relativizing to fitness, in one way or another" (Cummins and Roth 2009, 83).

So, why not take Cummins's suggestion and transmute the lead of interest relativity into the gold of objectivity simply by fixing the relativity to a certain current interest or goal, such as fitness or statistical deviation, yielding (pseudo) objectivity without reference to history? As Cummins admits, this strategy is just a cosmetic makeover that yields a make-believe objectivity that is a "thinly disguised" relativity, not the genuine objectivity that medical diagnosis requires. To take an analogy, if one believes that "good" relativistically means "good relative to a given culture's values," one cannot evade relativism and achieve value objectivity in any meaningful sense simply by stipulating that absolute good means "good relative to my culture." The question remains of whether there is an objective sense of "function" beyond the ad hoc maneuver of stipulating a fixed relational element.

As to Cummins's suggestion of using fitness as the objectifying interest, medicine was being pursued for over two millennia before the concept of fitness ascended to its current Darwinian explanatory perch, so that approach fails to get at what justifies the formation of the concept of "function." In any event, fitness or reproductive success in the current environment has complex relationships to biological design. As Murphy says, "Health and fitness are different concepts"; reducing fitness is not necessarily a disorder (if it was, then deciding not to have an additional child would be a disorder). Even if being blind or being unable to walk or being schizophrenic makes no difference to fitness and does not hinder reproduction in our current or future environment, nevertheless these conditions are objectively dysfunctions, that is, failures of parts to perform functions they were biologically designed to perform. Nor can one say that CR functions in the medical sense are those that support health, because health is absence of disorder, and disorder is harmful dysfunction, and dysfunction is—according to the present proposal—any component's causation of a reduced capacity for health, and thus there is a vicious circularity. In sum, you just can't get from CR functions to the objectivity of medical diagnosis that Murphy demands.

Can CR Functions Account for the Objectivity of Dysfunction?

How, then, does Cummins apply his CR-function approach to medical dysfunction and disorder, where there is a failure of biological function? Here is how: "Systematic accounts relativize failures to function properly to a target explanandum: component x is failing to function properly, relative to a capacity C of the containing system S, if (other things equal) S fails to have C (or has a relatively diminished capacity) because of what x is doing" (Cummins and Roth 2009, 79). They explain, "Thus, systematic accounts allow for a kind of relativized or instrumental normativity: what something needs to do for the containing system to exercise the target capacity" (79).

Thus, if one is interested in the effect of a certain infection (such as the "brain-eating" amoebic infections), and that type of infection almost always causes death, but in 1 out of 100 cases the infected individual survives due to idiosyncratic immunologic features, then in that case, the researcher would, according to Cummins, be justified in saying that the infected individual suffered from an immunological dysfunction that caused him or her to survive the infection. This view of CR dysfunction is a *reductio ad absurdum* of Cummins's view of functions as a plausible foundation for medicine.

Cummins further addresses the CR account of dysfunction in a discussion of blindness. Blindness is a medical disorder because the eyes are not capable of doing what they are biologically designed to do—that is, they are not capable of performing their natural function. However, Cummins and Roth (2009) state that the CR-function view cannot go along with this simple description because it cannot refer to natural functions that are by their nature historical, and the essence of CR functions is to eschew all reference to history:

> A perhaps more serious objection is that this sort of instrumental normativity—viz., the you-ought-to-do-x-to-achieve-g sense—will not accommodate the fact that a blind person's eyes are still for seeing. ... The objection is that since the eyes of blind people never perform the function of enabling sight, systematic accounts should deny that a blind person's eyes are for seeing (and, thus, deny that the eyes are not functioning properly). To us, this appears to rely on a type–token ambiguity. Eyes generally (the type) enable seeing. A blind person's eyes (here, the token) are not for anything in that individual. ... The sense that the eyes of a blind person are for seeing is simply the recognition that other humans do see, and that the eyes are an essential part of the human visual system. Thus, the blind person's eyes are not functioning properly (assuming here that the problem is really with the eyes) because they are not functioning in the way required for humans to see. (Cummins and Roth 2009, 79; a similar approach is taken by Boorse 2002)

These comments make it clear that CR functions, when applied to medicine, are not only not objective, but because they are ahistorical, they also must be essentially statistical and/or value based. Yet, the statistical and value views are precisely the views that must be rejected because they cannot answer the antipsychiatric challenge that has been faced by psychiatry for over a half century and would leave psychiatry without a solid conceptual foundation. The Soviet dissidents and runaway slaves and sexual Victorian women were statistically deviant and disapproved of and disvalued in their social contexts, yet were not disordered. Today, there are debates over many conditions as to their diagnostic status, yet the conditions are statistically deviant and disvalued (e.g., ADHD-type rambunctious behavior in schoolchildren). The CR-function approach simply abandons the project of making sense of a coherent and nonoppressive psychiatric medical specialty, which is the point of conceptual analysis of "medical disorder," to chase dubious philosophical ideological will-o'-the-wisps. The application of CR functions as a basis for medical diagnosis is a thoroughly value-laden approach that leaves no ultimate scientific ground for disputing interest-driven function claims and thus has nothing to say about opposed diagnostic-judgments grounded in different interests. In contrast, SE functions offer a solid value-free scientific foundation in evolutionary theory and factual claims about biological design. To call the CR approach more scientific than the SE approach is without foundation.

Bock and von Wahlert and the Biological Origins
of the CR- versus SE-Functions Distinction

One might ask: If Murphy's quest for an objective sense of CR dysfunction and the rejection of SE function cannot find a plausible foundation in Cummins's work, is such a rationale provided by some of the other prominent proponents of CR functions? I consider two of the most cited papers defending CR functions to show that they both accept SE functions and offer no solution to the medical objectivity challenge to CR functions.

Murphy heavily cites Amundson and Lauder's influential (1994) paper (which I will consider in due course), which in turn relies heavily on a classic paper by evolutionary biologists Walter Bock and Gerd von Wahlert (1965). That paper, despite not using the "CR" terminology (which, however, I will use in describing it), can be considered the origin of the contemporary CR-function notion. I believe that Bock and von Wahlert's position sometimes has been misunderstood as supporting Cummins's position, so I take some time to comment on it.

Bock and von Wahlert start from the position that there are two common uses of "function" in biology that need to be disambiguated: "A major source of ambiguity stems from the several meanings of function in biology. Function is used in the sense of the physical and chemical properties of the feature and in the sense of the role the feature has in the life of the organism. A review of the literature of functional anatomy will reveal that both meanings are employed. ... We feel that these two concepts must be separated sharply" (1965, 276–277).

In constructing their terminology, Bock and von Wahlert choose to use the term "function" to label all of a feature's physiological causal actions on any aspect of the organism: "Basically the function of a feature is its action or how it works...which include all physical and chemical properties arising from its form (i.e., its material composition and arrangement thereof)" (274). This use of "function" is emphatically independent of any selection-related or other teleological implications: "We wish to stress that the definition of function as given above does not involve any aspect of purpose, design, or end-directedness. Moreover, this definition of function is free, as it should be, of any form of teleology" (274).

As Amundson and Lauder (1994) point out, Bock and von Wahlert's treatment of CR function diverges from Cummins's approach in that there is no interest relativity of CR functions in their account. This is because they do not relativize their CR functions to a given analysis but rather simply encompass within that category every possible action under every possible circumstance, including highly artificial stressors that would not occur in a natural habitat. Otherwise, Bock and von Wahlert and Cummins are on the same page: "Apart from the issue of unutilized functions, Cummins's concept of function matches the anatomists'" (1994, 450).

In contrast to "functions" so defined, Bock and von Wahlert (1965) label as "biological roles" the traditional SE functions directly linked to natural selection: "The biological role of a faculty...may be defined as the action or the use of the faculty by the organism in the course of its life history....Each biological role of the faculty is under the influence of a set of selection forces" (278–279); "An evolutionary adaptation is...formed by a biological role coupled with a selection force....The interaction between the organism and its environment is through a couple formed by the biological role and the selection force" (296). The notion of biological role is closely linked to the central explanatory puzzle of biology, the organism's adaptation to its natural environment, which Bock and von Wahlert agree is an SE-type evolutionary notion: "Clarity of meaning would be increased if the general term 'adaptation' were restricted to evolutionary adaptation" (285).

Bock and von Wahlert diverge from Cummins in considering SE function, or "biological role," to be a scientifically central sense of "function" linked directly to explanation by natural selection, with CR functions an instrumentally useful step toward that goal. They thus consider CR and SE functions as complementary and not in competition. Their analysis implies that they would have rejected outright anything like the attempted purge of SE functions from biomedical theory that Cummins and Murphy propose. They allow that the SE-function "biological role" usage is traditional: "We agree that many biologists formulate functional statements in a teleological framework....Most workers discussing this problem probably use the term function in the sense of biological role" (274–275).

The functions that do not correspond to biological roles are considered nonutilized functions, and they, unlike functions with biological roles, have no SE functions: "Some of these faculties would be non-utilized ones corresponding to the non-utilized functions. Each utilized faculty of a feature is controlled by a different set of selection forces and hence each would have a separate evolution" (276). Thus, Bock and von Wahlert do not accept the Cummins zero-sum approach that SE functions are dispensable and "function" just means CR function. For them, SE functions are a central biological concept.

The distinction between function and biological role yields a division of labor within biological research between those doing laboratory work that may explore functions in dimensions never seen in the wild and those studying the natural life history of the organism:

> The function of a feature may be studied and described independently of the natural environment of the organism as is done in most studies of functional anatomy. The animal is placed in an experimental device which allows ascertainment of the functions of the feature with various degrees of precision. But the conditions are almost always highly artificial. In addition to these studies of pure function are investigations of biological anatomy in which the "function" (= biological role) of a structure is studied with the animal living freely in its natural habitat. Both types of studies are required to obtain different, but related sets of information which are prerequisites for the study of adaptation. (274)

The last sentence of this passage underscores that Bock and von Wahlert understand that the essential scientific challenge of biology concerns teleology and that, even for them, the study of CR functions ultimately is aimed at elucidating SE functions linked to adaptation and natural selection. By formulating the notion of CR functions, Bock and von Wahlert want to make the science of SE functions more effective. They argue that the focus on CR functions is valuable due to its epistemological usefulness in the pursuit of SE functions. Rather than the usual procedure of identifying a proposed SE function and then following it back to the causal actions of a feature that has that effect as its function, one can start with all "functions" (in the sense of causal actions) of the organism's features, devoid of premature teleological assumptions, and follow those effects forward, thereby discovering unsuspected biological roles: "Usually the biological roles of a feature are the guides to the function that are studied; however, this procedure may hinder the clarification of important functions of the feature which may be utilized in some or all cases" (n. 1, 274).

Thus, Bock and von Wahlert's point is not to eliminate or even downplay the importance of naturally selected biological roles of features. Rather, it is to provide a framework that allows biologists to be optimally open-minded in discovering biological roles by actually seeing which CR functions yield biological roles rather than either assuming from a CR function what the biological role must be ("the biological role of a feature cannot be predicted with any certainty from the study of the form and the function of the feature" [278]) or reasoning back from plausible biological roles to what CR functions are for.

Contrary to the usual impression, for Bock and von Wahlert, the analysis of CR functions is ultimately about identifying SE functions. But, what, then, is the importance of studying nonutilized CR functions, even ones that go beyond anything that occurs under usual conditions in the wild? The primary answer lies in Bock's interest in preadaptation, where, in response to changing environmental pressures, nonutilized CR functions are exploited in novel ways to support new biological roles. Formerly defined as "a structure is said to be preadapted for a new function if its present form which enables it to discharge its original function also enables it to assume the new function whenever need for this function arises" (292), they suggest that the definition can now be reformulated more clearly as "a feature is said to be preadapted when its present forms and functions (both utilized and non-utilized ones) allow ... [it] to acquire a new biological role ... whenever the need (= appearance of the selection force) for this new adaptation ... should arise" (292). They explain that, as a result, "preadaptation should not be construed of as a change in functions as has been expressed in earlier papers, but as a change in biological roles. With the origin of a new adaptation, a new selection force acts upon the feature" (292).

Bock and von Wahlert explain that discovery of biological roles justifies concern about CR functions: "A worker may consciously or unconsciously study functions of features that never occur during the life of the organism. ... These non-utilized functions cannot be ignored because we generally do not know which functions are utilized and which are not utilized by the organisms and because the non-utilized functions form an important basis of the phenomenon of preadaptation" (274). Bock and von Wahlert's notion of preadaptation is rightly equated by Amundson and Lauder with Gould's notion of "exaptation," but their analysis possesses a crystal clarity about the close relationship between preadaptation and natural selection that stands in sharp contrast to Gould's befuddled claims about exaptation somehow undermining natural selection explanations. (For discussion of Gould's confusions, see Wakefield 1999a, 2016a.)

There can be no solace in Bock and von Wahlert's analysis for Cummins's and Murphy's "competition" view of the relationship between CR and SE functions in biology or for Cummins's and Murphy's claims for the priority of CR functions. It is clear that Bock and von Wahlert's article is intended as a corrective to overly simplistic approaches to SE functions that they agree are at the center of biological theorizing and not at all as a critique of SE functions.

Amundson and Lauder's Defense of CR Functions

Murphy several times cites an influential article by Amundson and Lauder (1994), "Function without Purpose: The Uses of Causal Role Function in Evolutionary Biology," in support of his position that psychiatric diagnosis can be based wholly on CR functions. Amundson and Lauder's position in turn rests on Bock and von Wahlert's (1965) influential argument considered above but moves beyond it to address the CR versus SE function debate. Their paper has become the locus classicus of the defense of CR functions in biology, so I examine whether or not it supports Murphy's position.

The title of Amundson and Lauder's paper looks promising from Murphy's perspective because it seems to suggest that, even within natural selection's citadel of evolutionary biology, the CR formulation may hold sway. However, it turns out that the title alludes to a more modest claim. They want to dispute not the importance or necessity of SE functions but the claim that CR functions are eliminable in favor of SE functions or somehow subordinate to SE functions. Their paper does not primarily focus on medical diagnosis and is not a repudiation of the fact that there are domains within biomedical theory in which SE function is the primary function concept. They acknowledge that even functional anatomical studies are often guided by the desire to understand SE functions: "Functional anatomists typically choose to analyze integrated character complexes which have significant biological roles" (450).

When they do discuss medically related functional notions, Amundson and Lauder take a position directly opposed to Murphy's. They assert unequivocally that "purpose and dysfunction" are "concepts to which CR function doesn't apply" (451). That is, CR functions are objectively neutral between health and disorder.

Amundson and Lauder consider a related objection to CR functions that they call "the problem of pathological malformations of functional items" (452–453). The background to this discussion is that SE theorists have attempted to outflank CR-function arguments by claiming that categories of anatomical features are themselves SE-defined concepts, so that one cannot even conceptually define a type of organ (e.g., a heart) for CR functions without first specifying an SE-type natural function (e.g., pumping blood) that it was biologically designed to perform and that defines its category. That is, hearts just are organs for pumping blood, so SE functions logically precede anatomical generalizations that use CR functions. SE theorists generally argue that a major goal of a theory of function is to explain dysfunction, and that poses the problem of how we recognize pathological specimens (or for that matter radically different cross-species specimens) as the organs that they are, and the functional account is claimed to resolve this problem.

> According to these theorists, only SE function can categorize parts into their proper categories irrespective of variation and malformation. It does so by defining "function categories." CR function (like other non-historical theories) cannot define appropriate function categories, and so is unable both to identify diseased or malformed hearts as hearts, and to identify the same organ under different forms in different species.
>
> On pathology, Millikan points out that diseased, malformed, and otherwise dysfunctional organs are denominated by the function they would serve if normal. "The problem is, how did the atypical members of the category that cannot perform its defining function *get* into the same function category as the things that actually can perform the function?" A CR analysis of a deformed heart which cannot pump blood obviously cannot designate its *function* as pumping blood, since it doesn't have that causal capacity. On the other hand, even the organism with the malformed heart has a selective history of ancestors which survived because *their* hearts pumped blood. So the category "heart" which ranges over both healthy and malformed organs must be defined by SE, not CR, function. (453)

Amundson and Lauder argue that "SE functionalists are simply mistaken in this claim" that evolutionary history is conceptually prior to functional anatomy. They claim that rather than either SE or CR functions, "the classifications come from a third, non-functional source" (453). That source consists of anatomical, morphological, and histological evidence that allows identification of organs within and often across species, and it can identify both functional and dysfunctional instances of an organ:

> Even a severely malformed vertebrate heart, completely incapable of pumping blood (or serving any biological role at all), could be identified as a heart by histological examination.... Anatomical categorizations of biological items already embrace interspecies and pathological diversity without any appeal to purposive function. Anatomical distinctions are not normally based on CR function *either*, to be sure. Functional anatomists *per se* do not categorize body parts. Rather they study the capacities of anatomical complexes which have already been categorized by comparative anatomists. Causal role functional anatomy proceeds unencumbered by demands to account either for the categorization or the causal origins of the systems under analysis. (457–458)

Murphy reiterates Amundson and Lauder's point that "it is entirely possible to iden-tify anatomical units by anatomical considerations, regardless of proper function…on morphological and physiological grounds, regardless of history." On this point I agree; Amundson and Lauder do persuasively correct SE theorists' conceptual overreach in suggesting that anatomy must be based on SE-function categories. After all, anatomists were identifying hearts from obvious morphological features long before Harvey's dis-covery of the heart's function.

However, there is a serious problem with the sheer morphological solution that Amundson and Lauder downplay by placing it in a note. In discussing the problem of identifying hearts across very differently structured species in which histological, mor-phological, and homological comparisons may break down, Amundson and Lauder admit that there are limits to their account that leave an opening for the functional analysis:

> There is one felicitous application of Neander's claim about the inadequacies of morphological criteria to designate hearts. Since the category `heart' is used across major taxonomic differ-ences, a vertebrate taxonomist unfamiliar with mollusks might well not be able to use *verte-brate* morphological criteria to identify a *molluscan* heart. And, to get only slightly bizarre, it is possible to imagine discovering a new taxon of animals which has organs functionally identifi-able as hearts, but which fit the morphological criteria for hearts of no known taxon. We agree with the SE functionalist's point in this rather limited set of cases. (n. 4, 467)

This note appears to directly contradict Amundson and Lauder's contention that hearts are strictly anatomically identifiable across species and malformations. However, I believe one should resist fleeing back to the SE theorists' claims. Amundson and Laud-er's morphological argument remains compelling within a certain sphere. Moreover, the argument that hearts are by definition blood pumpers comes dangerously close to making it a conceptual truth that the function of hearts is to pump the blood, whereas that is one of the greatest empirical discoveries in the history of physiology. In addition, the problem of recognizing mollusk hearts may not lead quite as straightforwardly back to the SE position as it might seem. Davies (2001) argues that the SE approach to organ identification fares no better than the CR approach in regard to including malfunctions within the appropriate category because the functional category depends on a defini-tion in terms of the evolutionary history of hearts that did pump adequately. Thus, it is unclear how pathological hearts that do not pump adequately and did not contribute to that history get into the historically relevant set: it seems possible that a careful defini-tion of the historically determined set might overcome this obstacle, but Davies's point is that there is in fact a certain arbitrariness to the decision as to how to draw the bound-aries of that functionally defined historical kind and so an arbitrariness as to whether it includes malfunctioning instances (see Allen and Neal 2019; Sullivan-Bissett 2017).

To thread this needle, the account of organ categories may have to be more sub-tle than either a simple SE or simple morphological account allows. A compromise conceptualization using a black-box essentialist approach (Wakefield 1999b, 2000a, 2004) may be able to resolve these issues in a way that explains the intuitions of both SE and CR theorists. One can take seriously Amundson and Lauder's claim that "even a severely malformed vertebrate heart, completely incapable of pumping blood (or serving any biological role at all), could be identified as a heart by histological examination," while realizing that this is true of *some* deformed or malfunctioning hearts but not all (e.g., Amundson and Lauder's example of a deformed heart displaced to the knee). What the mollusk example shows is that despite the powerful anatomical considerations that can be brought to bear in recognizing hearts that are normal and abnormal or across species, there is a limit to that approach where we can be genuinely surprised that something not initially recognizable as a heart is indeed a heart on functional grounds. This sort of surprising extension of a theoretical category to new instances that do not share superficial features with standard cases is what the black-box essentialist account is designed to explain. Such an account would allow that we can initially identify a base set of hearts—normal and abnormal—by the morphological criteria described by Amundson and Lauder and use that morphologically defined base set to define a broader functional category. Thus, by "heart," we mean any organ across species that has the same natural function—defined in relation to the process of natural selection that led to the presence of *those* organs, both normal and abnormal—as the base set of hearts identified morphologically and histologically in the human species.

This black-box essentialist approach to organ definition allows that morphological criteria are sufficient for recognizing a base set of hearts in humans and analogous creatures without reference to SE functions, and this allows functional anatomy to get under way with no reference to natural selection. It then appropriately becomes an empirical discovery rather than a conceptual truth that the base set of human hearts has the natural function of—and, after Darwin, was naturally selected for—pumping blood, implying that hearts in general are organs naturally selected for pumping blood. These discoveries are not part of the concept of heart but are what is referred to indirectly in saying that "hearts are those anatomical parts with the same biological-design functional essence as the base set of morphologically recognizable hearts." The category of hearts can then be extended across species to very different creatures with hearts that are not at all morphologically like ours based on this understanding of the functional essence of hearts. And, contra Davies, this analysis gets both pumping and nonpumping instances of hearts into the base set and thus into the set to be explained by the essential SE function.

Can CR Functions Be Saved from the Promiscuity Objection?

A major objection to CR functions as interest-relative causal roles is that such attributions would seem to be applicable across the sciences, yet such function attributions commonly occur only in the few scientific domains with SE functions, namely, the biopsychosocial, medical, and artifactual domains. This apparent mismatch between the predicted "liberality" or "promiscuity" of CR functions and actual scientific practice suggests that CR functions in fact depend on a background framework of biological design, as, for example, Philip Kitcher (1993) argues:

> Without recognizing the background role of the sources of design, an account of the Cummins variety becomes too liberal. Any complex system can be subjected to functional analysis. Thus we can identify the 'function' that a particular arrangement of rocks makes in contributing to the widening of a river delta some miles downstream, or the "functions" of mutant DNA sequences in the formation of tumors—but there are no genuine functions here, and no functional analysis. The causal analysis of delta formation does not link up in any way with a source of design; the account of the causes of tumors reveals *dysfunctions*, not functions. (Kitcher 1993, 390)

Similarly, Millikan (1989) points out that the contributions of clouds to the rain cycle should qualify for CR functions, and Neander (1991) observes that the plate tectonics yielding earthquakes satisfy Cummins's criteria, yet clouds and tectonic plates don't literally have the natural function of producing rain or earthquakes.

Davies (2001) tries to save CR theory from falsification by arguing that SE domains are the only ones that are hierarchically organized, and CR functions are applied only to hierarchical organizations. However, function language was used long before a modern understanding of hierarchical systems, and in any event, there are subdomains within the SE domains that are not hierarchical but to which function language is still applied (see below).

Amundson and Lauder (1994) admit that "whimsical 'functional analyses'" of meteorological or geological systems "are indeed counterintuitive results" (448, 452) but initially dismiss the problem because "the criticism simply does not apply to the real world of scientific practice" (452), a response with which Murphy expresses some sympathy. This of course misses the point. The CR account of function predicts that scientists *should* be making these attributions, so the lack of such attributions—the very fact that they are "whimsical"—falsifies the CR analysis, rendering the CR theory itself whimsical.

Amundson and Lauder have a more substantive response to the promiscuity objection. Cummins puts forward criteria for what makes a good or interesting functional analysis, such as that the system is of interest, the analyzing capacities are simpler or different in type from the analyzed capacities, and the system is complex. Amundson and Lauder argue that the whimsical functions do not meet Cummins's criteria and thus do not occur: "By Cummins's own evaluative criteria (and given the facts of the real world) functional analyses of these systems would have no interest. Analyzing capacities would not be significantly simpler or different in type from analyzed capacities (are plate movements simpler than earthquakes?) nor would the system's organization be notably complex.... All of the interesting causal role functions have a history of natural selection.... Earthquakes and rainfalls... have no such history, and so no complex functional organization" (452).

The claim that causal analyses of earthquakes and the water cycle are of no interest and are not complex is implausible, to say the least. But, there is a more basic problem. To shore up their argument, Amundson and Lauder demonstrate how Cummins's guidelines for good functional analyses apply to a specific case:

> In a valuable functional analysis, the analyzing capacities will be simpler and/or different in type from the analyzed, and the system's discovered organization will be complex. Suppose the capacity to crush of the hypothetical jaw derives from the extremely simple fact that objects between the two bones are subjected to the brute force of muscle X forcing the bones together. Here the "organization" of the system is almost degeneratively simple, and the force of the muscle hardly simpler or different in kind from the crushing capacity of the jaw. A functional analysis of very low value. On the other hand, suppose that the jaw is a complex of many elements, muscle X is much weaker than the observed crushing capacity, the crushing action itself is a complex rolling and grinding, the action of muscle X moves one of its attached bones into a position from which the bone can support one of the several directions of motion, and that this action must be coordinated with other muscle actions so that it will occur at a particular time in the crushing cycle. Here X's function is much simpler than the analyzed capacity, is different in kind (moving in one dimension in contrast to the three dimensional motion of the jaw) and the organization of components which explains jaw action is complex indeed. A functional analysis of high value. (1994, 451)

This illustration inadvertently but decisively refutes Amundson and Lauder's reply to the promiscuity objection by revealing that function attributions in science do not at all depend on Cummins's criteria for "good functional analysis." In the example, Amundson and Lauder explain that the simple jaw's mastication muscle lacks all of the Cummins-specified properties, thus yielding a bad functional analysis or not being amenable to functional analysis. What they fail to observe is that that muscle still would be described unequivocally by any biologist—or nonbiologist—as having the biological function of enabling the chewing of food, and would be considered to have this function to no lesser degree than the muscle in the example of a "good" functional analysis. Consequently, the claimed low-value status of functional analyses in other scientific disciplines fails to explain away the lack of function attributions, and the promiscuity objection remains unaddressed.

For Amundson and Lauder's response to be persuasive, every function attributed to an organic or artifactual system must satisfy Cummins's "goodness" criteria to a greater degree than any system in any other domain, a claim that is not credible. For example, there is a little extendable piece of plastic on the output tray of my printer that is linked to absolutely nothing else, yet clearly has the function of stopping the pages of larger printed files from falling to the ground. This analysis does not fulfill any of the "good" complexity criteria, but it is still a clear instance of an item having a function because the aforementioned part is clearly designed to contribute to the printer's designed purpose of providing a convenient and clean printed outcome. There are many simple biological mechanisms as well that work directly to fulfill their attributed SE function and are less complex than the workings of plate tectonics or meteorological phenomena but can be recognized as designed, as Amundson and Lauder seem to acknowledge: "Given a simple trait with a known biological role, the evolutionist might feel justified in ignoring anatomical details" (450). In any event, even if one absurdly dismisses all the rest of science as being of less interest or not as systematically complex as biological systems, one cannot do the same with medical pathology. Pathological conditions often depend for their existence on systemic relationships every bit as complex as those in health, implying that we should be attributing functions—rather than dysfunctions—to disordered parts, contrary to scientific reality. The claim that functions have nothing to do with design and that it just so happens that the only systems complex enough to warrant function attributions are designed ones is just as ad hoc and spurious as it seems.

The promiscuity objection thus remains a perfectly effective objection that casts doubt on CR functions. I suspect that Cummins understands this situation better than his defenders do, for rather than trying to concoct a rationalization to explain why CR functions are not attributed in most domains of scientific research, Cummins, as we saw, accepts such counterintuitive cases as legitimate function attributions and suggests that we jettison out intuitions along with our standard scientific practices—an extraordinary degree of revisionism on which Murphy has no comment.

Biological Design as the Target Explanandum for Function Attributions

The black-box essentialist analysis of function addresses a further much-debated question, namely, the nature of the relationship between the concept of a natural function and Darwin's theory of natural selection. For convenience, in this reply, I have used the standard "SE" abbreviations for selected effects functions, but this misleadingly suggests that "function" just means "selected effect." Both Neander (1991) and Millikan (1989), in well-known papers, claim on different grounds that "function" means "naturally selected effect." Neander argues that this is what biologists and others commonly mean today by "function," and Millikan says it is simply a theoretical definition that has little to do with ordinary usage. Cummins, too, writes as if the SE account proposes that "function" *means* or is *theoretically defined as* "naturally selected" and in his arguments exploits the various paradoxes and confusions that result.

However, as I have argued elsewhere (Wakefield 2000a), "function" cannot mean "naturally selected effect," for two reasons of a type familiar from the natural-kind/

essentialist literature: (1) biologists have understood the concept of a natural function going back to Aristotle and Harvey but had no idea of the theory of evolution, and (2) it is an empirical discovery that natural functions are naturally selected effects and it could have turned out—indeed, in principle, it could still turn out—otherwise (e.g., we might find that the theists are right and that natural functions are determined by the intentions of a Divine Creator rather than evolution). Darwin did not redefine the concept of function that had existed since Aristotle and Harvey; he explained that natural functions are in fact naturally selected effects.

So, precisely how is "function" linked to naturally selected effect? "Function" is a shared concept based on prototypical examples of intuitively nonaccidental (biologically designed) beneficial effects like sight and on the idea that some common underlying process or processes must be responsible for such remarkable phenomena. These are notions shared by Aristotle, Harvey, and us. It is a scientific discovery, not a conceptual truth, that functions exist because of natural selection. So, function is not directly linked to natural selection either by a conceptual analysis or by a theoretical definition. The link consists instead of two steps: first, a conceptual analysis that identifies functions—as understood by Aristotle, Harvey, and us—as effects that share an essential explanatory process with prototypical nonaccidental benefits like sight and, second, the modern discovery that the essential process is natural selection.

Surprisingly, the black-box essentialist view fits well with the typical descriptions of the empirical, conceptual, and theoretical situation in the history of biology even by those who also support the option of attributing CR functions. For example, Bock and von Wahlert (1965) aptly summarize what amounts to a black-box essentialist account of biological function, which holds that biological design—or what they refer to as adaptation—is a fundamental observation that already presupposes teleology and that motivates the search for an account of how there can be teleological functions:

> The idea of a close correlation between the features of living organisms and the conditions of their environment predates by many years the general acceptance of any theory of organic evolution by biologists. Pre-evolutionary biologists understood the general notion and many of the details of this correlation between organisms and environment as well as we do today; what they lacked was a solid scientific explanation of the how and the why of adaptation. Rather than the notion of adaptation being a consequence of the acceptance of organic evolution, the search for an explanation of these observations was a major impetus in the development of a scientifically acceptable theory of organic evolution. (282–283)

Similarly, when discussing the homology of structures across species as the foundation of functional anatomy that does not rely on SE functions—instead relying on indicators such as similarity in structure, identical connections or position within an overall structural pattern, and common developmental origin in the embryo—Amundson and Lauder offer an analysis that fits well with the black-box essentialist analysis:

Comparative anatomy, morphology, and the concept of homology predate evolutionary biology. They provided Darwin with some of the most potent evidence for the fact of descent with modification. ... So the evolutionary definition of homology mentioned above is a theoretical definition. As with other theoretical definitions, it is subject to sniping from practitioners of conceptual analysis. A philosopher could argue (pointlessly) that "homology" cannot mean "traits which characterize monophyletic clades," since many 1840s biologists knew that birds' wings were homologous to human arms but disbelieved in evolution (and so disbelieved that humans and birds shared a clade). SE advocates' usual reply to the William Harvey objection is applicable here. Just as Harvey could see the marks of biological purpose without knowing the origin or true nature of biological purpose, preDarwinian anatomists could see the marks of homology without knowing the cause and true nature of homology itself. (1994, 454–455)

Amundson and Lauder here imagine a conceptual objection to the standard Darwinian nonfunctional definition of homology as common derivation, namely, that homology cannot mean anything that presupposes Darwinian theory of descent with modification because the concept of homology was understood and homologies were recognized by biologists well before Darwin wrote. Despite Amundson and Lauder's dismissive remarks about conceptual analysis (which flow from their earlier rebuttal of SE theorists' incorrect conceptual-analytic arguments), they seriously respond to this objection, revealing that the conceptual analyst's "sniping" is not all that "pointless" after all. They respond, "Just as Harvey could see the marks of biological purpose without knowing the origin or true nature of biological purpose," so "pre-Darwinian anatomists could see the marks of homology without knowing the cause and true nature of homology itself." Thus, what Amundson and Lauder, following Millikan, label the Darwinian "theoretical definition" of homology is not a definition at all but the empirical discovery of a hypothesized essential nature of a previously recognized phenomenon. The black-box essentialist analysis of "homology" would fit this account quite well. But, more to the point, their characterization of Harvey's recognition of biological design without knowing its Darwinian "true nature" or essence acknowledges what is best understood as a black-box essentialist structure to the notion of biological design.

Peter Godfrey-Smith (1993) versus the Harmful Dysfunction Analysis: Reply to the Editors

Finally, I need to briefly address support for Murphy's position that comes from an unexpected quarter. Despite my boundless gratitude to the editors of this volume, Denis Forest and Luc Faucher, I do want to disagree with them on one important claim they make in their introduction to this volume. In the course of discussing Cummins's causal-role (CR) model of function, they assert that "it is not impossible to derive an account of dysfunctions from this view of functions (Godfrey-Smith 1993)," thus agreeing with Murphy and citing Peter Godfrey-Smith's influential paper in support of their assertion. I too admire the clarity, perspicuity, and depth of insight that Godfrey-Smith consistently brings to topics in philosophy of biology and philosophy of science more generally. However, in this case, the editors' endorsement of Murphy's claim overlooks what I believe is the entirely vacuous nature of Godfrey-Smith's claim.

Here is what Godfrey-Smith says:

> On Cummins analysis, functions are not effects which explain why something is there, but effects which contribute to the explanation of more complex capacities and dispositions of a containing system. Although it is not always appreciated, the distinction between function and *malfunction* can be made within Cummins' framework, as well as within Wright's. If a token of a component of a system is not able to do whatever it is that other tokens do, that plays a distinguished role in the explanation of the capacities of the broader system, then that token component is malfunctional. The concept of malfunction is context dependent on Cummins' view, just as the concept of function in general is. (Godfrey-Smith 1993, 200)

Of course, one can always arbitrarily *stipulate* some interest-relative meaning of "malfunction" within a CR-function perspective. For example, one can stipulate that by "malfunction," one will mean whatever is statistically unusual, or whatever does not bring about the outcome that one is interested in studying, or whatever one doesn't want to happen. However, the standard problem in the function literature is whether, given that Cummins-type functions are explicitly relative to the interests of the observer (or "context dependent," as Godfrey-Smith describes it), there is an account of malfunction definable within the Cummins-style view of function that has a coherent relationship to the standard objective meaning of malfunction within psychiatric and medical diagnosis.

The problem is that the primary goal in characterizing malfunction or dysfunction is to make sense of medicine, and as we have seen above with various deployments of the CR notion, Godfrey-Smith's characterization of CR malfunction has no relationship to what we mean by malfunction in medicine. Godfrey-Smith states that a malfunction occurs when "a component of a system is not able to do whatever it is that other tokens do." This claim can be interpreted in various ways. It might mean that there is a malfunction in a component whenever there exists *any* other instance of the component that can do *anything* that the target component cannot do. However, on this interpretation, every instance of every mechanism would be "malfunctioning" simply in virtue of normal variation. Moreover, a cancerous cell can do things that a normal cell cannot do, so on this broad interpretation of Godfrey-Smith's criterion, the normal cell would be malfunctioning. Indeed, any genetic mutation that can cause disease would thereby render the normal genes malfunctioning.

One might try to fix this problem by more plausibly interpreting Godfrey-Smith as claiming that an instance of a component is malfunctioning only when it cannot do something that the *majority* of instances of the component can do. This is a common strategy among those trying to defend the CR function analysis. However, this notion of malfunction would be based purely on statistical deviance. If there is one thing on which there is a near-consensus among philosophers of psychiatry, it is that a purely statistical definition of dysfunction and disorder does not get at our intuitive medical concepts. Such an account does not adequately distinguish normal variation from malfunction, excellence from pathology, epidemics and statistically common disorders from normality, and so on. (The exception is Christopher Boorse's [1977] biostatistical theory, which does place its faith in statistical deviance and fails for this reason among others; see my reply to Lemoine in this volume.)

However, such statistical or technical attempts to save Godfrey-Smith's claim are beside the point due to a more basic problem, revealed at the end of the above passage: "The concept of malfunction is context dependent on Cummins' view, just as the concept of function in general is." That is, Godfrey-Smith acknowledges that because any capacity or disposition of a system that is of interest can be the target of a CR-functional analysis, the notion of CR malfunction must be interest relative as well. This is a claim that even CR defender Murphy (this volume) now belatedly questions as conflicting with the objectivity of medical dysfunctions.

As we have seen, Cummins himself (Cummins and Roth 2009) accepts that on his interest-relative systems or CR approach to function, dysfunction must be defined in interest-relative terms: "Systematic accounts relativize failures to function properly to a target *explanandum*. … Thus, systematic accounts allow for a kind of relativized or instrumental normativity: what something needs to do for the containing system to exercise the target capacity" (2009, 79). Cummins's analysis thus gives up any pretense to explaining the objectivity of medical diagnosis. Whether your heart ceasing to pump is a dysfunction in the medical sense is not dependent on your interests. Even if you are suicidal or tired of life, the heart's lack of pumping is a medical dysfunction. If you are a medical researcher and the capacities of certain genes or bodily conditions to cause diseases are what interest you (e.g., the capacity to form new tumors in certain forms of cancer; the capacity of the heart to cause edema in congestive heart failure), then whatever bodily component actions lead to that outcome will have that outcome as their CR functions, and within that context, the failure to cause the tumor formation or edema, respectively, becomes a malfunction. This implication constitutes a clear *reductio ad absurdum* of the CR notion of malfunction put forward by Godfrey-Smith, at least as a notion of malfunction relevant to medical diagnosis.

So, if the question is how one can start from CR functions and get to a conceptually adequate account of malfunction in the objective sense relevant to medicine, the answer is that you can't get there from here. The interest relativity of CR functions and CR dysfunctions, acknowledged by Godfrey-Smith as well as Cummins, makes it impossible for any attempted definition of CR malfunction to approximate the objective nature of the intuitive medical notion of malfunction.

In the same paper, Godfrey-Smith (1993) offers a way out of the problem posed by his passage above if "malfunction" is interpreted in its medical sense. He famously insists that CR and SE functions are two different kinds of functions that are dominant in different subdisciplines of biology, and they are not to be confused even while both are to be accepted as legitimate: "We should accept both senses of function, and keep them strictly distinct. All attempts to make one concept of function work equally for behavioral ecology and physiology are misguided. On this view, 'Wright functions' and 'Cummins functions' are both effects which are distinguished by their explanatory importance. The difference is in the type of explanation" (Godfrey-Smith 1993, 200–201).

Suppose that for the sake of argument, we accept Godfrey-Smith's famously proposed "consensus" that both SE and CR forms of functional explanation are real and legitimate ways of identifying functions. This consensus implies that the relevant question is not which approach is the superior one to adopt for all of the biomedical sciences (this is the unfortunate way that Murphy approaches the issue). Rather, the relevant question is which of the two approaches to function attributions, SE or CR, is the appropriate one specifically for the function and dysfunction attributions underpinning medical and psychiatric diagnosis of disorder versus normal variation. This approach obviates the need for a forced answer to how the CR approach can define malfunction, because malfunction in the medical sense can be a domain in which SE functions are the more appropriate of the two approaches.

Conclusion

Murphy accepts that medical judgments of dysfunction must be objective and acknowledges that CR functions on their face are not objective due to their interest relativity. So far, neither Murphy's own arguments nor Cummins's presentation nor the arguments and positions of the writers cited by Murphy—several of whom are biologists and ought to know—nor the biological literature itself support Murphy's contention that CR functions can and should supplant SE functions. Most important, there is no evidence in anything presented in Murphy's paper for his claim that CR functions can yield an appropriately objective sense of dysfunction of the kind that can support the practice of medical diagnosis in anything like the form it currently exists.

However, this does not entirely resolve the issue of whether such an explanation exists. Although putting forward no solution to this conundrum himself, Murphy in effect outsources the solution to the problem of dysfunction objectivity by citing philosophers Carl Craver and Marcel Weber as having put forward theories that can explain how CR functions can provide the foundation for objective medical judgments of dysfunction and disorder. Murphy thus suggests that my work "overlooks the extensive work done in recent years by philosophers of biology who have developed [the CR approach] into a causal-explanatory account."

Thus, to complete a fair assessment of Murphy's argument for CR functions as a foundation for medical diagnosis, it is necessary to go beyond the arguments laid out in

Murphy's chapter and directly consider—and not once again overlook—the work of the authors he cites as having the solutions he seeks. I therefore provide in a supplement to this reply a close examination of whether Craver's or Weber's analyses cited by Murphy provide the solution Murphy requires to warrant his CR-function approach to medicine.

References

Allen, C., and J. Neal. 2019. Teleological notions in biology. In *The Stanford Encyclopedia of Philosophy*, E. N. Zalta (ed.). https://plato.stanford.edu/cgi-bin/encyclopedia/archinfo.cgi?entry=teleology-biology.

Amundson, R., and G. V. Lauder. 1994. Function without purpose: The uses of causal role function in evolutionary biology. *Biology and Philosophy* 9: 443–469.

Ap, T. 2016. This is what reading is like if you have dyslexia. *CNN Health*. https://www.cnn.com/2016/03/05/health/dyslexia-simulation/index.html.

Armstrong, T. 2015. The myth of the normal brain: Embracing neurodiversity. *AMA Journal of Ethics* 17(4): 348–352.

Artigas-Pallarés, J. 2009. Dyslexia: A disease, a disorder, or something else? *Revue Neurologique* 48(suppl. 2): S63–S69.

Blanco, D. B. 2019. A molecule long thought harmless plays a role in pancreatic cancer, could hint at cure. *Discover*, June. http://blogs.discovermagazine.com/d-brief/2019/06/20/a-molecule-long-thought-harmless-plays-a-role-in-pancreatic-cancer-could-hint-at-cure/#.XbN5WZNKgWo.

Bock, W. J., and G. von Wahlert. 1965. Adaptation and the form-function complex. *Evolution* 19: 269–299.

Boorse, C. 1975. On the distinction between disease and illness. *Philosophy and Public Affairs* 5(1): 49–68.

Boorse, C. 1976. Wright on functions. *Philosophical Review* 85: 70–86.

Boorse, C. 1977. Health as a theoretical concept. *Philosophy of Science* 44: 542–573.

Boorse, C. 2002. A rebuttal on functions. In *Functions: New Essays in the Philosophy of Psychology and Biology*, A. Ariew, R. Cummins, and M. Perlman (eds.), 63–112. Oxford University Press.

Cummins, R. 1975. Functional analysis. *Journal of Philosophy* 72: 741–765.

Cummins, R. 2002. Neo-teleology. In *Functions: New Essays in the Philosophy of Psychology and Biology*, R. Cummins, A. Ariew, and M. Perlman (eds.), 157–173. Oxford University Press.

Cummins, R., and M. Roth. 2009. Traits have not evolved to function the way they do because of a past advantage. In *Contemporary Debates in Philosophy of Biology*, F. Ayala and R. Arp (eds.), 72–86. Blackwell.

Davies, P. S. 2001. *Norms of Nature: Naturalism and the Nature of Functions*. MIT Press.

Du Bois-Reymond, E. 1882. The seven world-problems. *Popular Science Monthly*. https://en.wikisource.org/wiki/Popular_Science_Monthly/Volume_20/February_1882/The_Seven_World-Problems. April 25, 2018.

Dyslexia has a language barrier. 2004. *The Guardian*, September 22. https://www.theguardian.com/education/2004/sep/23/research.highereducation2

Dyslexia is not a disease. n.d. Davis Dyslexia Association International. https://www.dyslexia.com/question/dyslexia-is-not-a-disease/.

Eisenberg, D. T. A., B. Campbell, P. B. Gray, and M. D. Sorenson. 2008. Dopamine receptor genetic polymorphisms and body composition in undernourished pastoralists: An exploration of nutrition indices among nomadic and recently settled Ariaal men of northern Kenya. *BMC Evolutionary Biology* 8: 173.

Engle, D. D., H. Tiriac, K. D. Rivera, A. Pommier, S. Whalen, E. T. Oni, et al. 2019. The glycan CA19–9 promotes pancreatitis and pancreatic cancer in mice. *Science* 364: 1156–1162.

First, M. B., and J. C. Wakefield. 2010. Defining 'mental disorder' in *DSM-V*. *Psychological Medicine* 40(11): 1779–1782.

First, M. B., and J. C. Wakefield. 2013. Diagnostic criteria as dysfunction indicators: Bridging the chasm between the definition of mental disorder and diagnostic criteria for specific disorders. *Canadian Journal of Psychiatry* 58(12): 663–669.

Gluckman, P., A. Beedle, and M. Hanson. 2009. *Principles of Evolutionary Medicine*. Oxford University Press.

Godfrey-Smith, P. 1993. Functions: Consensus without unity. *Pacific Philosophical Quarterly* 74: 196–208.

Habib, M. 2000. The neurological basis of developmental dyslexia: An overview and working hypothesis. *Brain* 123: 2373–2399.

Halbrook, C. J., and H. C. Crawford. 2019. Hiding in plain sight: A common biomarker of pancreatic disease has a functional role in pathogenesis. *Science* 364(6446): 1132–1133.

Harvey, W. 1628/1993. *On the Motion of the Heart and Blood in Animals*. Trans. R. Willis. Prometheus Books.

Horwitz, A., and J. C. Wakefield. 2007. *The Loss of Sadness: How Psychiatry Transformed Normal Sorrow into Depressive Disorder*. Oxford University Press.

Hubel, D. H., and T. N. Wiesel. 1959. Receptive fields of single neurones in the cat's striate cortex. *Journal of Physiology* 148: 574–591.

Hubel, D. H., and T. N. Wiesel. 1962. Receptive fields, binocular interaction and functional architecture in the cat's visual cortex. *Journal of Physiology* 160: 106–154.

Jorgenson, E., N. Matharu, M. R. Palmer, J. Yin, J. Shan, T. J. Hoffman, et al. 2018. Genetic variation in the SIM1 locus is associated with erectile dysfunction. *Proceedings from the National Academy of Sciences of the United States of America* 115(43): 11018–11023.

Josberger, E., P. Hassanzadeh, Y. Deng, J. Sohn, M. J. Rego, C. Amemiya, et al. 2016. Proton conductivity in ampullae of Lorenzini jelly. *Science Advances* 2(5): e1600112–21600112: 1–6.

Kareklas, K., D. Nettle, and T. V. Smulders. 2013. Water-induced finger wrinkles improve handling of wet objects. *Biology Letters* 9(2): 1–3.

Kingma, E. 2013. Naturalist accounts of mental disorder. In *The Oxford Handbook of Philosophy and Psychiatry*, K. W. M. Fulford, M. Davies, R. G. T. Gipps, G. Graham, J. Z. Sadler, G. Stanghellini, and T. Thornton (eds.), 363–384. Oxford University Press.

Kitcher, P. 1993. Function and design. *Midwest Studies in Philosophy* 18: 379–397.

Knoll, J. L., IV, and R. W. Pies. 2019. Cruel, immoral behavior is not mental illness. *Psychiatric Times*, August 19. https://www.psychiatrictimes.com/couch-crisis/cruel-immoral-behavior-not-mental-illness.

Lilienfeld, S. O., S. J. Lynn, J. Ruscio, and B. L. Beyerstein. 2010. Myth #17: The defining feature of dyslexia is reversing letters. In *50 Great Myths of Popular Psychology: Shattering Widespread Misconceptions about Human Behavior*, 37–38. John Wiley. https://www.psychologicalscience.org/media/myths/myth_17.cfm.

Lloyd, E. 2005. *The Case of the Female Orgasm: Bias in the Science of Evolution*. Harvard University Press.

Millikan, R. 1989. In defense of proper functions. *Philosophy of Science* 56: 288–302.

Murphy, D. 2006. *Psychiatry in the Scientific Image*. MIT Press.

Murphy, D., and R. L. Woolfolk. 2000. The harmful dysfunction analysis of mental disorder. *Philosophy, Psychiatry, and Psychology* 7(4): 241–252.

Neander, K. 1991. Functions as selected effects: The conceptual analyst's defense. *Philosophy of Science* 58(2): 168–184.

Payn, N. M., and J. C. Wakefield. 1982. The effects of group treatment of primary orgasmic dysfunction on the marital relationship. *Journal of Sex and Marital Therapy* 8: 135–150.

Protopapas, A., and R. Parrila. 2018. Is dyslexia a brain disorder? *Brain Sciences* 8(61): 1–18.

Protopapas, A., and R. Parrila. 2019. Dyslexia: Still not a neurodevelopmental disorder. *Brain Sciences* 9(9): 1–5.

Reason. 2019. In *Merriam-Webster.com*. https://www.merriam-webster.com/dictionary/reason.

Ribatti, D. 2009. William Harvey and the discovery of the circulation of the blood. *Journal of Angiogenesis Research* 1(3): 1–2.

Schneps, M. H. 2015. Dyslexia can deliver benefits. *Scientific American Mind*, January 1. https://www.scientificamerican.com/article/dyslexia-can-deliver-benefits/.

Smith, W. L., E. Everman, and C. Richardson. 2018. Phylogeny and taxonomy of flatheads, scorpionfishes, sea robins, and stonefishes (Percomorpha: Scorpaeniformes) and the evolution of the lachrymal saber. *Copeia* 106(1): 94–119.

Spitzer, R. L. 1997. Brief comments from a psychiatric nosologist weary from his own attempts to define mental disorder: Why Ossorio's definition muddles and Wakefield's "harmful dysfunction" illuminates the issues. *Clinical Psychology: Science and Practice* 4(3): 259–261.

Spitzer, R. L. 1999. Harmful dysfunction and the *DSM* definition of mental disorder. *Journal of Abnormal Psychology* 108(3): 430–432.

Steinberg, P. L., and Buoy Medical Review Team. 2019. 28 reasons for a light or severe headache and nausea: A comprehensive guide on headaches, whether it's a headache after eating, a workout, or due to an illness. *Buoy Health Blog*, March 8. https://www.buoyhealth.com/current/28-types-of-headaches-and-causes.

Sullivan-Bisset, E. 2017. Malfunction defended. *Synthese* 194(7): 2501–2522.

Symonds, D. 1979. *The Evolution of Human Sexuality*. Oxford University Press.

Szanto, A., V. Narkar, Q. Shen, I. P. Uray, P. J. A. Davies, and L. Nagy. 2004. Retinoid X receptors: X-ploring their (patho)physiological functions. *Cell Death & Differentiation* 11, S126–S143.

Taylor, C. 1964. *The Explanation of Behavior*. Routledge and Kegan Paul.

Tinbergen, N. 1963. On aims and methods of ethology. *Zeitschrift für Tierpsychologie* 20: 410–433.

Treiman, R., J. Gordon, R. Boada, R. L. Peterson, and B. F. Pennington. 2014. Statistical learning, letter reversals, and reading. *Scientific Studies of Reading* 18(6): 383–394.

Wakefield, J. C. 1992a. The concept of mental disorder: On the boundary between biological facts and social values. *American Psychologist* 47: 373–388.

Wakefield, J. C. 1992b. Disorder as harmful dysfunction: A conceptual critique of *DSM-III-R*'s definition of mental disorder. *Psychological Review* 99: 232–247.

Wakefield, J. C. 1993. Limits of operationalization: A critique of Spitzer and Endicott's (1978) proposed operational criteria of mental disorder. *Journal of Abnormal Psychology* 102: 160–172.

Wakefield, J. C. 1995. Dysfunction as a value-free concept: A reply to Sadler and Agich. *Philosophy, Psychiatry, and Psychology* 2: 233–46.

Wakefield, J. C. 1997a. Diagnosing *DSM-IV*, part 1: *DSM-IV* and the concept of mental disorder. *Behaviour Research and Therapy* 35: 633–650.

Wakefield, J. C. 1997b. Diagnosing *DSM-IV*, part 2: Eysenck (1986) and the essentialist fallacy. *Behaviour Research and Therapy*: 35: 651–666.

Wakefield, J. C. 1997c. Normal inability versus pathological disability: Why Ossorio's (1985) definition of mental disorder is not sufficient. *Clinical Psychology: Science and Practice* 4: 249–258.

Wakefield, J. C. 1997d. When is development disordered? Developmental psychopathology and the harmful dysfunction analysis of mental disorder. *Development and Psychopathology* 9: 269–290.

Wakefield, J. C. 1998. The *DSM*'s theory-neutral nosology is scientifically progressive: Response to Follette and Houts. *Journal of Consulting and Clinical Psychology* 66: 846–852.

Wakefield, J. C. 1999a. Evolutionary versus prototype analyses of the concept of disorder. *Journal of Abnormal Psychology* 108: 374–399.

Wakefield, J. C. 1999b. Mental disorder as a black box essentialist concept. *Journal of Abnormal Psychology* 108: 465–472.

Wakefield, J. C. 1999c. The concept of mental disorder as a foundation for the *DSM*'s theory-neutral nosology: Response to Follette and Houts, part 2. *Behaviour Research and Therapy* 37: 1001–1027.

Wakefield, J. C. 2000a. Aristotle as sociobiologist: The "function of a human being" argument, black box essentialism, and the concept of mental disorder. *Philosophy, Psychiatry, and Psychology* 7: 17–44.

Wakefield, J. C. 2000b. Spandrels, vestigial organs, and such: Reply to Murphy and Woolfolk's "The harmful dysfunction analysis of mental disorder." *Philosophy, Psychiatry, and Psychology* 7: 253–269.

Wakefield, J. C. 2001. Evolutionary history versus current causal role in the definition of disorder: Reply to McNally. *Behaviour Research and Therapy* 39: 347–366.

Wakefield, J. C. 2004. The myth of open concepts: Meehl's analysis of construct meaning versus black box essentialism. *Applied & Preventive Psychology* 11: 77–82.

Wakefield, J. C. 2006. What makes a mental disorder mental? *Philosophy, Psychiatry, and Psychology* 13: 123–131.

Wakefield, J. C. 2007. The concept of mental disorder: Diagnostic implications of the harmful dysfunction analysis. *World Psychiatry* 6: 149–156.

Wakefield, J. C. 2009. Mental disorder and moral responsibility: Disorders of personhood as harmful dysfunctions, with special reference to alcoholism. *Philosophy, Psychiatry, and Psychology* 16: 91–99.

Wakefield, J. C. 2011a. Darwin, functional explanation, and the philosophy of psychiatry. In *Maladapting Minds: Philosophy, Psychiatry, and Evolutionary Theory*, P. R. Andriaens and A. De Block (eds.), 143–172. Oxford University Press.

Wakefield, J. C. 2011b. *DSM-5* proposed diagnostic criteria for sexual paraphilias: Tensions between diagnostic validity and forensic utility. *International Journal of Law and Psychiatry* 34: 195–209.

Wakefield, J. C. 2014. The biostatistical theory versus the harmful dysfunction analysis, part 1: Is part-dysfunction a sufficient condition for medical disorder? *Journal of Medicine and Philosophy* 39: 648–682.

Wakefield, J. C. 2015. Psychological justice: *DSM-5*, false positive diagnosis, and fair equality of opportunity. *Public Affairs Quarterly* 29(1): 32–75.

Wakefield, J. C. 2016a. The concepts of biological function and dysfunction: Toward a conceptual foundation for evolutionary psychopathology. In *Handbook of Evolutionary Psychology*, D. Buss (ed.), 2nd ed., vol. 2, 988–1006. Oxford University Press.

Wakefield, J. C. 2016b. Diagnostic issues and controversies in *DSM-5*: Return of the false positives problem. *Annual Review of Clinical Psychology* 12: 105–132.

Wakefield, J. C. 2019. The harmful dysfunction analysis of addiction: Normal brains and abnormal states of mind. In *The Routledge Handbook of Philosophy and Science of Addiction*, H. Pickard and S. H. Ahmed (eds.), 90–101. Routledge.

Wakefield, J. C., and M. B. First. 2003. Clarifying the distinction between disorder and nondisorder: Confronting the overdiagnosis ("false positives") problem in *DSM-V*. In *Advancing DSM: Dilemmas in Psychiatric Diagnosis*, K. A. Phillips, M. B. First, and H. A. Pincus (eds.), 23–56. American Psychiatric Press.

Wakefield, J. C., and M. B. First. 2012. Placing symptoms in context: The role of contextual criteria in reducing false positives in *DSM* diagnosis. *Comprehensive Psychiatry* 53: 130–139.

Wakefield, J. C., D. Wasserman, and J. A. Conrad. 2020. Neurodiversity, autism, and psychiatric disability: The harmful dysfunction perspective. In *Oxford Handbook of Philosophy and Disability*, A. Cureton and D. Wasserman (eds.), 501–521. Oxford University Press.

Wang, C. 2017. Let me introduce you to "Asian fit" glasses. *Refinery29*. https://www.refinery29.com /en-us/asian-glasses.

Why Asian fit? It's not just for Asians. 2019. *TC Charton*. https://www.tc-charton.com/asian-fit -eyewear.aspx.

Wright, L. 1973. Functions. *Philosophical Review* 82: 139–168.

Ziegler, J. C., C. Perry, A. Ma-Wyatt, D. Ladner, and G. Körne-Schulte. 2003. Developmental dyslexia in different languages: Language-specific or universal? *Journal of Experimental Child Psychology* 86: 169–193.

15 Do the Works of Carl Craver or Marcel Weber Explain How Causal Role Functions Can Provide Objective Medical Judgments of Dysfunction? Supplementary Reply to Dominic Murphy

Jerome Wakefield

We have seen that Murphy fails to make his case that there is a way that CR functions can explain the objectivity of medical dysfunction in a way comparable to the objective account of the harmful dysfunction analysis (HDA; see the main reply to Murphy for references). However, he cites the works of Carl Craver and Marcel Weber as providing such an explanation. In this supplement to my reply to Murphy, I examine whether Craver's or Weber's work does provide such an explanation.

Carl Craver's (2007) Analysis of Mechanistic Explanation

Murphy prominently cites Carl Craver as a philosopher whose work can provide an explanation for how, despite interest relativity, CR functions can nonetheless provide the basis for an objective naturalist account of biological functions and thus a foundation for medical diagnostic judgments. In evaluating Murphy's claim, I will consider the book by Craver (2007) that Murphy cites as well as a related article by Craver (2001) that Craver cites in his book. I shall argue that Craver is not addressing, let alone solving, the problem of objectivity confronting Murphy's "function" claim. I hasten to add that this is not a criticism of Craver. Craver's work is precise, insightful, and illuminating regarding the problem he does address, which is the nature of an adequate CR mechanistic explanation.

Working within a broadly Cummins-inspired CR-function framework, Craver (2007) elaborates a "causal-mechanical model of constitutive explanation" in neuroscience—or simply "mechanistic explanation" (2007, 107): "Mechanistic explanations are constitutive or componential explanations: they explain the behavior of the mechanism as a whole in terms of the organized activities and interactions of its components" (2007, 128). His aim is to show how CR analysis "will have to be amended and revised if it is to offer a normatively adequate account of constitutive mechanistic explanation" (2007, 107). Explanatory adequacy is defined in comprehensive terms: "The central criterion of adequacy for a mechanistic explanation is that it should account for the multiple features of the phenomenon, including its precipitating conditions, manifestations, inhibiting conditions, modulating conditions, and nonstandard conditions" (2007, 139). In Craver's CR-inspired model, multilevel hierarchical, contextual, and etiological causal processes in the component parts of a mechanism combine to explain the full set of dispositional capacities conferred on the containing mechanism.

He thus embraces Wesley Salmon's (1984, 1998) causal-mechanical analysis of explanation, rejecting covering-law, unificationist, and prototype-activation accounts. He also rejects reductionist demands to formulate theories at one privileged ontological level, instead allowing multiple mechanism levels to enter into adequate explanations. Unlike Cummins, Craver's exclusive interest is in explanations of a system's capacities in terms of its components at various sublevels. In contrast, Cummins's account of functional analysis allows noncomponential causal stories as well, such as psychological explanations in which a capacity is analyzed in terms of other capacities at the same level (e.g., the capacity to bake a cake in terms of the capacity to look up the recipe, to follow directions, etc.; or the capacity for action in terms of the capacity to have belief and desire reasons for the action).

Now, with respect to Murphy's claims, Craver acknowledges what Murphy will not accept, that the essential interest relativity of CR functions means that mechanistic explanation applies equally to healthy and disordered conditions. Thus, CR functions offer no resources to make this foundational medical distinction in any objective way:

> If one is interested in explaining the behavior of a mechanism under diseased or industrial conditions, then one will be interested in componency relations under those conditions. Although we are often interested in states of health or features that have been selected for, there is no reason to insist upon this restriction. There is no way to know what constitutes the "appropriate" conditions without specifying the pragmatic context in which one is operating. (Craver 2007, 155–156)

Craver is quite explicit that functions in the CR sense can be purely destructive and pathological:

> My account of mechanistic role functions does not appeal to any sense of adaptiveness in an environment; instead it appeals only to roles in contextual systems. These contextual systems may be adaptive or destructive, and they need not even be the kinds of systems for which talk of adaptation is appropriate. Heart disease, high blood pressure, cardiac arrhythmia, and arterial hardening all have mechanisms that span multiple levels, and this three-tiered perspective is as useful in those contexts as in those that are adaptive. Descriptions of hierarchical mechanisms are always descriptions of the mechanisms for…something that one wants to understand (build, control, predict)…without necessarily being adaptive or maladaptive. (Craver 2001, 67)

Sometimes Craver seems for a moment to write as if there is an objective and naturalist CR distinction between health and pathology, but he then steps back and clarifies that the CR view rejects any such notion due to the relativization of function to investigator interests and values:

Finally, the component should be physiologically plausible. It should not exist only under highly contrived laboratory conditions or in otherwise pathological states. Of course, what constitutes a contrived condition or a pathological state varies across explanatory contexts. If one is trying to explain healthy functions, then pathological conditions might be considered physiologically implausible. If, on the other hand, one is trying to explain a disease process, one's explanation might be physiologically implausible if it assumes conditions only present in healthy organisms. What matters is that the parts' existence should be demonstrable under the conditions relevant to the given request for explanation of the phenomenon. (2007, 132)

In keeping with these views, Craver frequently provides examples of CR-type analysis in which the "functions" will be the production of a medically pathological condition: "A broken ... kidney's mechanistic role is then identified against the fixed backdrop of a description of the way the circulatory system generally works, or the way that it preferably works, or the way that it works in whatever (normal or pathological) mechanism that we seek to understand" (Craver 2001, 72): "We provide an etiological explanation of why John is a victim of heart disease when we blame his smoking and diet and, perhaps, the mechanisms by which smoking and diet produce heart disease" (2001, 69–70); "Some mechanistic explanations ... explain an event by describing its antecedent causes. Dehydration is part of the etiological explanation of thirst. Prion proteins are part of the etiological explanation of Creutzfeldt-Jacob disease. Excessive repetition of the CAG nucleotide pattern on the fourth chromosome is part of the etiological explanation for Huntington's disease" (2007, 107–108).

Given the interest relativity of the CR-mechanistic explanation, Craver conceptualizes an organ being "broken" as a deviation in how it works from any standard or class of entities one chooses. He rejects the statistical approach to brokenness because some CR functions concern statistically rare or manufactured phenomena. The baseline for judging what is broken can be what is statistically common, or what we prefer, or even a pathological trajectory in which we are interested. Thus, if one is studying the cause of progressive renal failure, a "broken" kidney might be one that spontaneously begins to function normally.

To the objection that one can define health within the mechanistic approach by simply identifying the organism's standard functioning, Craver makes clear that, given the interest relativity of all such analyses, what is normal or standard is not an independently definable notion but itself relative to the interests of the investigator. Sometimes that determining context might be the health of the organism, but that is an additional extra-CR concept imposed by the investigator and not defined by the functional analysis:

"Normal" and "standard" conditions amount to something like "the way that the mechanism behaves under the conditions that we consider most appropriate for our current explanatory purposes." Sometimes this is assessed in terms of the healthy and fit organism, and normal means something like "behavior consistent with or conducive to overall system health and function." Sometimes it is assessed in terms of evolutionary stories, and so means something like "behavior similar to that which preserved the trait in the population of organisms." Sometimes normalcy is assessed in terms of its utility for an experiment, and so means something like "behavior consistent with or conducive to manipulation and detection with my experimental protocol." There is no need to be more restrictive about this notion. "Normal" and "standard" are defined relative to an implied investigative context. (Craver 2007, n. 13, 127)

Given such choices due to the interest relativity of CR functions, Craver alludes to the inevitable issue of value intrusion and bias that can enter into CR function judgments:

Describing an item's mechanistic role is a perspectival affair. This perspectival take on functional ascription should be a reminder that what we take as functional descriptions can be tinged in a very direct way by our interests and biases. (Craver 2001, 73)

In the context of psychiatry, such perspectival neutrality on what is normal versus pathological can yield rationalization of social control of deviance. That is, like all Cummins-inspired views, Craver's analysis allows social values to determine what is of interest and thus to dictate functional hierarchies. This provides no protection from what Murphy portrays as the objection to diagnosis of the medical skeptic, who says that disorder judgments are just based on social value criteria. This approach is dangerously confusing when it comes to psychiatric diagnostic judgments of function and dysfunction. Suddenly, to use some standard examples, the interests of slaveholders in the antebellum South can allow for a legitimate "dysfunction" attribution to runaway slaves (the infamous diagnosis of "drapetomania"), and from the Soviet state's perspective, the Soviet dissidents can be legitimately considered to suffer from a mental dysfunction. We know that these are in fact illegitimate diagnoses because the "dysfunction" judgments underlying them are *false*, but that is a conclusion that cannot be reached objectively from a CR starting point that sees all capacities of the containing system as equally potential functions depending on the interests of the investigator. Relativizing notions of biological function and dysfunction is an assault on the legitimacy of disciplines like psychiatry that are already prone to confuse social undesirability and deviance with mental disorder. The objectivity of the function/dysfunction distinction makes medicine special and allows it to be more than a servant of social control. In effect, the CR approach yields a normative approach to disorder attribution by way of perspectival definition of function and dysfunction, yielding to Murphy's skeptic who says diagnosis is just about values. Murphy's attempt to reject the skeptic's position is undermined by his embrace of CR functions.

However, against some evolutionists, Craver obviously rejects the notion that SE functions aimed at explaining normality are the only kind of real functions. He insists on the need for CR mechanistic analyses that can be equally aimed at disordered or other anomalous features not amenable to SE explanation:

Some workers in the systems tradition assume or stipulate that all explanandum phenomena have been selected by evolution by natural selection or that the phenomena are otherwise adaptive (that is, the phenomenon is how something behaves when it is behaving properly). In the philosophy of biology, Cummins is best known for his attacks on Wright's adaptive view of functions. I side with Cummins. Neuroscientific explanations often focus on malfunctions, disease states, laboratory phenomena, pharmaceutical contrivances, and industrial and military applications (for example, how the vestibular system works in zero-gravity)....No doubt, some of the features of the brain have straightforward adaptive etiologies, but I do not want to presuppose for present purposes that all of them do. Either way, one still needs the more limited sense of role-functions, activities that make some crucial contribution to the behavior of a containing system. (2007, n. 10, 124)

In rejecting the claim that all neurobiological explanatory activity in every area should be in terms of SE functions, Craver here expresses a pluralism in which there are explanatorily rich SE functional explanations needed in some areas but where of course "more limited" CR functions are also needed. Note that he suggests that SE explanations are especially appropriate when one is interested in "how something behaves when it is behaving properly" (the medical notion of proper function or health) but that CR functions are especially needed to study departures from biologically designed functioning such as "malfunctions, disease states, laboratory phenomena, pharmaceutical contrivances, and industrial and military applications (for example, how the vestibular system works in zero-gravity)." I would say that in the end, both CR and SE analysis is necessary to understand both domains, but in particular that the disorder/nondisorder part of "behaving properly" in the objective adaptationist more-than-perspectival-interest sense is strictly and essentially dependent on SE functional analysis. Everything Craver says is consistent with this understanding.

In sum, Craver's work does not in any way support Murphy's view that CR functions can be naturalized in such a way as to support objective judgments of disorder and pathology. To the contrary, Craver is crystal clear that health and disorder are equally mechanistically explainable, are both of interest, and thus, relative to the mechanisms that produce them, are equally "functions" in the CR sense. He offers no account of how CR functions can objectively distinguish health from disorder and even implies that SE functions may well be needed for such a discrimination. Thus, he provides Murphy no lifeboat in which to escape the objections to his claim that CR functions are an adequate foundation for psychiatric diagnosis, given that Murphy accepts that disorder attributions must be objective judgments that something has gone wrong "under the hood" of the individual. Consequently, Craver's analysis offers no support for Murphy's contention that philosophers are resolving the problem of how CR functions can enable one to draw an objective naturalistic medical distinction between health and pathology.

Marcel Weber's Coherence Theory of Natural Function

I have been considering Murphy's response to a key objection to using CR functions as a basis for attribution of psychiatric and medical disorder. The objection, which he acknowledges as a serious one, is that CR functions, due to their being interest relative, cannot explain the objectivity of biological function and dysfunction as these concepts are applied in medical diagnosis. His response is to cite other philosophers who, he says, are formulating ways in which to construct relevant objective function judgments from CR functions. We have seen in my reply to Murphy and above that his citations of Bock and von Wahlert (1965), Amundson and Lauder (1994), and Craver do not support his point because they are pluralists about "function's" meanings who are not trying to do what Murphy describes.

However, Murphy's fourth and final citation to Marcel Weber's work on functional organization offers more hope for Murphy's point. Weber, in the course of a larger discussion of holism, explicitly frames his work in part as an attempt to explain how a CR-function approach can support a naturalist, objective account of biological function. I now consider whether Weber's approach succeeds in vindicating the ability of CR functions to explain biological functions without the addition of SE functions. Murphy cites an article (Weber 2005a) and a book (Weber 2005b) by Weber as supporting his point. My discussion is based on both, but I primarily focus on the article because Weber says that in it, he presents a "modified version" of his similar remarks in the relevant pages (35–39) of the book.

The main theme of Weber's article is, as Murphy suggests, to try to present an objective naturalistic account of biological functions within the constraints of the CR analysis of function. (Weber prefers to refer to CR functions as "Cummins functions" or as the "dispositional" concept of functions, and I use all three terms interchangeably here.) The challenge, as we have seen, is that CR functions are interest-relative and thus neither objective nor naturalist. Weber fully accepts this challenging starting point, characterizing Cummins's account of function as follows: "X's function in system S is φ exactly if X's capacity to φ is part of an adequate analytic account of S's capacity to ψ" (190). The choice of ψ is entirely unconstrained by this formula and depends on the interests of the investigator. Consequently, the fact that X's capacity to φ is part of an account of the outcome of interest ψ is sufficient for concluding that φ is a function of X within the system. Weber is also quite clear on how this CR approach to functions differs fundamentally from the SE approach: "What is crucial with this account is that function ascriptions according to this definition do not explain the *presence* of the function bearer in the system. In other words, the identification of something as a function entails nothing about why this thing is part of the system. In contrast, the etiological account of functions holds that this is precisely what a functional ascription explains" (190).

Given that any organismic capacity, healthy or disordered, can be explained causally by reference to the organism's parts, Weber acknowledges that the interest relativity of CR functions implies a prima facie mismatch between the CR account of function and a standard usage of "function" within certain areas of biology in which a function is not relative to the researcher's interests but an objective fact about the organism:

> Cummins…fully accepts the consequence that, on his account, the overall systems capacity is ours to choose, and it does not appear to be among his goals to naturalize functions. However, it seems to be a goal of biological science to identify the natural functions of some organ and structure. A biologist who says "I happen to be interested in blood circulation, therefore I see the heart's function in pumping blood" would appear rather unusual. Biologists want to discover what the function of some biological structure is, and they want their functional explanations to be made true by natural facts. Thus, Cummins' desiderata for functional analysis and those of a modern biologist appear to be different. (Weber 2005a, 191)

So, why doesn't Weber just adopt the etiological SE approach to biological functions as his objective approach? Clearly, as we shall see, Weber, like Cummins, is driven by a broader agenda related to philosophy of mind—in this case, the idea that forms of holism may be common to philosophy of mind and philosophy of biology. One might wonder if the rivalry in philosophy of mind between classic CR functionalism and Millikan's SE-function analysis of meaning has eventuated in what amounts to a proxy war in philosophy of biology!

Weber is clearly opposed to any etiological or historical loading of "function," and he does offer a couple of arguments against the SE view as a univocal approach:

> First, it will not admit anything as a function that has just arisen anew (for example, by spontaneous mutation) without having experienced the influence of natural selection yet. Second, biologists sometimes attribute functions without knowing the evolutionary past of some part or structure. (Weber 2005a, 191)

These are weak reasons to give up the use of natural selection in determining biological function. In the limit case of the initial occurrence of a novel spontaneous mutation that accidentally confers a new capacity, it is usual to say that the novel effect is not its natural function but a fortuitous benefit. People who, say, develop a chance mutation that makes them impervious to HIV infection are not said to possess a mutation that has the natural function of protecting them from HIV. Rather, by happy accident, they have a mutation that protects them from HIV and "functions to" (if you will) protect them.

As to the point that biologists often attribute functions without knowing the evolutionary past (a point made also by Murphy and by many other critics), of course they do. Even when there are attributions of function, they are generally based on inferences about biological design from circumstantial evidence rather than knowledge of evolutionary history. Evolution is an essentialist *theory* of natural functions, not the meaning of "function" (see my reply to Lemoine in this volume). One can do plenty of biological and psychiatric science without knowing evolutionary histories (see my reply to Kincaid in this volume) or even without knowing about evolution. The notion of a natural or biological function was understood long before Darwin and is understood today by those who reject or are ignorant of Darwinian theory. Aristotle did not need to know about evolution to judge that a function of the eyes is to enable one to see, of the hands to grasp, of fear to evade danger, or that teleology was somehow involved in acorns regularly turning into oak trees. Weber's argument that people judge functions without knowing evolutionary history, and therefore functions cannot be naturally selected effects, confuses sense and reference and is as fallacious as arguing people often judge liquids to be water without knowing chemistry, and therefore water cannot be H_2O. One does not have to know that water is H_2O to start a useful science of hydrology, and one does not have to know that biological functions are naturally selected effects to recognize natural functions and even to inaugurate a useful profession of medicine that tries to help people when something goes harmfully wrong with biologically designed functioning.

Note that in constructing his objective version of CR functions to match the standard objective usage he describes, Weber is not claiming that, if he can make his idea about objective CR functions work, then there is no need for some other objective notion such as SE functions. Like most other defenders of CR functions, Weber allows that "function" may be polysemous and that there is room for more than one meaning in different contexts. For example, he says that "to make sense of scientific practice it is necessary to give an account (or several accounts, should there be different concepts of function used in biology) that picks out those things as functions that biologists ascribe functions to" (191) and remarks that it is "questionable" if there is one standard usage of "function" in biology (191). This is the same openness to other than CR functions that we saw in many of the authors cited by Murphy.

I now turn to Weber's proposed solution to Murphy's question of how CR functions can finesse interest relativity and successfully mimic a naturalist account of biological functions without reference to natural selection or other etiological historical criteria. Weber attempts to do this by developing a position within functional biology that is analogous to coherentist views of the justifiability of beliefs in epistemology, where it is the internal coherence of a system of beliefs that allows one to judge it as "true." Analogously, Weber adds a "coherence" requirement to the CR account's function attributions that is intended to yield objective judgments without any reference to external criteria such as evolutionary history: "this account can be supplemented with a coherence condition in order to avoid a certain kind of relativity to the investigator's interest" (2005a, 190).

Weber argues that although there are an indefinite number of causal capacities of a mechanism that might be of interest, only certain of the mechanism's causal capacities are part of a larger interacting coherent system of capacities of various mechanisms that constitute the system's incredibly complex interacting system of functions, and it is those coherence-manifesting effects and only those that constitute a mechanism's biological functions: "the parts of a system have some of their characteristic properties—namely, their biological functions—only because they form a coherent system with other components that have biological functions" (200). This offers what Weber initially hopes is an objective and naturalistic way of establishing which of a mechanism's many effects on which of the organism's many capacities are the mechanism's natural functions.

The coherence analogy suggests to Weber that he can analyze functions by means of coherence: "X's function in system S is φ exactly if X's capacity to φ coheres with other capacities belonging to (parts of) S. The concept of coherence as understood here designates a complex relation between a large number of capacities. The basic relation on which this coherence relation is based consists in a capacity's contribution to another capacity. The exemplary case is the heart's contribution to the circulatory system's capacity to transport solutes and cells through the body" (192–193). Weber further explains the notion of coherence and illustrates it as follows:

> Let us say that a system of capacities is coherent if it contains a sufficiently complex net of such contributory relations between the various capacities, such that many capacities contribute to other capacities that contribute themselves to other capacities and so forth....Biological organisms contain an elaborate network of capacities that contribute to other capacities. Here is just a small section through such a network: The function of certain ion channels in nervous membranes is to regulate ion permeability because this capacity is part of an account of the nervous membrane's capacity to fire action potentials. But the nervous membrane's capacity to fire action potentials is part of an account of the nervous system's capacity to process information. Therefore, it is a function of nervous membranes to fire action potentials. Furthermore, the nervous system's capacity to process information is part of an analytic account of the organism's capacity to locate food and sexual partners. Therefore, it is a function of the nervous system to process information. The organism's capacity to locate food is part of an analytic account of its capacity to ingest energy-rich compounds and nutrients, which are part of analytic accounts of the liver's capacity to synthesize purines and pyriminides and of the muscles' capacity to transform chemical energy into motion. (193–194)

Weber observes,

> It is obvious that biologists could tell many endless stories like this one. Any organism of some complexity will reveal zillions of such explanatory relations; this is what it means to possess a functional organization (and perhaps, to be an organism). What I am suggesting here is that, if there is a unique way of laying such a coherent functional organization over an organism it is the place of a given capacity in such a coherent system that underwrites this capacity's status as a function, and not its selection history nor the investigator's interests. (193)

However, Weber is immediately forced to supplement the coherence account. The analogy to belief systems offers the first clue of trouble. To take the analogy further, the standard objection to the coherence theory of truth is that truth is objective, whereas there can be different mutually contradictory equivalently coherent systems of beliefs. Optimizing coherence of beliefs is thus not necessarily the same as optimizing the truth of beliefs. For example, for all we know, certain all-encompassing religious dogmatic belief systems or even some delusional systems or pathological belief systems may contain many false beliefs and yet may be as coherent as belief systems that contain many more truths. Against Weber's coherence theory of functions, one might raise a similar objection—in effect, an analog of Bertrand Russell's (1907) classic objection to the coherence theory of truth that there are equally coherent systems of belief that go along with a proposition and its negation, so coherence per se cannot constitute truth. Analogously, given a disease that does not reduce life expectancy, a causal relation and its negation may be part of equally coherent and self-maintaining systems of CR functions. The claim that health is more coherent than illness is not immediately persuasive given that there is no reason to think that maintaining a chronic disease state in a living human being involves any less causal pathways to organism features than does maintaining a healthy state. As Weber emphasizes, organisms are complex systems of interacting natural functions that have a remarkable coherence, and, interacting with parts of that coherent system, there can be equally remarkable coherent subsystems of dysfunctions induced during some disease processes that, for example, allow cancer to spread despite all the genetic safeguards, allow infections to persist despite the immune system, and allow parasites to coexist within us and adjust our internal environments to their own benefit. At the very least, the level of coherence in disease versus health is an empirical question, so a coherence view implies that it is an empirical question whether each disease is in fact a natural function, a position impossible to defend.

A second strike against the coherence theory is that it does not explain the continuity in the attribution of biological function over historical time. Weber's examples of coherence are all examples of the amazingly complex workings of the human body that we have come to understand relatively recently, as in the above quoted example. However, biologists identified objective functions long before they had an inkling of how complicated we are at the many levels we now understand. In this regard, it is worth comparing two explanations for why we judge the heart's function to be pumping the blood. Here is Weber's explanation, in which he presents a more convoluted version of Hempel's (1965) classic dilemma of why pumping the blood is the function of the heart, whereas making a sound is not:

> The heart has the capacity to pump blood, which contributes to the circulatory system's capacity to deliver oxygen and nutrients to all body cells. But the circulatory system does many other things: For example, it delivers signaling molecules such as hormones and removes metabolic waste from the cells for chemical decomposition in the liver or dialytic removal in the kidneys. It also carries platelets (for repair), antibodies and immune cells such as B- and T-lymphocytes through the body. For simplicity, let us treat these various activities of the circulatory system as one capacity, the transport capacity of the circulatory system. The question now is whether

biologists have chosen this capacity just so, because they happen to be interested in transport. This seems not right. Intuition prompts us to say that the transport capacity is the salient capacity of the circulatory system. The circulatory system also generates heat and carbon dioxide, uses up energy-rich compounds, makes noises, forms blood clots and hence causes disease and death, but these capacities are not salient.

But why is the transport capacity salient? An obvious answer is that the transport capacity is the circulatory system's function, while generating heat and carbon dioxide, using up energy-rich compounds, making noises and forming blood clots are not.... This raises the obvious question of what underwrites the functional status of the circulatory system's transport capacity. Perhaps it is the fact that the transport capacity contributes to a variety of other capacities that are also functions: cell respiration, immune defense, catabolic waste removal, metabolic coordination, sexual differentiation, and so on.

Now, what is salient about this passage is that we know that Sir William Harvey (1628/1993) identified pumping the blood as the function of the heart without knowing any of those other specifics. He knew nothing about coherence of the heart's pumping with the many other processes mentioned by Weber. So, why did he conclude, correctly, that pumping the blood (i.e., blood transport) is the function of the heart? No doubt, mostly biologists are trying to figure out how things work without worrying about strong function statements. Indeed, as Tinbergen (1963) famously noted, a mechanistic understanding of how things work is integral to an overall evolutionary explanation (I agree; see my reply to Gerrans in this volume). Indeed, one cannot really see the ways that functional attributions and explanations are needed until one has a grasp of the descriptive facts that allow one to conclude that there is a design-like quality that makes the existence of natural functions likely. For example, Harvey's discovery that the function of the heart is to circulate the blood is considered by many to be the greatest single medical discovery of all time (Friedland 2009) and took place more than 200 years before Darwin's discoveries. Yet it is clear that in attributing a primary function of pumping blood to the heart, Harvey was influenced by strong intuitions about biological design, although he did not yet know what explained biological design:

> From the symmetry and magnitude of the ventricles of the heart and of the vessels entering and leaving (since Nature, who does nothing in vain, would not have needlessly given these vessels such relatively large size), from the skilfull and careful craftsmanship of the valves and fibres and the rest of the fabric of the heart, and...how great the amount of transmitted blood...I began privately to think that it might rather have a certain movement, as it were, in a circle....It must therefore be concluded that the blood in the animal body moves around in a circle continuously and that the action or function of the heart is to accomplish this by pumping. This is the only reason for the motion and beat of the heart. (Harvey 1628/1993, as quoted in Ribatti 2009, 1–2)

Harvey focuses on certain features of form and causal power, as CR theorists insist, but, contrary to CR theory, he is not primarily interested in sheer causal or capacity attributions except as a path to understanding design. It is not the causal features and capacities for blood movement of the ventricles per se that capture his attention, but, in light of relatively simple and primitive observations of structure combined with the assumption of biological design ("Nature, who does nothing in vain, would not have needlessly given these vessels such relatively large size"), and from detailed observations of the nature of design-like features ("from the skilfull and careful craftsmanship of the valves and fibres and the rest of the fabric of the heart"; Harvey had experimented with the way the valves force blood in one direction), he concludes, first, mechanically and contrary to the standard thought of his day, that the blood "might rather have a certain movement, as it were, in a circle" before ultimately concluding with the stronger statement that "the action or function of the heart is to accomplish this by pumping," using "reason" as a term connoting the purpose for which the heart is there ("This is the only reason for the motion and beat of the heart"). In light of endless such historical examples (e.g., Aristotle had no understanding of the myriad causal linkages necessary to get from an acorn to an oak tree but nevertheless understood the production of the oak tree as the final cause, or function, of the acorn), it would appear that Weber's appeal to complex coherence relations is an ad hoc appeal to things we know now long after our notion of biological function became a regular part of biological theorizing.

To the degree that coherence seems likely in biologically designed organisms, Weber seems to have gotten the relationship between design and coherence backward. The history of the study of the heart illustrates that in our ignorance of mechanisms and their natural-selective history, coherence is generally implicitly assumed based on an assumed teleology, not the other way around. For example, we don't really know yet why we need to sleep (or at least we didn't until recently; there are some exciting developments in this area). Thus, we don't really know the degree to which sleep is all that coherent with the rest of our functions. Yet from circumstantial evidence, we assume that we are biologically designed to sleep and so it is normal, and we presume that likely it links to many other functions. This is despite the fact that sleep takes away a third of our lives, leaving us during that time largely unaware of our environment, functionally impaired, periodically hallucinating, and partially paralyzed. Yet sleep isn't considered a disorder. This would remain true even if we were to discover that sleep is not very linked to other functions but a unique one-off naturally selected adaptation that could be suppressed without harm (e.g., as is usually the case with our biologically designed capacity to develop a fever in response to an infection). A lack of high coherence of the kind Weber describes would not make our need for sleep any less normal given that it is biologically designed.

Furthermore, high degrees of coherence can be achieved by socially constructed functions that are not natural or biological functions. Indeed, cultures often support their ideologies by claiming that certain functions that have become "second nature" within that culture are natural to human beings, when in fact those functions have been locally constructed by the culture. Because such ideologies can serve as rationales for oppression of deviant individuals and misclassification of such individuals as disordered, drawing the distinction between biological functions and other forms of socially cultivated functioning is a major goal of an analysis of the concept of mental disorder. The coherence view fails to accomplish this goal because socially cultivated functioning can become integrated in overall functioning in a coherent fashion. For example, Kingma (2013) observes that a social invention such as reading can be so integrated with other functions that it can appear naturally selected until we recall that it is an invention.

The coherence account is also subject to counterexamples of a kind that might be called "function danglers." Surely there can be functions of specific single organismic features that have relatively isolated causal chains leading to their final result and so do not interact with many other features. Worms apparently have light-sensing cells on their tails, and thus one imagines perhaps that they feel a sense of satisfaction when finally fully underground, but that function of the light-sensitive cells may interact with nothing else on its way to reinforcing the safety of being underground. So, its level of coherence would be quite low. One can imagine even more extreme cases, such as external markings that have a function in terms of potential predators but do not interact at all with other features of the organism. Such "danglers" possess biological functions just as fully as the highly coherent ones described by Weber, yet they are not significantly coherent.

The Self-Reproduction Criterion

Weber recognizes that uniqueness of function is not assured by his coherence criterion, and he tries to obtain uniqueness by adding another criterion, "self-reproduction," by which he means the organism's continued existence over time. This criterion, borrowed from McLaughlin (2001), is intended to further whittle down the effects that define the privileged coherent system that equates to objective biological functions:

> The crucial question is obviously whether there is a *unique* coherent system of capacities. Doubts are in order; it is quite conceivable that there are many ways of knitting various causal dispositions of the parts of an organism into a coherent system in the manner just outlined. However, what seems less likely is that there are several systems that are *explanatorily equivalent*. It is possible that, for any type of organism, there exists exactly one coherent system of capacities that best explains how the organism can self-reproduce. By "self-reproduction" I mean not procreation, but the organism's capacity to maintain its form or identity for a certain appropriate duration (see McLaughlin 2001). This appears to be the most universal property in biology (note that not all organisms procreate!), and it is certainly the property that biologists ultimately want to understand. For these reasons, it is appropriate to take self-reproduction as the capacity that a system of functions must explain. (194)

In sum: "I conclude that a biological (role) function is a capacity that either contributes to a higher-level system capacity that is itself a role function or contributes directly to an organism's self-reproduction" (2005b, 40). Interestingly, the view that inspired Weber's use of self-reproduction is an etiological view, which he rejects, so he must amend it. Weber explains,

> A different kind of etiological account of functions has recently been developed by Peter McLaughlin (2001). On McLaughlin's view, ... A system can only have functions if it is capable of self-reproduction. By this, McLaughlin means the maintenance of an organism's form over time, which is not to be confused with ... procreation ... by constantly regenerating their parts. My body does not contain the same carbon atoms as it did 20 years ago, but the individual organism that I am sustains metabolic activities continually replacing all the atoms and molecules that make up my body. (2005b, 37)

Why is this an etiological account despite no involvement of natural selection? The basic idea is simply that if a mechanism in an organism contributes to the survival (or "self-reproduction") of the organism, then because the organism survives, the mechanism also survives within it, and thus there is a sense in which the mechanism's effect explains its own continued existence: "McLaughlin argues that there is a sense in which tokens of function bearers, by virtue of what they do, indirectly cause their own continuing presence in an individual organism, namely by contributing to the maintenance of the whole system (token). Thus, McLaughlin's account can be classified as etiological" (2005b, 37). Weber firmly abandons any etiological element of the self-reproduction account, distinguishing his use of self-reproduction from that of McLaughlin who inspired it: "It is important to appreciate that, on this account of functional explanation, the ascription of a function to a biological entity implies nothing about why tokens of this entity are present in the systems that are given a functional analysis. ... McLaughlin's version of the etiological function concept ... does not correctly capture the use of the term 'function' ... because, as I have argued, functional analysis does not at all attempt to explain why tokens of function bearers are present in a biological system" (40). Thus, it is McLaughlin's account of functions as CR contributors to self-reproduction without the explanatory element.

One might be dubious from the start that one can define the criterion of self-reproduction without a prior understanding of health and thus of function. What constitutes the acceptable perpetuation of the organism depends on the proper functioning of the organism's parts, or else any horrific disordered state that maintains life would qualify all the parts as functioning properly. This misunderstanding that one can analyze the functions of parts in terms of organismic maintenance goes all the way back to Hempel's (1965) classic paper on functions in which Hempel at one point proposed that an effect of an organ is a function if it "ensures the satisfaction of certain conditions ... which are necessary for the proper working of the organism" (305). As Cummins (1975) observes, this is circular as an analysis of "function" because "it seems clear that for something to be in working order is just for it to be capable of performing its functions, and for it to be in adequate or effective or proper working order is just for it to be capable of performing its functions adequately or effectively or properly" (753). "Self-reproduction" does not even seem to require self-reproduction in a properly working way and so is even more subject to Cummins's objection than is Hempel's claim.

These broader concerns aside, Weber's coherence account is not saved from ample counterexamples by the arbitrary addition of the self-reproduction filter to identify objective natural functions. One immediate set of counterexamples consists of those reproductive organs and features concerned solely with reproduction that do not contribute to self-reproduction and yet have functions. A second set of counterexamples involves those many serious illnesses that in our modern environment do not influence life expectancy and so on the basis of self-reproduction alone cannot be classified as disorders.

A third set of counterexamples, noted above, consists of the many ways that humans culturally exploit their natural mechanisms so that cultural practices become a seamless part of a coherent and interacting set of capacities supporting self-reproduction. In such cases, a capacity is part of the coherent system supporting self-reproduction but is not considered a biological function, yet Weber's account would classify it as a function. For example, the ability to learn to read is not a biological function of any human mechanism, yet it is difficult to imagine a capacity that enters into our lives in modern literate societies more coherently as part of a larger interacting system of capacities that keep us alive.

There are also mechanisms with biologically designed capacities that possess functions but are not currently contributing to self-reproduction due to changes in the environment. For example, the preference for fatty and sweet foods is the function of certain taste and hunger mechanisms, yet in our current environment, we spend our lives trying to minimize, distance ourselves from, and otherwise control that capacity from expressing itself in behavior because with our plentiful food supply, these tastes yield lower self-reproduction via disease causation. Yet other clear counterexamples to the self-reproduction view emerge from the theory of kin selection, which implies that some naturally selected functions may go against self-reproduction and encourage individuals to sacrifice themselves to save cofamilial individuals who have a sufficient share of the same genes, thus increasing the likelihood of gene perpetuation at the cost of ending self-reproduction. One can think here of the seemingly programmed non-self-reproduction of salmon after spawning that provides nutrients to offspring or the ready sacrifice of soldier ants.

I conclude that Weber's coherence account, even with the self-reproduction epicycle added, does not save CR functions from its fatal flaws as an account of what we mean by natural function in the context of biological design. The problem here is not the details of the particular proposals. The problem is the entire strategy of starting with the anemic CR account of function and trying through various restrictions to get the result to come out equivalent to the robust SE account of functions that accurately reflects the objective sense of biological function. Like analyzing "human being" as "featherless biped," one might get close to material equivalence, but one would still not be achieving an understanding of how we think about the concept, why it is objective, and why we take it so seriously.

Conclusion

The examination of the work of Craver and Weber that Murphy cites shows that in fact those sources fail to provide any solution to the problem of how CR functions can explain the objectivity of medical dysfunction. This means that Murphy fails to directly show or indirectly indicate how CR functions can undergird an objective sense of dysfunction and disorder in medicine and psychiatry. Murphy thus fails at his self-appointed task of showing how CR functions can explain when something has objectively gone wrong "under the hood" of the human being. The "scientific image" he creates of psychiatry based on CR functions is in fact unscientific and subject to all the abuses that the analysis of the concept of mental disorder was undertaken to address. And, the HDA remains the only scientifically grounded account that fulfills the objectivity criterion that he accepts.

References

Amundson, R., and G. V. Lauder. 1994. Function without purpose: The uses of causal role function in evolutionary biology. *Biology and Philosophy* 9: 443–469.

Bock, W. J., and G. von Wahlert. 1965. Adaptation and the form-function complex. *Evolution* 19: 269–299.

Craver, C. F. 2001. Role functions, mechanisms, and hierarchy. *Philosophy of Science* 68(1): 53–74.

Craver, C. F. 2007. *Explaining the Brain: Mechanisms and the Mosaic Unity of Neuroscience*. Oxford University Press.

Cummins, R. 1975. Functional analysis. *Journal of Philosophy* 72: 741–765.

Friedland G. 2009. Discovery of the function of the heart and circulation of blood. *Cardiovascular Journal of Africa* 20(3): 160.

Harvey, W. 1628/1993. *On the Motion of the Heart and Blood in Animals*. Trans. R. Willis. Prometheus Books.

Hempel, C. G. 1965. The logic of functional analysis. In *Aspects of Scientific Explanation and Other Essays in the Philosophy of Science*, 297–330. Free Press.

Kingma, E. 2013. Naturalist accounts of mental disorder. In *The Oxford Handbook of Philosophy and Psychiatry*, K. W. M. Fulford, M. Davies, R. G. T. Gipps, G. Graham, J. Z. Sadler, G. Stanghellini, and T. Thornton (eds.), 363–384. Oxford University Press.

McLaughlin, P. 2001. *What Functions Explain: Functional Explanation and Self-Reproducing Systems.* Cambridge University Press.

Ribatti, D. 2009. William Harvey and the discovery of the circulation of the blood. *Journal of Angiogenesis Research* 1(3): 1–2.

Russell, B. 1907. On the nature of truth. *Proceedings of the Aristotelian Society* 7: 228–249.

Salmon, W. S. 1984. *Scientific Explanation and the Causal Structure of the World.* Princeton University Press.

Salmon, W. S. 1998. *Causality and Explanation.* Oxford University Press.

Tinbergen, N. 1963. On aims and methods of ethology. *Zeitschrift für Tierpsychologie* 20: 410–433.

Wakefield, J. C. 2003a. The Chinese room argument reconsidered: Essentialism, indeterminacy, and strong AI. *Minds and Machines* 13: 285–319.

Wakefield, J. C. 2003b. Fodor on inscrutability. *Mind and Language* 18: 524–537.

Weber, M. 2005a. Holism, coherence and the dispositional concept of functions. *Annals of the History and Philosophy of Biology* 10: 189–201.

Weber, M. 2005b. *Philosophy of Experimental Biology.* Cambridge University Press.

16 The Developmental Plasticity Challenge to Wakefield's View

Justin Garson

Introduction

According to Jerome Wakefield's influential analysis of "disorder," part of what makes something a mental disorder is that it stems from an inner dysfunction. A trait is dysfunctional, in turn, when it cannot do what natural selection designed it for. Many of Wakefield's critics have raised the possibility that there could, in principle, be mental disorders that do not involve inner dysfunctions in this sense. Along these lines, I'm going to argue that some mental disorders might result from "developmental mismatches." This takes place when the environment that the fetus or child encounters is very different from its adult environment, and the kinds of strategies (physical traits, behaviors, or psychological dispositions) that the fetus or child used to master the early environment are maladaptive in the later environment. I argue that this would be a case of disorder without dysfunction, and I give some empirically plausible examples. To begin, however, I will discuss a concrete example of a developmental mismatch in the biological world.

The tiny crustacean of the genus *Daphnia* provides a remarkable example of developmental plasticity. One species, *Daphnia cucullata*, is about 3 millimeters in length and inhabits lakes across Europe. It has several invertebrate predators. If a *Daphnia* is raised in the vicinity of predators, it grows a tough, helmet-shaped head. This "helmet" is a boon as it makes it difficult for predators to swallow it. The helmet, I take it, is an adaptation designed by natural selection to protect the *Daphnia* in perilous waters. Other species of *Daphnia* have evolved equally impressive defenses, such as tail spines, "neckteeth," and crests (a kind of pointed head shape) (Tollrian and Dodson 1999). These are called "inducible" defenses as their appearance is triggered by the presence of kairomones, a kind of hormone released by the predator. They can also be epigenetically transmitted (Agrawal et al. 1999). If a female *Daphnia* is exposed to kairomones, her offspring are more likely to grow the helmet-shaped head even in the absence of predators.

There are some drawbacks to the "helmet" phenotype. First, helmets are metabolically expensive; they require more calories to maintain. Second, the large head reduces the *Daphnia*'s mobility. That is why natural selection gave the *Daphnia* a certain degree of morphological flexibility. It only grows the helmet if it needs to. Once a phenotype is selected—"helmet" versus "normal"—reversibility is limited. (Different defenses show different degrees of reversibility, from completely reversible to completely irreversible; the helmet phenotype is closer to the latter.) This is an example of developmental plasticity. Something inside the *Daphnia* encodes a conditional rule: "if predators, then helmet; if no predators, then no helmet."

Developmental plasticity is a subtype of phenotypic plasticity, and there are many different mechanisms for it (Pigliucci 2001). Imprinting is another such mechanism (see section I). At the most general level, developmental plasticity takes place when there are at least two distinct adult phenotypes the juvenile organism can grow into, and which phenotype it assumes depends on the contingencies of its formative context. When biologists talk about developmental plasticity, moreover, they typically imply that each adult phenotype represents an *adaptation* to that specific developmental context, that is, that the phenotype is "appropriate" to that context. Getting a permanent scar as a result of a playground accident is not an example of developmental plasticity.

Developmental plasticity has its risks. The big risk is a "developmental mismatch." Suppose we hatch some *Daphnia* eggs in a tank swarming with predators, and they grow the helmet-shaped head. Suppose we then remove the predators from the tank. Then the *Daphnia* experience only the disadvantages of the helmet phenotype and none of its perks. Their condition becomes *chronically maladaptive*. It would be acutely troublesome for them if we forced them to compete over limited resources with their "normal"-shaped counterparts, who need less food and can get to it faster.

Some biologists like to describe the risks inherent in developmental plasticity by using a gambling metaphor. The developing organism can be seen as making a kind of "prediction" about what its future world will be like, on the basis of its present conditions. In other words, it "samples" its present environment and extrapolates into the future. It then "selects" a phenotype that would maximize its fitness in that anticipated future environment. This is called a "predictive adaptive response" (Gluckman et al. 2009; Glover 2011). If its "prediction" turns out to be correct, it is rewarded with enhanced fitness; if it is incorrect, its fitness is reduced. The latter scenario is a "developmental mismatch."

Here is an intuition that I have. (Fortunately, I need not rely exclusively on intuition here, because I have a specific theory of function, one with strong independent credentials, that yields precisely this result. In the next section, I'll describe that theory.) It seems to me that talk of "dysfunction" is out of place when it comes to developmental mismatches. Let me clarify. Suppose there is a member of *Daphnia* that chose the "wrong" phenotype; that is, suppose it was raised in a tank with predators, it grew the helmet-shaped head, and later, the predators were removed. It exhibits a developmental mismatch and takes a fitness loss as a result. In my opinion, this does not represent an inner "dysfunction." Put metaphorically, nothing "went wrong" inside that *Daphnia*. Its developmental machinery is operating exactly as it is "supposed to." It is neither defective nor diseased; it's just unlucky. (Of course, the mismatch can *cause* a dysfunction, for example, if the *Daphnia* dies of malnutrition. But that sort of dysfunction is incidental to the mismatch; having a mismatch does not logically imply dysfunction.)

This brings me to the central question of the chapter. What if some of our current psychiatric ailments result from developmental plasticity, *rather than* dysfunction? In other words, what if, in certain individuals with bona fide mental disorders, the disorder represents a developmental mismatch, much like a helmet-shaped *Daphnia* in a predator-free environment (see Garson 2015, chap. 8)? Some psychiatric researchers take this possibility quite seriously (for a recent review, see Glover 2011). For example, they argue that some anxiety disorders, such as generalized anxiety disorder, might arise from a contrast between one's formative environment and one's adult environment. The "formative" environment can include both the prenatal "environment," as well as the postnatal environment of the infant or young child. Such mismatches can be chronically maladaptive for the individuals that possess them. This is not a bit of philosophers' speculation but an empirically plausible conjecture, one that should be accepted, or refuted, on empirical grounds. I do not know whether this budding research program—sometimes known as Developmental Origins of Health and Disease (DOHaD)—will ultimately be vindicated (for an overview, see Gluckman and Hanson 2006). But I think it represents an exciting new avenue for exploring the roots of major mental disorders.

This conjecture—that *some mental disorders are developmental mismatches*—raises a significant problem for Wakefield's "harmful dysfunction" (HD) analysis of mental disorder, which holds that all mental disorders stem from biological dysfunctions (e.g., Wakefield 1992, 1999a, 2011). I will lay out the developmental plasticity challenge in three stages. First, I will set out the underlying theory of biological function and dysfunction that Wakefield and I accept. An important upshot of this discussion is that there is a distinction between saying that a trait is *dysfunctional* and saying that it is *functioning normally in an unsuitable environment* (or, perhaps better, that it is unable to function *due to* an unsuitable environment). I will also raise the thorny issue of "function indeterminacy" and explain its relevance to my argument. Second, I will describe a line of criticism that Wakefield's opponents have repeatedly raised. It is called the "evolved mismatch critique." I raise it here because the logical structure of that argument mirrors, in some important ways, the logical structure of my own. I happen to believe that the evolved mismatch critique, when properly understood, undermines Wakefield's analysis, but I will not lean too heavily on that argument here. In the third part, I will explain the developmental plasticity challenge. I will also respond to potential objections against this challenge.

To give credit where credit is due, I should point out that two psychologists, John Richters and Stephen Hinshaw (1999, 442–443), raised a version of this "developmental plasticity challenge" against Wakefield's analysis. They ask us to consider a hypothetical example of a young boy who grows up in an abusive home and develops symptoms of conduct disorder as a result (e.g., aggressive behavior). Suppose that those symptoms were functional and adaptive in the abusive home and that he had those symptoms *because* they were useful to him. Suppose, finally, that when the boy moves to a new, nurturing home, he retains the symptoms of conduct disorder. The boy's "hostile world orientation" is now a fixed part of his young personality, much like the *Daphnia*'s helmet-shaped head. Richters and Hinshaw believe that, in this case, the boy has a mental disorder with no underlying dysfunction. In my terminology, this would be a "developmental mismatch." Richters and Hinshaw, however, raise the example in passing and not entirely persuasively (in section III, I will address Wakefield's response). Moreover, their paper makes numerous general claims about function and development that I do not accept. One way to think about my project is that it represents an attempt to illuminate, more clearly than they did, the logical structure of the argument underlying their example and to give a more plausible example to bolster their case.

I. What Are Functions? What Are Dysfunctions?

One of the perennial questions of the philosophy of psychiatry is, what are mental disorders? What do all of these diverse conditions, such as schizophrenia, bipolar disorder, and personality disorders, have in common—if anything—that makes them mental disorders? In Wakefield's view, disorders generally, whether mental or physical, are *harmful dysfunctions* (the "HD analysis"). This definition has two parts: *harm* and *dysfunction*. First, in order for something to be a disorder, it must be harmful as judged by prevailing social norms. Second, for something to be a disorder, it must stem from an inner dysfunction on the part of the individual. It can be a dysfunction on the part of the brain or nervous system, for example, or it can be a dysfunction on the part of the mind. The notion of *dysfunction* is what distinguishes disorders, per se, from socially deviant behavior (such as belonging to the American Nazi Party) and from psychological states that are merely unpleasant to have (such as stress about a job interview). The idea that the notion of *dysfunction* is somehow implicated at the core of mental disorders has been raised before (e.g., Spitzer et al. 1977; Klein 1978; American Psychiatric Association 1980, 6). Unfortunately, those authors did not provide a clear explanation of what "dysfunctions" were, so their attempts at definition left much to be desired.

What is it, then, for something to be a dysfunction? What are functions? Here, Wakefield relies on a certain conception of function that philosophers of science developed in the 1970s and 1980s, the *selected effects* theory of function (see Wright 1973; Millikan 1984; Neander 1991). There are several nuances here when it comes to distinguishing various forms of the theory, but roughly, the theory holds that *the function of a biological trait is whatever it was selected for by natural selection*. In other words, the function of a trait is the reason it evolved by natural selection. The reason my nose has the *function* of helping me breathe, and not the *function* of holding up glasses, is that the former benefit explains why people have noses (via appeal to natural selection). Traits that did not evolve by natural selection, such as birthmarks or freckles, do not have functions at all, even if they happen to benefit us from time to time. I accept the selected effects theory, and in the remainder of this chapter, I will take it for granted, and I urge the reader to do the same, at least for the sake of argument. (Garson [2016] defends the theory from several common criticisms.)

Now that we know what functions are, it would seem that defining "dysfunction" would be fairly easy. But we quickly encounter conceptual obstacles. In the remainder of this section, I will note some of those obstacles and develop a definition of "dysfunction" that resolves them. At first pass, it would seem that *something is dysfunctional just when it cannot perform its function*. The eyes of a person who is congenitally blind are dysfunctional because they cannot perform their function of seeing.

There are some details that are not entirely resolved, but it is not necessary to resolve them here. For example, most traits can exhibit various rates of functioning, and it is difficult to "draw a line" between those instances when a trait functions at a low but intuitively "acceptable" rate and those instances when it is dysfunctional (Wakefield 1999a, 379; also see Schwartz 2007; Garson and Piccinini 2014). Some of Wakefield's critics have raised this "line drawing problem" as a significant objection (e.g., Lilienfeld and Marino 1995, 414), but I do not consider it a deep problem. Rather, it reflects the standard sort of vagueness that most philosophical concepts possess. In my usage, to say a trait is "dysfunctional" implies either that it cannot perform its function at all (e.g., cardiac arrest) or that it can only perform its function at an unacceptably low rate. A trait is "nonfunctional" when it does not have a function (birthmarks or freckles).

Here is a more serious problem with our simplistic definition of dysfunction. Just because a trait cannot perform its function, that alone does not make it dysfunctional. In other words, the inability to perform a function (at an acceptable rate) is necessary, but not sufficient, for dysfunction. A simple example will prove the point. Suppose I am blindfolded. My eyes cannot perform their function of seeing. They are not, however, dysfunctional. So dysfunction is not just the inability to perform a function but something more. To say that something is dysfunctional implies that it cannot perform its function for intrinsic or constitutional reasons and not just because of an unsuitable environment (Dretske 1986; Neander 1995; Wakefield 1999a, 385). There are various ways we can describe the blindfold situation. One way is to say that my eyes are "functioning normally in an unsuitable environment." Another way is to say that my eyes are "unable to function *because* of an unsuitable environment." It does not really matter which way we describe the case. The important point is that it is not a dysfunction.

These considerations suggest that we should amend our definition to say that *something is dysfunctional just when it cannot perform its function, for "inner" or "constitutional" reasons, rather than because it's in an unsuitable environment.* But we are not quite out of the woods yet. There is a certain conceptual puzzle that has plagued the selected effects theory for decades and creates new trouble for defining "dysfunction." (In fact, it plagues most theories of function that tie function to evolution.) It is called the problem of function indeterminacy. (There are various forms of indeterminacy; here, I will describe the "hierarchical" form of indeterminacy.) The problem of indeterminacy, at the most general level, is that there are many ways of describing a trait's function, all of which are allowed by the selected effects theory. Is the function of the heart simply to *beat*? To *circulate blood*? To *bring nutrients to cells*? To *keep the organism alive*? All of these descriptions are acceptable because they are all effects that explain why the heart evolved by natural selection. (The issue is more complex, because the heart has other functions than merely beating; for example, it also regulates its rate of pumping in order to maintain a stable ratio of carbon dioxide to oxygen. I will set aside such details at present and simply focus on the heart's beating.)

Fortunately, in most cases, it does not matter how we describe the heart's function. In some cases, however, it matters quite a bit, particularly when we are trying to specify, in a rigorous and precise way, when something dysfunctions. That is because different ways of describing a trait's function may be more or less suggestive of "dysfunction." Suppose somebody's heart is beating at a relatively normal rate, but that person has a ruptured artery in his or her brain that prevents blood from circulating effectively. Is that person's *heart* dysfunctional? If we say that the function of the heart is simply to *beat* (i.e., engage in systole and diastole), then it is *not* dysfunctional. It is doing exactly what it is "supposed to" do. If we say that the function of the heart is to *circulate blood*, it *might* be dysfunctional (since, after all, it cannot do what it is "supposed to" do). It would depend on the details of our definition of dysfunction.

Different theorists have proposed different solutions to the problem, and I will not attempt to survey them all. I endorse a simple and plausible solution developed by Neander (1995), who also explores conceptual nuances that I do not have the space to explore here. Her solution stems from the following observation. In our example, the different descriptions of the heart form a certain series, that is, a hierarchy defined by cause and effect. By beating, the heart circulates blood. By circulating blood, the heart brings nutrients to cells. By bringing nutrients to cells, the heart keeps us alive. When we say that the function of the heart is simply *to beat*, we are describing the most "proximal" member of that chain. When we say that the function of the heart is to *keep us alive*, we are describing its most "distal" member. When we say that the function of the heart is to *bring nutrients to cells*, we are describing an "intermediate" member of that chain, somewhere between the most proximal and the most distal.

Her view is that a trait is dysfunctional only when it cannot perform its most proximal function. The heart is dysfunctional only when it cannot *beat*. There are two good reasons for accepting her solution. The first is that it is intuitively appealing. I think it gives the "correct" verdict in the example of the heart. The second is that it is, from a biomedical perspective, the most sensible solution. In the biomedical context, when we say that something is dysfunctional, we are indicating, in a pragmatic way, that it is an appropriate target of medical intervention (Buller 1997). But presumably, if the heart cannot circulate blood because of a ruptured brain artery, we should target the artery and not the heart! To say that the heart is dysfunctional seems contrary to good medical practice. Wakefield (1999a, 386) also describes the problem of indeterminacy (see his bacterium example), and he seems to accept the same solution.

My viewpoint about function indeterminacy informs my intuition about the *Daphnia* case. Let's assume, for the sake of simplicity, that there is a mechanism (M) in the *Daphnia* that obeys the following rule: "if predators, then helmet; if no predators, then no helmet." There are many ways of describing M's function. We could say that M's function is to trigger a certain developmental sequence (one that yields the helmet head) in response to kairomones. Perhaps it does this by releasing a certain hormone into the bloodstream. Then the function of M is to *release hormone H in response to kairomones*. Alternatively, we could say that M's function is to *protect the individual from predators*. The former is a more proximal way of describing its function and the latter a more distal way of describing its function. That is because the two descriptions form a series: the mechanism typically *protects the individual from predators* by *releasing hormone H in response to kairomones*.

Now, suppose we have a developmental mismatch. Is there any dysfunction? Described in the most proximal way, the answer is no. M fully and adequately discharged its function when it released hormone H in response to kairomones. Described in a more "distal" way, there could be a dysfunction. After all, if there are no predators around, M certainly cannot perform its function of protecting the individual from them. So, whether or not it is "dysfunctional" depends, in part, on how we describe it. I prefer the more proximal description for the reasons I gave above.

My discussion may seem to belabor the point, but there are cases where I think Wakefield is potentially inconsistent in his approach to function indeterminacy, and the way we describe the *Daphnia*-type case is pivotal to my argument. On one hand, Wakefield's (1999a, 386) explicit comments about indeterminacy seem to agree with my own, namely, that we should prefer the most "proximal" description of an item's function (as in the bacterium case). On the other hand, some of his specific examples seem to run contrary to that point. He discusses an example of filial imprinting gone awry, that is, where a gosling imprints on a passing porcupine (Wakefield 1999b, 468; 2000, 263). (Imprinting refers to a developmental "window" of time in which a juvenile organism forms a strong, lifelong preference. The function of filial imprinting in goslings is to cause them to form an attachment to their own mothers. The mechanism by which this works is that they form an attachment to the first large, suitably moving object that they encounter. Imprinting goes awry when the mechanism causes a gosling to imprint on an object that is not its mother.) The gosling now has an enduring inner disposition to follow around a porcupine. Wakefield says that this disposition is a dysfunction. I do not consider it a dysfunction (Murphy and Woolfolk [2000b, 279] have similar reservations about Wakefield's imprinting case). I think there would be a dysfunction if the gosling failed to imprint on a passing porcupine, so long as that porcupine moved about in the right sort of way and if that porcupine entered the gosling's visual field at just the right time. The gosling's disposition would be chronically maladaptive but not dysfunctional.

I suspect that the difference of opinion between Wakefield and myself traces back to the problem of function indeterminacy. For there are two ways of describing the function of the imprinting mechanism in the gosling's brain, and one is more proximal than the next. The first, most proximal description is to say M's function is to cause the gosling to form a strong attachment to the first large, suitably moving object it sees. The second, more distal description is to say M's function is to cause the gosling to have a disposition to follow its mother. The first is more proximal than the second because the mechanism typically causes the gosling to follow its mother *by* causing the gosling to form a strong attachment to the first large, suitably moving object it sees. If we stick with the first description in the porcupine case, we see there is no dysfunction. M has performed its job admirably. If we stick to the second description, we have some evidence of dysfunction (after all, M cannot discharge its function). I have given reasons for my preference for the more proximal description. I will come back to this issue in section III.

To summarize this rather abstract discussion: the function of a trait is the reason it evolved by natural selection, and *a trait is dysfunctional just when it cannot carry out its most proximal function, for constitutional reasons.*

II. The Evolved Mismatch Criticism of the HD Analysis

In this section, I present one long-standing objection against Wakefield's view, the "evolved mismatch" criticism. I raise it here because it forms a backdrop to my own argument (next section), and it has a very similar logical structure. What if some of our devastating psychiatric ailments, such as major depression, anxiety disorders, psychopathy, and so on, actually *benefited* our Pleistocene ancestors? What if, moreover, the *fact* that they benefited those ancestors partly explains why they are around today? Then, if we accept the selected effects theory of function, we would have to say that those disorders do not arise from "dysfunctions." They would be adaptations. Furthermore, if we accept the HD analysis, we would be forced to conclude that depression (say) is not actually a mental disorder. That strikes me as deeply counterintuitive. It seems to me that depression, particularly when severe enough to lead to hospitalization or suicide attempts, constitutes a paradigmatic mental disorder, regardless of how it happened to evolve. People who have raised this mismatch critique against Wakefield include Lilienfeld and Marino (1995, 416; 1999, 406), Richters and Hinshaw (1999, 442), Woolfolk (1999, 662), Bolton (2001, 194), Murphy and Stich (2000, 81), and Murphy and Woolfolk (2000a, 244).

Let me clarify what I take to be the strongest form of the evolved mismatch argument. I am *not* claiming that any particular mismatch hypothesis is true. Rather, the best argument is a modal one, and I will summarize it in four sentences: it is empirically plausible that some mental disorders represent mismatches, not dysfunctions. Therefore, it is logically possible that the same is true. But the HD analysis implies that this claim is logically impossible. So, the HD analysis is wrong.

Here is another way of putting the point, one that Wakefield sometimes opts for. To the extent that the HD analysis is a conceptual analysis of clinical usage, then Wakefield is committed to the following prediction: *if* researchers and clinicians were to generally accept that a certain condition (say, antisocial personality disorder) is an evolved mismatch, *then* they would stop labeling it a "disorder." Wakefield uses the example of fever to bolster his point. Medical researchers once considered fever to be a "disorder"; when they came to grasp its adaptive significance, they stopped calling it that (Wakefield 2000, 260; also see Wakefield 1999b, 468). I am not entirely convinced by this example, since what we discovered about fever is that it is beneficial for us. It is not a mismatch at all. So, I don't think we can use the fever example to draw inferences about an evolved mismatch case. Moreover, as I indicated above, it would be surprising to me if Wakefield's prediction were correct, because several researchers have endorsed mismatch hypotheses for various disorders, and they seem to believe, judging by their terminology, that the conditions they study are, in fact, "disorders" (or "pathologies," "diseases," etc.) (e.g., McGuire and Troisi 1998; Gluckman and Hanson 2006; Glover 2011). Nonetheless, I applaud Wakefield for being willing to make a risky prediction, and I wish more philosophers would do the same.

I will give a simple example to convey the style of an "evolved mismatch" explanation. One theory of depression is known as the "social competition" hypothesis (Price et al. 1994). In the Pleistocene era, when many of our cognitive mechanisms were being formed, there were numerous male-to-male conflicts over food, shelter, and sexual partners. Occasionally, one of the "disputants" must have been severely outcompeted by the other. Now, zoom in on a particular such conflict. Suppose the "underdog" had some gene mutation that caused him to feel depressed, rather than aggressive. Suppose his depressed mood made him bow out of the fight and to accept a lower status within the social hierarchy. Then, the depressed feelings would have conferred a fitness advantage (over individuals with no mutation), since it would have prevented him from getting killed or wounded in a pointless fight. The proponents of the social competition hypothesis believe that it explains various cognitive, behavioral, and neurochemical features of depression and that it has important implications for therapy.

Mismatch explanations are a subtype of adaptationist explanation. As such, they can, in the best-case scenario, be rejected or revised as fresh evidence surfaces. For example, Murphy (2005, 756) notes that the social competition hypothesis fails to explain a range of somatic symptoms associated with depression, but he acknowledges that other mismatch hypotheses may be superior. For example, some mismatch theorists have argued that depression does not result from competition, but it has a kind of signaling function to elicit help from parents or partners (Watson and Andrews 2002). Others have tried to synthesize the competition and signaling theories (see the "social risk" hypothesis of Allen and Badcock 2003; for a recent overview, also see Rottenberg 2014). (Of course, if there are different types of depression, then one would not expect a single mismatch theory to cover them all.) Others have criticized mismatch hypotheses for phobias (Murphy 2005; Faucher and Blanchette 2011). My point is that, even if one or another specific mismatch hypothesis fails, that does not undermine the credibility or coherence of mismatch hypotheses generally. By the same token, the failure of one or another adaptationist hypothesis does not undermine adaptationism as a research program. If anything, I think the general research program is gaining new momentum, particularly in light of the DOHaD.

Note that it is one thing to be critical of the way that clinicians overdiagnose depression, and it is another thing to deny that depression is a disorder. Horwitz and Wakefield (2007) eloquently argued that clinicians overdiagnose depression. But in saying this, they acknowledge that there is a genuine mental disorder (which they sometimes call "depressive disorder") and that, sometimes, psychiatrists correctly identify it. The claim I am making is this: what if, say, what they call "depressive disorder" turns out to be an evolved mismatch? Then, Wakefield would have to acknowledge that it is not a mental disorder, which is contrary to the view that he and Horwitz staked out in that book.

In the next section, I will explore a variant on the evolved mismatch argument, one that has been neglected in the literature surrounding the HD analysis. I call it the developmental plasticity challenge, and I think it raises additional problems for Wakefield's view.

III.   Developmental Mismatches and Dysfunctional Mechanisms

Suppose there were some condition (one that psychiatrists study) that proved to be a developmental mismatch, rather than an evolved mismatch. That is, suppose it were the outcome of developmental plasticity, but the environment changed, like the *Daphnia*'s helmet-shaped head in predator-free waters. Then, according to the HD analysis, it would not stem from a "dysfunction," and therefore, it would not be a mental disorder. I think there are empirically plausible cases of such developmental mismatches, and they constitute a problem for Wakefield's view.

Perhaps the most plausible example of a developmental mismatch is for the anxiety disorders, such as generalized anxiety disorder. When we talk about anxiety disorders, we are not talking about transient states of disturbance that accompany common stressors such as a job loss or a move. Those emotions, I take it, are normal, nondisordered responses to the vicissitudes of life. What I am talking about are more or less chronic, maladaptive conditions that seem disproportionate to any external "triggers." Generalized anxiety disorder is described as a chronic and uncontrollable state of worry that is disproportionate to external stressors and that can easily shift from one concern to another. It can be associated with restlessness, fatigue, and the inability to concentrate. Panic disorder is the condition of having recurring panic attacks. These are typically short-lived but extremely intense episodes of distress and discomfort (American Psychiatric Association 2013). If anything has a right to be called a mental disorder, these do.

Is it plausible to think that anxiety disorders, at least in some individuals, represent developmental mismatches—more or less irreversible adaptations to prenatal or early postnatal experiences? There is some suggestive evidence for the theory. The empirical basis for the theory is that fetuses, infants, and young children who are exposed to highly stressful environments are susceptible to anxiety disorders as adults (e.g., Heim and Nemeroff 2001; McGowan et al. 2009; Glover 2011). Perhaps that should not seem very surprising, but it leads to an intriguing conjecture: what if susceptibility to anxiety disorders is an example of developmental plasticity? That is, what if susceptibility represents a kind of adaptation to a high-stress developmental context? Then, those disorders would not, in fact, represent dysfunctions. They would have the exact same ontological status as the helmet-shaped head of the *Daphnia*. They would be adaptations. If that were the case, then, according to the HD analysis, they would not be disorders. That seems wrong.

One might wonder how having an anxiety disorder, like generalized anxiety disorder, could be beneficial or useful. In what context might those help us survive? The specific adaptationist hypothesis on offer is that anxiety is associated with enhanced vigilance to potential threats in one's environment (Glover 2011). People who are anxious tend to watch out for things that might hurt them. As a consequence, if there are real, genuine threats in one's formative environment, then it could very well pay to be anxious as an adult, in a kind of chronic, intense, way, not in a run-of-the-mill way. (I presume that Wakefield would agree that some level of anxiety is adaptive, but that extreme levels represent a dysfunction of those anxiety-generating mechanisms. But my point is that it is empirically plausible that "extreme" levels of anxiety could represent adaptations, too. That is the possibility I wish to explore here.) Similar sorts of arguments have been offered for other disorders such as attention-deficit/hyperactivity disorder and conduct disorder.

As a matter of logic, there are two ways that Wakefield could defend his theory, on the assumption that some mental disorders represent developmental mismatches. First, he could say that there is no dysfunction in those individuals, but there is no disorder either. Second, he could accept that, of those anxiety disorders that result from developmental plasticity, they are genuine mental disorders, but there *is* an underlying dysfunction. I will briefly summarize why both responses strike me as unsatisfying.

Wakefield (1999b, 468) explores both lines of argument in response to Richters and Hinshaw's (1999) example. Recall that, in their argument, we are asked to imagine a young boy who grows up in an abusive family environment and responds by developing symptoms of conduct disorder. They ask us to suppose that those symptoms are, at least initially, adaptations and that they are useful and valuable to him in that abusive environment. Later, the boy moves to a nurturing, nonabusive environment, but the symptoms of conduct disorder do not abate. They are a "fixed" part of his character, like the *Daphnia*'s helmet-shaped head. They argue that this would be an example of a disorder without a dysfunction. Wakefield entertains two different responses: the first that there is no dysfunction and no disorder either, and the second that there is both a disorder and a dysfunction.

3.1 No Dysfunctions, No Disorders

It seems to me that Wakefield's first line of response, which would deny that anxiety disorders are actually mental disorders, strays perilously close to resolving the issue by definitional fiat or stipulation. At the very least, I would like to be given an independent reason for thinking that, if some anxiety disorders result from plasticity, then they are not real disorders at all. Without any good independent reason, I worry that the HD analysis is something like a stipulative definition, rather than a conceptual analysis or a theoretical definition (e.g., Millikan 1989), and Wakefield clearly does not intend the HD analysis to be a piece of stipulation. Moreover, as I indicated above, the few people who have endorsed the claim that some mental disorders are developmental mismatches seem to describe those conditions as "disorders," "pathologies," and so on (as I indicated in the previous section; e.g., Gluckman and Hanson 2006). So I do not think this first line of response is entirely promising.

One line of evidence that Wakefield might adduce to support this move is to say that clinical intuitions are, in fact, overwhelmingly on his side and that my own linguistic intuitions are idiosyncratic. Interestingly, Wakefield and his colleagues have conducted some experiments that suggest that clinical intuitions tend to be consistent with his HD analysis of mental disorder (Wakefield et al. 2002; Wakefield et al. 2006). Those experiments went as follows. A large number of graduate students in mental health were presented with a series of vignettes. In one version of the story (the "negative environment" vignette), a teenager exhibits various symptoms of conduct disorder, but these symptoms are portrayed as having current usefulness (e.g., in response to current family abuse or gang activity). In another version of the story (the "internal dysfunction" vignette), a teenager exhibits the same symptoms, but nothing in the story would suggest that they are appropriate or useful responses to some current life situation. Graduate students tended to judge that the individual in the first vignette did *not* have a genuine mental disorder, but the individual in the second did. Wakefield interpreted this result to support his HD analysis, because there is clearly no "dysfunction" in the first.

I do not believe that these vignettes are relevant to this discussion, although they are fascinating in their own right. That is because they do not contrast "dysfunction" scenarios with "mismatch" scenarios. Rather, they contrast a scenario in which the condition has obvious current utility with one where it does not. Technically, a "mismatch" scenario would fall under the second type of vignette, where the trait in question does not have current utility. It would be interesting, however, to extend those sorts of experiments to investigate clinical intuitions regarding mismatch cases.

3.2 Both Dysfunctions and Disorders

The second way to respond is to say that, in the case I've described (where anxiety disorders result from developmental plasticity), the affected individuals do have mental disorders, but there *are* underlying dysfunctions. But where is the dysfunction? Wakefield entertains this response to the conduct disorder case. As he writes (1999b, 468), "If the mechanism's function is to shape personality specifically in response to the early broader environment (not the family environment, which evolutionarily is expected to be reasonably benign) to prepare for the later broader environment, then the 'accidental' setting of personality parameters by extreme (evolutionarily unexpectable) family abuse is a dysfunction." The idea is this. In the conduct disorder case, the child has a certain cognitive mechanism, M. The function of M is to sample the threat level in his formative environment and to shape his personality as a result, so as to prepare him for the types of encounters he might face in the future. Unfortunately, because of the abusive family environment, M is unable to adequately prepare him for his future environment. After all, the future environment (let us suppose) is relatively benign, which, of course, he couldn't have guessed from his abusive family life. So, M cannot fully discharge its function, and it is dysfunctional.

If this is the sort of response that Wakefield is committed to, then there is a substantive disagreement between Wakefield and myself regarding how to describe the conduct disorder case. Like the blindfold case or the *Daphnia* case, I would say that this is a situation where M is functioning normally in an unsuitable environment (or, perhaps, M is unable to function because of the unsuitable environment) and it is not dysfunctional. It seems to me that the function of this hypothetical cognitive mechanism is to "sample" the ambient level of threat in the formative environment and to adapt the child's personality as a result. It seems to me that the mechanism in question has discharged its function flawlessly, just like the *Daphnia*'s helmet head or like the gosling's imprinting on a passing porcupine. (Keep in mind, of course, that as a result of the anxiety disorders, various dysfunctions may ensue from time to time. Someone who is prone to panic attacks might form the false belief that heavy exercise will promote fresh panic attacks and refrain from exercise on that account, thereby increasing his or her risk for cardiovascular disease. But that sort of dysfunction would be incidental to the disorder; it would not be constitutive of it. Additionally, note that I am not claiming that, e.g., conduct disorder is actually an adaptation but that the empirical plausibility of that conjecture suffices to undermine Wakefield's analysis.)

As I indicated in section I, this disagreement has its root, I think, in the problem of function indeterminacy, which I described earlier. There are always two different ways to describe the function of some cognitive mechanism. First, we can describe it in "proximal" terms. Here, in the case of conduct disorders, the mechanism has the function of (say) sampling the threat level in the early environment and calibrating the lifetime level of aggressiveness accordingly. Second, we can describe it in "distal" terms. Here, the mechanism has the function of protecting the child from future threats. How should we classify the developmental mismatches? If we describe the mechanism in terms of its proximal function, it seems to me that there is no dysfunction. If we describe the mechanism in terms of its distal function, there can be. I believe that Wakefield describes the conduct disorder case in terms of "dysfunction" because he has latched onto the more "distal" description of the function, and I think this is inconsistent with his explicit remarks on indeterminacy, where he states that we should prefer the most "proximal" description of an item's function (again, see Wakefield's [1999a, 386] bacterium example). As a consequence, I do not believe that this particular line of response is available to him.

In the foregoing, I have raised a fairly novel critique of Wakefield's HD analysis, the developmental mismatch challenge. I have pointed out that my argument is, in essence, a modal one. It is empirically plausible, and hence logically possible, that *some mental disorders result from developmental mismatches,* but the HD implies that this is logically impossible, so the HD analysis is incorrect. The HD analysis also makes a prediction about clinical usage and I have given reasons for my skepticism about that prediction. I have explored two sorts of responses that Wakefield might give and discussed why I think they are unsatisfying.

Acknowledgments

I'm grateful to Robyn Bluhm, David Frank, Ginger Hoffman, Brent Kious, and Jonathan Tsou for comments and feedback on an earlier draft. I'm also grateful to the audience members of the 2015 meeting of the Association for the Advancement of Philosophy and Psychiatry in Toronto, where some of this material was presented.

References

Agrawal, A. A., C. Laforsch, and R. Tollrian. 1999. Transgenerational induction of defences in animals and plants. *Nature* 401: 60–63.

Allen, N. B., and P. B. T. Badcock. 2003. The social risk hypothesis of depressed mood: Evolutionary, psychosocial, and neurobiological perspectives. *Psychological Bulletin* 129(6): 887–913.

American Psychiatric Association. 1980. *Diagnostic and Statistical Manual of Mental Disorders.* 3rd ed. American Psychiatric Association.

American Psychiatric Association. 2013. *Diagnostic and Statistical Manual of Mental Disorders.* 5th ed. American Psychiatric Association.

Bolton, D. 2001. Problems in the definition of 'mental disorder.' *The Philosophical Quarterly* 51(203): 182–199.

Buller, D. 1997. Individualism and evolutionary psychology (or, in defense of "narrow" functions). *Philosophy of Science* 64(1): 74–95.

Dretske, F. 1986. Misrepresentation. In *Belief: Form, Content, and Function,* R. Bogdan (ed.), 17–36. Clarendon.

Faucher, L., and I. Blanchette. 2011. Fearing new dangers: Phobias and the cognitive complexity of human emotions. In *Maladapting Minds: Philosophy, Psychiatry, and Evolutionary Theory,* P. R. Adriaens and A. De Block (eds.), 33–64. Oxford University Press.

Garson, J. 2015. *The Biological Mind: A Philosophical Introduction.* Routledge.

Garson, J. 2016. *A Critical Overview of Biological Functions.* Springer.

Garson, J., and G. Piccinini. 2014. Functions must be performed at appropriate rates in appropriate situations. *British Journal for the Philosophy of Science* 65(1):1–20.

Glover, V. 2011. Prenatal stress and the origins of psychopathology: An evolutionary perspective. *Journal of Child Psychology and Psychiatry* 52(4): 356–367.

Gluckman, P., A. Beedle, and M. Hanson. 2009. *Principles of Evolutionary Medicine.* Cambridge University Press.

Gluckman, P., and M. Hanson (eds.). 2006. *Developmental Origins of Health and Disease.* Oxford University Press.

Heim, C., and C. B. Nemeroff. 2001. The role of childhood trauma in the neurobiology of mood and anxiety disorders: Preclinical and clinical studies. *Biological Psychiatry* 49(12): 1023–1039.

Horwitz, A. V., and J. C. Wakefield. 2007. *The Loss of Sadness: How Psychiatry Transformed Normal Sorrow into Depressive Disorder.* Oxford University Press.

Klein, D. F. 1978. A proposed definition of mental illness. In *Critical Issues in Psychiatric Diagnosis,* R. L. Spitzer and D. F. Klein (eds.), 41–71. Raven Press.

Lilienfeld, S. O., and L. Marino. 1995. Mental disorder as a Roschian concept: A critique of Wake-field's "harmful dysfunction" analysis. *Journal of Abnormal Psychology* 104: 411–420.

Lilienfeld, S. O., and L. Marino. 1999. Essentialism revisited: Evolutionary theory and the concept of mental disorder. *Journal of Abnormal Psychology* 108(3): 400–411.

McGowan, P. O., A. Sasaki, A. C. D'Alessio, S. Dymov, B. Labonte, M. Szyf, G. Turecki, and M. J. Meaney. 2009. Epigenetic regulation of the glucocorticoid receptor in human brain associates with childhood abuse. *Nature Neuroscience* 12(3): 342–348.

McGuire, M., and A. Troisi. 1998. *Darwinian Psychiatry*. Oxford University Press.

Millikan, R. G. 1984. *Language, Thought, and Other Biological Categories*. MIT Press.

Millikan, R. G. 1989. In defense of proper functions. *Philosophy of Science* 56(2): 288–302.

Murphy, D. 2005. Can evolution explain insanity? *Biology and Philosophy* 20(4): 745–766.

Murphy, D., and S. Stich. 2000. Darwin in the madhouse: Evolutionary psychology and the clas-sification of mental disorders. In *Evolution and the Human Mind: Modularity, Language, and Meta-Cognition,* P. Carruthers and A. Chamberlain (eds.), 62–92. Cambridge University Press.

Murphy, D., and R. L. Woolfolk. 2000a. The harmful dysfunction analysis of mental disorder. *Philosophy, Psychiatry, and Psychology* 7: 21–252.

Murphy, D., and R. L. Woolfolk. 2000b. Conceptual analysis versus scientific understanding: An assessment of Wakefield's folk psychiatry. *Philosophy, Psychiatry, and Psychology* 7(4): 271–293.

Neander, K. 1991. Functions as selected effects: The conceptual analyst's defense. *Philosophy of Science* 58(2): 168–184.

Neander, K. 1995. Misrepresenting and malfunctioning. *Philosophical Studies* 79(2): 109–141.

Pigliucci, M. 2001. *Phenotypic Plasticity: Beyond Nature and Nurture*. Johns Hopkins University Press.

Price, J., L. Sloman, R. Jr. Gardner, P. Gilbert, and P. Rohde. 1994. The social competition hypoth-esis of depression. *British Journal of Psychiatry* 164(3): 309–315.

Richters, J., and S. Hinshaw. 1999. The abduction of disorder in psychiatry. *Journal of Abnormal Psychiatry* 108(3): 438–445.

Rottenberg, J. 2014. *The Depths: The Evolutionary Origins of the Depression Epidemic*. Basic Books.

Schwartz, P. H. 2007. Defining dysfunction: Natural selection, design, and drawing a line. *Philoso-phy of Science* 74(3): 364–385.

Spitzer, R. L., M. Sheehy, and J. Endicott. 1977. *DSM-III*: Guiding principles. In *Psychiatric Diagno-sis,* V. M. Rakoff, H. C. Stancer, and H. B. Kedward (eds.), 1–24. Brunner/Mazel.

Tollrian, R., and S. I. Dodson. 1999. Inducible defenses in Cladocera: Constraints, costs, and mul-tiple environments. In *The Ecology and Evolution of Inducible Defenses,* R. Tollrian and C. D. Harvell (eds.), 177–202. Princeton University Press.

Wakefield, J. C. 1992. The concept of mental disorder: On the boundary between biological facts and social values. *American Psychologist* 47(3): 373–388.

Wakefield, J. C. 1999a. Evolutionary versus prototype analyses of the concept of disorder. *Journal of Abnormal Psychology* 108: 374–399.

Wakefield, J. C. 1999b. Mental disorder as a black box essentialist concept. *Journal of Abnormal Psychology* 108: 465–472.

Wakefield, J. C. 2000. Spandrels, vestigial organs, and such: Reply to Murphy and Woolfolk's 'The harmful dysfunction analysis of mental disorder.' *Philosophy, Psychiatry, and Psychology* 7: 253–269.

Wakefield, J. C. 2011. Darwin, functional explanation, and the philosophy of psychiatry. In *Maladapting Minds: Philosophy, Psychiatry, and Evolutionary Theory*, P. R. Adriaens and A. De Block (eds.), 143–172. Oxford University Press.

Wakefield, J. C., S. A. Kirk, K. J. Pottick, D. K. Hsieh, and X. Tian. 2006. The lay concept of conduct disorder: Do nonprofessionals use syndromal symptoms or internal dysfunction to distinguish disorder from delinquency? *Canadian Journal of Psychiatry* 51: 33–39.

Wakefield, J. C., K. J. Pottick, and S. A. Kirk. 2002. Should the *DSM-IV* diagnostic criteria for conduct disorder consider social context? *American Journal of Psychiatry* 159(3): 380–386.

Watson, P. J., and P. W. Andrews. 2002. Toward a revised evolutionary adaptation analysis of depression: The social navigation hypothesis. *Journal of Affective Disorders* 72(1): 1–14.

Woolfolk, R. L. 1999. Malfunction and mental disorder. *The Monist* 82(4): 658–670.

Wright, L. 1973. Functions. *Philosophical Review* 82: 139–168.

17 Does Developmental Plasticity Pose a Challenge to the Harmful Dysfunction Analysis? Reply to Justin Garson

Jerome Wakefield

I have learned much from Justin Garson's insightful writings on the concepts of biological function and dysfunction (e.g., Garson 2016; Garson and Piccinini 2014), and I am grateful to him for his contribution to this volume that pushes his thinking about these concepts in some fresh directions. His paper usefully opens up the area of evolutionary developmental biology (known as "evo-devo") as an additional empirical domain in which to explore the validity of my harmful dysfunction analysis (HDA) of medical, including mental, disorder. The HDA claims that "disorder" refers to "harmful dysfunction," where dysfunction is the failure of some feature to perform a natural function for which it is biologically designed by evolutionary processes and harm is judged in accordance with social values (First and Wakefield 2010, 2013; Spitzer 1997, 1999; Wakefield 1992a, 1992b, 1993, 1995, 1997a, 1997b, 1997c, 1997d, 1998, 1999a, 1999b, 2000a, 2000b, 2001, 2006, 2007, 2009, 2011, 2014, 2016a, 2016b; Wakefield and First 2003, 2012). There has been only minimal attention to this area in the discussion of the HDA; one earlier interchange on this topic between Richters and Hinshaw (1999) and me (Wakefield 1999b) is reconsidered below, and the field has grown dramatically since then. A detailed analysis of evo-devo's implications for the HDA is long overdue, and I welcome Garson's invitation to return to this topic.

Many prominent critics of the HDA's approach to medical disorder agree with the idea that a disorder involves a dysfunction but disagree with the HDA's evolutionary interpretation of biological function and dysfunction (e.g., see the papers by Murphy and Lemoine in this volume and my replies). In contrast, Garson agrees with me that the concepts of biological function and dysfunction are best understood in evolutionary terms and instead targets the claim that medical disorder presupposes biological dysfunction.

Like some other prominent critics of the HDA (e.g., see my reply to Cooper in this volume), Garson holds that disorders can be naturally selected. He thinks this is possible because when naturally selected features that were adaptive in earlier species environments are maladaptively mismatched to today's altered environment, the mismatch between our biologically designed nature and the environment is or can be a disorder, contradicting the HDA's dysfunction requirement. No doubt many of our problems are due to such mismatches. However, as I shall show, this is not how our concept of disorder works and for good reason if the concept is to form the foundation of a viable medical discipline of psychiatry that resists antipsychiatric critiques.

Garson's "mismatch" argument is multilayered. He presents the evolved mismatch objection in three somewhat different forms. I will disentangle and somewhat reassemble the various arguments and build up to his main argument in steps parallel to his three arguments.

First Version: The Evolutionary Mismatch Objection

Garson initially argues for a standard form of the mismatch objection to the HDA that he christens the "evolved mismatch critique." In general, the recent evo-devo literature characterizes evolutionary mismatches as arising "upon exposure to an entirely novel environment, or to an environment that is beyond the evolved physiology and adaptive capacity of the individual" (Low and Gluckman 2016, 69). Moreover, such exposure occurs regularly because, as an authoritative book in the field explains, one of the "fundamental principles of evolutionary medicine" is that "humans now live in very different ways and in different environments from those where the majority of selective processes affecting the modern human phenotype operated. In this respect we are biologically 'mismatched' to many aspects of our current environment" (Gluckman et al. 2016, 162). These authors describe the general idea of evolutionary mismatches as follows:

> Environmental factors acting during the phase of developmental plasticity interact with genotypic variation to change the capacity of the organism to cope with its environment in later life. Because the postnatal environment can change dramatically, whereas the intrauterine environment is relatively constant over generations, it may well be that much of humankind is now living in an environment beyond that for which we evolved. (Gluckman and Hanson 2006b, 4)

> Evolutionary change is slow and our social and physical environments have changed very fast through the broader processes of cultural evolution.... The biological processes that determined our present structure and function largely evolved in very different environments from those we now inhabit. Thus, the most common way in which evolutionary pathways are associated with ill-health is through the consequential mismatch that can arise... when an individual lives in an environment which is evolutionarily novel or where the individual's evolved capacity to adapt is exceeded. One example... is obesity and its associated morbidities. Another example is the mismatch between the evolved reproductive decline in women, starting in the fourth decade of life, and the pattern of reproduction shaped by cultural evolution and widely practiced in modern societies, with later pregnancies and resulting demand for fertility services. Scurvy represents a historical example of mismatch.... During human evolution there

was continual access to fruit, and thus the mutation which led to our inability to synthesize vitamin C was "neutral" until exposed by an evolutionary novelty produced by cultural evolution (i.e., boats capable of long sea voyages during which a dietary source of vitamin C was absent). ... Given that humans and our hominin ancestors survived as hunters and foragers for 99% of our existence, it can be argued that selection has driven our biology and metabolism to be better matched to the physical activity and diet that characterized the foraging way of life. From this perspective, the current global epidemic of metabolic disease can be understood, in part, as a result of a mismatch between our 'ancient' foraging-adapted genome and our rapidly changing modern diet and lifestyle. (Gluckman et al. 2016, 167, 210)

The objection to the HDA based on evolutionary mismatches is simply that problematic mismatches between an individual's naturally selected nature and environmental context are disorders, and thus dysfunction is not necessary for disorder. Garson notes that this is a "long-standing objection" that "Wakefield's opponents have repeatedly raised" and insists that "the evolved mismatch critique, when properly understood, undermines Wakefield's analysis." So, despite having addressed this objection before (Horwitz and Wakefield 2012; Wakefield 1999a, 2010), I consider the reasons for rejecting Garson's version of the mismatch thesis, which he poses as follows:

What if some of our devastating psychiatric ailments, such as major depression, anxiety disorders, psychopathy, and so on, actually *benefited* our Pleistocene ancestors? What if, moreover, the *fact* that they benefited those ancestors partly explains why they are around today? Then, if we accept the selected effects theory of function, we would have to say that those disorders do not arise from "dysfunctions." They would be adaptations. Furthermore, if we accept the HD analysis, we would be forced to conclude that depression (say) is not actually a mental disorder. That strikes me as deeply counterintuitive. It seems to me that depression, particularly when severe enough to lead to hospitalization or suicide attempts, constitutes a paradigmatic mental disorder, regardless of how it happened to evolve.

Evolutionary mismatches are of course real and important to understand. However, Garson applies this perspective not as a scientific causal hypothesis to explain some problem but as a conceptual thesis about the meaning of "disorder." The best evidence against such a conceptual evolutionary mismatch thesis is our actual disorder judgments. Known mismatches between our evolved natures and current environmental conditions, no matter how problematic, are not intuitively considered disorders. For example, the evolved desire for sex with people other than one's partner is mismatched with our monogamous social mores, the evolved desire for high-fat and sweet foods is harmfully mismatched with the overabundance of such foods in our environment, and our evolved aggressive and fight-or-flight impulses when stressfully interacting with others are mismatched with our dense, high-interaction, and often frustrating social environments, but none of these mismatches are in themselves considered disorders, although they are certainly *risk factors* for developing disorders. The early age of puberty is mismatched to the age of social maturity in our complex society, and the evolved age of optimal female fertility is mismatched to social pressures for later childbearing to meet demands for lengthy education and establishment of a career prior to childbearing, yet these evolved mismatches are not considered disorders. Sleep researchers believe that there is normal variation both between individuals and within an individual's life span in the nature of a person's synchronization of sleep with their circadian rhythm, such that some people are naturally (to put it colloquially) "morning people" and some are naturally "night people," and it is generally accepted that night people are painfully disadvantaged and mismatched to our 9-to-5 work culture and especially our school system that generally starts even earlier (adolescents are disproportionately night people), but this mismatch, which has no discernible benefit, is generally considered a normal variation and not a disorder. The natural tendency to be sedentary and an aversiveness to exercise when there is no immediate demand for activity is thought to have evolved to conserve energy but is maladaptive in our current environment in which there are few demands for vigorous physical activity, yielding excessive sedentariness, yet is not considered a disorder. To take an extreme case, even mass killers, whose wanton levels of aggression may have been adaptive in some earlier environment but are surely radically mismatched with our current social environment, are generally judged nondisordered (Knoll and Pies 2019).

Moreover, the intuitions expressed in public and professional controversies indicate that when someone believes a mismatch hypothesis, they tend to doubt the corresponding disorder attribution. In fact, a mismatch account is generally taken as strong evidence that there is not a disorder. For example, those who acknowledge that the symptoms associated with attention-deficit/hyperactivity disorder (ADHD) are seriously problematic in today's school environment but think that such childhood rambunctiousness and exploratory urges are part of the normal range of naturally selected childhood inclinations—and thus are not generally a dysfunction of impulse control and attentional mechanisms—do *not* tend to see such problematic behavior within our mismatched school environment as a disorder. Rather, they argue just the opposite, that if the problem is a mismatch between evolved childhood behavior and our educational practices, then we are oppressively diagnosing and medicating nondisordered children and should change the school system. This points to one reason why the difference between disorder and mismatch is fundamentally conceptually important—namely, they suggest different priorities or options for intervention.

The most troubling problem with the mismatch account of disorder is that it undermines one of the basic goals of an analysis of mental disorder, namely, to respond to the antipsychiatric critique by distinguishing socially deviant, disapproved, or undesirable conditions from legitimate psychiatric disorders. This goal is undermined because most mismatches between the evolved nature of individuals and the current environment that come to attention of mental health professionals are precisely the kinds of mismatches with current social demands and values that the antipsychiatrists accused psychiatry of pathologizing. Consequently, embracing mismatches as disorders elevates social demand into a potential arbiter of disorder. Many of the absurd diagnoses that we deride as oppressive historical misattributions of disorder would potentially become disorders under the mismatch hypothesis. Soviet dissidents diagnosed with "sluggish schizophrenia," runaway slaves diagnosed with "drapetomania," and masturbating or nocturnally emitting Victorian youths diagnosed with "spermatorrhea" were all engaging in evolutionarily normal behavior mismatched to their social environments and thus legitimately diagnosable as disordered according to the mismatch approach. The fact that confusing mismatches such as social deviance with disorder undermines the medical legitimacy of psychiatry is reflected in the *Diagnostic and Statistical Manual of Mental Disorders*'s (*DSM*'s) explicit statement in the definition of mental disorder that social deviance—a salient form of mismatch between evolved normal variation and social demands—is insufficient for disorder unless there is also a dysfunction: "Socially deviant behavior (e.g., political, religious, or sexual) and conflicts that are primarily between the individual and society are not mental disorders unless the deviance or conflict results from a dysfunction in the individual" (American Psychiatric Association 2013, 20).

Garson of course focuses specifically on evolutionary mismatches, because those offer potential counterexamples to the HDA. However, momentarily casting a wider net, it is worth noting that a general mismatch criterion for disorder makes no sense because mismatches between people's natures or their early learning and their current environments are unfortunately omnipresent in life—and in fact are not in themselves considered disorders. Immigrants who do not speak the local language, kids who are the first from their families to go to college and don't know the implicit social rules for that environment, people who need a job but don't have the required skills or personal attributes to successfully fill the available openings, people desirous of a relationship but unattractive by social standards, and individuals who have irreconcilable differences with their partners would all be considered disordered if mismatches alone warranted disorder attributions. Casting a wider net only casts further doubt on the mismatch account.

In sum, the thesis that evolved mismatches fall under the concept of disorder is incorrect conceptually as reflected in both lay and professional community judgments. It is also self-defeating in terms of the goal of understanding psychiatry as a legitimate medical discipline.

Second Version: The Modal Mismatch Argument

Garson's second version of the mismatch objection may initially look like just a more technically stated version of the first version, and it does build on some of the same points made in the first version's passage above, but it is quite different. After presenting the basic evolved mismatch argument above, he says,

Let me clarify what I take to be the strongest form of the evolved mismatch argument. I am *not* claiming that any particular mismatch hypothesis is true. Rather, the best argument is a modal one, and I will summarize it in four sentences: it is empirically plausible that some mental disorders represent mismatches, not dysfunctions. Therefore, it is logically possible that the same is true. But the HD analysis implies that this claim is logically impossible. So, the HD analysis is wrong.

This is a common objection to the HDA—namely, why couldn't we just empirically discover that some disorders are naturally selected nondysfunctions that are very harmful in our current environment, disproving the HDA's dysfunction requirement? There are two novel things to notice about this modal argument. First, as Garson indicates, relocating the objection to the modal realm allows him to remain entirely neutral on all factual matters, thus to avoid commitments regarding the existence of any specific actual mismatches, such as those presented above. Second, the modal argument can be understood as claiming not that problematic mismatches in general are classifiable as disorders (which is how I interpreted the first version, above) but rather that it is possible that *some* mental disorders are mismatches. Consequently, identifying mismatches that are not disorders, as I did above to obtain counterexamples to the general claim that mismatches are disorders, will not defeat Garson's modal argument. The question is not whether mismatches are generally disorders but whether, in association with certain other properties such as severity, some mismatches can be disorders.

When Garson says that "it is empirically plausible that some mental disorders represent mismatches, not dysfunctions," that appears to directly beg the question at issue. To be non-question-begging, it must mean that it is empirically plausible that *some conditions currently classified as mental disorders* represent mismatches rather than dysfunctions. If the baseline is *DSM-5* categories and diagnostic criteria, this is very likely true. Given our inability to directly identify most mental dysfunctions, some *DSM-5* symptom-based diagnostic criteria sets almost certainly pick out mixtures of dysfunctions and mismatches that have similar presentations. However, according to the HDA, the mismatches are false-positive diagnoses and not genuine psychiatric disorders, even if currently misclassified as disorders. So, the question in deciding between the HDA and mismatch accounts is whether conditions currently categorized as disorders that are identified as mismatches would continue to be considered disorders.

This line of thought reveals that there is a crucial suppressed premise in Garson's modal argument: *For at least some conditions that are currently considered mental disorders, if it were established that the condition is due to an evolutionary mismatch and not to a dysfunction, then the condition would continue to be considered a mental disorder.*

There are two ways that Garson's crucial suppressed premise can be secured, and Garson implicitly addresses both. One way is by arguing that some disorders are so obviously and manifestly disorders that they would not change in disorder status no matter what we found out about their etiology. The other way is by an empirical evaluation of what actually happens when we discover that purported disorders are mismatches. I consider the viability of each of these in turn.

The Theoretical Argument: Are There Bona Fide Mental Disorders That Would Continue to Be Classified as Mental Disorders No Matter What We Found Out about Their Etiology?

The theoretical approach to supporting Garson's suppressed premise is to claim that, of the conditions now considered disorders that could possibly turn out to be mismatches, some are so obviously disorders on grounds of their symptomatic phenomenology that they would continue to be considered disorders no matter what theory about their etiology we might come to hold. This move is implicit in Garson's specification that he is discussing only the most "severe" and "devastating psychiatric ailments" and when in the course of his argument he calls the conditions he is considering "bona fide disorders" and "paradigmatic disorders," thus suggesting their irreversible disorder status, and explicitly when, in discussing the example of depression, he asserts that "depression, particularly when severe enough to lead to hospitalization or suicide attempts, constitutes a paradigmatic mental disorder, regardless of how it happened to evolve." If so, and if some disorders might turn out to be mismatches and not dysfunctions (as I am agreeing they might), then his suppressed premise, his modal argument, and his anti-HDA conclusion are secured.

The problem with this claim is that it is plainly false. There are simply no conditions—not severe depression, not schizophrenia, not psychopathy—that are so indefeasibly considered disorders that no new information about their etiology could persuade us differently. Disorder judgments are inherently fallible etiological explanatory-sketch hypotheses postulating dysfunction. "Bona fide" or "paradigmatic" disorders can be understood as conditions for which it is most difficult to imagine the possibility of an etiological pathway that does not involve dysfunction. But when people do imagine such possibilities, they also imagine that the condition is not a disorder.

Garson's claim that there are "bona fide" or "paradigmatic" disorders" that are so clearly disorders that no discoveries about their evolutionary etiology could lead informed observers to question that they are disorders represents a lack of historical and cultural perspective. Even those conditions considered the most severe mental disorders, such as schizophrenia and severe depression, have been claimed by serious and thoughtful theorists to be nondisorders on the basis of views that denied the presence of internal dysfunction. (I leave aside here the mistaken claims of Thomas Szasz [1974] that mental disorders do not exist because dysfunctions must consist of physical lesions and no such lesions have been identified.) For example, both R. D. Laing (1968) and a school of thought in family dynamics (Bateson et al. 1956) famously claimed that schizophrenia is a normal response to an abnormal family environment or to "double-binding" family communication patterns, respectively, rather than a medical disorder. Many theoreticians have claimed that some or all depression is a biologically designed response and thus not a disorder (e.g., Andrews and Thompson 2009: "the impairments associated with depression are usually the outcome of adaptive tradeoffs rather than disorder" [623]; Nesse 2014: "Is depression an adaptation…or a pathological state?" [14]) (see also the discussion regarding depression in Garson's paper). Behavioral theorists, on the basis of their learning-based theories of psychological functioning, have often denied the existence of any genuine mental disorders in the medical sense on the grounds that the etiology of all behavioral conditions is normal learning, albeit sometimes occurring in abnormal environments or in ways that violate social rules and so yield problematic behaviors (e.g., Ullman and Krasner 1969).

Nor is it the case, as Garson's passage suggests, that the "severe" or "devastating" nature of a condition makes it a bona fide disorder. There are many devastatingly severe conditions that are not considered disorders simply because they are understood to be part of human biological design. Sleep is presumably the most overall disabling condition of the human species, taking away one-third of our lives in a state of incapacity, periodic hallucination, and partial paralysis; grief is one of the most devastating emotional pains one can suffer; fatigue with extended exertion costs us the ability to function effectively under continuing physical demand; childbirth pain is often claimed to be the worst pain women feel in their lives, and advanced pregnancy is extremely impairing of basic physical capacities; and infancy and young childhood entail almost total dependence on others. Yet, none of these "devastating" conditions are considered disorders because they are judged to be part of human biological design.

Garson cites suicidality as a compelling indicator of disorder, but that is because we implicitly take it as a compelling indicator of failure of normal biologically designed human functioning. When that link is cast into doubt, the inference to disorder is also cast into doubt. Suicide over disappointed love was surprisingly common in some periods of history, and suicide over issues of honor, pride, shame, or guilt continues to occur in many cultures, yet these are not necessarily considered mental disorders because we understand how normal human emotions within a certain kind of cultural background could generate such behavior without there being a failure of biological design anywhere in the causal chain. Suicidality can be a rational choice to escape from physical or emotional pain, an avoidance of the implications of a horrific medical diagnosis, a call for help, an altruistic act in defense of loved ones or one's country, or an inclusive fitness-motivated act analogous to an organismic-level form of cellular apoptosis. So, yes, it is *conceptually conceivable* that even severe suicidal immobilizing depression could be a nondisordered state, just like extreme immobilizing grief and just like the periodically immobilizing phenomenon of sleep—which leaves the individual unable to pursue survival and reproduction activities and vulnerable to predation—are nondisorders. Severe depression as a nondisorder of course strikes Garson—and most of the rest of us—as deeply counterintuitive because, unlike grief and sleep, our background knowledge is such that the idea that it is not a dysfunction appears absurd on its face, as it has to physicians since antiquity—but that is not to say it is evidentially indefeasible.

The Empirical Argument: When Bona Fide Mental Disorders Are Discovered to Be Mismatches and Not Dysfunctions, Are They Still Considered Mental Disorders?

The second way to try to support Garson's suppressed premise—that if conditions considered disorders were discovered to be mismatches, they would still be considered disorders—is by examining what actually happens in the rare instances that such switches of etiological theory occur. My claim—and the prediction that follows from the HDA—is that when a condition believed to be a disorder is found to be due to a mismatch, then—modulo inertia and pragmatic considerations—there will be a tendency to reclassify the condition as a nondisorder.

Garson acknowledges the admirable riskiness of this prediction: "I applaud that Wakefield is willing to make a risky prediction and I wish more philosophers would do the same." Nevertheless, he of course thinks my risky claim is false and tries to reveal its absurdity by formulating my prediction using one of the "severe" conditions that he mentioned earlier as an example: "Wakefield is committed to the following prediction: *if* researchers and clinicians were to generally accept that a certain condition (say, antisocial personality disorder) is an evolved mismatch, *then* they would stop labeling it a 'disorder.'"

Now, the standard example I have used in support of my claim is the recent history of thinking about fever, which illustrates that even a "paradigmatic" disorder is reclassified as a nondisorder if it is discovered to be naturally selected features. At one time, fever was thought to be a paradigmatic physical disorder that was caused by toxic products of infection. Indeed, infections of various inferred etiologies and origins were often simply distinguished as etiologies of fever as the prime pathology, as in "typhoid fever," "yellow fever," "scarlet fever," "Congo fever," "dengue fever," "Lassa fever," "San Joaquin Valley fever," "West Nile fever," "Rocky Mountain spotted fever," "Parrot fever," "cat-scratch fever," and literally scores of others. However, once it was discovered that the "bona fide" and paradigmatic" disorder of fever is in fact a sophisticated biologically designed defensive response to infection—the body's raised temperature during a fever is actually regulated to be at the higher level using complex feedback mechanisms just like normal temperature and will tend to return to the fever level if artificially lowered—fever was reclassified as a nondisordered reaction and the guidelines for management rethought.

However, Garson rejects the fever example as a proper test of my claim on the grounds that it is not a pure mismatch example because of fever's potential beneficial effects in fighting infection: "I am not entirely convinced by this example, since what we discovered about fever is that it is beneficial for us. It is not a mismatch at all. So, I don't think we can use the fever example to draw inferences about an evolved mismatch case." In fact, the degree of fever's actual benefit under most circumstances in our current pathogen environment remains unclear, and I would maintain that surely fever's clear status as a complexly biologically designed feature would be sufficient to eliminate it from the disorder category even if it had no current benefits, but Garson does have a point. Similarly, Garson rejects the empirical evidence generated by my studies of clinical judgment of conduct disorder (Wakefield et al. 2002; Wakefield et al. 2006), which showed that conditions that satisfy *DSM* diagnostic criteria for conduct disorder and are usually judged disorders are judged to be nondisorders when the symptoms are due to understandable reactions to circumstances rather than an internal dysfunction. Again, his rationale is that the environmental circumstances described in the clinical vignettes show that given those circumstances, the symptoms benefited the described youths, and thus the behavior was not a pure mismatch without benefit. Note, however, that even if Garson's argument that these are not pure mismatches is accepted, these examples of reversal of disorder judgments do at least show that paradigmatic disorders can be reclassified.

Suppose the fever example is rejected and we accept Garson's ground rule that conditions with significant ongoing benefits don't count as mismatches. Are there then any other examples of newly hypothesized pure mismatches by which we can test my risky claim?

Happily, there is now a more conclusive test of my claim in which my prediction has been confirmed in a natural conceptual experiment. Remarkably, this test involves the very same paradigmatic severe disorder that Garson uses to illustrate the unlikelihood that my prediction will be confirmed, namely, antisocial personality disorder or "psychopathy." In recent research, it has been argued that adolescent-onset conduct disorder—as opposed to early-onset conduct disorder—is due to a mismatch between budding adolescent development and our cultural rules regarding adolescents. Similarly, moderate adult psychopathy has been argued by some researchers to be a naturally selected human variant that was advantageous in the past but is mismatched with the current social environment, and researchers have empirically tested this evolutionary hypothesis. Note that these researchers agree that both conduct disorder and psychopathy are maladaptive in our present environment, so current benefit or current adaptation is not an issue here. In both the conduct disorder and psychopathy cases, researchers concluded that if the mismatch hypothesis is correct, then the condition is not in fact a mental disorder after all. In fact, researchers who study psychopathy basically see the mismatch and disorder accounts as conflicting rival hypotheses. (In my reply to Cooper in this volume, I review this research on conduct disorder and psychopathy.) To demonstrate the sharp distinction that researchers draw between disorder and mismatch hypotheses and the inclination of those who accept the mismatch theory to reverse the field's earlier disorder attribution, I offer the following series of quotes from various authors in the psychopathy literature:

(1) Adolescence-limited antisocial behavior is not pathological behavior.... The origins of adolescence-limited delinquency lie in youngsters' best efforts to cope with the widening gap between biological and social maturity. (Moffitt 1993, 692)

(2) Is sociopathy an adaptation or an abnormality?...Because a behavior, trait, or mechanism may have evolved for its adaptive value does not imply necessarily that it is still adaptive in the current environment....Thus, something may be an adaptation without being adaptive.... Sociopaths... clearly have both social and psychophysiological "deficits" if the standard we use is the nonsociopath.... If sociopaths are not a type designed by natural selection to fill a particular niche, then we could probably agree that they do not function normally; but if they are a type, then...the medical model is no longer appropriate. (Mealey 1995, 583–584)

(3) From an evolutionary perspective psychopathy seems to be an adaptation rather than a disease. (Kinner 2003, 67)

(4) Two models have guided the study of psychopathy. One suggests that psychopathy is a psychopathology, i.e., the outcome of defective or perturbed development. A second suggests that psychopathy is a life-history strategy of social defection and aggression that was reproductively viable in the environment of evolutionary adaptedness (EEA). These two models make different predictions. (Lalumiere et al. 2001, 75)

(5) On any such "selectionist" model, psychopaths are certainly different than the rest of us, biologically speaking. However, they are not, in any biological sense, disordered. (Reimer 2008, 187)

(6) The medical model attributes sociopathy to a "pathogen," in this case an emotional deficit that may be genetically rooted and physiologically expressed.... Framing sociopathy in evolutionary terms accordingly frees us from the explanatory constraints imposed by the medical model. (Machalek 1995, 564)

(7) Psychopaths routinely disregard social norms by engaging in selfish, antisocial, often violent behavior. Commonly characterized as mentally disordered, recent evidence suggests that psychopaths are executing a well-functioning, if unscrupulous strategy that historically increased reproductive success at the expense of others.... Mental disorder and adaptation accounts of psychopathy generate opposing hypotheses. These results stand in contrast to models positing psychopathy as a pathology, and provide support for the hypothesis that psychopathy reflects an evolutionary strategy. (Krupp et al. 2012, 1)

(8) In a recent study, we found a negative association between psychopathy and violence against genetic relatives... and argued that it failed to support the hypothesis that psychopathy is a mental disorder, suggesting instead that it supports the hypothesis that psychopathy is an evolved life history strategy. (Krupp et al. 2013, 1)

These experts take evolved mismatch to be in conflict with a pathology attribution, and their belief that psychopathy is likely a mismatch has caused them to reject the universal prior assessment of psychopathy as a disorder. This literature demonstrates that presumed disorders found to be due to evolutionary mismatches will be reconceptualized as nondisorders, and it decisively falsifies Garson's crucial suppressed premise using an example that Garson himself put forward. The HDA's risky prediction is thus confirmed in this test case. I assume that Garson will be even more admiring of my risky prediction now that it has been confirmed in an instance he set out as a test case.

There are other examples of dynamic reversals of disorder attribution when mismatch hypotheses are accepted. For example, ADHD would seem to be a paradigmatic disorder and its symptoms to have no benefit in our current constraining school environments. So, we might ask: What would happen if children with bona fide disorders of ADHD turned out to have a naturally selected gene for exploration and novelty seeking that is incompatible with contemporary school discipline but was adaptive in the nomadic environment in which humans evolved, thus indicating that in their cases the condition is a mismatch? Or, what if children who are the youngest in their school classes were found to get diagnosed at higher rates with ADHD, implying that the developmentally least mature students, who possess less inhibitory control than older children in the same grade as a matter of normal developmental variation, are being diagnosed with a disorder because this developmental variation is mismatched with school demands relative to older children in the same grade? These are both recently discovered forms of actual mismatch (Eisenberg et al. 2008; Evans et al. 2010; Zoega et al. 2012). As far as we know, there is no benefit in our current environment for these genetic or developmental variants that create problems in school. As the HDA predicts, those who made these discoveries and those who have accepted them as demonstrating mismatch rather than dysfunction tend to reject the notion that the children in question have a genuine mental disorder of ADHD, and some experts have publicly reversed their disorder attribution in such cases. (See my reply to De Vreese in this volume for further discussion of these examples and the response to them.)

In sum, the modal version of the evolved mismatch objection fails because its crucial suppressed premise—that conditions judged to be disorders will still be judged to be disorders if they are found to be due to evolved mismatches—is false.

Third Mismatch Version: The Developmental Mismatch Objection

I have responded above to the standard evolutionary mismatch objection to the HDA, to Garson's modal version of that objection, and to the modal argument's implied claim that once we have identified certain "bona fide" disorders, they will continue to be considered disorders no matter what we come to believe about their etiology. Although I will continue to comment on the evolutionary mismatch claims, I will now focus on Garson's primary innovation, his attempt to strengthen the mismatch objection by claiming that "developmental mismatches"—a concept to be explained shortly that has emerged from recent evo-devo theory in the area known as Developmental

Origins of Health and Disease (DOHaD)—provide intuitive counterexamples to the HDA that are endorsed by researchers. Garson repeatedly cites the publications of the leading DOHaD theorists, Gluckman and Hanson (2006a; Gluckman et al. 2016) and their colleagues, as expressing such anti-HDA intuitions. I focus primarily on their work and briefly consider other authors cited by Garson at the end.

Although Garson applies the modal argument and makes the "bona fide disorder" assumption in his discussion of developmental mismatches, I mostly leave those aspects aside as irrelevant here. The "bona fide disorder" notion has been adequately refuted above; disorder claims always involve etiological explanatory sketches and can be revised if etiological theories are revised. As to the modal argument, no such relocation to the realm of possible judgments is necessary because Garson claims that the DOHaD theorists he cites actually do judge developmental mismatches to be both naturally selected nondysfunctions and disorders. If he is portraying the literature correctly, then we are dealing here not with possibilities but with actual judgments that pose a conceptual challenge to the HDA, whether or not they turn out to be true.

Recall that Garson applauds my willingness to make risky predictions and that in the case of evolutionary mismatches, my risky prediction (that once a disorder was confirmed to be a mismatch, it would no longer be considered a disorder) was confirmed in the psychopathy and ADHD examples. Garson's further claim that leading DOHaD theorists consider developmental mismatches to be disorders demands an even more risky prediction. Rather than trying to explain away these pathbreaking experts' judgments as unreflective, confused, pragmatic, or otherwise spurious, I venture the prediction (perhaps foolishly given what I know of Garson's careful scholarship!) that Garson misinterprets his own sources. The cited DOHaD theorists, I hypothesize, do not in fact understand developmental mismatch as disorder and have views more consistent with the HDA than Garson suggests. I thus now turn to Garson's cited sources and closely examine the evidence for how they think about disorder and mismatch. Due to this unorthodox response, I amply document each of my findings with textual quotes.

What, then, are the basic claims of DOHaD theory, and what are developmental mismatches and how do they differ from the standard evolutionary mismatches considered earlier? The DOHaD literature concerns the fascinating phenomenon of biologically designed choice points in prenatal developmental programming that are oriented toward adapting to a predicted later environment. The idea is that there are naturally selected forms of early developmental plasticity in which the developing organism samples the environment and, based on what it finds, selects a developmental trajectory from among multiple potential trajectories that becomes irreversibly fixed once selected. The selected trajectory represents not just an adaptive reaction to the current environment but a predictive adaptive response (PAR) to that potential anticipated type of environment in the future: "We define PARs as a form of developmental plasticity that evolved as adaptive responses to environmental cues acting early in the life cycle, but where the advantage of the induced phenotype is primarily manifest in a later phase of the life cycle. The cue…induces changes in the developmental trajectory of form and function such that the organism presets its physiology in expectation of that physiology matching its future environment" (Gluckman, Hanson, and Spencer 2005, 527). The cues in the human case consist largely of maternal signals of nutrition and stress via placental inputs detected by the fetus: "The fetus predicts its postnatal environment based on maternal cues transduced via the placenta and sets its physiological homeostatic mechanisms to match that postnatal environment" (Gluckman, Hanson, Spencer, and Bateson 2005, 673). Each of the fetus's potential adult phenotypes represents a naturally selected adaptation to a specific anticipated adult environment (e.g., high vs. low nutrition), and once it is selected during a limited critical-period developmental window, the trajectory is permanently fixed irrespective of the actual nature of the later environment: "One part of the reaction norm may be associated with better survival in one type of environment, while another is better suited to a different environment. … Developmental plasticity can act early in life to change the course of development, leading to irreversible trajectories that manifest as different phenotypes. … There are critical windows for plasticity in different systems. … An environmental influence may have a lifelong impact if the cue acts during the critical developmental window, but will not have analogous effect if acting outside this window" (Gluckman and Hanson 2006c, 33–34).

DOHaD theorists emphasize that PAR mechanisms are naturally selected adaptive responses, not random events or dysfunctions resulting from developmental pathology: "These are not simply the effects of constraint in utero, but rather mechanisms by which the fetus uses an early environmental cue to 'predict its future' and adopts a developmental pathway that might best suit it to its expected postnatal or adult environment. … The evolution of the ability to mount a predictive and adaptive plastic response will probably depend on a number of features, such as the accuracy of the cue and the frequencies of the various environmental states, as well as the consequences of a mismatch and the intrinsic costs of plasticity itself" (Gluckman, Hanson, Spencer, and Bateson 2005, 673); "As the nutritional environment is the most critical for species survival, it is not surprising that the systems most likely to be programmed are those associated with metabolism, growth, reproduction and coping with stress. Provided that across a species the prediction is more often right than wrong, the genetic infrastructure of PARs…will be positively selected during evolution" (Gluckman and Hanson 2006c, 41); "In mammals, an adverse intrauterine environment results in an integrated suite of responses, suggesting the involvement of a few key regulatory genes, that resets the developmental trajectory in expectation of poor postnatal conditions" (Gluckman, Hanson, and Beedle 2007, 1).

To get the flavor of developmental plasticity and PARs, consider some fascinating examples of irreversible developmental trajectories selected early in life. The axolotl "chooses to be either aquatic or amphibious depending on the availability and size of fresh-water ponds during early development." In the tiger snake, "jaw size is matched to prey size, a feature determined not by genetics but by exposure during the neonatal phase to prey of different sizes." And, in the desert locust, "the choice of wing and metabolic phenotype is determined in the larval phase in response to a pheromonic signal from the mother at egg-laying about population density. The wing shape and metabolism will be set for a migratory form if the population density is high and for the solitary non-migratory form if the density is low" (Gluckman and Hanson 2006c, 34, 36).

Garson focuses on another example, a small lake-dwelling crustacean, *Daphnia*: "*Daphnia* provides a remarkable example of developmental plasticity.... If a *Daphnia* is raised in the vicinity of predators, it grows a tough, helmet-shaped head. This 'helmet' is a boon as it makes it difficult for predators to swallow it. The helmet, I take it, is an adaptation designed by natural selection to protect the *Daphnia* in perilous waters... triggered by the presence of kairomones, a kind of hormone released by the predator.... There are some drawbacks to the 'helmet' phenotype. First, helmets are metabolically expensive; they require more calories to maintain. Second, the large head reduces the *Daphnia*'s mobility. That is why natural selection gave the *Daphnia* a certain degree of morphological flexibility. It only grows the helmet if it needs to. Once a phenotype is selected—'helmet' versus 'normal'—reversibility is limited.... Something inside the *Daphnia* encodes a conditional rule: 'if predators, then helmet; if no predators, then no helmet.'"

When the PAR's "prediction" goes awry, this yields a *developmental mismatch* between organism and environment. Whereas the evolutionary mismatches considered earlier occur when our biologically designed nature that was adaptive in our species' earlier environment is confronted with a novel environment, a developmental mismatch occurs when the predicted environment that triggers the organism's PAR is not the actual environment that the organism comes to confront in adulthood. Developmental mismatches can occur for a great variety of reasons. The prediction can be inaccurate either because of maternal deviations from the existing environment (e.g., lower nutrition due to poverty), maternal pathology that alters placental input, or changes in the environment between the fetal and adult stages (e.g., extreme richness of the Western diet): "Predictions may be erroneous if the fetus is exposed to an impaired fetal environment and thus receives maternal/environmental cues that are not representative of the actual environment, leading to inaccurate predictions and adoption of an inappropriate developmental trajectory. In humans and other mammals, the causes of such an impairment may be pathological, for example due to maternal or placental disease, or physiological, involving factors such as poor maternal nutrition (e.g. a hypocaloric or low-protein diet), maternal stress, or maternal constraint.... The discordance between the predicted versus actual environment during later life, known as developmental mismatch, may lead to a physiology that is unsuited to coping with the mature environment. The fetus that predicts an energy-poor environment but grows up in an environment with an abundance of food may lack the capacity to adjust and hence be more vulnerable to disease development....The size of the adverse effects is dependent on the degree of mismatch and other determinants of variation" (Low, Gluckman, and Hanson 2012, 654). Moreover, the PAR mechanism is designed to work for a range of inputs and a range of environments that were common during the evolution of the organism's species and may not be able to adaptively respond to extreme inputs at the fetal stage or extreme later environments that are outside the expectable ranges.

We now finally come to Garson's formulation of a challenge to the HDA based on the possibility that standard mental disorders might be found to be developmental mismatches. First, here is how he describes the problem of developmental mismatch using his *Daphnia* example: "Suppose we hatch some *Daphnia* eggs in a tank swarming with predators, and they grow the helmet-shaped head. Suppose we then remove the predators from the tank. Then the *Daphnia* experience only the disadvantages of the helmet phenotype and none of its perks. Their condition becomes *chronically maladaptive*. It would be acutely troublesome for them if we forced them to compete over limited resources with their 'normal'-shaped counterparts, who need less food and can get to it faster."

Such developmental mismatches, Garson claims, are not dysfunctions and, if disorders, pose a challenge to the HDA:

> Here is an intuition that I have....It seems to me that talk of "dysfunction" is out of place when it comes to developmental mismatches. Let me clarify. Suppose there is a member of *Daphnia* that chose the "wrong" phenotype; that is, suppose it was raised in a tank with predators, it grew the helmet-shaped head, and later, the predators were removed. It exhibits a developmental mismatch and it takes a fitness loss as a result. In my opinion, this does not represent an inner "dysfunction." Put metaphorically, nothing "went wrong" inside that *Daphnia*. Its developmental machinery is operating exactly as it is "supposed to." It is neither defective nor diseased; it's just unlucky. (Of course, the mismatch can *cause* a dysfunction, for example, if the *Daphnia* dies of malnutrition. But that sort of dysfunction is incidental to the mismatch; having a mismatch does not logically imply dysfunction.)
>
> This brings me to the central question of the chapter. What if some of our current psychiatric ailments result from developmental plasticity, *rather than* dysfunction? In other words, what if, in certain individuals with bona fide mental disorders, the disorder represents a developmental mismatch, much like a helmet-shaped *Daphnia* in a predator-free environment....Such mismatches can be chronically maladaptive for the individuals that possess them....I do not know whether this budding research program—sometimes known as Developmental Origins of Health and Disease (DOHaD)—will ultimately be vindicated (see Gluckman and Hanson 2006a for an overview). But I think it represents an exciting new avenue for exploring the roots of major mental disorders. This conjecture—that *some mental disorders are developmental mismatches*—raises a significant problem for Wakefield's "harmful dysfunction" (HD) analysis of mental disorder, which holds that all mental disorders stem from biological dysfunctions.

So, Garson claims that developmental mismatches—either all or some—are not dysfunctions but are still disorders. As we saw earlier regarding the "bona fide disorder" notion, one cannot rely on the current classification of a condition as a disorder to establish how the condition would be considered if new discoveries were made about its etiology. So, to evaluate Garson's claim that developmental mismatches are non-dysfunctions that are disorders, we have to examine how DOHaD theorists actually consider their proposed mismatches.

Note that with respect to the one mismatch that Garson says the most about—namely, the *Daphnia* that develop burdensome helmets but then confront an adult environment without the predators from which the helmets are designed to protect them—it appears that Garson goes against his own claim and dismisses the condition as a nondisorder. Garson says that his intuition is that the maladaptive helmets are not a dysfunction because development proceeded as biologically designed, and I agree. Garson's argument against the HDA depends on such cases nonetheless being disorders, but in the *Daphnia* case, Garson does not say that. Instead, he says, "Put metaphorically, nothing 'went wrong' inside that *Daphnia*. Its developmental machinery is operating exactly as it is 'supposed to.' It is neither defective nor diseased; it's just unlucky." I take it that the phrase "neither defective nor diseased" is equivalent to "neither dysfunctional nor disordered." Garson's intuition here seems to be consistent with the HDA and seems right on its face: the *Daphnia* is normal but maladaptively mismatched to its environment, and that might cause a disorder but it is not a disorder. Garson notes that the *Daphnia* "takes a fitness loss" due to the mismatch, but a fitness loss is not a disorder. The DOHaD literature repeatedly cautions that reduced fitness in an environment is not the same as reduced health. Indeed, Gluckman et al. (2016) list as one of the "Fundamental Principles of Evolutionary Medicine" that "selection operates to enhance fitness, not primarily to enhance health or longevity" (162) and reiterate that "selection operates to enhance inclusive reproductive fitness, not necessarily health" (175). In sum, the same reasoning that Garson applies to the mismatched *Daphnia*—that it is neither dysfunctional nor disordered—should apply to all evolutionary and developmental mismatches.

The primary evidence Garson presents for his claim that developmental mismatches are or can be disorders—indeed, other than his own intuition, which he acknowledges might be idiosyncratic, the *only* evidence he presents—consists of his repeated assertion that leading theorists in the DOHaD field judge such mismatches to be disorders: "Some psychiatric researchers take this possibility [i.e., that some disorders are developmental mismatches] quite seriously. . . . Such mismatches can be chronically maladaptive for the individuals that possess them. . . . I do not know whether this budding research program—sometimes known as Developmental Origins of Health and Disease (DOHaD)—will ultimately be vindicated (see Gluckman and Hanson 2006 for an overview)"; "several researchers have endorsed mismatch hypotheses for various disorders, and they seem to believe, judging by their terminology, that the conditions they study are, in fact, 'disorders' (or 'pathologies,' 'diseases,' etc.) (e.g., McGuire and Troisi 1998; Gluckman and Hanson 2006a; Glover 2011)"; "Moreover, as I indicated above, the few people who have endorsed the claim that some mental disorders are developmental mismatches seem to describe those conditions as 'disorders,' 'pathologies,' and so on (as I indicated in the previous section; e.g., Gluckman and Hanson 2006a)." So, the most direct way to test Garson's claim is to examine whether leading DOHaD theorists do conceptualize developmental mismatches as disorders.

One might interpret Garson's claim in either of two ways. First, there is the stronger general claim that DOHaD theorists conceptualize developmental mismatch as itself conferring disorder status. Alternatively, one might make the weaker claim (along the lines of Garson's "bona fide disorder" argument) that DOHaD theorists would allow that when conditions already considered disorders are discovered to be mismatches, those are cases of developmental mismatches that are disorders. It is not entirely clear which thesis Garson is defending, so I address both.

There are three critical points that I document below in response to these claims. First, throughout their writings, DOHaD theorists consistently distinguish pathology from risk factors for developing pathology and insist that an evolutionary or developmental mismatch between organism and environment is not a pathology or disorder in its own right but a risk factor for developing pathology. Second, the available evidence indicates that these theorists hold that when a condition widely considered to be a disorder is found to be an evolutionary or developmental mismatch, the disorder label is a mistake and the condition should not continue to be medicalized but should be understood as a normal variation that is problematic only due to the mismatched environment in which it occurs. Third, there is a distinction between developmental mismatches due to evolved PAR mechanisms and mismatches due to various dysfunctions of development, and the DOHaD literature recognizes such true dysfunctions and refers to them as "disruptions." It is among disruptions—which are not naturally selected trajectories and thus classifiable as dysfunctions—that disorders may be found, and this approach is consistent with the HDA. Thus, there is nothing in the cited DOHaD theorists' writings that poses a basic challenge to the HDA. I will document these points with quotes from the DOHaD literature.

First, then, it is striking that throughout the DOHaD literature, it is made crystal clear that the result of an evolutionary or PAR-generated developmental mismatch that reduces fitness is not a disorder but a normal-range naturally selected variant that, due to the problematic interactions with the environment that result from the mismatch, can create a greater *risk* of developing a disorder. The development of an actual disorder, it is explained, requires a proximal cause that constitutes a dysfunction. These points are made consistently and repeatedly across publications, as in the following passages (I add emphases to the uses of "risk" and cognates): "The fundamental assumption underlying the DOHaD model is that environmental factors acting in early life have consequences which become manifest as an *altered disease risk* in later life" (Gluckman and Hanson 2006c, 33); "It should be emphasized that mismatch does not cause disease, but rather *increases the risk of disease* in later life" (Low, Gluckman, and Hanson 2012, 654); "In general, we are not arguing that evolutionary processes cause disease, rather that they have important effects on the *relative risk of developing symptoms or disease.* ... With respect to all that we consider in this book, it is important to think in terms of *variations or changes in disease risk* rather than viewing ultimate mechanisms as leading directly to causation of disease" (Gluckman et al. 2016, 161–162, 163); "In modern humans, such a *mismatch leads to a risk of disease.* ... Because the upper limit of the nutritional environment is rising globally, the *risk of disease due to mismatch* increases even for individuals who had normal early development" (Gluckman and Hanson 2004, 1735, fig. 3); "The model suggests that a mismatch between fetal expectation of its postnatal environment and actual postnatal environment contribute to later *adult disease risk*" (Gluckman, Hanson, and Pinal 2005, 130); "Where the prediction is incorrect, however, the organism is left with a postnatal physiology that is mismatched and inappropriate, putting it at increased *risk* from predation or disease" (Gluckman, Hanson, Spencer, and Bateson 2005, 673); "Critical periods in development result in irreversible changes; if the environment in childhood and adult life differs from that predicted during fetal life and infancy, the developmental responses may increase the *risk of adult disease*" (Godfrey 2006, 6); "Early life influences can alter later *disease risk*— the 'developmental origins of health and disease' (DOHaD) paradigm. ... Mismatch between the anticipated and the actual mature environment exposes the organism to *risk of adverse consequences—the greater the mismatch, the greater the risk*" (Gluckman, Hanson, and Beedle 2007, 1); "When there is a mismatch, the individual's ability to respond to environmental challenges may be inadequate and *risk of disease increases.* Thus, the degree of the mismatch determines the individual's *susceptibility to chronic disease*" (Godfrey et al. 2007, 5R, 6R); "Developmental factors play a considerable role in determining individual *disease risk* later in life. This phenomenon is known as the Developmental Origins of Health and Disease (DOHaD). ... In the event of a mismatch between the early and mature environment, such anticipatory responses may become maladaptive and lead to *elevated risk of disease*" (Low et al. 2012, 650); "Generally the practice of medicine focuses on the issues of *proximate* causation—namely the actual physiological and anatomical disruptions that lead to disease, because it is these pathological processes that inform most diagnostic and therapeutic choices. ... But what this book aims to demonstrate is ... ultimate, that is evolutionary, pathways that affect *the risk of developing disease*" (Gluckman et al. 2016, 161); "Evolutionary processes mediate *disease risk* via multiple pathways. ... The key role of evolutionary and developmental histories in influencing *disease risk* provides a framework for understanding the etiology of many noncommunicable diseases" (Low and Gluckman 2016, 69).

These passages make clear—in direct contradiction to Garson's claim—that the DOHaD paradigm is about how early influences alter disease risk, not disease itself, and that developmental mismatch is not itself a disease but rather exposes the organism to the risk of disease where "the greater the mismatch, the greater the risk"—*not* the greater the disorder. The DOHaD literature thus agrees with the HDA that because the PAR-triggered alterations are evolutionarily selected options and are not dysfunctions, they are not disorders even if mismatched. Only dysfunctional conditions that arise from them are considered disorders.

If the strong general thesis that maladaptive evolutionary or developmental mismatches are disorders is rejected by DOHaD theorists, do they at least allow the weaker thesis, which Garson seems at times to be defending, that some mismatches that are not dysfunctions are nonetheless disorders? No doubt some evolutionists talk this way for a variety of reasons (see below). However, the evidence from the writings of leading DOHaD theorists suggests that they understand that developmental mismatch is not disorder when there is only maladaptation to an environment and no dysfunction. That is, when confronted with conditions that are widely considered disorders but that are in fact evolutionary or developmental mismatches, leading DOHaD theorists tend to argue that this is a conceptual confusion and that the condition should not be classified as a disorder. On the other hand, confronted with a disruption of development that can be construed as a dysfunction, they tend to accept that a resulting problematic condition is a disorder. Here are some examples including both developmental and evolutionary mismatches, as well as both nondisorders and disorders.

Both the earlier and later DOHaD anthologies (Gluckman and Hanson 2006a; Gluckman et al. 2016) use the condition of lactose intolerance, an evolutionary mismatch, to lay out the case that mismatches can be mistaken for disorders but should not be so considered—and the logical point would seem to apply to both evolutionary and developmental mismatches. I quote from the authors' later version of this illuminating example at some length:

> Consider a young man who presents with abdominal pain, bloating, and diarrhea. He is a recent immigrant from Southeast Asia with no history of these symptoms. He reports that yesterday he shared lunch with work colleagues during which he consumed a couple of glasses of milk and had a plate of ice cream. This was unusual for him, but his colleagues, who are of European ethnicity, were unaffected. Why is this young man made ill by ingesting a normal foodstuff?
>
> Cows' milk, like the milk of most mammals, is rich in the disaccharide lactose. The sugar transporters in the human gastrointestinal tract cannot move intact lactose across the gut wall, but babies can digest lactose because of the presence of the enzyme lactase, which breaks down lactose into easily absorbable glucose and galactose. In most humans, lactase expression in the intestine disappears after weaning, but human populations with a history of pastoralism—mostly people of northern European or East African origin—have a high prevalence of

mutations in the promoter region of the lactase gene, causing the enzyme to be expressed within the intestinal tract throughout life. This enables them to consume milk throughout their lives.

But this young man of Asian origin does not carry the persistence mutation and therefore does not express lactase in his duodenum... his symptoms arise from a mismatch between his genetic origin—from a population where, historically, consumption of milk after weaning was unknown and lactase persistence is rare—and his current environment where milk is easily available and widely consumed.

...This example is central to the purpose of this book, because Western medical textbooks often define the inability to absorb lactose as a metabolic *disorder*—adult hypolactasia—but from an evolutionary point of view this man's inability to digest lactose is *normal* and is shared with 70% of the world's population. It has only become manifest in an environment distinct from that to which he is adapted.... This concept of an organism *matched* or *mismatched* with its environment is fundamental to both evolutionary biology and evolutionary medicine, where mismatch... may lead to pathology.... The World Health Organization classifies such 'lactose intolerance' as a metabolic disorder, although in fact this trait represents the normal and ancestral human condition. (Gluckman et al. 2016, 5–6)

I take it the point is that, although the stomach problems resulting from drinking milk may be a disorder in virtue of the digestive dysfunction, this individual's inherent condition of lactose intolerance is not itself a disorder even though it is mismatched to and maladaptive in his current environment, because it is how he was biologically designed. This is analogous to Garson's *Daphnia* that was perfectly designed for an environment that unfortunately it does not inhabit—which even Garson judges to be nondisordered. The passage provocatively makes clear that the criterion of dysfunction takes precedence over maladaptation in a given environment and thus that the World Health Organization's classification of lactose intolerance in itself as a disorder should be rejected—although the manifestation of that condition in digestive dysfunction would of course remain a disorder.

Turning to developmental dysfunction, a clear example of how DOHaD theorists react to the medicalization of a mismatch with considerable psychological ramifications is provided in papers considering the trend in Western countries toward earlier puberty, especially among girls. Although the papers acknowledge that some cases of early puberty involve developmental disruptions that are true dysfunctions (e.g., brain lesions, hormonal disorders) and therefore disorders, DOHaD authors argue that the broader trend toward early puberty among girls in the developed world is due to developmental plasticity responding to various fetal influences, with an outcome that is severely mismatched to current social demands. These authors routinely and emphatically distinguish medical disorder from mismatch in their discussion of early puberty and make clear that the mismatch itself should not be confused with medical disorder. In fact, they take pains to correct what they see as a mistake by others in assuming there is a disorder when in fact there is a developmental mismatch, as in the following passages from two articles: "We will argue that there is a risk that early puberty is being inappropriately perceived as a medical issue rather than recognizing that there is mismatch between biological reality and the increasingly complex society in which young people live" (Gluckman and Hanson 2006d 26); "Recent decades have exposed a mismatch between the age of biological maturation and the age of psychosocial competency.... We must be careful not to inappropriately medicalize early puberty. The use of the term 'precocial puberty' to describe early puberty which does not have a pathological basis is inappropriate" (Gluckman and Hanson 2006d, 30); "In the past few decades, as puberty has advanced, biological maturation has come to precede psychosocial maturation significantly for the first time in our evolutionary history. Although this developmental mismatch has considerable societal implications, care has to be taken not to medicalize contemporary early puberty inappropriately" (Gluckman and Hanson 2006e p. 7); "There is...increasing awareness of the consequences of the psychosocial 'mismatch' which arises from early biological reproductive competence in societies in which young women do not obtain psychological or social maturity until at least their late teens. Generally, a medical approach is taken to early menarche. Here, we review evidence suggesting that the timing of puberty...can be better understood by reference to evolutionary principles. These considerations...challenge the concept that it is necessarily pathological" (Gluckman and Hanson 2006e, 7); "We have suggested that an evolutionary perspective...argues for more careful use of the term 'precocious puberty'. This term implies pathology...the vast majority of young women undergoing menarche at increasingly younger ages have normal physiology and progression of puberty; their physiology has been simply determined by their distant ancestors" (Gluckman and Hanson 2006d, 11).

Another indicator that these theorists clearly distinguish disorder from developmental mismatch occurs in the title of an inserted text box that explores various adaptive and maladaptive features of posttraumatic stress disorder (PTSD). The box is titled, "Post-traumatic Stress Disorder: Adaptive or Pathological?" (Gluckman et al. 2016, 274). By "adaptive" here, they mean adaptive not in the immediate environmental sense but in the sense that applies to PAR reactions—namely, it was naturally selected as adaptive in our species' environments of evolutionary adaptation (EEA). Their conclusion seems to be that PTSD has components that by themselves are naturally selected, but the overall configuration is a dysfunction and thus a disorder. The point is that they unblinkingly contrast adaptive with pathological, implying that naturally selected features are assumed to be nonpathological and on that basis raising the question whether PTSD should be considered a genuine disorder.

In case I am giving the contrary impression, it should be emphasized that despite the nondisorder status of mismatched PAR conditions, there is ample room for dysfunction and disorder within the developmental mismatch approach. Leading DOHaD authors distinguish normal-range environmental circumstances to which the plastic response is biologically designed from more extreme or pathological environmental inputs that they term developmental "disruptions" and roughly correspond to dysfunctions. They understand that this distinction is conceptually fundamental, and it is repeatedly emphasized, "These [PAR] factors act through the processes of developmental plasticity...and can be distinguished from developmental disruption" (Gluckman, Hanson, and Pinal 2005, 130); "Normal development may be disrupted by early environmental influences; individuals that survive have to cope with the damaging consequences" (Gluckman, Hanson, Spencer, and Bateson 2005, 671); "A key issue is to distinguish between factors that disrupt development and which are not regulated and those that are based on the processes of developmental plasticity and may have adaptive value....We have to accept that some environmental exposures...simply disrupt the normal pattern of development" (Gluckman and Hanson 2006b, 2); "Extreme developmental environments lead to developmental disruption....Within the normal range of variation...maximal fitness is conferred by the action of predictive adaptive responses" (figure 3.1 legend, Gluckman and Hanson 2006c, 37); "Not all environmental factors act during early development through these plastic processes. Some environmental influences are clearly pathological and lead to disruption of development rather than channeling development. Teratogenesis is the most obvious manifestation of pathology....Developmental disruption may also occur at a less overt level. The change may not be in gross structure, leading to a malformation, but in the substructure or function of the organ. This change in structure or function has no adaptive value at any stage in the organism's life" (Gluckman and Hanson 2006c, 34); "Environmental factors acting during the phase of developmental plasticity can either act to disrupt the normal program of development or to modulate it. Developmental disruption may be overtly teratogenic...or may be much more subtle. Clearly, such disruptive responses cannot be considered adaptive" (Gluckman and Hanson 2006b, 3); "Developmental plasticity, which has an adaptive origin, must be distinguished from developmental disruption, which does not" (Gluckman et al. 2016, 96).

The many forms of disruption yield many pathways to developmental disorder: "Errors in prediction might arise either because the postnatal environment has shifted or because the foetus has received faulty information on which to base its prediction. The latter is most likely to happen in the presence of maternal disease or placental dysfunction, but also as a result of exaggerated maternal constraint....Developmentally disruptive events in response to environmental stimuli irreversibly interfere with embryonic development and, depending on their nature, may have deleterious effects either in utero and/or after birth. Generally, such cues act by interfering with a developmental process during periods of vulnerability, such that structural deficits emerge. The stimulus may be a drug, ionizing radiation, a major environmental shift such as hyperthermia or hypoxia, disease, or a gross nutritional disruption" (Gluckman, Hanson, Spencer, and Bateson 2005, 672); "The fidelity of the prediction is influenced by…pathophysiological factors, such as maternal or placental disease or changes in maternal nutrition.…Fetal growth patterns can be affected by maternal nutritional balance within the normal absolute-intake range" (Gluckman and Hanson 2006c, 44–45); "It is possible, for example, that the mechanism which increases…vigilance in offspring becomes maladaptive when it causes a disabling level of phobia in some individuals. In light of findings that genetic changes in many different loci appear to contribute to the risk of schizophrenia, it may be that such traits generally improve cognitive fitness, but at some point reach a cliff-edge and failure" (Glover 2011, 358); "Predictions may be erroneous if the fetus is exposed to an impaired fetal environment and thus receives maternal/environmental cues that are not representative of the actual environment, leading to inaccurate predictions and adoption of an inappropriate developmental trajectory. In humans and other mammals, the causes of such an impairment may be pathological, for example due to maternal or placental disease, or physiological, involving factors such as poor maternal nutrition (e.g. a hypocaloric or low-protein diet), maternal stress, or maternal constraint" (Low, Gluckman, and Hanson 2012, 654).

This is an area in which the complexity leads to ambiguity. As Gluckman and Hanson (2006b) observe, "Evaluating whether a response is adaptive or disruptive may be difficult" (5). Even if the HDA is accepted as the correct analysis of disorder, one might find legitimate disagreement about whether, say, environmentally induced myopia or conduct disorder in response to abuse is or is not a dysfunction and thus is or is not a disorder (see the comment on indeterminacy, below). DOHaD theorists offer some more esoteric examples: "For example, is the reduction in nephron number in sheep after maternal exposure to very high doses of glucocorticoids in early gestation (Wintour et al., 2003) a process where the steroid has disrupted the normal pattern of nephron differentiation, or is it part of some adaptive process mimicking a normal situation where the fetus responds to maternal glucocorticoids crossing the placenta under situations of maternal stress? Similarly, is the continuous relationship between maternal vitamin A intake and nephron number in the rat a dose-dependent disruptive effect or does it have adaptive value?" (Gluckman, Hanson, and Beedle 2007, 5). I believe that answering these types of questions sometimes leads us to the limits of functional thinking and also may bring us to confront issues of indeterminacy of function, as Garson suggests. However, where there are reasonably firm intuitions once details are filled in, they also can illuminate the structure and scope of our concept.

Other Authors Cited by Garson

I have surveyed above the writings of the leading school of DOHaD theorists, sifting the evidence regarding Garson's claims versus the HDA as a way to explain their intuitions. Garson cites some other publications not addressed above that he thinks are congenial to his view, and they deserve comment. First, it should be kept in mind that in considering whether mismatches are considered disorders, one can easily be misled by the literature's casual usage of "disorder." When DOHaD theorists address conditions generally labeled disorders and especially mental disorders, they often describe the conditions as "disorders" even when discussing potential evolutionary and developmental mismatches. However, this is more terminological than conceptual. Given the great fanfare and controversy surrounding each revision of the *DSM*, and given that the *DSM* and *International Classification of Diseases* (*ICD*) are considered official listings, it is potentially confusing and no small thing to suggest that a condition listed as a mental disorder is in fact not a disorder. It is easier and safer in anything other than a conceptual-analytic context to use "disorder" just to mean "whatever is listed as a disorder in *DSM* (or *ICD*)" and proceed with one's etiological theorizing.

Other than Gluckman and his colleagues, Garson cites two references regarding mismatches being considered disorders, and both of them take this terminological route. Garson cites McGuire and Troisi's (1998) book in which they make a case for evolutionary theory as an integrating framework for psychiatry. However, this book has nothing much to say about the concept of mental disorder and takes no stand on whether developmental mismatches are disorders. Instead, the authors explicitly state that in using the term "disorder," they will simply abide by the *DSM-IV*'s listing of conditions as disorders: "We will use the term ... *disorder* when we are referring to disorders specifically as they are described in the fourth edition of the American Psychiatric Association's *Diagnostic and Statistical Manual of Mental Disorders* (*DSM-IV*, 1994)" (1998, 13). Consistent with this orthodox perspective, when they later confront the question of "how disorders are defined," they simply note, "As most readers will be aware, there is no generally accepted definition. ... We will not dwell on this point but will settle for the definition used in *DSM-IV*" (1998, 14) and quote the *DSM-IV* definition. So, this book's disorder attributions offer no support for Garson's conceptual claims. Note that in quoting the *DSM-IV* definition, McGuire and Troisi omit the conceptually crucial "dysfunction" sentence ("Whatever its original cause, it must currently be considered a manifestation of a behavioral, psychological, or biological dysfunction in the individual" [1994, xxi–xxii]). This omission anticipates Troisi's (2006) later identification of disorder with reduced fitness independent of dysfunction: "A maladaptive psychological or behavioral syndrome that impacts negatively on the individual's inclusive fitness. ... A dysfunctional mechanism underlying the syndrome is neither necessary nor sufficient for a diagnosis of mental disorder" (Troisi 2006, 328). This is the very position rejected as obviously wrong by leading DOHaD theorists, and it is a position that renders psychiatry helpless to respond to antipsychiatric critiques because almost any socially disapproved feature can be made fitness-reducing through social sanctions. Indeed, on Troisi's analysis, being a member of a severely oppressed minority could be a disorder.

Garson also cites Glover (2011). Glover's paper is a review that suggests that the DOHaD paradigm as developed by Gluckman and colleagues might be systematically extended to a broad range of psychodiagnostic variables. Glover does not directly address the nature of the disorder/nondisorder boundary and relies on *DSM* categories to label as disorders the mismatched conditions she discusses. However, Glover's reliance on *DSM* classifications to identify mismatches with disorders seems to be justified only by misidentifying maladaptiveness with disorder: "A mismatch between what was adaptive in an earlier environment and the world in which we now live can lead to pathology. Thus the outcomes which can be increased by prenatal stress or anxiety and their potential adaptive value in our ancestral environment…can be quite maladaptive in our modern environment. For example, we are not usually exposed to the type of danger for which extra vigilance (anxiety) or readily distracted attention (ADHD) would be helpful, and these symptoms can both be distressing and impede formal learning" (359). Moreover, Glover hints at lurking conceptual questions about such labels when she says things like: "The evolutionary perspective can add a new viewpoint in trying to understand the long-term effects of prenatal stress. Fetal programming may help explain why some forms of developmental psychopathology have persisted in the population. It could be of evolutionary benefit to have a minority of individuals who are more vigilant (anxious), impulsive or with readily distracted attention (ADHD), or willing to break the rules or be aggressive (conduct disorder). In times of stress it may be adaptive to have a higher proportion of the population with these traits" (364); "An evolutionary perspective may give a different understanding of children in our society with these symptoms.…The type of cognitive deficits observed after prenatal stress…may be those which were adaptive in a past environment" (356); and "Gluckman et al. (2009) make the case that concepts of health and disease are altered by taking an evolutionary perspective. Our understanding of an individual's health may depend on knowledge of their evolutionary origin and how that interacts with the modern world" (Glover 2011, 359). It is difficult to believe that when Glover says, "Thus some of the altered outcomes observed after prenatal stress may well, in their milder forms, have been adaptive in more primitive conditions" (357), that if pushed, she would insist that nonetheless these are medical disorders—but ones that could be "cured" by placing the individual in a more threatening environment! In sum, Glover's paper, like McGuire and Troisi's book, explores evolutionary perspectives on the conditions currently classified as mental disorders without stopping to reflect on the concept of disorder itself. It thus offers no serious grounds for resolving the issues raised by Garson one way or the other. The only sources cited by Garson that take this issue seriously are the ones by Gluckman and colleagues cited extensively above.

Thus, the evidence of the texts cited by Garson goes against his claims and supports the HDA. Garson demands that "at the very least, I would like to be given an independent reason for thinking that, if some…disorders result from plasticity, then they are not real disorders at all." I have provided that reason—namely, this is the best interpretation of the views of the leading theorists in the DOHaD field, and the evidence Garson cites to support his case is entirely based upon but mischaracterizes those views. He also says, "The HD analysis also makes a prediction about clinical usage and I have given reasons for my skepticism about that prediction." I showed in earlier comments that his skepticism about my "fever" example can be addressed by presenting other even more persuasive examples, and above I have now also shown that DOHaD theorists confirm my prediction as well, for example, in their suggesting that lactose intolerance and early puberty, both medicalized conditions, should be demedicalized because they are mismatches, and more generally in their reasoning behind those claims.

References

American Psychiatric Association. 2013. *Diagnostic and Statistical Manual of Mental Disorders*. 5th ed. American Psychiatric Association.

Andrews, P. W., and J. A. Thomson Jr. 2009. The bright side of being blue: Depression as an adaptation for analyzing complex problems. *Psychological Review*, 116(3): 620–654.

Bateson, G., D. D. Jackson, J. Haley, and J. Weakland. 1956. Toward a theory of schizophrenia. *Behavioral Science* 1: 251–264.

Dodge, K. A., J. E. Bates, and G. S. Pettit. 1990. Mechanisms in the cycle of violence. *Science* 250: 1678–1683.

Eisenberg, D. T. A., B. Campbell, P. B. Gray, and M. D. Sorenson, M. D. 2008. Dopamine receptor genetic polymorphisms and body composition in undernourished pastoralists: An exploration of nutrition indices among nomadic and recently settled Ariaal men of northern Kenya. *BMC Evolutionary Biology* 8: 173.

Evans, W. N., M. S. Morrill, and S. T. Parente. 2010. Measuring inappropriate medical diagnosis and treatment in survey data: The case of ADHD among school-age children. *Journal of Health Economics* 29: 657–673.

First, M. B., and J. C. Wakefield. 2010. Defining 'mental disorder' in *DSM-V*. *Psychological Medicine* 40(11): 1779–1782.

First, M. B., and J. C. Wakefield. 2013. Diagnostic criteria as dysfunction indicators: Bridging the chasm between the definition of mental disorder and diagnostic criteria for specific disorders. *Canadian Journal of Psychiatry* 58(12): 663–669.

Glover, V. 2011. Prenatal stress and the origins of psychopathology: An evolutionary perspective. *Journal of Child Psychology and Psychiatry* 52(4): 356–367.

Gluckman, P. D., A. Beedle, T. Buklijas, F. Low, and M. Hanson. 2016. *Principles of Evolutionary Medicine*. 2nd ed. Oxford University Press.

Gluckman, P., A. Beedle, and M. Hanson. 2009. *Principles of Evolutionary Medicine*. Cambridge University Press.

Gluckman, P. D., and M. A. Hanson. 2004. Living with the past: Evolution, development, and patterns of disease. *Science* 305(17): 1733–1736.

Gluckman, P. D, and M. A. Hanson (eds.). 2006a. *Developmental Origins of Health and Disease.* Oxford University Press.

Gluckman, P. D., and M. A. Hanson. 2006b. The developmental origins of health and disease: An overview. In *The Developmental Origins of Health and Disease,* P. D. Gluckman and M. A. Hanson (eds.), 1–5. Cambridge University Press.

Gluckman, P. D., and M. A. Hanson. 2006c. The conceptual basis for the developmental origins of health and disease. In *The Developmental Origins of Health and Disease,* P. D. Gluckman and M. A. Hanson (eds.), 33–50. Cambridge University Press.

Gluckman, P. D., and M. A. Hanson. 2006d. The evolution of puberty. *Molecular and Cellular Endocrinology* 254–255: 26–31.

Gluckman, P. D., and M. A. Hanson. 2006e. Evolution, development and timing of puberty. *Trends in Endocrinology and Metabolism* 17(1): 7–12.

Gluckman, P. D., M. A. Hanson, and A. S. Beedle. 2007. Early life events and their consequences for later disease: A life history and evolutionary perspective. *American Journal of Human Biology* 19(1): 1–19.

Gluckman, P. D., M. A. Hanson, and C. Pinal. 2005. The developmental origins of adult disease. *Maternal & Child Nutrition* 1(3): 130–141.

Gluckman, P. D., M. A. Hanson, and H. G. Spencer. 2005. Predictive adaptive responses and human evolution. *TRENDS in Ecology and Evolution* 20(10): 527–553.

Gluckman, P. D., M. A. Hanson, H. G. Spencer, and P. Bateson. 2005. Environmental influences during development and their later consequences for health and disease: Implications for the interpretation of empirical studies. *Proceedings of the Royal Society B: Biological Sciences* 272(1564): 671–677.

Godfrey, K. 2006. The 'developmental origins' hypothesis: Epidemiology. In *The Developmental Origins of Health and Disease,* P. D. Gluckman and M. A. Hanson (eds.), 6–32. Cambridge University Press.

Godfrey, K. M., K. A. Lillycrop, G. C. Burdge, P. D. Gluckman, and M. A. Hanson. 2007. Epigenetic mechanisms and the mismatch concept of the developmental origins of health and disease. *Pediatric Research* 61(5, pt. 2): 5R–10R.

Kinner, S. 2003. Psychopathy as an adaptation: Implications for society and social policy. In *Psychological Dimensions to War and Peace. Evolutionary Psychology and Violence: A Primer for Policymakers and Public Policy Advocates,* R. W. Bloom and N. Dess (eds.), 57–81. Praeger/Greenwood.

Knoll, J. L., IV, and R. W. Pie. 2019. Cruel, immoral behavior is not mental illness. *Psychiatric Times,* August 19. https://www.psychiatrictimes.com/couch-crisis/cruel-immoral-behavior-not-mental-illness.

Krupp, D. B., L. A. Sewall, M. L. Lalumière, C. Sheriff, and G. T. Harris. 2012. Nepotistic patterns of violent psychopathy: Evidence for adaption? *Frontiers in Psychology* 3: 1–8.

Krupp, D. B., L. A. Sewall, M. L. Lalumière, C. Sheriff, and G. T. Harris. 2013. Psychopathy, adaption, and disorder. *Frontiers in Psychology* 4: 1–5.

Laing, R. D. 1967. *The Politics of Experience*. Penguin Books.

Lalumière, M. L., G. T. Harris, and M. E. Rice. 2001. Psychopathy and developmental instability. *Evolution and Human Behavior* 22(2): 75–90.

Low, F., and P. D. Gluckman. 2016. Evolutionary medicine III: Mismatch. In *Encyclopedia of Evolutionary Biology*, R. M. Kilman (ed.), 69. Academic Press.

Low, F. M., P. D. Gluckman, and M. A. Hanson. 2012. Developmental plasticity, epigenetics and human health. *Evolutionary Biology* 39(4): 650–665.

Machalek, R. 1995. Sociobiology, sociopathy, and social policy. *Behavioral and Brain Sciences* 18(3): 564.

McGuire, M., and A. Triosi. 1998. *Darwinian Psychiatry*. Oxford University Press.

Mealey, L. 1995. Primary sociopathy (psychopathy) is a type, secondary is not. *Behavioral and Brain Sciences* 18(3): 579–599.

Moffitt T. E. 1993. Adolescence-limited and life-course-persistent antisocial behavior: A developmental taxonomy. *Psychological Review* 100: 674–701.

Neander, K. 1995. Misrepresenting and malfunctioning. *Philosophical Studies* 79: 109–141.

Nesse, R. M. 2000. Is depression an adaptation? *Archives of General Psychiatry* 57(1): 14–20.

Reimer, M. 2008. Psychopathy without (the language of) disorder. *Neuroethics* 1(3): 185–198.

Richters, J., and S. Hinshaw. 1999. The abduction of disorder in psychiatry. *Journal of Abnormal Psychiatry* 108: 438–445.

Spitzer, R. L. 1997. Brief comments from a psychiatric nosologist weary from his own attempts to define mental disorder: Why Ossorio's definition muddles and Wakefield's "harmful dysfunction" illuminates the issues. *Clinical Psychology: Science and Practice* 4(3): 259–261.

Spitzer, R. L. 1999. Harmful dysfunction and the *DSM* definition of mental disorder. *Journal of Abnormal Psychology* 108(3): 430–432.

Szasz, T. S. 1974. *The Myth of Mental Illness: Foundations of a Theory of Personal Conduct*. Rev. ed. Harper & Row.

Troisi, A. 2015. The evolutionary diagnosis of mental disorder. *WIREs Cognitive Science* 6: 323–331.

Troisi, A., and M. McGuire. 2002. Darwinian psychiatry and the concept of mental disorder. *Neuroendocrinology Letters* 23(suppl. 4): 31–38.

Ullman, L. P., and L. Krasner. 1969. *A Psychological Approach to Abnormal Behavior*. Prentice-Hall.

Wakefield, J. C. 1992a. The concept of mental disorder: On the boundary between biological facts and social values. *American Psychologist* 47: 373–388.

Wakefield, J. C. 1992b. Disorder as harmful dysfunction: A conceptual critique of *DSM-III-R's* definition of mental disorder. *Psychological Review* 99: 232–247.

Wakefield, J. C. 1993. Limits of operationalization: A critique of Spitzer and Endicott's (1978) proposed operational criteria of mental disorder. *Journal of Abnormal Psychology* 102: 160–172.

Wakefield, J. C. 1995. Dysfunction as a value-free concept: A reply to Sadler and Agich. *Philosophy, Psychiatry, and Psychology* 2: 233–46.

Wakefield, J. C. 1997a. Diagnosing *DSM-IV*, part 1: *DSM-IV* and the concept of mental disorder. *Behaviour Research and Therapy* 35: 633–650.

Wakefield, J. C. 1997b. Diagnosing *DSM-IV*, part 2: Eysenck (1986) and the essentialist fallacy. *Behaviour Research and Therapy*: 35: 651–666.

Wakefield, J. C. 1997c. Normal inability versus pathological disability: Why Ossorio's (1985) definition of mental disorder is not sufficient. *Clinical Psychology: Science and Practice* 4: 249–258.

Wakefield, J. C. 1997d. When is development disordered? Developmental psychopathology and the harmful dysfunction analysis of mental disorder. *Development and Psychopathology* 9: 269–290.

Wakefield, J. C. 1998. The *DSM's* theory-neutral nosology is scientifically progressive: Response to Follette and Houts. *Journal of Consulting and Clinical Psychology* 66: 846–852.

Wakefield, J. C. 1999a. Evolutionary versus prototype analyses of the concept of disorder. *Journal of Abnormal Psychology* 108: 374–399.

Wakefield, J. C. 1999b. Mental disorder as a black box essentialist concept. *Journal of Abnormal Psychology* 108: 465–472.

Wakefield, J. C. 2000a. Aristotle as sociobiologist: The "function of a human being" argument, black box essentialism, and the concept of mental disorder. *Philosophy, Psychiatry, and Psychology* 7: 17–44.

Wakefield, J. C. 2000b. Spandrels, vestigial organs, and such: Reply to Murphy and Woolfolk's "The harmful dysfunction analysis of mental disorder." *Philosophy, Psychiatry, and Psychology* 7: 253–269.

Wakefield, J. C. 2001. Evolutionary history versus current causal role in the definition of disorder: Reply to McNally. *Behaviour Research and Therapy* 39: 347–366.

Wakefield, J. C. 2006. What makes a mental disorder mental? *Philosophy, Psychiatry, and Psychology* 13: 123–131.

Wakefield, J. C. 2007. The concept of mental disorder: Diagnostic implications of the harmful dysfunction analysis. *World Psychiatry* 6: 149–156.

Wakefield, J. C. 2009. Mental disorder and moral responsibility: Disorders of personhood as harmful dysfunctions, with special reference to alcoholism. *Philosophy, Psychiatry, and Psychology* 16: 91–99.

Wakefield, J. C. 2011. Darwin, functional explanation, and the philosophy of psychiatry. In *Maladapting Minds: Philosophy, Psychiatry, and Evolutionary Theory*, P. R. Andriaens and A. De Block (eds.), 143–172. Oxford University Press.

Wakefield, J. C. 2014. The biostatistical theory versus the harmful dysfunction analysis, part 1: Is part-dysfunction a sufficient condition for medical disorder? *Journal of Medicine and Philosophy* 39: 648–682.

Wakefield, J. C. 2016a. The concepts of biological function and dysfunction: Toward a conceptual foundation for evolutionary psychopathology. In *Handbook of Evolutionary Psychology*, D. Buss (ed.), 2nd ed., vol. 2, 988–1006. Oxford University Press.

Wakefield, J. C. 2016b. Diagnostic issues and controversies in *DSM-5*: Return of the false positives problem. *Annual Review of Clinical Psychology* 12: 105–132.

Wakefield, J. C., and M. B. First. 2003. Clarifying the distinction between disorder and nondisorder: Confronting the overdiagnosis ("false positives") problem in *DSM-V*. In *Advancing DSM: Dilemmas in Psychiatric Diagnosis*, K. A. Phillips, M. B. First, and H. A. Pincus (eds.), 23–56. American Psychiatric Press.

Wakefield, J. C., and M. B. First. 2012. Placing symptoms in context: The role of contextual criteria in reducing false positives in *DSM* diagnosis. *Comprehensive Psychiatry* 53: 130–139.

Zoega, H., U. A. Valdimarsdottir, and S. Hernandez-Diaz. 2012. Age, academic performance, and stimulant prescribing for ADHD: A nationwide cohort study. *Pediatrics* 130: 1012–1018.

18 Biological Function Hierarchies and Indeterminacy of Dysfunction: Supplementary Reply to Justin Garson

Jerome Wakefield

A considerable amount of Garson's chapter is taken up with issues concerning indeterminacy of biological function. The issues he raises about indeterminacy are important to address but take us into some general territory that I think is better dealt with separate from his main argument. In this supplementary section on the indeterminacy issue, I first explain why Garson raises this issue as part of his anti–harmful dysfunction analysis (HDA) developmental mismatch argument and then explain why his indeterminacy-related moves fail to save his argument from my reply. I then offer some tentative comments critiquing the solution to indeterminacy challenges that he borrows from Neander (1995). Finally, I reply to indeterminacy-based critiques Garson offers of some of examples I have put forward of dysfunctions. Note that the problem of indeterminacy of biological function tends to be discussed in relation to teleosemantic theories that attempt to derive mental contents from biological functions because in such theories, ambiguities about function can yield problems in determining mental content. However, here I am concerned only with biological functions themselves and ignore whether or how they impact on teleosemantics.

The specific form of indeterminacy Garson considers arises from the fact that selected mechanisms generally possess not just one function but a hierarchical set of functions. As Garson explains, "The problem of indeterminacy ... is that there are many ways of describing a trait's function, all of which are allowed by the selected effects theory. Is the function of the heart simply to *beat*? To *circulate blood*? To *bring nutrients to cells*? To *keep the organism alive*? All of these descriptions are acceptable because they are all effects that explain why the heart evolved by natural selection." A key insight is that these functions are organized in a cause-effect hierarchy, in which the performance of one function combines with some expectable environmental circumstances to bring about the performance of another function: "In our example, the different descriptions of the heart form a certain series, that is, a hierarchy defined by cause and effect. By beating, the heart circulates blood. By circulating blood, the heart brings nutrients to cells. By bringing nutrients to cells, the heart keeps us alive. When we say that the function of the heart is simply *to beat*, we are describing the most 'proximal' member of that chain. When we say that the function of the heart is to *keep us alive*, we are describing its most 'distal' member. When we say that the function of the heart is to *bring nutrients to cells*, we are describing an 'intermediate' member of that chain."

This multiplicity of functions poses a question about when to say that a feature is dysfunctioning because some of its functions might be performed and others not for varying kinds of reasons. Clearly, the simple failure of a function to be performed is intuitively insufficient for dysfunction. For example, Garson observes that if a stroke prevents blood from flowing through the brain and thus causes the heart to fail in its function of circulating the blood, that is intuitively not a heart dysfunction even though a function of the heart fails to be performed. Similarly, consider the ocean bacterium that has a magnetosome mechanism that orients its motion in such a way as to guide it to the deeper deoxygenated water that it requires for survival (Dretske 1986; Wakefield 1999a). The magnetosome has a hierarchy of functions: it orients the bacterium's motion toward prevailing north in the local magnetic field; by doing so, it orients the bacterium's motion toward the earth's true magnetic north, which is almost always the same as local north under standard oceanic conditions, and by doing so, it orients the bacterium's motion toward deeper water away from deadly surface oxygen. (It works this way only for the Northern Hemisphere bacteria considered here, where the magnetic field's lines are such that magnetic north indicates deeper water; in the Southern Hemisphere, the corresponding bacteria are biologically designed to orient toward south.) Now, in the highly unlikely event that a bacterium happened to live near an enormous rock outcropping that distorted the local magnetic field so that local north was in fact true south, the magnetosome's most proximal function of detecting and orienting motion toward local magnetic north is being performed and so there is no dysfunction there, but its other two functions of orienting motion toward true north and deeper water are failing to be performed, perhaps leading the bacterium to swim dangerously close to the surface. Yet, there is no dysfunction because the failure of the bacterium's functions is entirely due to the unusual nature of its environment, not to anything that goes wrong internally with its magnetosome.

So, there is a question of how and when to translate failures of a feature's various functions into an attribution of dysfunction. Before presenting Garson's solution to this problem, it is worth clarifying: why does Garson raise the hierarchy-of-functions and indeterminacy-of-dysfunction issue to begin with? The answer is that he thinks he needs to address this problem in order to fill a gap in his anti-HDA argument. Garson's central argument is that when a "bona fide" disorder is due to a developmental mismatch, it is a disorder without a dysfunction and thus a counterexample to the HDA. To make this argument work, he needs to establish that there is no dysfunction in a developmental mismatch. He uses his *Daphnia* example to support the intuition that the initial predictive adaptive response in which a developmental choice is made based on sampling the environment during early development is not a dysfunction of the developmental mechanism that triggered it. Recall that in the example, a *Daphnia* has a mechanism, M, that is triggered during an early critical developmental period by its detection of predators' kairomones in the water of the *Daphnia*'s lake, and if triggered, M causes the irreversible development of a "helmet"-like structure that markedly increases the *Daphnia*'s chances for survival in a lake with predators but markedly decreases its survival chances if there are no predators, and it is burdened with this extra structure. So, this naturally selected developmental trigger is based on an implicit "prediction" that if predators are present in the lake during development, they are likely to be present in the same lake during adulthood. However, suppose that after M is triggered by detection of kairomones and the helmet develops, the *Daphnia*'s lake subsequently empties of predators and the helmet becomes seriously maladaptive, so there is a developmental mismatch (this is my naturalized version of Garson's example of his intentionally emptying a pool of all its predators after the *Daphnia* develops a helmet). Garson defends his intuition that, no matter what happens later, M is not dysfunctional when it triggers the helmet's development because at that point, M is doing precisely what it is biologically designed to do: "Here is an intuition that I have. ... It seems to me that talk of 'dysfunction' is out of place when it comes to developmental mismatches ... a member of *Daphnia* that chose the 'wrong' phenotype ... exhibits a developmental mismatch and it takes a fitness loss as a result. In my opinion, this does not represent an inner 'dysfunction.'"

I agree with Garson's intuition that when the *Daphnia* develops a helmet in response to detected predators' kairomones, that is not a dysfunction even if the helmet is later mismatched to the environment and disadvantageous. So far, there is no dysfunction.

Nonetheless, in light of function hierarchies and indeterminacy considerations, Garson realizes that this does not quite give him the premise his anti-HDA argument requires, because he needs to be able to assert that there is *no* dysfunction in a developmental mismatch, whereas so far he can only say the initial triggering of helmet development is not a dysfunction. Garson observes that there are in fact two hierarchically organized functions of M, a proximal function to develop a helmet upon detection of kairomones and a distal function to increase the *Daphnia*'s later survival by triggering the helmet's development. In fact, the distal function is not performed when there are later no predators. Garson realizes that whether this failure of distal function allows one to say there is a dysfunction—and thus whether his anti-HDA argument works—depends on how one resolves the indeterminacy of dysfunction challenge:

> My viewpoint about function indeterminacy informs my intuition about the *Daphnia* case. Let's assume ... a mechanism (M) in the *Daphnia* that instantiates the following rule: "if predators, then helmet; if no predators, then no helmet." There are many ways of describing M's function. We could say that M's function is to trigger a certain developmental sequence (one that yields the helmet head) in response to kairomones ... by releasing a certain hormone into the bloodstream. ... Alternatively, we could say that M's function is to *protect the individual from*

predators. The former is a more proximal way of describing its function and the latter a more distal way.... That is because the two descriptions form a series: the mechanism typically *protects the individual from predators* by *releasing hormone H in response to kairomones.*

Now, suppose we have a developmental mismatch. Is there any dysfunction? Described in the most proximal way, the answer is no. *M* fully and adequately discharged its function when it released hormone *H* in response to kairomones. Described in a more "distal" way, there could be a dysfunction. After all, if there are no predators around, *M* certainly cannot perform its function of protecting the individual from them. So, whether or not it is "dysfunctional" depends, in part, on how we describe it.

So, Garson needs a solution to the indeterminacy of function issue that blocks describing the failure of *M*'s distal function of increasing the *Daphnia*'s later survival as a dysfunction. To block such a reply, Garson cleverly adopts Neander's (1995) proposed solution to the indeterminacy of dysfunction problem, which seems tailor-made for his purposes. Neander proposes what I will call the "proximal-function thesis," that one can only attribute dysfunction to failures of the most proximal function in a mechanism's hierarchy. Garson explains, "I endorse a simple and plausible solution developed by Neander (1995).... Her view is that a trait dysfunctions only when it cannot perform its most proximal function. The heart is dysfunctional only when it cannot *beat.*" If correct, the proximal-function thesis certainly does block citing the failure of *M*'s distal function of increasing later survival as a dysfunction and thus blocks the most obvious reply to Garson, and so Garson embraces the proximal-function thesis for what potentially can be described as a dysfunction: "I prefer the more proximal description for the reasons I gave above... the way we describe the *Daphnia*-type case is pivotal to my argument." To ensure the result he wants, Garson actually incorporates the proximal-function thesis into the final version of his analysis of the meaning of dysfunction: "the function of a trait is the reason it evolved by natural selection, and *a trait dysfunctions just when it cannot carry out its most proximal function, for constitutional reasons.*"

Garson needn't have gone to all this trouble. In my reply above, I did not mount the kind of reply that he anticipated in which one tries to find some distal level of dysfunction of *M* to counter his claimed nondysfunction-disorder counterexample. My response was based not on the claim that developmental mismatches involve distal dysfunctions of developmental mechanisms but rather on the claim that *developmental mismatches are not disorders to begin with.* A careful examination of the Developmental Origins of Health and Disease (DOHaD) texts that Garson cited as support for his approach revealed that those very DOHaD texts maintain that a developmental mismatch is not a disorder. His own sources indicate that, if a condition that is considered a disorder turns out to be a developmental mismatch, then it is not really a disorder. By showing that the disorder ascription is incorrect, I rendered Garson's indeterminacy of dysfunction analysis moot because his point about lack of distal dysfunctions is only relevant to his anti-HDA argument in the context of a disorder. My counterargument negated Garson's hypothesis that developmental mismatches can be disorders without dysfunctions and did so in a way that arguments about indeterminacy of dysfunction can't fix.

I now want to examine further the proximal-function thesis and dispute Garson's embrace of the thesis. I will argue that at a minimum, the thesis has explanatory limits and is subject to exceptions; it works for a wide range of examples of a certain kind, but it fails under other conditions.

To prepare the way to some of these counterexamples to the proximal-function thesis, let me first back up for a moment and clarify a point about the definition of "dysfunction." Before he incorporated the proximal-function thesis into the definition of dysfunction, Garson offered a simpler definition that "something is dysfunctional just when it cannot perform its function, for 'inner' or 'constitutional' reasons, rather than because it's in an unsuitable environment." A useful tweak to this definition is to explicitly specify that a feature is dysfunctional only if it is incapable of performing a function *under the conditions for which it was selected to perform that function*. For example, as Christopher Boorse (2002) points out, it is not a dysfunction of your blood-clotting mechanisms if they never actually perform the function of causing your blood to clot, if the reason is that you never are injured. Moreover, it is the internal structure of the clotting mechanisms that prevents them from performing their function of causing clotting when there is no injury; that is part of their design. Nonetheless, there is no dysfunction as long as the clotting mechanisms are capable of performing their function should the appropriate conditions occur for which the clotting capacity was selected, namely, an injury. Or, for example, erectile dysfunction is not the lack of an erection, and it is not the incapability of having an erection under current conditions but the incapability of having an erection when confronted with the standard appropriate environment in which erection is the biologically designed response—say, a sexually desired and responsive partner (for how Masters and Johnson managed to go wrong on this very elementary point, see Wakefield 1988). So, we might say: *a dysfunction is the inability of a mechanism to perform its function for internal reasons even under the appropriate circumstances for which it was selected to perform that function.*

Now, I agree with Garson that the distal failure to perform the function of greater fitness in the case of the *Daphnia*'s helmet's developmental mismatch with its later environment is not a dysfunction, and most such developmental mismatches are not dysfunctions. However, the reason is actually quite simple and can be stated without any need to invoke the proximal-function thesis: to have a dysfunction, a mechanism must be incapable for internal reasons of performing its function under the appropriate circumstances, but the *Daphnia* suffers from no such incapacity and thus no distal dysfunction from developmental mismatch. When the *Daphnia* is grown, although the helmet is highly maladaptive in the actual circumstances in which the *Daphnia* finds itself, the helmet is perfectly capable *under the appropriate circumstances* of performing its function of protecting against predators and increasing the *Daphnia*'s survival—namely, the (predicted) environment for which the helmet was selected, a lake with predators. So, there is no reason to attribute a dysfunction, quite independently of any indeterminacy considerations, because the cause of the failure of *M*'s function is in the environment, not in anything internal to *M*. The fact that the distal fitness function of *M* fails to be performed sheerly because of the unsuitable environment lacking predators in which the *Daphnia* finds itself is no more a developmental dysfunction than, say, it is a sexual dysfunction to find oneself in an environment without any potential sexual partners.

Consider the heart example. The heart beats, thereby pumps the blood, and thereby nurtures the cells throughout the body, and here again the distal functions are accomplished by the proximal function in combination with certain environmental conditions. If the environmental conditions do not occur—for example, if there is a blockage of blood vessels that keeps the blood from reaching cells throughout the body—the distal function of nurturing may not be performed, but that is not a heart dysfunction because the failure is due to the environment rather than to something internal to the heart, and in the right environmental circumstances (i.e., should the vessels be unblocked), the heart is still perfectly capable of performing the distal function. So, again, the proximal-function solution is not needed to explain our intuition that the heart does not have a dysfunction in virtue of having a stroke. These examples suggest that for a class of cases, the modified definition of dysfunction has sufficient explanatory power to render the addition of the proximal-function thesis superfluous.

Another problem with the proximal-function thesis is that it is contradicted by a class of cases in which there is a clear dysfunction at the proximal level that by itself and without further environmental vicissitudes makes failures to perform further distal functions inevitable. In such cases, we often feel perfectly comfortable attributing distal dysfunctions as well, contrary to the proximal-function thesis. For example, if the heart ceases beating within normal range, then it is not only a dysfunction that the heart is not capable of beating adequately but also a dysfunction that the heart is failing to propel the blood with vigor through the blood vessels, as well as a dysfunction that the heart is not adequately causing nurturance to reach the cells throughout the body. This is presumably because once the heart has a proximal beating dysfunction, it becomes incapable of performing those distal functions under standard conditions as well.

Similarly, imagine a (Northern Hemisphere) bacterium with a magnetosome that is malformed so that when it detects the local magnetic field, it orients the bacterium's motion toward local south, thus failing in its function of orienting the motion toward local magnetic north. That is surely a dysfunction, and it is just as surely a dysfunction that the magnetosome fails to perform its distal functions of orienting motion toward true north and toward the safe deeper water. This is so because the malformation in the magnetosome makes it incapable under standard oceanic conditions of performing any of these functions.

Despite these problems, the proximal-function solution does reflect the reality of a certain kind of case. Generally, if a mechanism performs its most proximal function, it will not have a dysfunction at any level because if it fails to perform a distal function, the failure will be due to an unexpectable environment, thus not a dysfunction. This is because in the causal "by means of" relations that create the hierarchy of functions, the most common situation is that each "by means of" link involves just two factors: the previous function being fulfilled and the presence of standard environmental circumstances. If the prior function is performed, it is only the expectable environmental facts that are left to go wrong and cause a failure, but that means that under the standard circumstances, the mechanism would be capable of performing the distal function, so there is no dysfunction. Thus, the proximal-function thesis reflects the reality that generally speaking, when there is no proximal dysfunction, there will be no distal dysfunction.

However, I now want to claim that there are cases that falsify the proximal-function thesis even when the proximal function is successfully performed. I believe that Garson pointed the way to understanding how this can occur by his emphasis on predictive adaptive responses (PARs) and developmental mismatches, for such cases do have properties that open the way to a persuasive domain of counterexamples to the proximal-function thesis. We saw above that DOHaD theorists have the concept of a developmental disruption, in which the input to a developmental mechanism is outside of the range for which it biologically designed to be adaptively responsive. Disruption is at the core of my hypothesis.

My hypothesis is the following: when there is irreversible developmental disruption in the performance of a proximal function that makes it impossible for internal mechanisms to accomplish downstream distal functions even under appropriate environmental circumstances, those failures of distal functions can be said to truly be dysfunctions. First, developmental disruption can be thought of as an input to developmental mechanisms that is outside of the range for which the developmental mechanisms were biologically designed, meaning roughly that it is outside the range of inputs that exerted the selective pressures that led to the mechanism's selection. If such a disruption in some developmental process occurs during a critical developmental window, it may permanently and irreversibly alter the subsequent trajectory of development in a way that was never selected for. This notion surely has many ambiguities and obscurities that warrant examination, but developmental disruption is a notion that is relied on throughout developmental theory and, as we saw, is amply discussed in the DOHaD literature, so I accept it as a working concept of adequate credentials for the sake of this analysis. Should such a disruption occur that permanently alters the mechanism's responses, at that point there may be internal reasons why the mechanism is incapable of performing subsequent distal functions even in the appropriate environment and thus dysfunctional. None of the examples used by Garson satisfy these criteria, and that is why it seems to him that mechanisms can never have distal dysfunctions, but in fact that appearance is due to an accidental feature of the examples rather than a correct general principle. The best way to test my hypothesis that true distal dysfunctions due to irreversible developmental disruption falsify the proximal-function thesis is by examples, to which I now turn.

Consider a somewhat different kind of magnetosome example than those above, more along the lines of Garson's PARs and developmental-mismatch focus. Consider a cousin species of the above bacterium species that evolved so that, rather than the magnetosome continually orienting the bacterium's movement, the magnetosome samples the environment once during an early critical developmental period and, based on its detection of local magnetic north during that period, permanently and irreversibly fixes the bacterium's direction of motion toward local north. There is still a hierarchy of functions during the critical period: the magnetosome performs the function of permanently and irreversibly fixing motion toward local north and, by doing so, performs the function of permanently and irreversibly fixing motion toward true north and, by doing so, performs the function of permanently and irreversibly fixing motion away from surface water. (This is not wholly implausible given that these three functions almost always coincide and this bacterium saves considerable energy costs of continual magnetosome sampling of the environment.)

Now, suppose that this bacterium happens to be near the magnetic rock outcropping described earlier at the very time of the magnetosome's crucial developmental window in which the bacterium's orientation of motion becomes permanently and irreversibly fixed. The magnetosome perfectly performs its proximal function of detecting local magnetic north and accordingly fixing motion. However, in doing so, it fails to perform its distal functions of fixing motion toward true north and away from the surface. But this time, there is a crucial difference from the earlier bacterium that happened to be near the rock outcropping. If the other bacterium just moved away from the rock outcropping that was distorting the magnetic field, in the standard environment, it would be fine. In contrast, the present bacterium, once its critical period has occurred, has a fixed internal structure such that even if it is placed away from the outcropping and into a standard oceanic magnetic environment—the appropriate environment for which its mechanisms were naturally selected—the bacterium will still swim relentlessly toward the surface and its death.

My intuition is that there is now something wrong with this bacterium and that there is a clear dysfunction of the magnetosome. That dysfunction of the magnetosome is not a failure of its proximal function, which is to direct the bacterium toward whatever was local north at the time of the critical period. The dysfunction is due to the failure of the magnetosome's distal functions of directing the bacterium to true north and away from the surface, which it is now incapable of doing even under ideal conditions due to the internal fixation of its motion orientation. This example of a case with no proximal dysfunction but clear distal dysfunction falsifies the proximal-function thesis. Developmental plasticity, especially critical periods of the sort studied by DOHaD, change the nature of the dysfunction picture quite dramatically in a way that leads to conclusions in conflict with Neander's analysis.

The above analysis in which a developmental disruption during a critical developmental window causes a distal dysfunction also explains a second example, which is an example of mine that Garson criticized as a violation of the proximal-function thesis. Richters and Hinshaw (1999) present an example of an abused child who gets a fixed idea about the threat posed by the environment and responds aggressively and so becomes conduct disordered. This can be construed as an early developmental mismatch type example, based to some degree on the findings of Dodge (1990) that internalized cognitions of threat seem to be the vehicle by which abuse is carried from childhood to adulthood. Richters and Hinshaw's point, parallel to Garson's *Daphnia* argument, was that this youth has a disorder—a "bona fide" disorder of conduct disorder, one might say—but there is no dysfunction because the child's learning was a calibrated response to its early environment, and thus this is a counterexample to the HDA. Garson notes that I provided two possible answers to this proposed counterexample. One possibility is that the described processes are within the expectable range that shaped the natural selection of personality traits and thus part of normal learning and personality formation, and then there is no dysfunction and no disorder even though the outcome is socially undesirable. Indeed, *Diagnostic and Statistical Manual of Mental Disorders* (*DSM-5*) backs me up on the claim that even where the conduct disorder symptoms are present, there is not necessarily a disorder if normal learning or normal personality formation took place in a high-threat general environment: "Conduct disorder diagnosis may at times be potentially misapplied to individuals in settings where patterns of disruptive behavior are viewed as near-normative (e.g., in very threatening, high-crime areas or war zones). Therefore, the context in which the undesirable behaviors have occurred should be considered" (American Psychiatric Association 2013, 474).

The other possibility is that the familial abuse took the early environment outside of the expectable range and, in DOHaD language, was a developmental disruption. Familial abuse is plausibly an evolutionarily unexpectable environment that interferes with the evolutionary point of the developmental mechanism, which is to make a reliable PAR based on detection of the likely level of threat in the general environment. In this case, given the disruption and irreversible fixation of threat sensitivity outside of the selected range, there is a developmental dysfunction and so the subsequent traits are a disorder.

My either/or response to Richters and Hinshaw was in fact strictly in keeping with the later DOHaD view documented above. We saw that the DOHaD literature admitted that it is often difficult to tell whether an early environmental input is within the range for which responses have been naturally selected or is a disruption. This is especially the case when there is a continuous variable (such as threat sensitivity) that at some extremes is no longer within the evolution-relevant range.

Another example of mine that Garson disputes on the basis of Neander's proximal-function thesis is my gosling example. I argue that a gosling who accidentally imprints on a passing fox (or, in earlier renditions, a porcupine) has both a dysfunction and a disorder. In this example, the claimed dysfunction is the failure not of the most proximal function, which is presumably imprinting on whatever creature is first observed upon hatching. I agree with Garson's comment that if the gosling did not imprint on the fox, that would be a dysfunction. However, this is not an either/or situation; each function's status must be evaluated on its merits. I think in this case there is a failure and dysfunction of a distal function, namely, imprinting on the mother. (Interestingly, as I argue elsewhere, there is nothing wrong with the gosling at the brain-descriptive level, for the problem is a matter not of brain functioning per se but of the reference or meaning of the image stored in its brain, a psychological-level mental-content construct, so that we have here an example of a psychological dysfunction that is not a brain dysfunction.)

Here is Garson's full critique of my gosling example:

There are cases where I think Wakefield is potentially inconsistent in his approach to function indeterminacy, and the way we describe the *Daphnia*-type case is pivotal to my argument. On the one hand, Wakefield's (1999a, 386) explicit comments about indeterminacy seem to agree with my own, namely, that we should prefer the most "proximal" description of an item's function (as in the bacterium case). On the other hand, some of his specific examples seem to run contrary to that point. He discusses an example of filial imprinting gone awry, that is, where a gosling imprints on a passing porcupine (Wakefield 1999b, 468; 2000, 263). (Imprinting refers to a developmental "window" of time in which a juvenile organism forms a strong, lifelong preference. The function of filial imprinting in goslings is to cause them to form an attachment to their own mothers. The mechanism by which this works is that they form an attachment to the first large, suitably moving object that they encounter. Imprinting goes awry when the mechanism causes a gosling to imprint on an object that is not its mother.) The gosling now has an enduring inner disposition to follow around a porcupine. Wakefield says that this disposition is a dysfunction. I do not consider it a dysfunction (Murphy and Woolfolk [2000b, 279] have similar reservations about Wakefield's imprinting case). I think there would be a dysfunction if the gosling failed to imprint on a passing porcupine, so long as that porcupine moved about in the right sort of way and if that porcupine entered the gosling's visual field at just the right time. The gosling's disposition would be chronically maladaptive but not dysfunctional.

I suspect that the difference of opinion between Wakefield and myself traces back to the problem of function indeterminacy. For there are two ways of describing the function of the imprinting mechanism in the gosling's brain, and one is more proximal than the next. The first, most proximal description is to say M's function is to cause the gosling to form a strong attachment to the first large, suitably moving object it sees. The second, more distal description is to say M's function is to cause the gosling to have a disposition to follow its mother. The first is more proximal than the second because the mechanism typically causes the gosling to follow its mother *by* causing the gosling to form a strong attachment to the first large, suitably moving object it sees. If we stick with the first description in the porcupine case, we see there is no dysfunction. M has performed its job admirably. If we stick to the second description, we have some evidence of dysfunction (after all, M cannot discharge its function). I have given reasons for my preference for the more proximal description.

It will be seen from the above passages that Garson rests his case against my gosling example completely on his prior acceptance of the proximal-function thesis. However, we have seen that that thesis cannot be given full confidence to reflect our intuitions in various kinds of cases. In fact, the structure of the example fits my "developmental disruption" schema, and the example seems to succeed in illustrating my point and falsifying the proximal-function thesis.

Garson's commentary misses the crucial fact that the imprinting process permanently and irreversibly locates an image of the target of the imprinting in the brain, and so once that occurs, the subsequent failures of function are due not to events in the environment but to the internal state of the gosling. Once the imprinting on the fox takes place, the gosling is incapable even under ideal circumstances—for example, in the presence of its mother—of performing basic functions that are developmentally essential and for which the mother alone is primed to provide a complementary interactor.

In a true developmental disruption, the subsequent trajectory is influenced in ways that are not consistent with selective pressures. This is what happens in the developmental sequence that befalls the gosling. The gosling following its mother triggers many other developmental programs and expectable inputs as the gosling watches its mother hunt for and share food, warm and shelter the gosling with her feathers, protect the gosling from predators, and help the gosling learn and recognize species-specific behaviors and vocalizations, as well as recognize conspecifics so that the gosling can eventually select an appropriate mate. Of course, all this could fail due to a deviant environment where the mother is not available. However, in the misimprinting example, it is not the environment that makes all these later developmental performances impossible. Rather, it is an internal structure in the gosling that makes the gosling incapable of responding to these various stimuli, namely, the permanent and irreversible developmental disruption that occurred when, in the critical window for imprinting, the gosling imprinted on a passing fox rather than its mother. My intuition is that this is a clear dysfunction of the imprinting process despite not being the most proximal function.

Lastly, while my hypothesis does not depend on it, it would be of interest if the above analysis predicted a way that our intuitions about dysfunction in Garson's own *Daphnia* example might be flipped. Here is a possibility: imagine that in a lake without predators, there is pesticide runoff pollution, and it happens that the pollutants have the same chemical signature used by the *Daphnia* to detect the presence of the predators' kairomones. (Note that in actuality, contrary to Garson's characterization, it is not detection of the kairomones that is the most proximal function of the *Daphnia*'s mechanism *M* but detection of the chemical signature by means of which the *Daphnia* detects the kairomones.) So, the most proximal function—detecting a certain chemical signature—is successfully performed. Yet, these *Daphnia* then develop helmets despite the lack of predators during the developmental period and are then severely disadvantaged by the helmets in surviving in the predator-free lake in adulthood. My intuition is that in this case, something has gone wrong and the mechanism *M* suffers a dysfunction in mistaking the pollutant for kairomone. In this case, a distal function—detecting kairomone—fails to be performed and is a dysfunction.

I conclude, first, that Garson's and Neander's proximal-function hypothesis does not fit common intuitions about dysfunction. And, second, the examples I have used in which there are distal dysfunctions despite successful proximal functions, despite being inconsistent with the proximal-function thesis, are entirely in keeping with common intuitions given the special situations of irreversible disruption on which they are based. It is the proximal-function thesis and not my examples that needs fixing.

References

American Psychiatric Association. 2013. *Diagnostic and Statistical Manual of Mental Disorders*. 5th ed. American Psychiatric Association.

Boorse, C. 2002. A rebuttal on functions. In *Functions*, A. Ariew, R. Cummins, and M. Perlman (eds.), 63–112. Oxford University Press.

Dodge, K. A., J. E. Bates, and G. S. Petti. 1990. Mechanisms in the cycle of violence. *Science* 250(4988): 1678–1683.

Dretske, F. 1986. Misrepresentation. In *Belief: Form, Content, and Function*, R. Bogdan (ed.), 17–36. Clarendon.

Neander, K. 1995. Misrepresenting and malfunctioning. *Philosophical Studies* 79: 109–141.

Richters, J., and S. Hinshaw. 1999. The abduction of disorder in psychiatry. *Journal of Abnormal Psychiatry* 108: 438–445.

Wakefield, J. C. 1988. Female primary orgasmic dysfunction: Masters and Johnson versus *DSM-III-R* on diagnosis and incidence. *Journal of Sex Research* 24: 363–377.

Wakefield, J. C. 1999a. Evolutionary versus prototype analyses of the concept of disorder. *Journal of Abnormal Psychology* 108: 374–399.

Wakefield, J. C. 1999b. Mental disorder as a black box essentialist concept. *Journal of Abnormal Psychology* 108: 465–472.

19 Harmful Dysfunction and the Science of Salience: Adaptations and Adaptationism

Philip Gerrans

Jerome Wakefield has proposed a definition of psychiatric disorder as involving an "inability of some internal mechanism to perform its natural function, wherein a natural function is an effect that is part of the evolutionary explanation of the existence and structure of the mechanism" (Wakefield 1992, 384).

The idea is that in psychiatric disorder, a mechanism is not performing the function it was selected for: either because of mechanistic malfunction or perhaps because current environmental conditions are too different from the environment that exerted selective pressure, causing a previously adaptive mechanism to have harmful effects (as when the human preference for high-calorie foods, which evolved as a response to scarcity, leads to diabetes in an environment of abundance). Wakefield is right to say that if we want psychiatric classification to reflect causation, we need to ensure that evolutionary considerations are theoretically incorporated in ways that help reveal underlying neural and cognitive mechanisms. There are, however, different ways to do this.

For strong adaptationists, the surface syndrome that confronts the clinician results from a problem with a cognitive adaptation whose nature can be inferred from the deficit. This, for example, is the aspiration of strong modular theory of mind deficit explanations of autism. The idea here is that some core deficits in social cognition characteristic of autism can be explained in terms of a developmental deficit in a modular capacity for mindreading that evolved as an adaptation for negotiating the social world (Cosmides and Tooby 1994; Baron-Cohen 1996).

It will, however, rarely be the case that a psychiatric disorder can be explained in terms of the (mal)function of a single well-defined cognitive adaptation. Patterns at the surface level, of behavior, belief, or experience, rarely directly reflect the operations of a single domain-specific cognitive system. More often, such patterns result from a cascade (often a developmental cascade) of events that ramify through the cognitive system (Karmiloff-Smith 1994, 1998; Stevens and Price 2000; Gerrans 2002, 2007; Stone and Gerrans 2006; Gerrans and Stone 2008). For this reason, strong adaptationist versions of evolutionary psychiatry are unlikely to succeed in directing us to cognitive or neural mechanisms. They are too "top down" in their analysis of the problem.

This is obvious in the case, for example, of theories that postulate an adaptive problem for which schizophrenic delusions represent a solution (Stevens and Price 2000; Dubrovsky 2002), but the point generalizes.

Once we abandon the strong adaptationist approach in favor of a cognitive neuroscience informed by evolutionary theorizing, psychiatric classification requires substantial revision. Wakefield's approach, I suggest, ultimately leads to abandoning the current *Diagnostic and Statistical Manual of Mental Disorders (DSM)* approach in favor of that that recommended by Dominic Murphy (2006)—namely, to allow classification and psychiatric practice to reflect the architecture of the mind disclosed by cognitive neuroscience. I make my argument via a case study of a, perhaps the, classic psychiatric phenomenon: delusion. Once we focus on mechanistic explanation, the primary role of evolutionary theory will be in the explanation of mechanistic functioning rather than the definition of syndromes.

I.   Mechanisms of Belief Fixation?

It is especially difficult to preserve a taxonomic role for evolutionary theory in the case of psychiatric disorders like delusion, whose classification involves the concept of belief. This is so even though the human cognitive phenotype does show entrenched patterns of belief fixation in specific domains, and some psychiatric disorders can be characterized in terms of typical abnormalities in those patterns (e.g., social cognition is a specific domain and autism is characterized by deficits of belief fixation in that domain). However, those patterns are produced by low-level neurocognitive mechanisms that produce an upward cascade of effects ultimately expressed as patterns of belief fixation. It makes no sense to see these neurocognitive mechanisms, which regulate things like the allocation of cognitive resources to salient information, the anticorrelation of hemispheric activity, and ocular saccades, as cognitive mechanisms selected for forming particular classes of beliefs, although they do have drastic consequences for the type and content of beliefs we are able to form. Rather, they are mechanisms that enable processing of information at specific levels of cognitive complexity, and we can make progress on determining their nature by tracing their evolutionary history at the correct level of cognitive resolution.

Depression illustrates why classifying psychiatric disorders in terms of characteristic patterns of belief abstracts too far from mechanisms. Of course, the *DSM* does not characterize depression in terms of patients' beliefs (although it does refer to ideas, thoughts, and feelings, all "surface-level" phenomena), but the relationship between beliefs and ultimate causes of depressive disorder exemplifies the point I want to make. The patterns of beliefs of severely depressive patients are typically self-accusing, introjective, and profoundly negative, and they express an experience and expectation of failure and hostility in the social world. This is not, however, because of the malfunction of a system designed to produce positive beliefs (perhaps by introducing positive bias into a domain-specific social reasoning system) about personal functioning. Rather, the beliefs of depressive patients express the life experience of someone whose engagement with the world has been disrupted by changes to very low-level cognitive systems (Gerrans and Scherer 2013).

Catherine Harmer and colleagues have examined the relationship between cognitive processing and mood following the administration of selective serotonin reuptake inhibitors (SSRIs) to depressive patients. They found that after one week's administration of serotonin, which changes the balance of norepinephrinergic and serotoninergic activity in the amygdala, patients' amygdala response to masked fearful faces was reduced, and the responses of their facial fusiform areas to happy faces were increased. Patients' explicit judgments about emotional expressions also changed accordingly. Patients were more likely to correctly identify positive emotional expressions, for example. Memory for positive words also increased (for a discussion, see Harmer et al. 2009). These effects have now been demonstrated repeatedly (Harmer 2008; Harmer et al. 2009; Di Simplicio et al. 2012; McCabe et al. 2011). Crucially, these effects occur well below the threshold of explicit awareness. Mood, however, does not remit so quickly, suggesting to Harmer that "antidepressants are able to modify behavioral and neural responses to emotional information without any change in subjective mood. Moreover the changes in emotional processing can be seen across different stimuli types and extend outside conscious awareness" (Harmer et al. 2009, 105).

The point is that the ultimate mechanisms here (or at least those positively affected by treatment) are subcortical systems involved in things like the scanning of faces to extract emotionally salient information. These mechanisms no doubt were selected for, since for humans, the eye region especially transmits information vital to reproductive success. A human who cannot automatically detect and process information about conspecifics' intentions and attitudes is at a huge social disadvantage. Not only that, but when these mechanisms fail to perform their normal role, the psychology of the patient changes drastically. Typically, her experience changes and her beliefs about the world and herself also change to reflect that experience, leading to the profile characteristic of depression. But it is not correct to say that those changes result from changes in a mechanism selected to form beliefs about the patient's prospects in the world.

The more we learn about the deep causal and cognitive structure of many psychiatric disorders, the more we discover about problems with this type of processing. Schizophrenic patients and patients with severe personality disorder also exhibit abnormalities of gaze tracking and face scanning (Green et al. 2000; Green et al. 2003).

These types of mechanisms seem to be precisely the entities described by Wakefield. They are mechanisms selected to perform fundamental aspects of social cognition. However, they appear nowhere in the characterization of depression in the *DSM*, and it is unobvious how their role in producing symptoms could be incorporated as part of the definition of the disorder without a complete reconceptualization of the nature of psychiatric classification.

II. Delusion and the *DSM*

I now turn to the case of delusion, which I shall argue presents similar challenges once we focus on the causally relevant mechanisms. The explanation of delusion requires understanding the selective history of relevant mechanisms, but the properties of those mechanisms have little to do with the concept of belief used in its definition. The *DSM-5* defines delusion as follows:

> Delusions are fixed beliefs that are not amenable to change in light of conflicting evidence. . . . The distinction between a delusion and a strongly held idea is sometimes difficult to make and depends in part on the degree of conviction with which the belief is held despite clear or reasonable contradictory evidence regarding its veracity. (American Psychiatric Association 2013)

This redefinition departs considerably from the definition in *DSM-IV*:

> A false belief based on incorrect inference about external reality that is firmly sustained despite what almost everyone else believes and despite what constitutes incontrovertible and obvious proof or evidence to the contrary. . . . When a false belief involves a value judgment, it is regarded as a delusion only when the judgment is so extreme as to defy credibility. (American Psychiatric Association, 2000)

Philosophers, as well as clinicians, have pointed out problems with the *DSM* definitions. For philosophers and cognitive scientists, the issue is highly salient in debates about the rationality constraint on belief ascription and the relationship between that constraint and theories of cognitive architecture (Stein 1996; Bortolotti 2005, 2009). Clinicians remain acutely interested in a closely related question: whether the difference between delusional and nondelusional belief is a matter of degree or kind. On some views, delusions are toward the end of a continuum of beliefs, which range from accurate beliefs impeccably produced according to canons of procedural rationality to psychoses (Maher 1988, 1999). On other views, delusions are the "hallmark of madness" radically discontinuous with normal beliefs (David 2013). The question of continuity of course matters in the clinic because treatment will vary according to etiology. The problem is complex because delusions are heterogeneous phenomena, ranging from the circumscribed and monothematic neuropsychological delusions to delusions associated with mood disorders and the grandiose and paranoid fantasies of schizophrenia. Thus, the *DSM* term really names a syndrome whose symptoms need to be explained on a case-by-case basis.

This syndrome aspect is exacerbated by the fact that delusions are defined as beliefs. The concept of "belief" itself refers to a syndrome: a pattern of behavior and thought, which, as Ryle put it, "hang together on the same propositional hook" (1949, 135).

There is no reason a priori to think that two believers of the same proposition, delusional or not, would acquire their beliefs in the same way. Testimony, experience, explicit reasoning, and intuition based on tacit cognitive processes can all produce beliefs, and the same belief can issue in different behavior depending on context. Thus, delusional and nondelusional patients can both believe the same proposition; it is the way it is believed that renders a belief a delusion.

Thus, the aim of a theory of delusion is a precise characterization of the difference between delusional and nondelusional subjects in the *way they believe*. And both *DSM* definitions direct us to a crucial feature of the difference: conviction in the face of obvious counterevidence. The idea is that nondelusional people would revise that particular belief in the face of readily available evidence.

The *DSM-IV* and *DSM-5* definitions characterize this doxastic rigidity differently. The *DSM-IV* explicitly invokes the notion of "false belief" and "incorrect inference." The *DSM-IV* thus suggests that the delusional subject is making a reasoning mistake of some kind. The nature and extent of such a mistake, and the validity of importing normative epistemic notions into the characterization of delusion, have been subjects of controversy in cognitive neuropsychiatry and philosophy for three decades now. A recent example is the revived discussion of the applicability of Bayesian principles to the understanding of delusion.

The *DSM-5* potentially sidesteps the problems raised by explicit reliance on normative notions of rational belief fixation, even though it uses the concept of insensitivity to change in the light of "conflicting evidence," which does lend itself to Bayesian theorizing and the project of conceiving delusion as a (possibly degenerate) form of abductive inference (Coltheart et al. 2010). The reason is that there is no essential need to involve normative epistemic concepts in explaining the tenacity of delusional belief. Perhaps the tenacity can be explained in psychological, cognitive, or neurobiological terms without reference to failure of reasoning or hypothesis testing.

Faced with these problems, one can see why one might opt for an evolutionary explanation: perhaps delusional beliefs are produced by malfunction of a module or group of modules designed by evolution to allow us to form beliefs on specific topics? After all, delusions do seem to cluster thematically: erotomania, grandeur, reference, control, paranoia, and so on. Perhaps this domain specificity has an evolutionary explanation. Very likely it does, but inference from delusional content to cognitive architecture will not get it right.

This type of adaptationist approach inherits the goal of evolutionary psychology to render belief fixation cognitively tractable by conceiving of the mind as a set of domain-specific reasoning devices. The mind does not have to search across all hypotheses to explain evidence provided by perception but restricts the search to a small set of hypotheses wired in by evolution. Thus, for example, we are evolved to explain conspecific behavior in terms of (most likely) intentions directed at us. This makes sense. The most relevant information for hominids is social, and false positives have small cost compared to mistakes. Paying too much attention to potentially relevant social signals such as gaze or posture is a benign misallocation of cognitive resources, but missing signs of aggression, alliance, or care can be disastrous.

The problem for adaptationism about belief rather than about domain-specific perceptual systems is that belief, as evidenced by what people say and do, is the output of the integrated functioning of a complex hierarchy of cognitive systems rather than the product of a single specialized system. The construction of abstract representations of reality that integrate sensory or perceptual information with background knowledge is a quintessentially domain-general ability.

In recent literature, we find concepts such as "reality testing" and "belief evaluation" proposed as descriptions of cognitive functions compromised in delusion (Gerrans 2013). These descriptions in effect restate fundamental principles of domain-general rational belief fixation as candidates for cognitive processes that have gone awry in delusion. As such, they are not incorrect: it is true to say that people with delusions are not testing their beliefs against reality or evaluating them for consistency with other beliefs. However, such analyses are really perspicuous redescriptions, rather than theoretical proposals, precisely because they cleave to the language of belief.

The same is true of another recent proposal, the "doxastic shear pin" hypothesis, which in effect proposes a mechanism for what Jaspers referred to as the fundamental reorganization of psychic life produced by delusion (McKay and Dennett 2009). Something that struck Jaspers and early asylum psychiatrists, which is missing from contemporary cognitive accounts, is the peculiar experience of the delusional state and the mesmeric effect it exerts. It seems that (some) delusions are compelled by experiences that, despite their implausibility, are so intense and absorbing that the subject reorganizes her mental life to fit the experience (Jaspers 1968). The idea behind the shear pin hypothesis is that perceptual or sensory processes generate experiences that are so overwhelming that higher-level processing simply cannot cope in the normal manner by trying to make them consistent with rest of the information available to the mind: "The delusion disables flexible, controlled conscious processing from continuing to monitor the mounting...error during delusional mood and thus deters cascading toxicity. At the same time, automatic habitual responses are preserved, possibly even enhanced" (Mishara and Corlett 2009, 531). The delusion is like a safety switch triggered by the mind to deal with a power surge of confusing and distressing information that threatens to short out higher-level processing.

The difficulty with all these proposals is not that they get the phenomena wrong but that they all rely on the language of belief, which is intrinsically agnostic about mechanisms.

III.   Mechanisms and Salience

In fact, however, quite a lot is known about mechanisms implicated in delusion, in the sense that some neural correlates have been identified. However, until the cognitive role played by those correlates is explained and linked to delusion, correlation cannot be transformed into causation.

For schizophrenic delusions, at least, dopaminergic activity has been strongly implicated. Dopamine synthesis during psychosis is abnormal; antipsychotic drugs such as haloperidol are dopamine agonists, and schizophrenic and neurotypical brains differ in the distribution and action of dopamine receptors as well as the activity of dopamine projections from the brainstem to cortical areas (Grace 1991; Murphy et al. 1996; Goldman-Rakic 1997; Gurden et al. 1999; Moore et al. 1999; Jay 2003; Seamans and Yang 2004; Howes and Kapur 2009). So the idea that dopaminergic activity has a causal role to play in the explanation of delusion is irresistible. But we need a theory that links the molecular and neural events to the inability to let go of beliefs triggered by highly anomalous experiences. The *DSM* definition does not help.

At this point, a Wakefieldian might appeal to the idea of an evolved system not performing the function it was selected for: but surely the dopaminergic system did not evolve under selective pressure to produce accurate beliefs. Dopamine regulatory systems exist in all chordates and precursors exist in nonchordates. In the mammalian central nervous system, the dopamine (DA) neurotransmitter systems are diversified. Yamamoto and Vernier note that

> DA acts to modulate early steps of sensory perception in the olfactory bulb and the retina, motor programming, learning, and memory, affective and motivational processes in the forebrain, control of body temperature, food intake, and several other hypothalamic functions as well as chemosensitivity in the area postrema and solitary tract, to cite only the main of the DA-controlled functions. Dysfunction of DA neurotransmission was initially shown in Parkinson's disease.... In addition, DA has now been shown to significantly contribute to the pathophysiology of several psychiatric disorders such as schizophrenia, addiction to drugs, or attention deficit with hyperactivity. (Yamamoto and Vernier 2011, 1)

This is just to point out that a simple adaptationist explanation of the role of DA in delusion, which implicates malfunction in a domain-specific belief fixation system, would be misleading. In fact, it would be a case of psychiatry trying to link neural correlates to symptoms via "the extensive (and expensive) [search] for … non-existent entities" (Halligan and Marshall 1996, 5).

Nonetheless, the dopaminergic system provides a paradigm case of the relevance of evolutionary theory to the explanation of cognition and psychiatric disorder. It also provides a poster child for the successful integration of formal learning theory, computational approaches to the mind, and neuroscience. Explanation of the role of the dopaminergic system invokes two key concepts from computational theory as well as evolutionary ideas: predictive coding and salience (Egelman et al. 1998; Braver et al. 1999; Braver and Cohen 2000; Durstewitz and Seamans 2002).

Predictive coding theories treat the mind as a hierarchically organized cognitive system that uses representations of the world and its own states to control behavior. All levels of the cognitive hierarchy exploit the same principle: error correction (Gottfried et al. 2003; Clark 2013; Hohwy 2013a). Each cognitive system uses models of its domain to predict its future informational states, given actions performed by the organism or its subsystems. When those predictions are satisfied, the model is reinforced; when they are not, the model is revised or updated, and new predictions are generated to govern the process of error correction. Discrepancy between actual and predicted information state is called *surprisal* and represented in the form of an error signal. Error signals are referred to as higher-level supervisory systems. These systems generate an instruction whose execution will cancel the error and minimize surprisal (Friston 2003; Hohwy et al. 2008). The process iterates until error signals are canceled by suitable action.

Thus, on the predictive coding model, the role of cognition is to detect and correct prediction error. When the world and the model of the world being used by the organism (or subsystemic component) match, there is no need to take further action, cognitive or behavioral. This principle applies universally across species (even those with rudimentary control systems we might hesitate to call minds). Even unicellular organisms need to navigate toward nutrients and away from toxins, as well as to learn and remember optimal behavior.

Thus, the most important information for the mind is signals of surprisal or prediction error. Such information is the most *salient* for any cognitive system since it signals misalignment between what the organism is trying to do and what it is actually doing. Not only that, but once the error is corrected, the organism needs to remember that solution and update its model of the world accordingly.

This framework has proved essential to the interpretation of the functioning of the human DA system. The DA system is essentially a salience system: it signals which information is relevant and needs to be the focus of activity. It does so by selectively enhancing activity in neural circuits, which represent salient information, allowing that information to dominate control functions, until an adaptive response is produced (Kapur 2003).

A crucial aspect of DA function is that it solves a problem, formally demonstrable in learning theory and predictive coding models, which recurs urgently in the wild: the problem of *reward prediction*. Consider a foraging squirrel faced by two trees, an oak and a pine. Climbing is exhausting, and only oaks have acorns. Eating acorns is intrinsically rewarding; climbing is not. So the squirrel does not need a reward to learn to eat acorns, any more than humans need to learn to enjoy mother's milk or high-calorie food. As it explores its environment, it needs to learn which trees are worth climbing and install the right, intrinsically unrewarding, instrumental behavior—namely, oak tree foraging. Were we to plant electrodes in the brain of a foraging squirrel, we might initially see activity in salience systems amplifying activity in sensory neural circuits activated by eating acorns. Over time, this activity would be replaced by activity in the salience system amplifying initiation of successful foraging. Ultimately, we would see a spike in the DA system when the squirrel saw an oak tree followed by a lesser spike when it found an acorn and no spike at all if no acorns were found after the climb. The role of a salience system is not to reward success but to *predict reward* for an organism (Schultz et al. 1997; Berridge and Robinson 1998; Gottfried et al. 2003; Heinz and Schlagenhauf 2010; McClure et al. 2003; Egelman et al. 1998; Smith et al. 2006).

In animals like rodents, this type of behavioral biasing is called *incentive salience* since it makes potentially rewarding object motivational magnets (Schultz et al. 1997; Berridge and Robinson 1998, 2003; Braver et al. 1999; Tobler et al. 2005; Kapur 2003; McClure et al. 2003; Smith et al. 2006). Human cognition uses the same dopaminergic salience system at all levels to target cognitive function by selectively enhancing activity in neural circuits processing potentially rewarding information (Braver et al. 1999; Braver and Cohen 2000; Abi-Dargham et al. 2002; Durstewitz and Seamans 2002; Egelman et al. 1998; Goldman-Rakic 1997; Grace 1991).

At the level of brute mechanism, DA enhances the signal-to-noise ratio (SNR) between communicating neural circuits. It does so via the interaction of at least two types of DA action. Phasic DA, delivered in short bursts, binds to D2 receptors on the postsynaptic membrane. It is rapidly removed by reuptake from the synaptic cleft and acts quickly. It is described as producing gating effects: determining which representations are allowed to interrupt and enter controlled processing. Gating is a spatial metaphor; "entry into controlled processing" refers to levels of activation sufficient to capture and retain attention, as well as to monopolize working memory and executive functions. A pattern of neural activation amplified and reinforced by phasic dopamine activity dominates other patterns of activation.

Tonic DA, which acts over longer time scales, accumulates in the synaptic cleft and binds to presynaptic DI autoreceptors triggering reuptake. This contrast between tonic and phasic activity is a ubiquitous neuroregulatory strategy. Tonic levels of a neurochemical are delivered and maintained at steady levels by slow, regular pulses of activity. Phasic activity is intense, staccato, and short-lived, interrupting the ongoing activity maintained by tonic levels.

Phasic and tonic DA are thus antagonists and have different effects on the circuits they afferent. Phasic DA, acting on prefrontal cortical (PFC) posterior circuits, produces a gating effect. It allows new activation patterns in the PFC-posterior circuitry to be formed, allowing representations of new stimuli. Tonic DA maintains an occurrent activation pattern, allowing a process to be sustained against interference or competition. Together, phasic and tonic dopamine provide a mechanism for the updating and maintenance of representations in working memory and thereby bias higher-level information processing adaptively (Arnsten 1998). The hypothesis follows and is consistent with neural network models that the balance of tonic and phasic DA is responsible for the rate of turnover of representations in the PFC-posterior networks (Grace 1991) that represent information required for higher-level cognitive processes. "Tonic DA effects may increase the stability of maintained representations through an increase in the SNR of background versus evoked activity patterns. In contrast, phasic DA effects may serve as a gating signal indicating when new inputs should be encoded and maintained" (Braver et al. 1999, 317).

This reward prediction framework tells us that the balance of tonic and phasic dopamine delivery would modulate the salience of representations at different levels, influencing learning, memory, planning, and decision and motivation. Furthermore, since unpredicted activity, which constitutes surprisal, is most salient and likely to be referred to as controlled processing, phasic dopamine activity that interrupts ongoing activity should be associated with novelty.

These predictions are borne out in single neuron studies of the ventral tegmentum area (VTA) of rats in a variety of paradigms. For example, in a conditioning paradigm, in the learning phase, dopamine neurons fire for the reward (Waelti et al. 2001; Montague et al. 1996; Schultz et al. 1997). As the association is learned, firing for the reward is reduced, and dopamine neurons fire for the instrumental behavior. In other words, they predict reward (Waelti et al. 2001, 43). Firing of dopamine neurons is modulated by nonarrival of predicted reward "in a manner compatible with the coding of prediction errors" (Waelti et al. 2001, 43). These neurons also respond to novel attention-generating and motivational stimuli.

In other words, it seems that the role of the dopamine system is to focus cognition on relevant stimuli. Events consistent with predictions produce less phasic activity in the dopamine system than novel (i.e., unpredicted) and affectively valenced (good or bad for the organism) events. Not only that, but once the associations are learned, dopamine functions as a reward prediction system, increasing firing for instrumental activity but reducing firing if the reward does not arrive.

As new cortical systems were layered over older ones, enabling higher levels of control and more abstract forms of representation, they inherited the same problems of resource allocation and adopted preexisting mechanistic solutions. In fact, we can see higher cognition as cognitive foraging: a search through representational space for relevant information. Thinking about lying on the beach is time wasting in the office but a vital use of cognitive resources at the travel agency deciding between holidays in Tahiti and Phuket. Imagining dying of skin cancer is ridiculous time wasting in the office but sensible cognitive resource allocation at the beach.

Higher levels of cognition face the same problems of adaptive biasing and exploit the same ancient mechanisms (Gottfried et al. 2003) to recapitulate the temporal structure of reward prediction. For example, neurons in the ventromedial prefrontal cortex, a structure implicated in almost all personal higher-level cognitive processes, are innervated by the dopamine system and exhibit the same patterns of interaction with it in learning tasks as lower-level systems.

IV. Dopamine and Delusion

The idea that the mind is a hierarchical control system using predictive coding principles, which depend crucially on salience systems, has an important implication for the explanation of delusion. Those experiences that signal surprisal will naturally dominate high-level cognition since it evolved to enable adaptive responses to problems that exceed the processing capacities of lower-level systems. The salience system will interact with the neural circuits that refer these problems, amplifying their activity (increasing the "gain" is the technical term in neural network theory) and thereby making them the focus of attention.

Against this background, the explanation of the role of the dopamine system in delusion turns out to be not so much a discrete psychological puzzle but a piece in the larger puzzle of understanding the relationships between lower- and higher-level control systems and the salience systems that modulate them. A brief survey of recent work shows just how far a deep understanding of delusion in terms of the processing of salient information takes us away from its characterization in terms of beliefs.

Recent work on the dopamine hypothesis of schizophrenia has concentrated on the role of dopamine in the salience system, comparing levels of phasic dopamine delivery in conditioning and learning paradigms to that of normal subjects. The basic idea is that in psychosis, the "wrong" representations become salient, and relevant novel information is not processed. At low levels, this is reflected in attentional deficits; at higher levels, it is reflected in failure to allocate metacognitive function appropriately. At all levels, what counts as surprisal (prediction error) is different for the schizophrenic mind as a consequence of abnormalities in the way the salience system works. Summarizing a range of studies, Heinz and Schlagenhauf express a developing consensus: "The blunted difference between relevant and irrelevant stimuli and outcomes may reflect chaotic attribution of salience to otherwise irrelevant cues, an interpretation that is in accordance with the idea that chaotic or stress-induced dopamine firing can interfere with salience attribution in schizophrenia" (2010, 477).

The salience interpretation of the dopamine system theory provides a unifying explanation of features of schizophrenia, including the characteristic phenomenology of the prodromal period in which subjects feel that events or objects are extremely significant and/or that they are hypersensitive. As Heinz and Schlagenhauf (2010, 474) put it, dopamine dysfunction may be particularly prominent during the early stages of schizophrenia before delusional mood is transformed into fixed and rigid patterns of delusion.

Transient episodes of felt significance are not abnormal, but in delusional subjects, dopamine dysregulation ensures that their hypersalience gives representations of objects or scenes a halo of significance and ensures that they continue to dominate attention working memory and executive function (Di Forti et al. 2007; Moore et al. 1999; Abi-Dargham et al. 2002; Grace 1991; Howes and Kapur 2009; Braver et al. 1999; Broome et al. 2005).

Following Laruelle and Abi-Dargham (1999), Kapur describes dopamine as "the wind of psychotic fire" (Kapur 2003, 14), which ensures that activity in circuits referring and processing delusion-related information increases to levels that make reallocation of resources to nondelusional information impossible for the psychotic subject.

A delusion is a response to that constant referral of surprisal, a "top-down cognitive phenomenon that the individual imposes on these experiences of aberrant salience in order to make sense of them" (Kapur 2003, 15). Once adopted, the delusion "serves as a cognitive scheme for further thoughts and actions. It drives the patients to find further confirmatory evidence—in the glances of strangers, the headlines of newspapers, and the tiepins of newsreaders" (Kapur 2003, 16). The effect of hypersalience is to entrench the delusion.

Mishara and Corlett (2009) wed this idea to the doxastic shear pin hypothesis, suggesting that prediction error signals from sensory systems are generated, amplified, and referred up the control hierarchy in delusion in a way that simply floods the executive systems with hypersalient information they cannot deal with (Hohwy and Rajan 2012; Hohwy 2013b):

> Delusions…involve a "reorganization" of the patient's experience to maintain behavioral interaction with the environment despite the underlying disruption to perceptual binding processes.…The delusion disables flexible, controlled conscious processing from continuing to monitor the mounting distress of the wanton prediction error during delusional mood and thus deters cascading toxicity. At the same time, automatic habitual responses are preserved, possibly even enhanced. (Mishara and Corlett 2009, 531)

Conclusion

Clearly, this is not the place to evaluate the neuroscience of schizophrenia, only to note that recent research converges on the idea that one important symptom (delusion) can be explained in terms of aberrant activity in the salience system, which amplifies and refers prediction errors that high-level control systems cannot cancel.

Wakefield is surely right that the explanation of this phenomenon involves the functioning of a salience system "designed" by evolution, which is either malfunctioning (making the wrong information salient) or, if it is functioning correctly (referring prediction error in the form of anomalous experience), warping the functioning of other systems with which it interacts. The explanation of salience outlined above makes use of evolutionary ideas all the way through.

Assuming that the science of salience is on track, how should the classification of psychiatric disorders involving the salience system proceed? It is worth noting, for example, that the salience system is implicated not only in delusion but also in addiction and attention-deficit/hyperactivity disorder. We could, in principle, reclassify these psychiatric disorders as members of a family of *disorders of the salience system*.

My own view is that Wakefield, by directing attention to mechanistic functioning and evolved cognitive architecture, may be advocating a far more radical approach to classification than he thought—one in which the everyday or folk conception of psychiatric phenomena is replaced entirely. Or perhaps, if not replaced, it will survive as something like the Mendelian concept of a gene: a bit of folk shorthand useful for introducing an entity in terms of its phenomenology but ultimately not part of scientific understanding. I think that the right approach here is the radical one: a complete reconceptualization of the phenomenon using the vocabulary of cognitive neuroscience, informed by, but not necessarily invoking, evolutionary theory.

References

Abi-Dargham, A., O. Mawlawi, I. Lombardo, R. Gil, D. Martinez, Y. Huang, D. R. Hwang, J. Keilp, L. Kochan, R. Van Heertum, J. M. Gorman, and M. Laruelle. 2002. Prefrontal dopamine D1 receptors and working memory in schizophrenia. *Journal of Neuroscience* 22(9): 3708–3719.

American Psychiatric Association. 2000. *Diagnostic and Statistical Manual of Mental Disorders*. 4th ed (text revision). American Psychiatric Association.

American Psychiatric Association. 2013. *Diagnostic and Statistical Manual of Mental Disorders*. 5th ed. American Psychiatric Association.

Arnsten, A. F. T. 1998. Catecholamine modulation of prefrontal cortical cognitive function. *Trends in Cognitive Sciences* 2(11): 436–447.

Baron-Cohen, S. 1996. *Mindblindness: An Essay on Autism and Theory of Mind*. MIT Press.

Berridge, K. C., and T. E. Robinson. 1998. What is the role of dopamine in reward: Hedonic impact, reward learning, or incentive salience? *Brain Research Reviews* 28(3): 309–369.

Berridge, K. C., and T. E. Robinson. 2003. Parsing reward. *Trends in Neurosciences* 26(9): 507–513.

Bortolotti, L. 2005. Delusions and the background of rationality. *Mind and Language* 20(2): 189–208.

Bortolotti, L. 2009. Delusion. In *The Stanford Encyclopedia of Philosophy*, E. N. Zalta (ed.), Winter 2013. http://plato.stanford.edu/archives/win2013/entries/delusion/. August 18, 2014.

Braver, T. S., D. M. Barch, and J. D. Cohen. 1999. Cognition and control in schizophrenia: A computational model of dopamine and prefrontal function. *Biological Psychiatry* 46(3): 312–328.

Braver, T. S., and J. D. Cohen. 2000. On the control of control: The role of dopamine in regulating prefrontal function and working memory. In *Control of Cognitive Processes: Attention and Performance XVIII*, S. Monsell and J. Driver (eds.), 713–737. MIT Press.

Broome, M. R., J. B. Woolley, P. Tabraham, L. C. Johns, E. Bramon, G. K. Murray, C. Pariante, P. K. McGuire, and R. M. Murray. 2005. What causes the onset of psychosis? *Schizophrenia Research* 79(1): 23–34.

Clark, A. 2013. Whatever next? Predictive brains, situated agents, and the future of cognitive science. *Behavioral and Brain Sciences* 36(3): 181–253.

Coltheart, M., P. Menzies, and J. Sutton. 2010. Abductive inference and delusional belief. *Cognitive Neuropsychiatry* 15(1–3): 261–287.

Cosmides, L., and J. Tooby. 1994. Beyond intuition and instinct blindness: Toward an evolutionarily rigorous cognitive science. *Cognition* 50(1): 41–77.

David, T. 2013. Delusions: Not on a continuum with normal beliefs. In *Imperfect Cognitions: Blog on Delusional Beliefs, Distorted Memories, Confabulatory Explanations, and Implicit Biases*, L. Bortolotti and E. Sullivan-Bissett (eds.). http://imperfectcognitions.blogspot.com.au/2013/10/delusions-are-hallmark-of-madness.html. August 20, 2014.

Di Forti, M., J. M. Lappin, and R. M. Murray. 2007. Risk factors for schizophrenia: All roads lead to dopamine. *European Neuropsychopharmacology* 17(suppl. 2): S101–S107.

Di Simplicio, M., R. Norbury, and C. J. Harmer. 2012. Short-term antidepressant administration reduces negative self-referential processing in the medial prefrontal cortex in subjects at risk for depression. *Molecular Psychiatry* 17(5): 503–510.

Dubrovsky, B. 2002. Evolutionary psychiatry: Adaptationist and nonadaptationist conceptualizations. *Progress in Neuro-Psychopharmacology and Biological Psychiatry* 26(1): 1–19.

Durstewitz, D., and J. K. Seamans. 2002. The computational role of dopamine D1 receptors in working memory. *Neural Networks* 15(4–6): 561–572.

Egelman, D. M., C. Person, and P. R. Montague. 1998. A computational role for dopamine delivery in human decision making. *Journal of Cognitive Neuroscience* 10(5): 623–630.

Friston, K. 2003. Learning and inference in the brain. *Neural Networks* 16(9): 1325–1352.

Gerrans, P. 2002. The theory of mind module in evolutionary psychology. *Biology and Philosophy* 17(3): 305–321.

Gerrans, P. 2007. Mechanisms of madness: Evolutionary psychiatry without evolutionary psychology. *Biology and Philosophy* 22(1): 35–56.

Gerrans, P. 2013. Delusional attitudes and default thinking. *Mind & Language* 28(1): 83–102.

Gerrans, P., and K. Scherer. 2013. Wired for despair: The neurochemistry of emotion and the phenomenology of depression. *Journal of Consciousness Studies* 20(7–8): 254–268.

Gerrans, P., and V. E. Stone. 2008. Generous or parsimonious cognitive architecture? Cognitive neuroscience and theory of mind. *British Journal for the Philosophy of Science* 59(2): 121–141.

Goldman-Rakic, P. S. 1997. The cortical dopamine system: Role in memory and cognition. *Advances in Pharmacology* 42: 707–711.

Gottfried, J. A., J. O'Doherty, and R. J. Dolan. 2003. Encoding predictive reward value in human amygdala and orbitofrontal cortex. *Science* 301(5636): 1104–1107.

Grace, A. A. 1991. Phasic versus tonic dopamine release and the modulation of dopamine system responsivity: A hypothesis for the etiology of schizophrenia. *Neuroscience* 41(1): 1–24.

Green, M. J., L. M. Williams, and D. Davidson. 2003. Visual scanpaths to threat-related faces in deluded schizophrenia. *Psychiatry Research* 119(3): 271–285.

Green, M. J., L. M. Williams, and D. R. Hemsley. 2000. Cognitive theories of delusion formation: The contribution of visual scanpath research. *Cognitive Neuropsychiatry* 5(1): 63–74.

Gurden, H., J.-P. Tassin, and T. M. Jay. 1999. Integrity of the mesocortical dopaminergic system is necessary for complete expression of in vivo hippocampal–prefrontal cortex long-term potentiation. *Neuroscience* 94(4): 1019–1027.

Halligan, P. W., and J. C. Marshall (eds.). 1996. *Method in Madness: Case Studies in Cognitive Neuropsychiatry*. Psychology Press.

Harmer, C. J. 2008. Serotonin and emotional processing: Does it help explain antidepressant drug action? *Neuropharmacology* 55(6): 1023–1028.

Harmer, C. J., G. M. Goodwin, and P. J. Cowen. 2009. Why do antidepressants take so long to work? A cognitive neuropsychological model of antidepressant drug action. *British Journal of Psychiatry* 195(2): 102–108.

Heinz, A., and F. Schlagenhauf. 2010. Dopaminergic dysfunction in schizophrenia: Salience attribution revisited. *Schizophrenia Bulletin* 36(3): 472–485.

Hohwy, J. 2013a. *The Predictive Mind*. Oxford University Press.

Hohwy, J. 2013b. Delusions, illusions and inference under uncertainty. *Mind and Language* 28(1): 57–71.

Hohwy, J., and V. Rajan. 2012. Delusions as forensically disturbing perceptual inferences. *Neuroethics* 5(1): 5–11.

Hohwy, J., A. Roepstorff, and K. Friston. 2008. Predictive coding explains binocular rivalry: An epistemological review. *Cognition* 108(3): 687–701.

Howes, O. D., and S. Kapur. 2009. The dopamine hypothesis of schizophrenia: Version III—the final common pathway. *Schizophrenia Bulletin* 35(3): 549–562.

Jaspers, K. 1968. The phenomenological approach in psychopathology. *British Journal of Psychiatry* 114(516): 1313–1323.

Jay, T. M. 2003. Dopamine: A potential substrate for synaptic plasticity and memory mechanisms. *Progress in Neurobiology* 69(6): 375–390.

Kapur, S. 2003. Psychosis as a state of aberrant salience: A framework linking biology, phenomenology and pharmacology in schizophrenia. *American Journal of Psychiatry* 160(1): 13–23.

Karmiloff-Smith, A. 1994. Beyond modularity: A developmental perspective on cognitive science. *International Journal of Language & Communication Disorders* 29(1): 95–105.

Karmiloff-Smith, A. 1998. Development itself is the key to understanding developmental disorders. *Trends in Cognitive Sciences* 2(10): 389–398.

Laruelle, M., and A. Abi-Dargham. 1999. Dopamine as the wind of the psychotic fire: New evidence from brain imagining studies. *Journal of Psychopharmacology* 13(4): 358–371.

Maher, B. A. 1988. Anomalous experiences and delusional thinking: The logic of explanation. In *Delusional Beliefs: Interdisciplinary Perspectives,* T. E. Oltmanns and B. A. Maher (eds.). Wiley.

Maher, B. A. 1999. Anomalous experience in everyday life: Its significance for psychopathology. *The Monist* 82(4): 547–570.

McCabe, C., Z. Mishor, N. Filippini, P. J. Cowen, M. J. Taylor, and C. Harmer. 2011. SSRI administration reduces resting state functional connectivity in dorso-medial prefrontal cortex. *Molecular Psychiatry* 16(6): 592–594.

McClure, S. M., N. D. Daw, and P. R. Montague. 2003. A computational substrate for incentive salience. *Trends in Neurosciences* 26(8): 423–428.

McKay, R. T., and D. C. Dennett. 2009. The evolution of misbelief. *Behavioral and Brain Sciences* 32(6): 493–510.

Mishara, A. L., and P. Corlett. 2009. Are delusions biologically adaptive? Salvaging the doxastic shear pin. *Behavioral and Brain Sciences* 32(6): 530–531.

Montague, P. R., P. Dayan, and T. J. Sejnowski. 1996. A framework for mesencephalic dopamine systems based on predictive Hebbian learning. *Journal of Neuroscience* 16(5): 1936–1947.

Moore, H., A. R. West, and A. A. Grace. 1999. The regulation of forebrain dopamine transmission: Relevance to the pathophysiology and psychopathology of schizophrenia. *Biological Psychiatry* 46(1): 40–55.

Murphy, B. L., A. F. Arnsten, P. S. Goldman-Rakic, and R. H. Roth. 1996. Increased dopamine turnover in the prefrontal cortex impairs spatial working memory performance in rats and monkeys. *Proceedings of the National Academy of Sciences* 93(3): 1325–1329.

Murphy, D. 2006. *Psychiatry in the Scientific Image.* MIT Press.

Ryle, G. 1949. *The Concept of Mind.* Hutchinson.

Schultz, W., P. Dayan, and P. R. Montague. 1997. A neural substrate of prediction and reward. *Science* 275(5306):1593–1599.

Seamans, J. K., and C. R. Yang. 2004. The principal features and mechanisms of dopamine modulation in the prefrontal cortex. *Progress in Neurobiology* 74(1): 1–58.

Smith, A., M. Li, S. Becker, and S. Kapur. 2006. Dopamine, prediction error and associative learning: a model-based account. *Network: Computation in Neural Systems* 17(1): 61–84.

Stein, E. 1996. *Without Good Reason: The Rationality Debate in Philosophy and Cognitive Science.* Oxford University Press.

Stevens, A., and J. Price. 2000. *Evolutionary Psychiatry: A New Beginning.* 2nd ed. Routledge.

Stone, V. E., and P. Gerrans. 2006. What's domain-specific about theory of mind? *Social Neuroscience* 1(3–4): 309–319.

Tobler, P. N., C. D. Fiorillo, and W. Schultz. 2005. Adaptive coding of reward value by dopamine neurons. *Science* 307(5715): 1642–1645.

Waelti, P., A. Dickinson, and W. Schultz. 2001. Dopamine responses comply with basic assumptions of formal learning theory. *Nature* 412(6842): 43–48.

Wakefield, J. C. 1992. The concept of mental disorder: On the boundary between biological facts and social values. *American Psychologist* 47(3): 373–388.

Yamamoto, K., and P. Vernier. 2011. The evolution of dopamine systems in chordates. *Frontiers in Neuroanatomy* 5(21): 1–21.

20   Are Cognitive Neuroscience and the Harmful Dysfunction Analysis Competitors or Allies? Reply to Philip Gerrans

Jerome Wakefield

I thank Philip Gerrans for his lucid and fascinating exploration of the developing interface between cognitive neuroscience and psychiatric nosology as seen through the prism of salience theory and related cognitive neuroscientific theories, and for his assessment of the relationship of these developments to my harmful dysfunction analysis (HDA) of medical, including mental, disorder. The HDA claims that "disorder" refers to "harmful dysfunction," where dysfunction is the failure of some feature to perform a natural function for which it is biologically designed by evolutionary processes and harm is judged in accordance with social values (First and Wakefield 2010, 2013; Spitzer 1997, 1999; Wakefield 1992a, 1992b, 1993, 1995, 1997a, 1997b, 1997c, 1997d, 1998, 1999a, 1999b, 2000a, 2000b, 2001, 2006a, 2007, 2009, 2011, 2014, 2016a, 2016b; Wakefield and First 2003, 2012).

I am excited by Gerrans's attempt in his work on the salience system to bring together an understanding of neurocognitive mechanisms with the phenomenological quality of lived experience, a long overdue but elusive synthesis. Although I sympathize with much of Gerrans's position and aspirations, I focus here on some areas of possible disagreement—"possible" because Gerrans writes with a light rhetorical touch that sometimes leaves his claims ambiguous. I see three primary areas of possible disagreement: the demoted heuristic role rather than conceptually fundamental role that Gerrans suggests for biological design and evolution and thus for the HDA in a neuropsychiatric theory of psychopathology, the sharp dichotomy Gerrans sees between what he calls "evolutionary psychology" or "strong adaptationism" and cognitive neuroscience, and the notion that there is a radical discontinuity between the sorts of insights he pursues and the aspirations of the *Diagnostic and Statistical Manual of Mental Disorders* (*DSM*). In exploring these claims, I will also make reference to the related views of Dominic Murphy, whom Gerrans cites.

Mechanical-Causal and Biological-Design Analyses as Complementary in a Theory of Disorder

First, then, is mechanical-causal analysis enough for a theory of psychopathology? Despite agreement that evolutionary theory is relevant to the theory of psychopathology, there seems to be a fundamental divergence between Gerrans and me on the nature of the role of evolutionary theory in an account of psychopathology. Gerrans agrees that evolutionary analysis applies to the neuroscientific salience systems he describes:

> Wakefield is surely right that the explanation of this phenomenon involves the functioning of a salience system "designed" by evolution, which is either malfunctioning (making the wrong information salient) or, if it is functioning correctly...warping the functioning of other systems with which it interacts. The explanation of salience outlined above makes use of evolutionary ideas all the way through.

On first glance, this passage seems to suggest an HDA approach. However, Gerrans also distances himself from the HDA's view that evolutionary theory provides a unique and essential conceptual foundation for disorder judgments. He construes evolutionary insight rather as a useful heuristic for constructing neuroscientific causal-mechanical explanations of symptoms:

> Wakefield is right to say that if we want psychiatric classification to reflect causation, we need to ensure that evolutionary considerations are theoretically incorporated in ways that help reveal underlying neural and cognitive mechanisms. There are, however, different ways to do this....Once we abandon the strong adaptationist approach in favor of a cognitive neuroscience informed by evolutionary theorizing, psychiatric classification requires substantial revision....I think that the right approach here is the radical one: a complete reconceptualization of the phenomenon using the vocabulary of cognitive neuroscience, informed by, but not necessarily invoking, evolutionary theory.

I will get to "different ways to do this," "strong adaptationism," and why classification "requires substantial revision" later. For now, observe that evolutionary considerations are important to Gerrans because they can "help reveal underlying neural and cognitive mechanisms." Evolution is thus demoted from the HDA's requirement that biological design must be explicitly or implicitly invoked in identifying a neurocognitive condition as psychopathology (more on this in a moment, too) to a consideration in which cognitive neuroscience is merely "informed by" evolutionary theorizing as a perspective that can yield additional insights in hypothesizing mechanisms, a vague and noncommittal relationship with no conceptual bite.

So far as I can tell, the reason that Gerrans—like Dominic Murphy, whom he cites—distances himself from the HDA's evolutionary framework for disorder judgments is that he believes that the HDA's evolutionary perspective is somehow in tension with or an alternative to the neuroscience agenda, rather than a complement to it. However, the idea that the HDA favors evolutionary explanation *over* mechanistic neuroscientific explanation confuses the conceptual-analytic and scientific-theory domains. It makes no sense on its face because an evolutionary explanation is based on and supported by a detailed understanding of the design-like characteristics of mechanisms, neurocognitive or otherwise, and their causal interactions. Even Tinbergen's (1963) classic list of four necessary components of an evolutionary explanation includes a mechanistic-causal understanding of how an evolved system works as essential to any such undertaking. More recently, the HDA was reportedly an inspiration for the National Institute of Mental Health's (NIMH's) Research Domain Criteria (RDoC) project to identify brain circuitry dysfunctions underlying psychopathology (see my reply to Demazeux in this volume), which suggests that NIMH understands the implications of the HDA better than do Gerrans and Murphy. In any event, for practical clinical interventive purposes, a mechanistic understanding of disorders is obviously of overwhelming importance. So, *of course* we should seek a mechanistic-causal understanding, including relevant cognitive neuroscientific mechanisms, that explains disorder symptoms. Such an analysis is totally consistent with, encouraged by, and complementary to the HDA.

It is true that often we can tell from superficial symptoms that something is going wrong with biologically designed processes, thus that there exists some dysfunction, long before we have the slightest idea of the nature of the relevant mechanisms and their functions and dysfunctions. Thus, it may misleadingly appear that evolutionary theorizing can proceed without the need for understanding of underlying neural mechanisms, when in fact an eventual combination of evolutionary and mechanistic-causal explanation is essential to understanding psychopathology.

In discussing delusions and other mental disorders, Gerrans repeatedly uses the language of dysfunction of biologically designed mechanisms ("dopamine dysfunction"; "dopamine dysregulation"; "hypersalience"; "abnormal"; "aberrant activity"), clearly placing his discussion within the domain of psychopathology. However, given that all neurocognitive functioning, whether normal or disordered, can be mechanistically characterized, what makes a neuroscientifically analyzed condition pathological and thus justifies applying the disorder/nondisorder distinction to the described conditions? Gerrans's notion that the discovery of mechanical causal principles is "informed by" evolution misses the fundamental nature of the biological-design analysis, which is to justify disorder attribution. There is no way to draw the disorder/nondisorder distinction among mechanistically described systems without an evolutionary perspective that allows one to judge whether something has gone wrong with their biologically designed functioning.

For example, certain patterns of neuronal firing in the mouse brain cause a male mouse to sexually mount a receptive female, certain patterns of firing of nearby neurons cause the same mouse to attack an encroaching male, and yet a third pattern of firing involving an overlapping region causes the mouse to attack a receptive female

(Anderson 2012; Lin et al. 2011). These are all equally good mechanical neuroscientific elaborations of causal relations. However, two of them are plausibly normal behavior and the other is plausibly pathological. To make this distinction, an evolutionary perspective on biological design must be imposed on the causal grid. Gerrans (and Murphy) ignore this additional step and thus cannot turn a mechanical-causal theory into a medical conceptualization of disorder versus nondisorder. (For further comments on this point, see my reply to Murphy in this volume.)

In a recent article (see also his chapter in this volume), Dominic Murphy seems to edge toward recognizing that a sheerly neurobiological causal description does not by itself validly distinguish disorder from nondisorder and that some additional factual criterion is needed:

> There is an important sense in which diagnoses cannot be validated at all, if by "validation" we mean "shown to be a real disorder." All validation can do is show that a pattern of behaviour deemed to be clinically significant depends on a physical process. Whether that pattern of behaviour is really pathological—rather than immoral or harmlessly odd—is another matter. ... It requires that judgements of pathology be like findings of positive charge, i.e. scientifically grounded, rather than judgements of ugliness, i.e. human responses. If so, there has to be some natural fact of the matter about whether some physical system is dysfunctional. If this cannot be done, then predictions about physical states can be validated, but disorders cannot be. (Murphy 2017, 4–5)

The solution to the conundrum posed by Murphy in this passage—the need for an extra fact beyond all the neuroscientific facts to warrant a scientifically objective attribution of dysfunction—is simply that a dysfunction is the failure of a naturally selected function. This is a historical fact about the biological design of the described neurobiological system in relation to its current performance, so it is an additional fact beyond all the cross-sectional neurobiological descriptive facts. Indeed, of two identically describable mechanical systems, one can be properly functioning and the other dysfunctioning given divergent evolutionary histories (Wakefield 1999a). The HDA and neuroscientific mechanical-causal elucidation are necessarily complementary elements in the analysis of mental disorder.

Neuroscience versus Evolutionary Psychology in the Quest for Dysfunctions

Although receptive to bringing evolutionary considerations into the theory of mental disorder, Gerrans notes that there are various ways one might do this, and he has several concerns about what he thinks is the HDA's specific approach to evolutionary explanation. Gerrans apparently equates the HDA's evolutionary understanding with two approaches that he calls "evolutionary psychology" and "strong adaptationism" and rejects both of the latter views. Additionally, he is particularly skeptical of evolutionary psychological explanations of pathological belief fixation.

First, then, regarding evolutionary psychology, both in his paper in this volume and in his broader work (e.g., Gerrans 2002, 2007; Gerrans and Stone 2008; Stone and Gerrans 2006), Gerrans emphasizes the fallibility of commonsense inferences shaped by folk-psychological constructs from the nature of overt symptoms to the postulation of dysfunctions in specific dedicated neurocognitive mechanisms that fit our folk-theoretic schemas. Thus, it is all too easy to postulate "sadness regulating mechanisms," "jealousy regulating mechanisms," "self-esteem regulating mechanisms," and so on. However, the brain works its wonders in mysterious ways that evolved under obscure fitness pressures constrained by unknown earlier adaptations, so, Gerrans argues, surface psychological phenomena are often no royal road to elucidating the structure of the deeper levels of processing that give rise to them.

Gerrans's prototypical example of the evolutionary psychology fallacy is the inference from autistic individuals' difficulty understanding others' intentional states to the postulation of a dedicated "theory of mind" module that is dysfunctional, when in fact the difficulty may be due to dysfunctions in deeper and much more general neurocognitive mechanisms that happen to manifest in theory-of-mind difficulties. It is the hypothesizing of such symptom-close dedicated cognitive modules formulated in terms of folk-psychological experienced variables that Gerrans labels "evolutionary psychology." He contrasts evolutionary psychology with explanation in terms of a combination of both deeper neuroscientific mechanisms (e.g., the salience mechanisms he describes at length that might amplify the salience of certain ideas to the point of delusion) and perceptual-surface neuroprocessing levels (e.g., automatic facial interpretation mechanisms that might bias toward seeing disapproval and thus toward depression) that he considers to be less folk-psychologically inspired and to constitute a more scientific "cognitive neuroscience." (I tend to understand "evolutionary psychology" less narrowly as a general discipline that encompasses all evolutionary understanding of psychological processes, but I will stick to Gerrans's usage here.)

Gerrans rebukes evolutionary psychology, and (I surmise) by implication the HDA, as follows:

> It will, however, rarely be the case that a psychiatric disorder can be explained in terms of the (mal)function of a single well-defined cognitive adaptation. Patterns at the surface level, of behavior, belief, or experience, rarely directly reflect the operations of a single domain-specific cognitive system. More often, such patterns result from a cascade (often a developmental cascade) of events that ramify through the cognitive system.

Any identification by Gerrans of the HDA with his target of evolutionary psychology in the above passage is a mistake. There is nothing in the HDA that says that the cognitive adaptations that constitute psychological functions must be "single, well-defined" or "single, domain-specific" adaptations or mechanisms, nor that the nature of mechanisms and their functions and dysfunctions must be able to be specifiable by directly reading them off from the "surface level, of behavior, belief, or experience." There is nothing in the HDA that precludes that a dysfunction can result from or even be constituted by a "cascade ... of events." (That comment by Gerrans seems to leave the door open to something going wrong with salience mechanisms that percolates higher and causes a more specific dysfunction in a particular "evolutionary psychology" middle-level regulating system.) I have argued elsewhere that dysfunctions can even occur in pathological-level interactions between mismatched individual mechanisms that are each individually performing within their normal ranges (Wakefield 1999a, 2006b). The HDA only asserts that to be a disorder, the explanation must attribute the harmful symptoms to *some* dysfunction of biologically designed mechanisms.

My extensive explanations of why dyslexia is considered a disorder despite reading not being selected for make clear that there need be no commonsense relationship between the function of the inferred dysfunctional mechanism and the nature of the consequent symptoms, other than a causal one. An inference from symptoms to the presence of a dysfunction that supports a provisional disorder judgment can be so weak as to be a sheerly existential hypothesis that a dysfunction exists in some mechanism, based on circumstantial evidence and remaining noncommittal on the kinds of mechanisms, functions, and dysfunctions involved. After that, it is scientific open season to theorize about the nature of the mechanisms, their function, and their dysfunctions. This takes time; in physical medicine, it was over 2,000 years from the time Hippocrates inferred a series of diagnostic categories to a scientific understanding of the mechanisms, functions, and dysfunctions underlying many of his categories. A measure of the surprising strength of the circumstantial evidence that supports such dysfunction inferences is that Hippocrates's speculative theories about etiology were wildly wrong, yet virtually every category he baptized has turned out to consist of what we still consider genuine disorders, although of course reorganized and relabeled as etiological knowledge increased.

Gerrans is surely correct that the facile inference from symptoms to the existence of a certain type of underlying biologically designed domain-specific middle-range modular brain mechanism and a certain kind of dysfunction of that mechanism can all too often be an unsupported projection of folk-theoretic notions, giving rise to infamous "just-so stories." For this reason, I tend to exert restraint and entertain skepticism about many evolutionary psychological explanations until adequate potentially falsifying testing occurs, and this is one reason why, throughout my work, I rarely discuss or endorse specific evolutionary psychological or cognitive neuroscientific hypotheses. Yet, it should also be kept in mind that the "just-so story" problem is a general one, and most science-based theorizing initially gets things wrong. Clever and ruthless potentially falsifying testing of theories leading to revisions that correct detected errors, not a priori specification of what kinds of hypotheses are allowable, is what makes science powerful and progressive.

If there is the sort of rivalry between "evolutionary psychology" and "cognitive neuroscience" that Gerrans portrays, the HDA is neutral on the outcome. The HDA mainly predicts the relationship between background beliefs about causation and consequent disorder attribution (see my reply to De Vreese in this volume for further elaboration of this point). Thus, in arguing for the HDA, I generally attempt to show that beliefs about biological design shape judgments about disorder versus nondisorder. So, my examples often cite current theories as examples of background beliefs. However, the theories' correctness or incorrectness is not relevant, except when I go beyond conceptual analysis and argue for substantive claims about what is and is not a disorder, as Allan Horwitz and I did in arguing for the invalidity of *DSM*'s major depression category in *The Loss of Sadness* (2007). Thus, whether or not the theory-of-mind module theory of autistic pathology turns out to be correct, it supports the HDA because those who believe the theory-of-mind modular account believe that autism is the harmful effect of a dysfunction in the hypothesized biologically designed module and consequently judge it a disorder. Equally supportive of the HDA are "neurodiversity" accounts of autism that are opposed to the "theory-of-mind" account, because they deny that autism is a disorder and thus are forced to argue that it is not due to a dysfunction (see my reply to Forest in this volume for a discussion of neurodiversity and autism from the HDA perspective). The HDA predicts not which theory is correct but that the judgment of disorder is consistently rationalized by a corresponding theory about biological design.

Sometimes, when discussing dysfunction hypotheses in a conceptual-analytic context, I might use abstract descriptions of postulated underlying mechanisms that are meant to be neutral on the kinds of mechanisms involved. For example, I might attribute major depression to a dysfunction of "sadness-generating mechanisms." This could easily be misconstrued as a commitment to middle-level dedicated mechanisms as the locale of the primary dysfunction. True, I do believe that in the case of sadness and other major emotions, there likely are such middle-level mechanisms, and their dysfunctions do play a role in emotion-related mental disorders. However, in such locutions, I mean to refer to *whatever* mechanisms are responsible for generating and regulating sadness responses (given the assumption that such basic emotions do have an evolutionary undergirding), whatever they may turn out to be. Gerrans makes the entirely correct point that, even if such mechanisms exist, it need not be that this is where the deepest or most crucial dysfunction is occurring in depression. Gerrans suggests instead that dysfunctional deeper neurocognitive processes may be feeding problematic information into a middle-range module, causing it to no longer function within the parameters for which it was biologically designed. If so, I agree that the etiology and diagnosis would have to reflect this deeper level of dysfunction that is disrupting downstream functions, perhaps yielding his proposed megacategory of "disorders of the salience system." Yet, Gerrans mentions that delusions tend to form into groups (e.g., grandiosity, jealousy, paranoia), suggesting the need for an explanation of this clumping in terms of middle-level adaptive mechanisms downstream from the salience system.

Neuroscience, Strong Adaptationism, and the HDA

Gerrans continues with a critique of what he calls "strong adaptationism":

> For this reason, strong adaptationist versions of evolutionary psychiatry are unlikely to succeed in directing us to cognitive or neural mechanisms. They are too "top down" in their analysis of the problem. This is obvious in the case, for example, of theories that postulate an adaptive problem for which schizophrenic delusions represent a solution (Stevens and Price 2000; Dubrovsky 2002), but the point generalizes.

However, I am not a "strong adaptationist" as that position is generally understood, and neither is strong adaptationism equivalent to the middle-range modular "evolutionary psychology" approach to which Gerrans seems to equate it. Strong adaptationists think that virtually all human features can be understood as adaptations and tend to explain disorders as adaptations to circumstances in the environment of evolutionary adaptation (EEA). I think, to the contrary, that things really can go wrong with almost any biologically designed system in ways that were never biologically designed to happen, and so there are dysfunctions that are not part of design, and those are what conceptually undergird the category of disorder. Thus, I claim that strong adaptationism about medical disorder is not only false but conceptually incoherent. In various publications, I have explained the fallacies involved in strong adaptationists' attempts to explain disorders as adaptations (Wakefield 2016; also see my reply to Cooper in this volume).

In any event, as Gerrans observes, the interestingly complex explanatory mechanisms identified by cognitive neuroscience are presumably not accidents but quite design-like and thus, barring alternative "spandrel"-type explanations, may be presumed to be biologically designed forms of brain circuitry. Cognitive neuroscience is adaptationist "all the way through" not as an ideology but as an empirical claim. As to Stevens and Price, their attempt to explain the prevalence of psychotic symptoms as the result of natural selection for charismatic leaders initially may appear to be an example of strong adaptationism about disorder, but a careful reading reveals that they in fact explain selection only for risk factors that are themselves adaptive but that in certain unselected combinations yield disorder (for further discussion of Stevens and Price, see my reply to De Block and Sholl in this volume).

Neuroscience, Belief Fixation, and the HDA

It appears that a further reason that Gerrans sees a tension between the HDA and mechanistic explanation is that he understands *DSM* diagnoses as well as the HDA as concerned with contents like beliefs, and he sees belief fixation as not subject to direct neuropsychological explanation in terms of naturally selected mechanisms. Writing of the very inadequate *DSM* criteria for delusion, he says,

> It is especially difficult to preserve a taxonomic role for evolutionary theory in the case of psychiatric disorders like delusion, whose classification involves the concept of belief.... The difficulty with all these proposals is not that they get the phenomena wrong but that they all rely on the language of belief, which is intrinsically agnostic about mechanisms.

However, these proposals are purposely agnostic because, rather than attempting to identify mechanisms, they are elaborating the surface descriptive phenomenology of delusions that tells us that something is going wrong *somewhere*, thus identifying the phenomenon that requires explanation by underlying mechanisms.

Moreover, the language of belief is not intrinsically agnostic about mechanisms describable at that level. Although belief mechanisms must have realizations in brain mechanisms, the belief-system level can possess emergent mechanisms that may have then exerted natural selection force on underlying brain mechanisms. Jerry Fodor observes, "Roughly, if you start out with a true thought, and you proceed to do some thinking, it is very often the case that the thoughts that the thinking leads you to will also be true. This is, in my view, the most important fact we know about minds" (Fodor 1994, 9). He thus refers to a mechanism at the belief level (or an idealization of a mechanism), namely, valid reasoning from premises to conclusion. One does not have to understand deeper processes to formulate a provisional theory of how the reasoning mechanism works at the belief level, as Aristotle already attempted.

Gerrans holds this position on belief fixation because he thinks that, although humans are adapted to engage in belief-related ideational behaviors, the relevant mechanisms belong to lower-level neurocognitive functioning rather than the ideational level:

> The human cognitive phenotype does show entrenched patterns of belief fixation in specific domains, and some psychiatric disorders can be characterized in terms of typical abnormalities in those patterns (e.g., social cognition is a specific domain and autism is characterized by deficits of belief fixation in that domain). However, those patterns are produced by low-level neurocognitive mechanisms that produce an upward cascade of effects ultimately expressed as patterns of belief fixation. It makes no sense to see these neurocognitive mechanisms... as cognitive mechanisms selected for forming particular classes of beliefs.... Rather, they are mechanisms that enable processing of information at specific levels of cognitive complexity, and we can make progress on determining their nature by tracing their evolutionary history at the correct level of cognitive resolution.

I cannot find in Gerrans's paper a cogent defense of this unlikely thesis. He is suggesting that, say, pathological jealousy involves neither dysfunction in any belief-close dedicated jealousy-belief-fixation mechanism or process, nor grandiosity in a belief-close dedicated self-esteem belief-fixation mechanism or process, nor depressive hopelessness in a belief-close loss-response belief-fixation mechanism or process. Of course, as Gerrans explains, belief fixation involves complex contextual background understanding and thus certainly interacts with general cognitive processing of the belief system that is not strictly modularized. But, that generic background processing does not preclude final-pathway canalization by specific mechanisms that account for the recognizable distinctions among primary emotions or major areas of cognition. The situation is no different in physical functioning; liver function involves a complex cascade of general bodily functions such as blood circulation and homeostatic thermo-regulation to provide an appropriate context, but that doesn't mean that there are no liver-specific mechanisms or that there is no such thing as a liver disorder.

Neuroscience, the *DSM-5*, and the HDA

Regarding the implications of cognitive neuroscience for psychiatric nosology, Gerrans concludes the following:

> Once we abandon the strong adaptationist approach in favor of a cognitive neuroscience informed by evolutionary theorizing, psychiatric classification requires substantial revision. Wakefield's approach, I suggest, ultimately leads to abandoning the current *DSM* approach in favor of that that recommended by Dominic Murphy (2006)—namely, to allow classifica-tion and psychiatric practice to reflect the architecture of the mind disclosed by cognitive neuroscience.

The supposed conflict suggested by this passage between *DSM* and the neuroscien-tific elucidation of mental disorder etiology is a strawman. Gerrans's suggestion that attention to neuroscientific explanations will correct a deep flaw in *DSM* of address-ing only a more superficial level ignores the circumstances in which *DSM*'s modern approach came about and the understanding of its project within which it was born.

The nosological problem facing psychiatry before *DSM-III*, among many other seri-ous problems such as diagnostic unreliability and reliance on psychoanalytic constructs, was not that too little attention was being paid to causal mechanisms by psychiatrists but that too many unestablished causal theories prematurely were being taken seri-ously, and thus there was a fragmentation of the field along theoretical lines. Every one of those theoretical approaches, ranging from neurobiological, behavioral, and cognitive theories to social stress and family dynamics theories as well as five flavors of psychoanalytic theory, felt they had fresh, illuminating, scientifically valid insights into the sources of mental disorder just as neuroscientists do now. Research was pur-sued by each school using different diagnostic criteria, so research samples could not be compared and the knowledge base was not cumulative. *DSM-III*'s solution was to propose criteria that were agreed on across theoretical perspectives to identify classes of mental disorders and thus create a level playing field for the demonstration of etiological hypotheses. There are many problems with the *DSM* system and how it has evolved, and I have spent a good deal of effort pointing to some of them. However, in no way is the system meant to be some sort of syndromal conceptual account of the nature of mental disorder (contrary to Murphy's [2017] portrayal). The syndromes are markers for likely underlying dysfunction (First and Wakefield 2013), and, as the *DSM's* definition of mental disorder makes clear, it is causation of harmful symptoms by a dysfunction that makes a condition a disorder. Thus, the goal of the *DSM* is to provide the initial step in bootstrapping to eventually cash out the reference to an inferred dysfunction for actual knowledge of etiological dysfunctions. The *DSM's* logic does not dictate or prejudge the nature of those dysfunctions.

But you don't need to take my word for it; precisely this point of the provisional nature of *DSM* symptomatic criteria awaiting etiological understanding was explained by Robert Spitzer in his introduction to *DSM-III* at the inauguration of the current descriptive system:

> *Descriptive Approach.* For some of the mental disorders, the etiology or pathophysiological processes are known....For most of the *DSM-III* disorders, however, the etiology is unknown. A variety of theories have been advanced, buttressed by evidence—not always convincing—to explain how these disorders come about. The approach taken in *DSM-III* is atheoretical with regard to etiology or pathophysiological process except for those disorders for which this is well established and therefore included in the definition of the disorder. Undoubtedly, with time, some of the disorders of unknown etiology will be found to have specific biological etiologies, others to have specific psychological causes, and still others to result mainly from a particular interplay of psychological, social and biological factors.
>
> The major justification for the generally atheoretical approach taken in *DSM-III* with regard to etiology is that the inclusion of etiological theories would be an obstacle to use of the manual by clinicians of varying theoretical orientations....For example, Phobic Disorders are believed by many to represent a displacement of anxiety resulting from the breakdown of defensive operations for keeping internal conflict out of consciousness. Other investigators explain phobias on the basis of learned avoidance responses to conditioned anxiety. Still others believe that certain phobias result from a dysregulation of basic biological systems mediating separation anxiety....Clinicians can agree on the identification of mental disorders on the basis of their clinical manifestations without agreeing on how the disturbances come about. (Spitzer 1980, 6–7)

The *DSM* states that it is atheoretical—that is, it does not include a theory of etiology in the diagnostic criteria—because "for most of the *DSM-III* disorders, however, the etiology is unknown." This is a pragmatic, epistemologically based compromise, not a conceptual or ontological statement about the concept of disorder. This atheoretical stance, we are told, applies "except for those disorders for which [etiology] is well established and therefore included in the definition of the disorder." The clear implication of this passage is that symptom syndromes, as in physical medicine, are understood not as ontological foundations but as transient epistemological necessities until etiological knowledge is established, at which time etiological criteria will supplement or replace syndromal criteria. Syndromes are the best that can be done at present to individuate disorders, but they are intended as provisional indicators on the way to more scientifically sophisticated and validated etiological disorder identification. Spitzer's example of multiple theories of phobia illustrates that the problem is not lack of attempts to identify causes but rather lack of established knowledge. The situation has not changed all that much today, to the consternation of many in the field.

Gerrans again cites Murphy in support of his claim that the *DSM* embraces a syndromal conception of disorder that needs to be overthrown for a causal conception. So, I briefly consider Murphy's view of *DSM*. It is useful to compare the above statement from *DSM-III* explaining its descriptive nosology with the following excerpts from Murphy's account of what he calls "the *DSM* Conception of Mental Illness" (references are deleted; consult the original for them):

> The *DSM* treats mental disorders as syndromes.…The previous version of the *DSM* assumed that each diagnosis represented malfunction in some mental, physical or behavioural trait or capacity (*DSM-IV-TR*, xxi). However, the diagnoses were listed without worrying about what that underlying malfunction might be, and in most cases there was (and remains) no agreement about what causes what. *DSM-5* defines mental disorders as syndromes comprising clinically significant disturbances of cognition, emotion or behaviour that reflect underlying dysfunctions. These…cannot be diagnosed if the behaviour is culturally normal or merely socially deviant, unless it reflects a dysfunction.…There are plenty of students of psychopathology who argue that the neglect of causal structure in psychopathology is getting in the way of science.…
>
> The *DSM* approach is often called "neo-Kraepelinian." But Kraepelin…saw classification by clinical description as an interim measure.…Kraepelin's preferred basis for classification and inquiry actually rested on his less well-remembered belief that "pathological anatomy promises to provide the safest foundation" for classification of mental illness in a mature psychiatry. He considered the correct taxonomy would be one in which clinical description, etiology and pathophysiology coincided.…
>
> There is a substantial difference between thinking of clinically-based, syndromic classification in this way and thinking of it as the *DSM* does. The *DSM* classification…is not advertised as the jumping-off point for a mature system of causally organised classification and practice. (Murphy 2017, 5)

Murphy concludes that the *DSM* is committed to syndromal classification and does not see itself as a starting point for development of a more mature etiologically based causal system of diagnoses. As we saw, *DSM-III* clearly indicates precisely the opposite; atheoretical definitions are to be used "except for those disorders for which [etiology] is well established," and it is expected that "with time, some of the disorders of unknown etiology will be found to have specific…etiologies" and then the etiology will be "included in the definition of the disorder." In his next-to-last sentence, Murphy asserts that Kraepelin's view that syndromes are used for initial classification as a stepping stone to etiological discovery is a substantially different way of thinking about syndromal diagnosis than the *DSM*'s, but in fact it is identical to the view enunciated by Spitzer in *DSM-III*. Murphy explains that Kraepelin sees "classification by clinical description as an interim measure," and, contrary to Murphy's portrayal, *DSM-III* sees it in exactly the same way. Kraepelin's model was general paresis, initially defined by syndrome and course, gradually distinguished phenomenologically from symptomatically similar conditions through syndromal analysis, and then, when eventually it was discovered to be caused by syphilitic brain infection, the etiology replaced the syndromal diagnostic approach. The hope was that *DSM*-based diagnosis would give rise to similar progress. The *DSM*, like Kraepelin, uses syndromes to try to pick out unknown dysfunctions, and the different possible symptom presentations of a given disorder, sometimes nonoverlapping, are united in being thought to pick out the same or a similar dysfunction. The quest to identify dysfunctions also explains many other features of the *DSM*'s diagnostic criteria sets, such as number of symptoms and durational thresholds (First and Wakefield 2013) and contextual exclusions (Wakefield and First 2012). All these features are aimed at trying to align the criteria with the target dysfunction(s).

Murphy's account confuses the epistemology of diagnosis with the ontology of mental disorder. The problem seems to be in part a matter of the limitations of Murphy's theory of concepts. As the above passage indicates, Murphy tends to see either syndromes or explicit, known causal etiologies as exhausting conceptual logic. Thus, he can ignore the *DSM* "dysfunction" clause because "the diagnoses were listed without worrying about what that underlying malfunction might be, and in most cases there was (and remains) no agreement about what causes what." This misses the basic point that a syndrome is being used to pick out an unknown but inferred dysfunction, the presence of which is conceptually essential, and this is precisely the conceptual feature that looks beyond the syndrome and awaits elucidation as the etiology of the symptoms. This structure is analogous to what I call "black-box essentialist" concepts, as elaborated in psychology by Medin and Ortony (1989) and in philosophy by Putnam (1975) and Kripke (1980), in which an essential factor unifying a category is unknown but is picked out by way of an observable "base set" of instances. The necessity of the reference to a known or inferred dysfunction in an analysis of "medical disorder" is a crucial insight that took Spitzer half a decade to come to, and without it, one gets the watered-down implausible syndromal view of disorder that Murphy mistakenly attributes to the *DSM*.

Murphy reports that many writers criticize the *DSM* for a "neglect of causal structure in psychopathology," but neglect is different from lack of scientific success despite great effort. *DSM-III* does not neglect causal structure; it is a compromise with the fact that we don't yet know causal structures. This is illustrated by Spitzer's phobia example; those who criticize the *DSM* for neglect of etiology are not in agreement about what the appropriate causal structures should be. If Gerrans (or anyone else) were actually to present psychiatry with serious *consensually persuasive* scientific evidence for mental disorder etiology—mere excitement at novel proposals by a subdiscipline's enthusiasts after some initial testing is *not* the same as established, persuasive scientific fact—the *DSM-5.1* committee would likely jump at it.

Murphy's skewed reading of the *DSM* leads to the sort of misunderstanding we saw in Gerrans. Rather than opposing or radically altering the *DSM*'s program, neuroscientific theories of disorders would advance and even vindicate the *DSM* program of starting from syndromes and bootstrapping to underlying dysfunctions and reorganized etiologically coherent syndrome categories. In fact, the *DSM-5* Task Force completely *agreed* with Gerrans and Murphy that we should move beyond the descriptive system, and early on, they infamously declared that *DSM-5* would be a "paradigm shift" (cf. Gerrans's "radical" change) in favor of brain circuitry and biomarkers, with eventual rectification with RDoC sure to follow. So, why didn't it happen? The goal was abandoned late in the revision process simply because there were no adequately confirmed brain-mechanism theories of disorder to put into the manual as diagnostic criteria. (Yes, there are lots of findings of group-level differences, but not ones that adequately distinguish disorder from normality to be used diagnostically.) This humiliating and disruptive late admission of failure could have been avoided by a good literature search at the outset of the *DSM-5* process, but the salience of the vision of what would be desirable blinded the task force to seeing what is.

Rather than disagreeing with *DSM*, Gerrans and Murphy are agreeing with *DSM* aspirations but making the same mistake of confusing wishes and aspirations with current reality. The problem is with reality, not with *DSM* doctrine. Despite Gerrans and Murphy being gripped by the enormous salience of advances in neurocognitive research, sobering pitfalls likely lie ahead for cognitive neuroscientific explanations of psychopathology as they did for every earlier salient research approach (Paulus and Thompson 2019). Gerrans's own theory of delusion as "salience overshoot" suggests that scientific ardor may be a constructive quasi-delusion and that caution is warranted. The difficult truth is that we are just not there yet.

References

First, M. B., and J. C. Wakefield. 2010. Defining 'mental disorder' in *DSM-V*. *Psychological Medicine* 40(11): 1779–1782.

First, M. B., and J. C. Wakefield. 2013. Diagnostic criteria as dysfunction indicators: Bridging the chasm between the definition of mental disorder and diagnostic criteria for specific disorders. *Canadian Journal of Psychiatry* 58(12): 663–669.

Fodor, J. A. 1994. *The Elm and the Expert: Mentalese and Its Semantics*. MIT Press.

Gerrans, P. 2002. The theory of mind module in evolutionary psychology. *Biology and Philosophy* 17(3): 305–321.

Gerrans, P. 2007. Mechanisms of madness: Evolutionary psychiatry without evolutionary psychology. *Biology and Philosophy* 22(1): 35–56.

Gerrans, P., and K. Scherer. 2013. Wired for despair: The neurochemistry of emotion and the phenomenology of depression. *Journal of Consciousness Studies* 20(7–8): 254–268.

Gerrans, P., and V. E. Stone. 2008. Generous or parsimonious cognitive architecture? Cognitive neuroscience and theory of mind. *British Journal for the Philosophy of Science* 59(2): 121–141.

Horwitz, A., and J. C. Wakefield. 2007. *The Loss of Sadness: How Psychiatry Transformed Normal Sorrow into Depressive Disorder*. Oxford University Press.

Kripke, S. A. 1980. *Naming and Necessity*. Harvard University Press.

Levy, N. 2017. Hijacking addiction. *Philosophy, Psychiatry, and Psychology* 24(1): 97–99.

Medin, D. L., and A. Ortony. 1989. Psychological essentialism. In *Similarity and Analogical Reasoning*, S. Vosniadou and A. Ortony (eds.), 179–196. Cambridge University Press.

Murphy, D. 2006. *Psychiatry in the Scientific Image*. MIT Press.

Murphy, D. 2017. Philosophy of psychiatry. In *The Stanford Encyclopedia of Philosophy*, 1–31, E. N. Zalta (ed.). https://plato.stanford.edu/archives/spr2017/entries/psychiatry/. April 7, 2019.

Paulus, M. P., and W. K. Thompson. 2019. The challenges and opportunities of small effects: The new normal in academic psychiatry. *JAMA Psychiatry* 76(4): 353–354.

Putnam, H. 1975. The meaning of meaning. In *Mind, Language, and Reality: Philosophical Papers*, H. Putnam (ed.), 215–271, vol. 2. Cambridge University Press.

Spitzer, R. L. 1980. Introduction. In *Diagnostic and Statistical Manual of Mental Disorders*, 1–12. 3rd ed. American Psychiatric Association.

Spitzer, R. L. 1997. Brief comments from a psychiatric nosologist weary from his own attempts to define mental disorder: Why Ossorio's definition muddles and Wakefield's "harmful dysfunction" illuminates the issues. *Clinical Psychology: Science and Practice* 4(3): 259–261.

Spitzer, R. L. 1999. Harmful dysfunction and the *DSM* definition of mental disorder. *Journal of Abnormal Psychology* 108(3): 430–432.

Stone, V. E., and P. Gerrans. 2006. What's domain specific about theory of mind. *Social Neuroscience* 1(3–4): 309–319.

Tinbergen, N. 1963. On aims and methods of ethology. *Zeitschrift für Tierpsychologie* 20: 410–433.

Wakefield, J. C. 1992a. The concept of mental disorder: On the boundary between biological facts and social values. *American Psychologist* 47: 373–388.

Wakefield, J. C. 1992b. Disorder as harmful dysfunction: A conceptual critique of *DSM-III-R*'s definition of mental disorder. *Psychological Review* 99: 232–247.

Wakefield, J. C. 1993. Limits of operationalization: A critique of Spitzer and Endicott's (1978) proposed operational criteria of mental disorder. *Journal of Abnormal Psychology* 102: 160–172.

Wakefield, J. C. 1995. Dysfunction as a value-free concept: A reply to Sadler and Agich. *Philosophy, Psychiatry, and Psychology* 2: 233–46.

Wakefield, J. C. 1997a. Diagnosing *DSM-IV*, part 1: *DSM-IV* and the concept of mental disorder. *Behaviour Research and Therapy* 35: 633–650.

Wakefield, J. C. 1997b. Diagnosing *DSM-IV*, part 2: Eysenck (1986) and the essentialist fallacy. *Behaviour Research and Therapy*: 35: 651–666.

Wakefield, J. C. 1997c. Normal inability versus pathological disability: Why Ossorio's (1985) definition of mental disorder is not sufficient. *Clinical Psychology: Science and Practice* 4: 249–258.

Wakefield, J. C. 1997d. When is development disordered? Developmental psychopathology and the harmful dysfunction analysis of mental disorder. *Development and Psychopathology* 9: 269–290.

Wakefield, J. C. 1998. The *DSM*'s theory-neutral nosology is scientifically progressive: Response to Follette and Houts. *Journal of Consulting and Clinical Psychology* 66: 846–852.

Wakefield, J. C. 1999a. Evolutionary versus prototype analyses of the concept of disorder. *Journal of Abnormal Psychology* 108: 374–399.

Wakefield, J. C. 1999b. Mental disorder as a black box essentialist concept. *Journal of Abnormal Psychology* 108: 465–472.

Wakefield, J. C. 2000a. Aristotle as sociobiologist: The "function of a human being" argument, black box essentialism, and the concept of mental disorder. *Philosophy, Psychiatry, and Psychology* 7: 17–44.

Wakefield, J. C. 2000b. Spandrels, vestigial organs, and such: Reply to Murphy and Woolfolk's "The harmful dysfunction analysis of mental disorder." *Philosophy, Psychiatry, and Psychology* 7: 253–269.

Wakefield, J. C. 2001. Evolutionary history versus current causal role in the definition of disorder: Reply to McNally. *Behaviour Research and Therapy* 39: 347–366.

Wakefield, J. C. 2006. What makes a mental disorder mental? *Philosophy, Psychiatry, and Psychology* 13: 123–131.

Wakefield, J. C. 2007. The concept of mental disorder: Diagnostic implications of the harmful dysfunction analysis. *World Psychiatry* 6: 149–156.

Wakefield, J. C. 2009. Mental disorder and moral responsibility: Disorders of personhood as harmful dysfunctions, with special reference to alcoholism. *Philosophy, Psychiatry, and Psychology* 16: 91–99.

Wakefield, J. C. 2011. Darwin, functional explanation, and the philosophy of psychiatry. In *Maladapting Minds: Philosophy, Psychiatry, and Evolutionary Theory*, P. R. Andriaens and A. De Block (eds.), 143–172. Oxford University Press.

Wakefield, J. C. 2014. The biostatistical theory versus the harmful dysfunction analysis, part 1: Is part-dysfunction a sufficient condition for medical disorder? *Journal of Medicine and Philosophy* 39: 648–682.

Wakefield, J. C. 2016a. The concepts of biological function and dysfunction: Toward a conceptual foundation for evolutionary psychopathology. In *Handbook of Evolutionary Psychology*, D. Buss (ed.), 2nd ed., vol. 2, 988–1006. Oxford University Press.

Wakefield, J. C. 2016b. Diagnostic issues and controversies in *DSM-5*: Return of the false positives problem. *Annual Review of Clinical Psychology* 12: 105–132.

Wakefield, J. C., and M. B. First. 2003. Clarifying the distinction between disorder and nondisorder: Confronting the overdiagnosis ("false positives") problem in *DSM-V*. In *Advancing DSM: Dilemmas in Psychiatric Diagnosis*, K. A. Phillips, M. B. First, and H. A. Pincus (eds.), 23–56. American Psychiatric Press.

Wakefield, J. C., and M. B. First. 2012. Placing symptoms in context: The role of contextual criteria in reducing false positives in *DSM* diagnosis. *Comprehensive Psychiatry* 53: 130–139.

21 Autistic Spectrum, Normal Variation, and Harmful Dysfunction

Denis Forest

> If I could snap my fingers and be nonautistic, I would not. Autism is part of what I am.
> —Grandin (2006)

Introduction

Since the pioneering work of Leo Kanner (Kanner 1943), the diagnosis of autism has been based on the so-called autistic triad, that is, the reunion of three types of features: impairment of social development, impairment of communication, and display of rigid and repetitive behavior (Baron-Cohen 2008). This mix of deficiency and oddity has been the basis on which autism has been identified as a developmental *disorder*. Research on autism has not only increased our knowledge on this condition in innumerable ways but also resulted in a more problematic picture of it. First, instead of a sharp contrast between autistic and nonautistic people, research has pointed out the presence of autistic features within some parts of the nonautistic population—which has led to the introduction of the notion of a broader autistic phenotype (Piven et al. 1997). Second, we have now good reasons to recognize a marked heterogeneity within what is called, since the work of Allen (1988) and Wing (1997), the autistic spectrum: high-functioning autism, where general intelligence is preserved, is quite different from "classic autism," and specialists are not unanimously convinced that the term "disorder" applies to it.[1] This evolution toward a greater recognition of preserved (or even enhanced) abilities of individuals in high-functioning autism has coincided with the development of the neurodiversity movement, which developed in the 1990s through the activity of online groups of high-functioning autistic persons (Ortega 2009; Jaarsma and Welin 2011).[2] The advocates of neurodiversity claim that nonautistic or, as they call them, "neurotypical" people have a negative bias against autistic persons and that we should stop confusing mere difference with genuine deficiency. So we have moved from a world where autism was a relatively well-defined medical category to a different universe marked by clinical heterogeneity, elusive boundaries, numerous first-person accounts of how autistic persons experience the world (Grandin 2006, 2009), and finally, controversy about the very application of the term "disorder" to autism.

According to Jerome Wakefield, "a disorder is a harmful dysfunction, wherein harmful is a value term based on social norms, and dysfunction is a scientific term referring to the failure of a mental mechanism to perform a natural function for which it was designed by evolution" (Wakefield 1992a, 373). Purely normative views of mental disorders, according to Wakefield, fail to recognize that function and malfunction are independent from our values, norms, and preferences; they miss the crucial point that there are objective, natural facts that ground our medical judgments. In this chapter, I want to confront the harmful dysfunction view (mentioned hereafter as HD analysis) and the contemporary debate about autism that revolves around two key questions: how should we explain autism, and should we think of it in terms of difference and normal variation, on one hand, or deficiency and disorder, on the other hand?

In a very thorough examination of HD analysis (Poland 2002), Jeffrey Poland has made a useful distinction between two projects that, according to him, coexist within the HD analysis: one is a descriptive project, "to reconstruct as accurately as possible the commitments of contemporary mental health practice regarding the concept of mental disorder," and a normative project, "to identify a set of conceptual commitments that ought to inform contemporary mental health practice." The descriptive project deals with scientific psychiatry as it is, the normative project, with scientific psychiatry as it should be. The content of this chapter will echo this distinction, and I shall answer two different questions. First, there is the descriptive issue: is research about autism and its explanation concerned with the discovery of dysfunctional mechanisms, where "dysfunctional" has the precise meaning that is attached to it within the framework of HD analysis, and are dysfunctions currently described independently from background normative judgments? The answer I intend to provide is negative: in the literature, with few exceptions, "dysfunction" of psychological or neural mechanisms is not understood as their failure to perform what they have been "designed" to do (section I). Moreover, factual judgments about impaired performance and dysfunction are usually inseparable from implicit evaluative claims (section II). My second question is as follows: is the definition of disorders as harmful dysfunctions helping us to settle the debate about deficiency versus diversity, by providing us a standard for the application of the notion of disorder?[3] To this second question, my answer will also be negative, especially because in the context of developmental disorders like autism, what counts as "harm" is less dependent on "social values" than what is required by HD analysis (section III). The suggestion that goes with these negative answers is offered as revisionary rather than radical: I do not suggest that we should give up the core of HD analysis (combining dysfunctions and their harmful consequences) but rather that we should analyze functional talk and harm in a different way. In a nutshell, I shall advocate a more mechanistic view of dysfunctions and an understanding of harm in terms of diminished ability.

I. Psychological Theories of Autism: What Is Dysfunctional, and in What Sense?

If we analyze some of the cognitive theories of autism that have been the most widely discussed in recent years, it seems to be an easy task to reconcile their construal of autism with HD analysis. My reason to start with psychological theories is that their common ambition has been to go *beyond* mere diagnostic criteria and to characterize underlying psychological *mechanisms*, that is, to offer causal explanations of autism involving some kind of disturbance at the psychological level. These theories are the mindblindness theory (Baron-Cohen 1995), the weak coherence theory (Frith 1989; Frith and Happé 1994), and the executive dysfunction theory (Ozonoff et al. 1991; Hill 2004)—for the sake of simplicity, I shall leave aside the empathizing-systemizing theory (Baron-Cohen 2009) that refines on the mindblindness theory.

1. According to the *mindblindness theory*, what is central to autism is the inability to ascribe correctly beliefs and desires to people in order to explain and predict their behavior or, as it is often said, to "read their minds." In its stronger form, the theory postulates that there is a mental mechanism dedicated to the ascription of mental states to others that takes the form of a cognitive module (a psychological faculty with its own cognitive domain and its specific operations, which entails the possibility of its own internal breakdown). This capacity is called in the literature the theory of mind (ToM) module (Baron-Cohen 1995). The idea is roughly that in the autistic mind, because of a defective ontogenetic history that does not lead to its proper development, the ToM module is not working the way it is supposed to.

2. According to the *executive dysfunction theory*, to understand autism, we have to focus on what is called executive function, that is, the ability to control action—where action may be the movements of the body but also the thoughts of the subject. The creation and execution of plans, the ability to stay focused on a given topic or to shift attention, presuppose the integrity of the executive system. Concerning autistic disorders, the executive dysfunction theory aims, in particular, at explaining repetitive behaviors and narrowed interests.

3. According to the *weak coherence theory*, there is a standard human form of information processing that is crucial to the construction of complex structures; it makes possible both to build and to recognize organized wholes, to memorize complex patterns (rather than their discrete elements). Autistic people would be specifically impaired in these information-processing mechanisms, and their levels of performances in all sorts of cognitive tasks (pattern recognition, memory of meaningful sentences, parsing of sentences) would be evidence of that.

In each case, what is postulated by the theory is that there is a psychological mechanism that fails to perform its function, whether it is the function of controlling action, of ascribing beliefs and desires to others, or of integrating details within coherent wholes. Accordingly, autism would be based on the dysfunction of some kind of psychological mechanism, and in each case, the dysfunction would produce *harmful* results (because one values the ability to control one's actions, the understanding of others as well as related social skills, or the ability to process information in a coherent manner). Explaining autism would consist in identifying the underlying dysfunction(s) that lead(s) to clinically significant, harmful consequences. Of course, advocates of each theory underline that there is much more to the symptoms of autism than what a rival theory can account for, but all such theories and their more recent counterparts share the same goals.

Objections that can be raised against this type of explanation are not necessarily a problem for HD analysis. For instance, concerning the mindblindness theory, the reduced social interactions of autistic children could be explained by a low-level deficit in the perception of social cues, rather than by a higher-level deficit in mentalizing per se (Gerrans 2002). It would be the lack of relevant input, rather than the dysfunction of a dedicated mechanism, that would carry the burden of the explanation: the theory of mind module, then, would become an unnecessary theoretical construct. But HD analysis is not committed to the prediction that, for any mental disorder, the underlying dysfunction is the dysfunction of a specialized mental mechanism (Wakefield 2000). If we give up the theory of mind module, this does not by itself compromise the application of the harmful dysfunction view to autism. However, this kind of immunity to refutation may be a sign of epistemic weakness, rather than a strength. The notion of a dysfunctional "mental mechanism" that would have been "designed" reflects the conviction that first, there must be some objective basis of mental disorders that is independent from our values and expectations and, second, that mental mechanisms are the product of evolution, like other biological mechanisms. Speaking of dysfunction, then, is rejecting relativism and being committed to the idea that mental disorders have a biological nature, but it is not much more than that.

Now, to use Poland's distinction quoted above, is it legitimate to say that mental disorders are currently defined in terms of harmful dysfunctions where "dysfunction" refers to the failure of a mental mechanism to perform "a natural function for which it was designed by evolution"? Mindblindness theory of autism can be (and has been) construed within an evolutionary framework.[4] It is possible to give to "dysfunction" the kind of meaning that *befits* HD analysis. But as it has been pointed out several times by critics of Wakefield's views (Murphy and Woolfolk 2000; Poland 2002; Murphy, this volume), functional talk can have a different meaning, and functional ascriptions may answer different kinds of explanatory purposes. Cummins's view of functions (Cummins 1975) according to which the function F of a component C is its contribution to the explanation of a capacity of the system in which C is embedded seems appropriate for psychological as well as physiological mechanisms. When a scientist tries to explain perseverations and narrowed interests in terms of the dysfunction of an executive system (which would usually monitor and controls action planification), the function of such a system is not seen as the reason why such a system has been recruited by natural selection. In more mechanistic terms (Machamer et al. 2000), its function is the contribution it makes to the behavioral and psychological repertoire of similar individuals belonging to the same species. The ascription of a dysfunction is not based on Darwinian speculation but on the contrast between a shared ability and an (intriguing) disability. So when we think of an "executive dysfunction theory of autism," we do not (have to) care about the past contribution of this system to the reproductive success of our ancestors. Research related to the executive function theory does not even try to address these issues. What counts is the explanatory value of a functional analysis that postulates an executive system and how the dysfunction of such a system (its failure to do what it usually does in humans, not what it has been designed to do) is able to help us to understand where autistic features come from. Even the mindblindness theory is, in practice, a theory of the *ontogeny* of mental mechanisms (Baron-Cohen 1995). Evolutionary psychologists can speculate about the origins of the theory of mind module, but this entity is useful in cognitive psychology only if it fits in a plausible mechanistic decomposition of the mind. The reference to an evolutionary background remains quite idle in this context.

Moreover, to be able to distinguish between functioning and malfunctioning in Wakefield's sense, we would have to know *when* an evolved mechanism is not doing what it has been designed to do and what the corresponding normal range of variation is in terms of level of performance (Schwartz 2007). Talking about failure and disability leads us to ignore the fact that cognitive tests usually do not offer evidence of a complete *lack* of ability in autistic persons, even for tasks where they are known to be at a disadvantage. For instance, in a task of sentence comprehension for which autistic and nonautistic subjects were tested (Just et al. 2004), error rates were only slightly different: error rates were 8% and 13% for the autistic group (for active and passive sentences), when they were 5% and 7% for the control group. We can interpret this result as the sign of a cognitive dysfunction as evidence of an impaired linguistic ability. But we could also consider (as the different pattern of brain activation in the autistic group suggests) that autistic people use a different cognitive strategy that is quite effective in a *majority* of cases: where shall we find reasons to justify our claim that an error rate of 5% indicates a level of performance that deserves to be called normal (the mind, then, is working "as designed") and that an error rate of 8% is equivalent to a cognitive dysfunction? There is a danger of circular reasoning here, because tests are there to determine what is impaired in the autistic mind, but the slight difference in the results is interpreted as a sign of disturbance *because* the subjects are known to be autistic and their faculties are presumed to be impaired. Adding evolutionary considerations will not help us to break this kind of circle.

To sum up, it is true that occasionally, the dysfunction of the theory of mind module has been conceived in the literature on autism as "the failure of a mental mechanism to perform a natural function for which it was designed by evolution." But on one hand, we have to remain cautious about the kind of just-so stories that proliferate in evolutionary psychology (Richardson 2010). And on the other hand, concerning the cognitive explanations of autism in general, there is no systematic reference to such an evolutionary background, and more important, such a background plays no special role when the merits and flaws of these cognitive explanations are discussed. We could add that what is true of psychological explanations would also be true of neurocognitive accounts of autism, like the so called broken-mirror view (Ramachandran 2011): it is quite easy to speculate both on the evolutionary history of mirror neurons and on the cognitive impact of the disruption of the mirror system, but in the end, all that matters is how relevant the functioning of the mirror system is to the causal explanation of autistic symptomatology (Hickok 2014).

II. Normality and High-Functioning Autism

In the previous section, I have tried to establish that cognitive explanations of autism are developed without being integrated to an evolutionary framework where dysfunction has the precise meaning that Wakefield is ascribing to it. But now I would like to follow a different strategy. Let us suppose that, in conformity with HD analysis, what mental mechanisms usually or typically do in the general population is what they have been designed to do. In nonautistic people, key mental mechanisms would function as designed, and in autism, the same mechanisms would fail to do what they are designed to do. Does it help us to solve the difficult problems linked today to the autistic phenotype in its wide diversity?

Let us take, for instance, the weak coherence theory. As we have seen, it links key aspects of autism with a definite kind of malfunction of psychological mechanisms. We could call its main hypothesis the central coherence view of cognitive processing (CCV). CCV is explicitly presented as a view of "*normal* [emphasis added] information processing" (Frith and Happé 1994). The meaning of "normal" here is statistical: when Frith and Happé mention, for instance, "the ease with which we recognize the contextually appropriate sense of many ambiguous words used in everyday speech," *they* clearly refers to what *most of us* are able to do *most of the time*. In the same paper, central coherence is even called a "universal feature of human information processing." But here normal has also, obviously, an *evaluative* character: processing information the way we do yields special benefits; it enables us to construct complex representations, to get the meaning of a joke, to memorize a meaningful sentence, and so on. Central coherence is not only the standard way of information processing; it is supposed to be the *right* way. Ascribing impaired or *dysfunctional* cognitive capacities to autistic people presupposes a given account of what it is like to be normal. In this case, humans would have evolved an ability for information processing along a principle of central coherence that is intrinsically *adaptive*. In the spirit of HD analysis, then, failure to reach central coherence would be a cognitive dysfunction.

However, one key discovery about autistic people has been that weak coherence, that is, relying on an alternative mode of information processing, instead of being always a source of impairment, may yield marked benefits in several contexts. There are now numerous examples of the "unusual strength" of autistic children on a large number of cognitive tasks: perception of detail, memory for word strings (rather than meaningful sentences), memory for unrelated items, recognition of upside-down faces, and so on (Frith and Happé 1994; Happé and Vital 2009). Looking for what is dysfunctional in autistic children, cognitive research on psychological mechanisms has revealed that in some areas, autism is not causing any form of obvious harm, as it may be a source of ability, excellence, or talent.

These results have several important implications. They mean, first, that coherence comes at a price (as in the case of neglected details) and that we have to contextualize success and failure. For instance, it is well known that there are side effects to the context sensitivity of cognitive processing that is typical of "central coherence." In the Titchener Illusion (see figure 21.1), when asked to compare the respective size of two (identical) circles, nonautistic people are mistakenly influenced by the size of other adjacent figures, while autistic people are not (Happé 1999). This means that autistic people, in a given

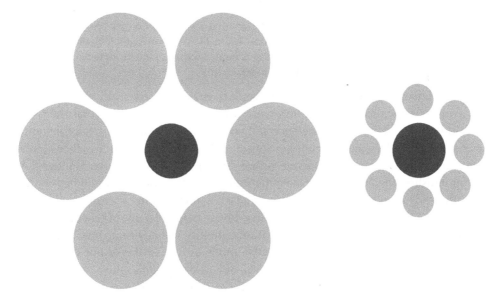

Figure 21.1
The Titchener Illusion. Context sensitivity leads to errors of judgments (the circles at the center are judged to have a different size). Autistic people do not succumb to this illusion (Happé 1999).

context, may make a perceptual judgment that is *correct* just because they *do not* rely (or not preferably) on the central coherence mode of information processing. Not succumbing to an illusion is hardly a clear sign of disturbance and impairment.

These results also mean that instead of thinking in terms of cognitive deficits in autism, we may have to think in terms of cognitive style (Happé 1999) and a different trade-off between abilities that are impaired and other abilities that may be enhanced, at least in high-functioning autism. This blocks any narrow, chauvinistic view of normality because if we look for dysfunctions and impairments on the sole basis of diminished performance, then an alternative view should be considered: autistic persons could label nonautistic people "coherentists" (with a pejorative meaning). They would dig in the scientific literature to list all the tasks where coherentists are clearly at a disadvantage to justify their own claims: strong coherence is a clear sign of a (widespread) abnormality. And in fact, this characterization of nonautistic people *has* been suggested. See this definition of the neurotypical syndrome (NT, that is, nonautistic people) that mimics and mocks the scientific description of autistic disorders:

> Definition of NT:—Neurotypical syndrome is a neurobiological disorder characterized by preoccupation with social concerns, delusions of superiority, and obsession with conformity... Neurotypical individuals often assume that their experience of the world is either the only one, or the only correct one....NT is believed to be genetic in origin. Autopsies have shown the brain of the neurotypical is typically smaller than that of an autistic individual and may have overdeveloped areas related to social behaviour. How common is it?—Tragically, as many as 9625 out of every 10,000 individuals may be neurotypical....There is no known cure for Neurotypical Syndrome. However, many NTs have learned to compensate for their disabilities and interact normally with autistic persons. (Posted on the website of the Institute for the Study of the Neurologically Typical, quoted by Brownlow 2010)

It is, then, extremely difficult to tell if "weak central coherence" can be understood in terms of *dysfunction* in Wakefield's sense. One possibility would be that there is a continuum between central coherence and weak coherence and that weak coherence as it is manifested in high-functioning autism and autistic talent is an instance of normal variation in human populations with a different trade-off between abilities that are diminished and abilities that are enhanced. Another possibility would be that the cognitive phenotype of high-functioning autism is in fact an instance of *harmless dysfunction*: the autistic mind deviates from an evolved, adaptive mode of functioning that corresponds to central coherence, but within current social environments, in the case of high functioning autism, this alternative mode of functioning is not detrimental and does not by itself cause significant harm. But, as significant as this alternative may seem in terms of conceptual analysis, we do not seem to be in a position to choose between these two very different descriptions of what high-functioning autism is. In particular, substituting brain mechanisms to psychological mechanisms to ground the ascription of a "dysfunction" would be a helpless move, because objective differences within the autistic brain, which do not resemble the focal lesions of traditional neuro-psychology (Baron-Cohen and Belmonte 2005), can be understood as the basis of an alternative mode of cognitive functioning: to distinguish what is dysfunctional and what is atypical, all will depend on the way we describe what the autistic brain does. For instance, "*reduction* in the connectivity between specialized local neural networks in the brain and possible *overconnectivity* within the isolated individual neural assemblies" (Rippon et al. 2007) is one way of characterizing the specific features of the autistic brain. But "overconnectivity within the isolated individual neural assemblies" could also be the basis on which, for instance, attention to detail supervenes (Grandin 2009, 1439–1440). One central problem of the research on the autistic brain is to go beyond what is merely plausible (Machamer et al. 2000) and to offer evidence that brain findings are *actually* related to the clinical picture. But it is also that we need to disentangle what is related to autism in general and what is related to the most unwelcomed aspects of severe autism. Pointing at overconnectivity, without further qualification, offers no evidence of natural dysfunction.

What counts for mental medicine is how we draw the line between a type of weak coherence (or more broadly an autistic phenotype) that counts as harmful and another that does not and how we explain the difference between the two. Talking of mental or neural mechanisms that perform or fail to perform their evolved function does not seem to help us much in that.

III. Harm without Values

In his seminal paper "The Concept of Mental Disorder" (Wakefield 1992a), Wakefield claims that "only dysfunctions that are socially disvalued are disorders," and it is quite obvious that autism today is a social problem as well as a purely medical question. As we have seen above, the claim of the neurodiversity movement has been that we should stop thinking of autism as a pervasive developmental disorder, waiting for a cure, and rejecting the very notion of an underlying dysfunction. The idea of dysfunction is linked to the decomposition of a whole into components among which one or several is (are) unable to perform its (their) function. This is precisely what has been challenged by activists like Jim Sinclair in his famous essay "Don't Mourn for Us" when he denies that autism is something that people *have* (they would *have*, for instance, an impaired theory of mind comparable to a broken leg or a cardiovascular disease) and that there would be "a normal child behind the autism" that, in principle, could be freed from its problem (Sinclair 1993). From the viewpoint of neurodiversity advocates, the "pervasive" character (to use Sinclair's word) of autism is assumed to be, not the simultaneous impairment of several cognitive areas, but a different mode of feeling and thinking "that colors every experience, every sensation, perception, thought, emotion, and encounter, every aspect of existence" (Sinclair 1993). Such a shift from a medical view to a different perspective where support and recognition of autistic people become crucial outside of medical institutions has important consequences. As statistics show that autists often confront problems like massive unemployment and low income, companies like the Danish society Specialisterne and networks like the Autistic Self Advocacy Network vindicate the application of the principle of equality of opportunities. The question, then, is social justice rather than medical explanation. And if we read recent studies and reports, it is quite obvious that the climate is changing: some major, global companies have specifically targeted people with autism in their recruitment policy (Erbentraut 2015). The underlying philosophy is not only that diversity (including "neurodiversity") is essential to innovation. It is also that people with autism have specific assets: they can be outspoken, which is perceived as a good thing in a context where constructive criticism may be attenuated by office politics. And, interestingly, what has been seen as defects, oddities, and the result of cognitive impairments in clinical contexts is redescribed in terms that underline the positive aspect of the same well-known features and their potential benefit in terms of professional achievement (Walsh et al. 2014). What was called narrow interests is now perceived as the ability to stay focused on a given task. Attention to detail is not presented as the inability to grasp large, coherent wholes but as the perception of elements that will be missed by the ordinary viewer. People with autism are at a disadvantage in the context of standard job interviews: but this tells us something about the standard of job interviews, not against people with autism. As a result, there may be an ongoing change in the appraisal of autism: in a different social setting, it seems to be *valued* as it has never been before. According to the proponents of neurodiversity, autism would be harmful only in some circumstances and for external reasons—because of the negative attitudes that are the product of deeply rooted prejudices. It may *cause* harm, then, in a society that mistakenly perceives it as a disorder and a source of impairments, but it is not harmful in itself. Is there a way to reconcile the medical view and the claims of neurodiversity? And how does the HD view relate to this debate? I suggest we give a closer look to the relations between disorders, values, and harm.

First, even if this changing attitude toward autism is confirmed, a reappraisal has not in itself the power to transform a disorder into a nondisorder, as if functions and dysfunctions were dependent on our values. In this I would side with Wakefield: more positive attitudes toward autism in general do not change the boundaries of what disorders are, even if they may change the *representation* of disorders. These attitudes coincide with the outcome of scientific research that has unveiled *facts* that were previously neglected: autistic talent has been "unmasked" by scientific research and by the exposure of exceptional cases. But this does not prove wrong the view that in many cases autism may be harmful. This means also that the claims of the neurodiversity movement suffer from the same flaw that plagues the traditional, medical view: claiming that all forms of autism are instances of normal variation is just another brand of essentialism. Advocating the rights of autistic persons in general is compatible with the recognition of the wide disparities within the autistic spectrum and of the vulnerability and disabilities that are the consequences of severe autism, which make the medical research as important as it has ever been. The reasonable, narrow view of neurodiversity—high-functioning autism is an instance of normal variation—does not entail the broad view—any kind of autism is a form of normal variation (Jaarsma and Welin 2011). Progress in terms of social integration does not offer evidence that the medical view is wrong in itself and that in all cases, disability is nothing more than a disvalued difference.

But then, what is needed is a view of harm that is more factual and not dependent on "social values." The deprivation of something that is both widespread and useful is in itself harmful, in this narrow sense, because it is a source of disadvantage. For a given subject, dysfunctions result in harm when they reduce significantly and repeatedly his autonomy, the range of his opportunities, or the probability of success of his actions (Forest and Le Bidan 2016). Jerome Wakefield acknowledges this sense of harm from time to time as in the example of kidneys (Wakefield 1992a, 384) when he says that "a dysfunction in one kidney often has no effect on the overall well-being of a person and so is not considered to be disorder": in this case, clearly, the absence of harm (and, as a consequence, the absence of a disorder) has little to do with "present cultural standards" but only with the lack of detrimental effects of the dysfunction on the ordinary life of the individual. To say that "to be considered a disorder, the dysfunction must also cause significant harm under present circumstances and according to present cultural standards" leaves open the possibility of the presence of harm under present circumstances *without* reference to cultural standards, as in the case of kidney dysfunction. In the very same sense, impairing language acquisition in a neurodevelopmental disorder is causing significant harm because in this case, the range of opportunities is severely reduced and results in a disadvantage for the child. And to know this, we don't need an evolutionary scenario about the benefits of language mechanisms. And we don't need to think of social values, because we cannot figure out a society where failing to learn how to speak would not be intrinsically detrimental to a human child.

Then, it is both true that only harmful dysfunctions matter to medicine (because of their significant consequences) and false that the presence or the absence of a disorder depends on "social values." To see this, we can make the following thought experiment. Let us imagine that in a given (imaginary) society, children who meet the criteria for classical autism (difficulties with language acquisition, reduced social interactions, and repetitive behavior) receive a most favorable treatment, because they are supposed to have been chosen for some kind of higher, spiritual purpose. According to religious beliefs that shape the attitudes of members of this society, the (apparent) deficiencies of autistic children are only the sign of their (hidden) supernatural powers. But in this case, we still have the underlying cognitive dysfunctions and the reduced abilities. And we have every reason to believe that in this case, classical autism is still a disorder, even if the child is placed in a most favorable environment. It does not seem possible, then, to claim that, underlying dysfunctions being kept constant, the presence or the absence of a mental disorder depends on social values. In many cases at least, whatever values we adopt or reject, the harmful consequences, in the sense above defined, are there to stay.

Conclusion

Hempel used to underline that functional talk presupposes a certain standard of what the "normal functioning" or the functional integrity of the corresponding system may be, and he insisted on the necessity of making such standards as explicit as it is possible (Hempel 1965). In medicine and psychiatry, in particular, it is not possible to make claims about function and dysfunction without sensible background assumptions relative to the integrity of the individual. And what psychiatry lacks, too often, is a theory of what mental health would be. Having no standard of integrity at all would lead us nowhere, but we have to be especially careful not to define these standards in an excessively narrow way and to remain sensitive to what we could call the *varieties* of mental health. One popular version of our evolutionary history is that what makes humans special is their mindreading ability, an ability that allows us, in particular, to navigate within large social groups. Another version would be our ability to construct abstract, coherent wholes and to decompose them into their elements. Autism, then, would be a disorder not just because autistic behavior is odd, or because autistic children fail to do several things, but because autistic persons deviate from a certain standard to which we give a special importance for theoretical reasons. It is, as a consequence, especially important that just-so stories that flourish in evolutionary psychology do not introduce bias in our representation of what mental disorders are. If, as I have suggested above, for a given subject, dysfunctions result in harm when they reduce significantly and repeatedly his autonomy, the range of his opportunities, the quality of his well-being, or the probability of success of his actions, we have, very roughly, a standard to judge when autism is a kind of normal variation (associated with different abilities and opportunities) and when it is a source of impairment that requests medical concern. Again, dysfunction, in this sense, is not defined in reference to an evolutionary background, and harm is not judged according to social values.

Notes

1. Baron-Cohen, 2008: "The official terminology is to use the acronym ASD, for autism spectrum disorder. I prefer the acronym ASC [Autistic Spectrum Condition], since individuals in the high-functioning subgroup are certainly different [....] but it is arguable whether these differences should be seen as a disorder" (p. 14).

2. To my knowledge, the first occurrence of the word "neurodiversity" in a publication is Blume, 1998.

3. About the second question, I want to stress that what I have in mind is not reducible to the "imprecise boundary objection" against which Jerome Wakefield has already vindicated his views (Wakefield, 1999). In his answer to Lilienfeld and Marino, he has claimed that the HD analysis, as an instance of conceptual analysis, is not aimed at resolving the question of the boundary of disorders, but aimed at "explaining shared judgments about a range of important cases that fall on one side or the other of the boundary" (379). But clearly, high-functioning autism is not a limited set of rare and exceptional, boundary cases, it covers a large part of the autistic spectrum. And as judgments about high-functioning autism are contradictory, and not "shared," the question is how to take sides in the debate in a non-arbitrary manner.

4. See the foreword by evolutionary psychologists Leda Cosmides and John Tooby to Baron-Cohen, 1995.

References

Allen, D. 1988. Autistic spectrum disorders: Clinical presentation in preschool children. *Journal of Child Psychology* 3 (suppl.): 48–56.

Baron-Cohen, S. 1995. *Mindblindness, an Essay on Autism and Theory of Mind*. MIT Press.

Baron-Cohen, S. 2008. *Autism and Asperger Syndrome*. Oxford University Press.

Baron-Cohen, S. 2009. Autism: The empathizing-systemizing (E.-S.) theory. *The Year in Cognitive Neuroscience Annals of the New York Academy of Sciences* 1156: 68–80.

Baron-Cohen S., and M. K. Belmonte. 2005. Autism: A window onto the development of the social and analytic brain. *Annual Review of Neuroscience* 28: 109–126.

Blume, H. 1998. Neurodiversity: On the neurological underpinnings of geekdom. *The Atlantic*, September 30, 1998. https://www.theatlantic.com/magazine/archive/1998/09/neurodiversity/305909.

Brownlow, C. 2010. Re-presenting autism: The construction of NT syndrome. *Journal of Medical Humanities* 31(3): 243–256.

Cummins, R. 1975. Functional analysis. *Journal of Philosophy* 72: 741–764.

Erbentraut, J. 2015. How these four companies are tackling the autism unemployment rate. *Huffington Post*, June 1, 2015. http://www.huffingtonpost.com/2015/05/07/autism-employment_n_7216310 .html.

Forest, D. and M. Le Bidan. 2016. In search of normal functions: BST, Cummins functions, and Hempel's problem. In *Naturalism in Philosophy of Health: Issues, Limits and Implications*, E. Giroux and M. Lemoine (eds.), 39–51. Springer Verlag.

Frith, U. 1989. *Autism: Explaining the Enigma*. Wiley-Blackwell.

Frith, U., and F. Happé. 1994. Autism: Beyond 'theory of mind.' *Cognition* 50(1–3): 115–132.

Gerrans, P. 2002. The theory of mind module in evolutionary psychology. *Biology and Philosophy* 17(3): 305–321.

Grandin, T. 2006. *Thinking in Pictures and Other Reports from My Life with Autism*. Bloomsbury.

Grandin, T. 2009. How does visual thinking work in the mind of a person with autism? A personal account. *Philosophical Transactions of the Royal Society B* 364: 1437–1442.

Happé, F. 1999. Autism: Cognitive deficit or cognitive style? *Trends in Cognitive Science* 3(6): 216–222.

Happé, F., and P. Vital. 2009. What aspects of autism predispose to talent? *Philosophical Transactions of the Royal Society B* 364: 1369–1375.

Hempel, C. 1965. The logic of functional analysis. *Aspects of Scientific Explanation and Other Essays in the Philosophy of Science*, 297–330. Free Press.

Hickok, G. 2014. *The Myth of Mirror Neurons*. Norton.

Hill, E. L. 2004. Executive dysfunction in autism. *Trends in Cognitive Sciences* 8(1): 26–32.

Jaarsma, P., and S. Welin. 2011. Autism as a natural human variation: Reflections on the claims of the neurodiversity movement. *Health Care Analysis* 20(1): 20–30.

Just, M. A., V. L. Cherkassky, T. A. Keller, and N. J. Minshew. 2004. Cortical activation and synchronization during sentence comprehension in high-functioning autism: Evidence of underconnectivity. *Brain* 127(pt 8): 1811–1821.

Kanner, L. 1943. Autistic disturbances of affective contact. *Nervous Child* 2: 217–250.

Machamer, P., L. Darden, and C. Craver. 2000. Thinking about mechanisms. *Philosophy of Science* 67(1): 1–25.

Murphy, D., and R. Woolfolk. 2000. The harmful dysfunction view of mental disorders. *Philosophy, Psychiatry, and Psychology* 7(4): 242–252.

Ortega, F. 2009. The cerebral subject and the challenge of neurodiversity. *Biosocieties* 4: 425–445.

Ozonoff, S., B. F. Pennington, and S. J. Rogers. 1991. Executive function deficits in high-functioning autistic individuals: Relationship to theory of mind. *Journal of Child Psychology and Psychiatry* 32: 1081–1105.

Piven, J., P. Palmer, D. Jacobi, D. Childress, and S. Arndt. 1997. Broader autistic phenotype: Evidence from a family history study of multiple-incidence autism families. *American Journal of Psychiatry* 154(2): 185–190.

Poland, J. 2002. *Whither Mental Disorders*. Unpublished manuscript.

Ramachandran, V. S. 2011. *The Tell-Tale Brain: A Neuroscientist's Quest for What Makes Us Human*. William Heinemann.

Richardson, R. C. 2010. *Evolutionary Psychology as Maladapted Psychology*. MIT Press.

Rippon, G., J. Brock, C. Brown, and J. Boucher. 2007. Disordered connectivity in the autistic brain: Challenges for the new psychopathology. *International Journal of Psychophysiology* 63(2): 164–172.

Schwartz, P. H. 2007. Defining dysfunction: Natural selection, design, and drawing a line. *Philosophy of Science* 74: 364–385.

Sinclair, J. 1993. Don't mourn for us. *Our Voice* 1(3). https://www.autreat.com/dont_mourn.html.

Wakefield, J. C. 1992a. The concept of mental disorder: On the boundary between biological facts and social values. *American Psychologist* 47(3): 373–388.

Wakefield, J. C. 1992b. Disorder as harmful dysfunction: A conceptual critique of *DSM-III-R*'s definition of mental disorder. *Psychological Review* 99(2): 232–247.

Wakefield, J. C. 1999. Evolutionary versus prototype analyses of the concept of disorder. *Journal of Abnormal Psychology* 108: 374–399.

Wakefield, J. C. 2000. Spandrels, vestigial organs and such: Response to "The harmful dysfunction view of mental disorders." *Philosophy, Psychiatry, and Psychology* 7(4): 253–269.

Walsh, L., S. Lydon, and O. Healy. 2014. Employment and vocational skills among individuals with autism spectrum disorder: Predictors, impact, and interventions. *Review Journal of Autism and Developmental Disorders* 1(4): 266–275.

Wing, L. 1997. The autistic spectrum. *Lancet* 350(9093): 1761–1767.

22 Do the Challenges of Autism and Neurodiversity Pose an Objection to the Harmful Dysfunction Analysis? Reply to Denis Forest

Jerome Wakefield

In his chapter in this volume, my friend Denis Forest presents a provocative overview of the increasing complexities and controversies surrounding the diagnosis of autism, including the neurodiversity movement's arguments against psychiatric labeling of autism as a disorder. He argues that in considering these developments, difficulties lie in wait for my harmful dysfunction analysis (HDA) of medical, including mental, disorder (First and Wakefield 2010, 2013; Spitzer 1997, 1999; Wakefield 1992a, 1992b, 1993, 1995, 1997a, 1997b, 1997c, 1997d, 1998, 1999a, 1999b, 2000a, 2000b, 2001, 2006, 2007, 2009, 2011, 2014, 2016a, 2016b; Wakefield and First 2003, 2012), especially regarding the key question of whether autism should be understood as normal variation or disorder. He argues that the "data" of the autism controversy, although not fundamentally disconfirming the HDA, require modification of both its dysfunction and harm components: "In a nutshell, I shall advocate a more mechanistic view of dysfunctions and an understanding of harm in terms of diminished ability." I will consider Forest's critique of the dysfunction criterion and most of his concerns about the harm requirement. I'll address other harm-related concerns in my reply to Cooper.

The diagnosis of autism emerged from observations of a triad of syndromally associated severe symptoms, including impairment of social development, impairment of communication, and display of rigid and repetitive behavior. The *Diagnostic and Statistical Manual of Mental Disorders (DSM-5)* officially expanded classic autism into an autistic spectrum of conditions varying in severity, engulfing the former milder diagnosis of Asperger's disorder. *DSM-5* also reduced the triad to a dyad of dimensions by combining impairment of social communication and impairment of social development into one overarching dimension of deficits in social communication and social interaction.

Forest observes that autism was recognized as a developmental disorder from the earliest days of its identification, but he does not try to explain why it seemed, and still seems, so obvious to almost everyone (other than those arguing for the most extreme neurodiversity position) that the initially identified severe condition—which, like Forest, I will refer to as "classic autism"—is a disorder rather than an unusual variant of normality. (I will return to this question below.) Instead, Forest focuses on recent developments that, he says, have clouded the initial picture of clear disorder. Newly recognized phenomena such as the autistic spectrum (Wing 1997), high-functioning autism with preserved general intellectual abilities, the broader autistic phenotype (BAP) consisting of personality traits that are mild versions of autistic-like symptoms, subthreshold cases satisfying one rather than both autistic dimensional criteria, and isolated but sometimes quite dramatic special talents in otherwise seriously impaired autistic individuals complicate the classic picture and make the category of autism increasingly problematic as to disorder status, he suggests.

It is this complex of autistic conditions that, Forest thinks, poses a challenge to the HDA. Based on his account of autism and the neurodiversity movement, Forest lodges three objections to the HDA. First, its reliance on the evolutionary model of dysfunction fails to reflect how dysfunction is actually used by researchers. Second, its analysis in terms of dysfunction is unhelpful in guiding disorder attributions in difficult cases within the autism category. Along with these first two objections, Forest presents several subsidiary concerns about the dysfunction requirement, such as that it is subject to "just-so" stories and that it fails to help us appreciate the many varieties of normality. Third, Forest argues that the harm criterion is too narrow in virtue of its being mistakenly linked to social values—a point that, as noted, I will partly address here and return to elsewhere in this volume. I focus here mainly on Forest's two objections to the "dysfunction" requirement as opposed to the "causal role" approach preferred by Forest, as well as his subsidiary criticisms of the dysfunction requirement.

First, then, Forest challenges whether HDA's evolutionary approach actually guides research on autism: "Is research about autism and its explanation concerned with the discovery of dysfunctional mechanisms, where 'dysfunctional' has the precise meaning that is attached to it within the framework of HD analysis?" Forest surveys three of the main theories of autism—mindblindness, executive dysfunction, and weak coherence— and concludes that only mindblindness theorists explicitly refer to evolutionary considerations. He thus concludes, "The answer…is negative: in the literature, with few exceptions, 'dysfunction' of psychological or neural mechanisms is not understood as their failure to perform what they have been 'designed' to do."

If not a failure of biologically designed function, what, then, is a dysfunction? Forest suggests that what is at work instead of the HDA is a concept of dysfunction that combines Robert Cummins's (1975) causal-role model with a normative component that determines which causes are dysfunctions: "Cummins's view of functions (Cummins 1975) according to which the function F of a component C is its contribution to the explanation of a capacity of the system in which C is embedded, seems appropriate for psychological as well as physiological mechanisms"; "Moreover, factual judgements about impaired performance and dysfunction are usually inseparable from implicit evaluative claims." That is, for Forest, a dysfunction in an internal component of the organism occurs when the component causes a species-atypical negative condition in the organism.

Forest's argument—that because some theorists who study autism do not explicitly couch their theories in terms of evolution, and therefore "dysfunction" must have no essential connection to failure of biological design—is invalid. True, some theories of autism are not explicitly evolutionary, but, even if the HDA is correct, why should they be? No reference to evolution is necessary for doing studies of the proximal causes and potential treatments of autism, which, as Forest observes, is all that matters from a practical perspective in most autism research. Even Tinbergen's (1963) list of four basic features of evolutionary explanation includes proximal causal explanation as a component. When researchers pursuing mechanistic causal understanding assume that autism is a disorder, something beyond a mechanistic understanding must be involved, for a mechanistic causal explanation can equally be given for disorders and nondisorders. That implicit additional assumption, the HDA claims, is that something has gone wrong with the organism in the sense that there is a failure of biological design. This implicit assumption need not be made explicit in most causal research.

To take an analogy, the science of water, hydrology, was around long before anyone understood let alone stated that water is H_2O. The Nile was dammed about 4000 BC for agricultural irrigation reasons, and other ancient civilizations, including the Greeks, Romans, and Chinese, manipulated water with irrigation canals, aqueducts, and flood-control structures. They did not have any trouble identifying, studying, and manipulating the liquid they were aiming to control despite not knowing it was H_2O. Theories of the water precipitation cycle existed in ancient times and began to be quantified in the seventeenth century, whereas the chemical constitution of water as two parts hydrogen and one part oxygen was identified by Henry Cavendish in 1781. Surely neuroscientists have similarly ample grounds for recognizing certain homologous structures as causative of autism and devising ways to intervene without knowing or explicitly stating the evolutionary history that explains the existence and natural function of that kind of mechanism, although to some degree, assumptions about natural functions are presupposed in theorizing about what is going wrong.

Against the evolutionary view, Forest raises the usual complaint that evolutionary explanations can be "just-so" stories. This is true of all theorizing; there are endless "just-so" stories in every domain of human thought, and sifting through the theories and establishing which is correct is precisely what science is about. In any event, this is an objection to being overly gullible in accepting superficially appealing evolutionary explanations, not an objection to the conceptual claim that biological design is integral to the concept of disorder. One must not mistake the evolutionary framework for any particular theory of biological design. Incorrect theories of human nature— often promoted socially to provide an objective veneer to social values—yield incorrect theories of normality and disorder. When an unsatisfactory theory of human nature is used to support an oppressive diagnostic regime, the way to attack it is not, absurdly, to deny that human nature has anything to do with what is normal and disordered, but rather to provide evidence that the specific theory is a flawed account of human nature. Finally, this concern violates parity of reasoning because Forest fails to raise the same objection to the often implausible "just-so" stories of the neurodiversity movement itself that suggest, for example, that because there is some occasional highly specific feature of autism that is potentially useful under some specific modern circumstances, autism was adaptive and naturally selected as a normal variation earlier in our species history.

Returning to an earlier question, why was classic autism perceived as a disorder? It cannot simply be, as Forest's causal-role view would have it, that classic autism has negative statistically uncommon symptoms caused by an internal state. That criterion is hopelessly invalid and would mistakenly imply that illiteracy, criminal behavior, marital infidelity, and many other clearly nondisordered normal-range problematic conditions are disorders as well. The HDA explains the judgment that classic autism is judged a disorder by a combination of two judgments about autism: that the condition is harmful (to this extent, it is like illiteracy, criminal behavior, etc.) and that it is likely caused by a dysfunction, that is, by a failure of some internal mechanism to perform its biologically designed function (in this respect, it is unlike illiteracy, etc.). Though we cannot directly observe dysfunctions of internal mechanisms and have virtually no valid biomarkers for mental disorders and so the judgment that there is a dysfunction remains inferential and fallible, in the case of classic autism, this inference appears justified in virtue of the gross failure of presumptively biologically designed human capacities to socially interact, detect others' mental states, flexibly regulate one's actions, and communicate effectively. It is the strong circumstantial evidence of a dysfunction in classic autism that caused it to be classified as a disorder.

Forest's second objection is that the HDA does not help to guide us in resolving the many nosological questions that arise about autism given the series of expansions of the autism category noted above: "My second question is as follows: is the definition of disorders as harmful dysfunctions helping us to settle the debate about deficiency versus diversity, by providing us a standard for the application of the notion of disorder? To this second question, my answer will also be negative."

I believe that the HDA account is essential to achieving the explanatory discriminations that Forest requests. Of course, no analysis of the concept of medical disorder alone will tell us how to explain the phenomenon of autism or whether autism is a normal variant or a disorder, for these are factual matters that must be empirically investigated. Given the complexities of research on the brain and mind, no quick answers are to be expected. However, in terms of guidance with regard to the schematic form that such an explanation should take, the HDA implies that Forest's two questions are intimately related; whether autism is a disorder or a normal variant will depend in part on how it is explained. Part of the explanation, as Forest emphasizes, must be a mechanical causal explanation of how various autistic conditions come about. However, as noted, all normal and disordered conditions have mechanical explanations, so the causal-role analysis is at best necessary but not sufficient. The HDA implies that whether a given form of autism is a disorder versus a normal variation will depend on how the causal explanation relates to our species' history of biological design and specifically whether the explanation involves a dysfunction. The HDA further implies that if the explanations of various conditions comprising the autistic spectrum differ with regard to the involvement of dysfunction, then the judgments of whether the conditions are disorders or normal variants will also differ.

Thus, the HDA suggests that the answers to Forest's questions may differ depending upon where along the spectrum one focuses. This sort of differentiated view may eventually undo the confusion that has resulted from the premature expansion of the classic notion of autism into the autistic spectrum and beyond. This expansion has followed legitimate scientific pathways of generalization, locating classic autism and other prima facie clearly disordered autistic conditions within a broader context that can yield fresh scientific insight. However, these expansions, while scientifically and clinically useful, have been accomplished without adequate attention to the conceptual underpinnings of the concept of medical disorder, leading to an inevitable confusion of broader autism-related normal variation and autistic disorder. The HDA can serve as a corrective to the uncritical expansion of the autism category that ignores the requirements for disorder. This is a service that the causal-role model cannot provide because both normal variants and disorders can be mechanistically explained, statistically infrequent, and problematic. Moreover, in offering this guidance, the HDA provides a provisional explanation of how it is that people on various sides of the neurodiversity dispute can hold opposed views about the diagnostic status of high-functioning autism while knowing the same basic facts about the condition: the dispute is over whether the described conditions allow one to plausibly infer that they are caused by dysfunctions and over whether they are harmful or not.

In a comment on one potentially problematic addition to the autism category, Forest says, "Instead of a sharp contrast between autistic and nonautistic people, research has pointed out the presence of autistic features within some parts of the nonautistic population—which has led to the introduction of the notion of a broader autistic phenotype (Piven et al. 1997)." So, there is a puzzle and some disagreement in the literature about how to think about BAP. It is difficult to see how Forest can even begin to address the BAP puzzle with his account of dysfunction. The causal-role model of dysfunction can be applied equally to classic autism, high-functioning autism, and BAP. In contrast, this extension of autism-related conditions poses no real problem for HDA classification. Prima facie, the BAP concerns normal variation in personality. Even Piven and colleagues, who were pioneers in this area and developed the scale most frequently used to measure BAP, protest that BAP is not a disorder and that the scale they devised to measure it should not be used to identify pathology of any kind, let alone autism (Piven and Sasson 2014). Moreover, based on emerging evidence, BAP is most plausibly considered at this time not to be based on dysfunctions. There is evidence that single milder autistic traits are advantageous and have been positively selected, and it is only certain confluences of them that for unknown reasons become deleterious (Polimanti and Gelernter 2017). On this theory, BAP, although statistically infrequent and perhaps sometimes causing mild harm in our social environment—and thus potentially misclassified as a disorder according to the causal-role account—is not in fact a disorder but a normal variation.

More generally, the fact that features of a disorder show up in more moderate levels in population personality dimensions without constituting disorders is absolutely routine for virtually all symptoms, even psychotic ideation. Even if such extensions introduce a degree of fuzziness to the category, this need have no implication for the disorder status of many clear cases. The existence of some boundary fuzziness does not imply the illegitimacy of an overall distinction that has clear cases on both sides of the boundary. Orange versus red, night versus day, and adult versus child are legitimate distinctions with clear cases on both sides, even though there are not the "sharp contrasts" at the boundaries between these categories that Forest might desire. The developments cited by Forest do raise important conceptual questions about boundary setting, but prima facie, they do not cloud the picture regarding many clear cases, including classic autism.

According to the HDA, the question of whether various forms of autism are disorders remains an empirical question, and the question can be raised and answered differently about various subgroups currently engulfed by the autism label. One obvious reason why the diagnostic status of various forms of autism is problematic is that we just don't know much about the causes of each of the varieties of autism. With further research and theory, and with interpretation of the results guided by the HDA, many problems of diagnosis of the sort raised by Forest can be put to rest. That is, according to the HDA, there are possible empirical routes to resolving issues of dysfunction versus function and thus of disorder versus nondisorder. (Harm poses different challenges.) For example, recently, evidence has emerged in animal models of autism for a specific kind of dysfunction in which genetic functioning in certain areas of the genome becomes constricted due to the chromatin being packed too tightly and the genes prevented from expression by closing them off from the cell's transcriptional machinery (Qin et al. 2018). In the animal model, when those constricting structures were loosened and the genes allowed to function, social capacities of the sort impaired in autism were restored (Qin et al. 2018). Now, suppose that it should turn out that this form of harmful dysfunction is at the heart of classic autism (or some forms of classic autism) and that we then discovered that high-functioning autism is due to milder levels of this same dysfunction. This would then support the conclusion that high-functioning autism, if judged harmful, is a mild form of autistic disorder. Alternatively, we could discover that high-functioning autism is not caused by this same process at all and is in fact a separate naturally selected variant due to advantages it confers and thus not a disorder. Or, we could find that high-functioning autism is due to a different type of dysfunction and is some disorder other than autism. Guided by the discriminating ability of the HDA's evolutionary dysfunction component, these issues can be addressed through evidence and theory.

Essentialist Confusions in the Extension of Diagnostic Categories

Aside from sheer ignorance of the empirical facts, there is a deeper source of confusion about the diagnostic status of autism that also applies to many other disorders and generally afflicts nosology these days. The puzzlement to which Forest refers is due to a subtle conflation of concepts that often occurs in dimensionalizing what start out as presumed disorder categories. Although for convenience we might choose syndromal language at times that refers to any conditions with certain symptoms, in the long run, we gravitate toward essentialist meanings and concepts in which categories of disorder are understood as determined by etiologies that amount to a specific type of dysfunction. Most disorder categories start out as essentialist concepts defined using some (presumptively, but defeasibly) clearly disordered base set that is syndromally manifested in harmful symptoms that are provisionally assumed to be due to the same etiology based on the same dysfunction (or possibly multiple dysfunctions that eventually can be distinguished and separated into multiple distinct disorders). The idea is, roughly, that the disorder is the etiologically homogeneous category consisting of the base set *and any other harmful condition that has the same dysfunction as its etiology*. Thus, as science advances, disorders tend to be extended in accordance with shared dysfunction etiology, not shared symptoms. This is why symptomatically, quite diverse conditions presumed to indicate the same dysfunction can fall under the same disorder and symptomatically similar conditions presumed to involve different dysfunctions can fall under different disorders.

However, the essence of the syndromal base set can be theorized in many different ways. How one extends essentialist concepts given the many properties possessed by a base set depends on two things. First, there are empirical or theoretical discoveries about the underlying nature of the base set. Second, there is the choice of a semantic or ontological marker to indicate the kind of category one intends to formulate and thus which kinds of features of the base set are relevant to guiding the extension of the category to new instances. Each base set can be generalized in many different ways based on different properties, so the ontological marker that one is defining as a presumptive disorder is crucial to the process of defining a nosological category.

For example, for water, the base set is the clear liquid in the familiar lakes and rivers, so "water" means "whatever is essentially like the clear liquid in the familiar lakes and rivers." However, without an ontological marker, this formula remains ambiguous in the extreme. That base set has many properties that might serve as an essence for a larger category depending on the ontological marker. Water is H_2O if the ontological marker is "same substance," but water is H_2O-that-also-has-the-essence-of-liquidity if the marker is "same liquid," and if the ontological marker is "matter (versus energy)," then the essence is different from either of these and is something like "composed of elementary particles." Which of these senses one is using matters pragmatically. A glass of ice is not a glass of water in the intended sense when asking for a glass of water in a restaurant, but it may be a glass of water in the relevant sense when asked for in a chemistry lab.

This point about specifying the ontological marker is often taken for granted, but it is where confusion about disorder categories can occur. In the case of autism, the initial base set consists of severe classic autism, and in principle, the category is extended from there in accordance with a postulated common etiology (or etiologies) of the base set. However, if the category is being essentialistically defined as a category of disorder, then, given that "disorder" means "harmful dysfunction," the essence must consist of a dysfunction, and the included conditions must be harmful. The ontological marker of "same disorder as" determines these constraints on how the category is extended. Anything falling outside of these regulative principles is not autism in the intended sense of a pathology in the same category as the identified base set of presumed pathological conditions. If this is the intended meaning of "autism," and if BAP and certain forms of high-functioning individuals with some autistic traits are in fact not suffering from disorders, then, with apologies to those whose identities may be tied up with this term, they are not autistic (in this historically anchored semantic sense). It was just a mistake by overreaching nosologists to ever apply this term to them based on the mistaken view that they are mild cases of the harmful dysfunction underlying classic autism. Such mistakes are not uncommon; for example, whales were thought of as fish for millennia until a deeper understanding of biology revealed that the kind of thing we refer to as fish do not share a deep biological nature with whales, which thus turn out not to be classifiable as fish after all. Some similar analysis may well apply to what we call "high-functioning autism"; it may not be autism at all.

However, very often, the greatest insight into a category of disorder can come from casting a broader research web and seeing the disorders as part of a larger category not constrained by harm or even by dysfunction and looking at all those conditions falling within the broader category, whether they are disorders or not. To take a very simple example, it is scientifically extraordinarily illuminating and explanatorily potent, and yields multiple fruitful lines of research, to consider what gives rise to the sickle cell gene and how the gene functions, despite the fact that, at least in malaria-endemic locations, having a single sickle gene is not necessarily a medical disorder. In effect, there is a three-point dimensional variable ranging from zero to two sickle cell genes that defines a scientifically important target of study, and it is only through studying that broader dimensional domain—and thus identifying the adaptive malaria-resistance properties of having a single sickle cell gene (the precise causal-role workings of which are still being explored and yielding surprising and potentially useful scientific insights) that we have come to a fuller understanding that sickle cell disease, like many genetic disorders, is the result of the genetic lottery leading to an individual having too many genes of a kind that are adaptive and selected for in more moderate amounts but that together yield a nonselected and harmful dysfunction. In malaria-endemic areas, a single sickle cell gene need yield neither dysfunction nor harm, yet it lies within a crucial domain of study that includes the disorder of sickle cell anemia.

Disorder is often, as in this case, the accidental confluence of selected features that, when occurring together, yield dysfunction (meaning a zone of outcome never selected for). Indeed, there is recent evidence that autism is precisely this sort of disorder in which individually advantageous genes that were naturally selected for cognitive and social advantages occur in specific combinations that for as yet unknown reasons shift to being jointly deleterious and causing dysfunction (Polimanti and Gelernter 2017). If this is correct, then the argument for studying a broader domain that includes, for example, the BAP and high-functioning autism should have some weight as a potentially fruitful pathway to new insights. However, this research strategy and the use of the term "autism" for the dimensional expression of features associated with the disorder must not be confused with the expansion of the domain of disorder. If "autism" is extended from classic autism with the ontological marker not being "the same disorder" but rather something like "some of the same cognitive or personality traits as in the triadic syndrome at varying levels of severity" (which encompasses both high-functioning autism and the broader autism phenotype), there is then no implication that something that falls under "autism" in this sense must be a disorder, any more than something that falls under "water" with the ontological marker of "same substance" must be a liquid. Scientists may want to study dimensions defined the former way to gain general understanding about variables linked to autism-the-disorder, but that does not mean they are studying autism-the-disorder.

The issue with autism, as with many categories of pathology, is that scientists like dimensions. They like the dimensions to be as encompassing as possible so that they can formulate the most perspicuous theories and do the most decisive statistical tests of data. Consequently, our initial clearly pathological categories are regularly generalized into dimensions. This has now confusedly gotten inflated into a supposed dimensional approach to pathology. Such dimensional generalizations often ignore the fact that if the marker for "same disorder" is cast aside and other features without that constraint are seen as essences and the category extended in accordance with those features, then generalization may occur in ways that are unrelated to pathological status. The larger more all-encompassing categories that result may socially still cling to their "disorder" status as a result of being tied to the original base set by which the relevant disorder category term was defined but may no longer represent the intended ontological constraint of pathology. It would be like extending "water" based on the H2O theory to all oxides and calling that much larger set of chemical substances "water."

Varieties of Health

With all the varied conditions now collected under "autism," Forest expresses the quite legitimate concern that "we have to be especially careful not to define these standards in an excessively narrow way and to remain sensitive to what we could call the *varieties* of mental health." Contrary to Forest's implication, this goal is entirely consistent with and best served by the HDA's evolutionary approach to human normality. Indeed, the misidentification of varieties of normal-range mental health as purported disorders is one of the primary ways I have deployed the HDA in my extensive work on false positives in psychiatric diagnosis. The HDA gives one a place to stand in formulating such critiques. Variation within normality is a routine and essential feature of evolutionary thinking across almost all human features. A focus on how human beings are biologically designed—as opposed to a focus on what is locally useful or culturally valued—leads to a critical examination of proposed expansions of diagnostic categories, and such skepticism can liberate us from diagnostic oppression. Without the in-principle objective touchstone of how human beings are in fact biologically shaped to be, diagnosis can and often does run amok in the direction of greatly overdiagnosing disorder as a tool of socialization and social control (Wakefield, Lorenzo-Luaces, and Lee 2017).

It is difficult to see how, without the HDA's biological design constraint, Forest proposes to recognize unusual varieties of health, including statistically deviant and socially disvalued varieties. Forest's causal-role approach to function and dysfunction offers no coherent account of function and dysfunction that might help here. Every condition, from "sluggish schizophrenia" (applied to political dissidents in the Soviet Union) to female clitoral orgasm in Victorian England (seen as a disorder by many physicians), could be analyzed as potential dysfunctions on a statistical-infrequency account, and they certainly have mechanical explanations that in the causal-role account can be translated into "dysfunctions." (Whether there is truly harm in these conditions despite the social disapproval is of course another matter; see the discussion of harm below and in my reply to Cooper in this volume.) So, where is the standard that tells us that we are dealing here not with dysfunctions but with "varieties of mental health"? For that, you need the HDA's evolutionary conceptualization of the enormous variation within normal-range human biological design.

Is Autism a Trade-off for Savant Talents and Thus a Normal Variation?

A further argument Forest puts forward against the HDA's explanatory powers concerns both autistic special talents and the "weak coherence" theory of autism. Here, he considers that the fact that a significant percentage of autistic individuals have been found to have unusual specific abilities within such spheres as memory, calculation, drawing, or music, or in attention to detail, has been used as an argument that autism is not a disorder. However, sometimes, features that are desirable come into existence as side effects of disorders that are in themselves harmful. As Forest ultimately concedes, "Autistic talent has been 'unmasked' by scientific research and by the exposure of exceptional cases. But this does not prove wrong the view that in many cases, autism may be harmful." The question is whether the HDA can illuminate how to think about this issue.

Regarding the isolated special abilities sometimes found in autistic individuals, Forest says, "These results also mean that instead of thinking in terms of cognitive deficits in autism, we may have to think in terms of cognitive style (Happé 1999) and a different trade-off between abilities that are impaired and other abilities that may be enhanced, at least in high-functioning autism." However, many disorders have some positive effects, but mostly these are either accidental side effects (e.g., cowpox inoculates against smallpox) or compensatory changes in response to the disorder (e.g., enhanced echolocation in blindness). The fact that a negative condition causes this sort of positive side effect or compensatory adjustment does not undo the disorder attribution to the negative condition. Forest's argument that autism may not be a disorder because its negative features are a trade-off for special talents depends on a stronger sense of "trade-off." His use of that term and his provisional limitation of his point to high-functioning autism indicate that he is considering the following hypothesis: perhaps the autistic individual's distinctive cognitive functioning is a normal variant that occurs as a result either of the random normal distribution of cognitive strengths and weaknesses in the population (as, for example, Einstein's extraordinary development of spatial ability may have been a normal-variational brain-developmental trade-off for early language learning) or as a biologically designed trade-off in which the autistic individual's weaknesses are the inevitable side effect of naturally selected strengths (as, for example, the negative features of pregnancy such as diminished physical agility in late stages of pregnancy and pain during childbirth are trade-offs for the naturally selected process of pregnancy). Such a trade-off account appears prima facie implausible for classic autism given that the severe global challenges would not seem to be even remotely offset by or required by the potential for isolated talents. The trade-off hypothesis makes most sense when applied to high-functioning autism or BAP.

However, there is simply no evidence that the savant skills of autistic individuals are naturally selected with social and emotional impairments as necessary trade-offs.

Several considerations weigh against such a hypothesis. First, savant skills do not appear regularly and they vary enormously. Estimates of the percentage of autistic individuals having any such skill range from classic studies suggesting 10% to around 25% up to as high as 63% to 88% (Happé 2018; Meilleur, Jelenic, and Mottron 2015) depending on the range of skills and perceptual acuities measured and the methodology used. However, specific skills do not exist in a substantial number of cases and in any event are highly varied, not always functionally meaningful, and sometimes transient. Moreover, savant skills are often extremely narrow (e.g., calendar calculations, jigsaw puzzle solving), placing in doubt their adaptive significance as the basis for a naturally selected trade-off. In no study does autism emerge as regularly accompanied by some uniform set of talents for which it might be hypothesized to be a side effect or trade-off, making it problematic as to how the negative autistic features could be explained as trade-offs for these skills. Finally, we know that a trade-off theory is not necessary to explain the occurrence of autism's advantageous isolated talents because certain brain disorders, including brain trauma and frontotemporal dementia, can occasionally yield the same sorts of talents, and in these cases, there is no question that the skills are the side effect of pathology, perhaps where some brain areas become disinhibited due to damage elsewhere.

Forest also suggests a second form of trade-off argument in which it is not savant talents in general but the characteristically decontextualized, detail-oriented cognition characteristic of many autistic individuals, sometimes called "weak coherence" (Frith 1989; Frith and Happé 1994), that may be a benefit of such magnitude that impairments in social skills may be a biologically designed or biologically normal-range trade-off for it. The claim is that, under some circumstances, a decontextualized focus on detail can yield divergent insights or perceptions that elude those with greater context sensitivity.

However, sensitivity to context seems to be a sophisticated normal-range biologically designed developmental achievement. Along with autistic individuals, children in general are not yet fully sensitive to context. For example, with their immature perceptual systems, children, like autistic individuals, are more resistant than neurotypical adults to optical illusions that result from context sensitivity (Doherty, Campbell, Tsuji, and Phillips 2010). Forest emphasizes that some companies are hiring autistic individuals with potential strengths in mind, such as being outspoken or attending to details that others might miss. This may be a step forward in terms of social justice, but lack of contextual sensitivity could render potential strengths ineffective because one requires a contextual understanding to know when speaking out or bringing disparate details to the attention of others is useful rather than distracting. Further serious dangers of lack of contextual sensitivity are revealed in numerous reports of autistic people experiencing such tragedies as drowning (e.g., McLaughlin and Sutton 2018; Sanchez 2018) or needless violent interactions with the police leading to imprisonment (Furfaro

2018) because of lack of sensitivity to relevant contextual cues. Overall, diminution in context sensitivity, whatever its marginal advantages, must be considered a serious intrinsic harm and not a plausible basis for a trade-off against other negative features of autism.

Neurodiversity versus Neurotypicality

Forest quotes a much-cited neurodiversity-inspired definition of the neurotypical syndrome (NT) that characterizes nonautistic individuals in a way that mimics the supposedly invalid description of autistic individuals as pathological. For example, it defines "neurotypical syndrome [as] a neurobiological disorder characterized by preoccupation with social concerns, delusions of superiority, and obsession with conformity. ... Tragically, as many as 9,625 out of every 10,000 individuals may be neurotypical." Forest implies that perhaps the HDA is stymied by how to interpret such descriptions.

Humor aside, what is actually wrong with the neurotypicality-mocking passage quoted by Forest? First, it suggests that neurotypicality is privileged for the vacuous reason that it just happens to be statistically typical. However, neurotypicality is privileged not because it is statistically normal but because it is inferred to be functionally normal. Many statistically infrequent problematic conditions, ranging from illiteracy to criminality, are not considered disorders, and many statistically normal conditions, such as dental caries and periodontal disease (which characterize roughly 80% of people's gums worldwide), are considered disorders. Statistical normality is at best a fallible indicator of functional normality when it comes to disorder judgments. Second, the passage suggests that not all aspects of neurotypicality are beneficial or desirable. However, health is not simply a matter of whether a condition is positive or negative. Most people would prefer not to be anxious at an upcoming test and not to experience the pain of grief, yet these negatively valued features are not considered disorders because they are functionally normal in terms of human biological design. All of his makes sense within the HDA framework. (For further discussion of autism and the HDA, see Wakefield et al. 2020.)

Does the Harm Criterion Need to Be More Factual?

Finally, Forest accepts the need for a harm criterion for disorder but, like many critics (see Cooper, this volume, for a similar objection and see my reply to Cooper for a fuller response), objects that the HDA's reliance on social values to determine harm is problematic and would prefer that values be more factual: "what counts as 'harm' is less dependent on 'social values' than what is required by HD analysis. ... What is needed is a view of harm that is more factual and not dependent on 'social values.'" Forest thinks that socially defining harm unduly restricts disorder judgments that could be based on harm "in itself": "The deprivation of something that is both widespread and useful is in itself harmful … because it is a source of disadvantage. For a given subject, dysfunctions result in harm when they reduce significantly and repeatedly his autonomy, the range of his opportunities, or the probability of success of his actions."

Forest is basically right in suggesting that the "social values" addendum to the "harm" requirement cannot be a general and absolute requirement. If harm can be understood independently of social values, it still satisfies the HDA's harm requirement. The social values addendum cannot be general and absolute because the HDA applies to all organisms that can become disordered, including to creatures that are nonsocial and, even if social, do not possess social values as a filter through which harm is understood. Thus, the social-values codicil to the harm requirement of the HDA ought to be read analogously to "dysfunction," where evolutionary theory offers the best empirical framework for understanding the concept.

Though desirable, and in principle consistent with the HDA, a theory of harm that would apply universally to the human case is elusive and philosophically highly controversial. Moreover, in the human case, the appeal to a culture-transcendent standard for harm that resembles current Western philosophical views but is to be applied universally in medical diagnosis raises worrisome issues of implicit Western triumphalism and of turning medicine into another battlefield in culture wars in which some people's needs are ignored because their condition is not deemed to be truly harmful (for an example of this danger, see Powell and Scarffe 2019; Wakefield and Conrad 2019). I tend to think that the social values addendum suitably broadly interpreted remains relatively benign and useful, that what are claimed by critics to be culture-transcendent "factual" human values are implicit in every human cultural value system, and that many of the harms human beings suffer are *pro tanto* harms related to their social roles and expectations. (Further reasons why I added the social values codicil in the human case on which my analysis has focused are detailed in my reply to Cooper in this volume, and I will not repeat them here.) So, I will briefly try to explain or defend here the social-values addendum from Forest's arguments for a more factual criterion.

It is true that some values are deeper, more presupposed by other values, and more widely embraced across cultures, and in this sense, one might say they are more "factual" than others. However, their factuality is not something independent of what actual human beings in actual cultures value but simply an expression of a more general valuing of them across human cultures. However, it is almost always true that the realization of such values will vary across cultures based on local more specific values and practices that will influence the evaluation of harm in medical diagnosis. A simple extrapolation of what we specifically value to the criterion of harm for all human cultures smacks of Western triumphalism.

For example, in terms of the above passage, surely usefulness is valued universally, but whether a specific feature is useful is culturally relative. Similarly, values such as *advantage, autonomy, opportunity,* and *success* are virtually universal cultural values, but the nature of their fulfillment is heavily culturally loaded. There is also some variation in social attitudes toward even such seemingly "factual" values. At moderate levels, autonomy may be a common value, but some societies, it is well known, disvalue high autonomy and instead value group devotion and cohesion, whereas those in the West tend to place autonomy and development of the unique aspects of the self at the highest level of desirability. While success in some sense is a universal human goal valued in all cultures, what actually constitutes success varies enormously among cultures and times. Similarly, opportunity in the form of access to social roles as a form of justice and self-realization exists in advanced liberal industrialized states with highly differentiated work roles that include some scarce and coveted positions but is not readily applicable to the way most human nomadic hunter-gatherer groups lived throughout history, so its deprivation would not constitute a disorder in that context. In my view, Forest's substantive value considerations fall comfortably within the HDA's social values–based harm component.

Forest further asserts, "Impairing language acquisition in a neurodevelopmental disorder is causing significant harm because in this case, the range of opportunities is severely reduced and results in a disadvantage for the child. And to know this, we don't need an evolutionary scenario about the benefits of language mechanisms. And we don't need to think of social values, because we cannot figure out a society where failing to learn how to speak would not be intrinsically detrimental to a human child."

According to the HDA, of course Forest is correct that we don't need evolution to know whether impaired language is harmful, because only dysfunction, and not harm, is evaluated relative to a baseline of biological design. More important, the claim that we don't need to refer to social values in judging the cited harms is immediately contradicted by the evidence Forest offers on its behalf, namely, that the reason it is clearly harmful is that it is harmful according to the values of every human culture because in every such culture, lack of linguistic ability is manifestly detrimental.

In a final argument, Forest offers a thought experiment in which a culture reveres classical autism as a sign of being chosen by the gods for a higher spiritual purpose, with the symptoms seen as trade-offs for supernatural powers. (This hypothetical is reminiscent of reports of schizophrenic individuals with their delusional symptoms being deified in certain cultures.) Forest argues that, according to the culture's social values, there is no harm to these children, but yet objectively, "we still have the underlying cognitive dysfunctions, and the reduced abilities. ... Classical autism is still a disorder, even if the child is placed in a most favorable environment." Forest concludes that "it does not seem possible, then, to claim that, underlying dysfunctions being kept constant, the presence or the absence of a mental disorder depends on social values."

This example does not seem to me to support Forest's point. Forest agrees with the HDA that there is a dysfunction, whatever the community thinks: "we still have the underlying cognitive dysfunctions. ... A reappraisal has not in itself the power to transform a disorder into a nondisorder, as if functions and dysfunctions were dependent on our values. In this I would side with Wakefield." (I would caution that in this last passage, Forest appears to be running together dysfunction and disorder; a reappraisal cannot change a dysfunction into a nondysfunction, but if the altered appraisal implies a lack of harm, then it can change a disorder into a nondisorder.)

Is there harm to these children according to the community's social values? Forest says that the community theorizes that the children's deficiencies are in fact divinely caused trade-offs for their unusual powers. That very theory implies that the children's deficiencies are generally seen by the community as *pro tanto* harms and are not seen as harmful in this instance only because of the theory that there is a trade-off. However, that theory is incorrect. Forest observes, "We still have the underlying cognitive dysfunctions, and the reduced abilities. ... Whatever values we adopt or reject, the harmful consequences, in the sense above defined, are there to stay." True, and the community would presumably agree, if it did not believe its false theory. The community positively values cognitive and other abilities, and their loss is a real harm by the community's own lights. However, due to an incorrect theory, they mistakenly think that in this particular case, the limitations result from a purposeful trade-off for a greater good, and so there is no harm of the sort relevant to disorder attribution. Consequently, in reality, given that the trade-off theory is false, the classic autism symptoms are harmful to these children *as judged by the community's own value system* even if that is not the belief of the community members. Once the situation is made explicit, I do not see any divergence here between harm and social values of the sort Forest suggests. (For the reader interested in further discussion of the sorts of objections raised by Forest to the harm criterion, see my reply to Cooper in this volume.)

References

Doherty, M. J., N. M. Campbell, H. Tsuji, and W. A. Phillips. 2010. The Ebbinghaus illusion deceives adults but not young children. *Developmental Science* 13(5): 714–721.

First, M. B., and J. C. Wakefield. 2010. Defining 'mental disorder' in *DSM-V*. *Psychological Medicine* 40(11): 1779–1782.

First, M. B., and J. C. Wakefield. 2013. Diagnostic criteria as dysfunction indicators: Bridging the chasm between the definition of mental disorder and diagnostic criteria for specific disorders. *Canadian Journal of Psychiatry* 58(12): 663–669.

Frith, U., and F. Happé. 1994. Autism: Beyond 'theory of mind'. *Cognition* 50: 115–132.

Happé, F. 1999. Autism: Cognitive deficit or cognitive style? *Trends in Cognitive Science* 3(6): 216–222.

Happé, F. 2018. Why are savant skills and special talents associated with autism? *World Psychiatry* 17(3): 280–281.

McLaughlin, E. C., and J. Sutton. 2018. Autistic man who went overboard on Carnival cruise was traveling with special needs group. *CNN*, December 20. https://www.cnn.com/2018/12/20/us/autistic-man-overboard-carnival-cruise/index.html.

Meilleur, A.-A. S., P. Jelenic, and L. Mottron. 2015. Prevalence of clinically and empirically defined talents and strengths in autism. *Journal of Autism and Developmental Disorders* 45: 1354–1367.

Piven, J., P. Palmer, D. Jacobi, D. Childress, and S. Arndt. 1997. Broader autistic phenotype: Evidence from a family history study of multiple-incidence autism families. *American Journal of Psychiatry* 154(2): 185–190.

Piven, J., and N. J. Sasson. 2014. On the misapplication of the broad autism phenotype questionnaire in a study of autism. *Journal of Autism and Developmental Disorders* 44: 2077–2078.

Polimanti, R., and J. Gelernter. 2017. Widespread signatures of positive selection in common risk alleles associated to autism spectrum disorder. *PLoS Genetics* 13(2): e1006618.

Powell, R., and E. Scarffe. 2019. Rethinking "disease": A fresh diagnosis and a new philosophical treatment. *Journal of Medical Ethics* 45(9): 579–588.

Qin, L., K. Ma, Z.-J. Wang, Z. Hu, E. Matas, J. Wei, and Z. Yan. 2018. Social deficits in *Shank3*-deficient mouse models of autism are rescued by histone deacetylase (HDAC) inhibition. *Nature Neuroscience* 21: 564–575.

Sanchez, R. 2018. An autopsy report says a missing North Carolina boy with autism likely drowned. *CNN*, November 29. https://www.cnn.com/2018/11/29/us/maddox-ritch-autistic-boy-death/index.html.

Spitzer, R. L. 1997. Brief comments from a psychiatric nosologist weary from his own attempts to define mental disorder: Why Ossorio's definition muddles and Wakefield's "harmful dysfunction" illuminates the issues. *Clinical Psychology: Science and Practice* 4(3): 259–261.

Spitzer, R. L. 1999. Harmful dysfunction and the *DSM* definition of mental disorder. *Journal of Abnormal Psychology* 108(3): 430–432.

Tinbergen, N. 1963. On aims and methods of ethology. *Zeitschrift für Tierpsychologie* 20: 410–433.

Wakefield, J. C. 1992a. The concept of mental disorder: On the boundary between biological facts and social values. *American Psychologist* 47: 373–388.

Wakefield, J. C. 1992b. Disorder as harmful dysfunction: A conceptual critique of *DSM-III-R*'s definition of mental disorder. *Psychological Review* 99: 232–247.

Wakefield, J. C. 1993. Limits of operationalization: A critique of Spitzer and Endicott's (1978) proposed operational criteria of mental disorder. *Journal of Abnormal Psychology* 102: 160–172.

Wakefield, J. C. 1995. Dysfunction as a value-free concept: A reply to Sadler and Agich. *Philosophy, Psychiatry, and Psychology* 2: 233–246.

Wakefield, J. C. 1997a. Diagnosing *DSM-IV*, part 1: *DSM-IV* and the concept of mental disorder. *Behaviour Research and Therapy* 35: 633–650.

Wakefield, J. C. 1997b. Diagnosing *DSM-IV*, part 2: Eysenck (1986) and the essentialist fallacy. *Behaviour Research and Therapy*: 35: 651–666.

Wakefield, J. C. 1997c. Normal inability versus pathological disability: Why Ossorio's (1985) definition of mental disorder is not sufficient. *Clinical Psychology: Science and Practice* 4: 249–258.

Wakefield, J. C. 1997d. When is development disordered? Developmental psychopathology and the harmful dysfunction analysis of mental disorder. *Development and Psychopathology* 9: 269–290.

Wakefield, J. C. 1998. The *DSM*'s theory-neutral nosology is scientifically progressive: Response to Follette and Houts. *Journal of Consulting and Clinical Psychology* 66: 846–852.

Wakefield, J. C. 1999a. Evolutionary versus prototype analyses of the concept of disorder. *Journal of Abnormal Psychology* 108: 374–399.

Wakefield, J. C. 1999b. Mental disorder as a black-box essentialist concept. *Journal of Abnormal Psychology* 108: 465–472.

Wakefield, J. C. 2000a. Aristotle as sociobiologist: The "function of a human being" argument, black box essentialism, and the concept of mental disorder. *Philosophy, Psychiatry, and Psychology* 7: 17–44.

Wakefield, J. C. 2000b. Spandrels, vestigial organs, and such: Reply to Murphy and Woolfolk's "The harmful dysfunction analysis of mental disorder." *Philosophy, Psychiatry, and Psychology* 7: 253–269.

Wakefield, J. C. 2001. Evolutionary history versus current causal role in the definition of disorder: Reply to McNally. *Behaviour Research and Therapy* 39: 347–366.

Wakefield, J. C. 2006. What makes a mental disorder mental? *Philosophy, Psychiatry, and Psychology* 13: 123–131.

Wakefield, J. C. 2007. The concept of mental disorder: Diagnostic implications of the harmful dysfunction analysis. *World Psychiatry* 6: 149–156.

Wakefield, J. C. 2009. Mental disorder and moral responsibility: Disorders of personhood as harmful dysfunctions, with special reference to alcoholism. *Philosophy, Psychiatry, and Psychology* 16: 91–99.

Wakefield, J. C. 2011. Darwin, functional explanation, and the philosophy of psychiatry. In *Maladapting Minds: Philosophy, Psychiatry, and Evolutionary Theory*, P. R. Andriaens and A. De Block (eds.), 143–172. Oxford University Press.

Wakefield, J. C. 2014. The biostatistical theory versus the harmful dysfunction analysis, part 1: Is part-dysfunction a sufficient condition for medical disorder? *Journal of Medicine and Philosophy* 39: 648–682.

Wakefield, J. C. 2016a. The concepts of biological function and dysfunction: Toward a conceptual foundation for evolutionary psychopathology. In *Handbook of Evolutionary Psychology*, D. Buss (ed.), 2nd ed., vol. 2, 988–1006. Oxford University Press.

Wakefield, J. C. 2016b. Diagnostic issues and controversies in *DSM-5*: Return of the false positives problem. *Annual Review of Clinical Psychology* 12: 105–132.

Wakefield, J. C., and J. A. Conrad. 2019. Does the harm component of the harmful dysfunction analysis need rethinking? Reply to Powell and Scarffe. *Journal of Medical Ethics* 45(9): 594–596.

Wakefield, J. C., and M. B. First. 2003. Clarifying the distinction between disorder and nondisorder: Confronting the overdiagnosis ("false positives") problem in *DSM-V*. In *Advancing DSM: Dilemmas in Psychiatric Diagnosis*, K. A. Phillips, M. B. First, and H. A. Pincus (eds.), 23–56. American Psychiatric Press.

Wakefield, J. C., and M. B. First. 2012. Placing symptoms in context: The role of contextual criteria in reducing false positives in *DSM* diagnosis. *Comprehensive Psychiatry* 53: 130–139.

Wakefield, J. C., L. Lorenzo-Luaces, and J. J. Lee. 2017. Taking people as they are: Evolutionary psychopathology, uncomplicated depression, and the distinction between normal and disordered sadness. In *The Evolution of Psychopathology*, T. K. Shackleford and V. Zeigler-Hill (eds.), 37–72. Springer.

Wakefield, J. C., D. T. Wasserman, and J. A. Conrad. 2020. Neurodiversity, autism, and psychiatric disability: The harmful dysfunction perspective. In *Oxford Handbook of Philosophy and Disability*, D. T. Wasserman and A. Cureton (eds.), 501–521. Oxford University Press.

Wing, L. 1997. The autistic spectrum. *Lancet* 350: 1761–1766.

23 Naturalism and Dysfunction

Tim Thornton

Introduction: Disorder and Naturalism

The concepts of illness, disease, and disorder all share a prima facie normative character. Even Robert Kendell, who defended a plainly factual account, conceded that appearance in his 1975 paper, "The Concept of Disease and Its Implications for Psychiatry." He writes,

> Before we can begin to decide whether mental illnesses are legitimately so called we have first to agree on an adequate definition of illness; to decide if you like what is the defining characteristic or the hallmark of disease.... By 1960 the 'lesion' concept of disease... had been discredited beyond redemption, but nothing had yet been put in its place. It was clear, though, that its successor would have to be based on a statistical model of the relationship between normality and abnormality.... But... [a statistical model] fails to distinguish between deviations from the norm which are harmful, like hypertension, those which are neutral, like great height, and those which are positively beneficial, like superior intelligence. (Kendell 1975, 309)

The normative aspect of disease is suggested in this passage by the dimension spanning harm to benefit. This is a distinction beyond mere degree of difference from a statistical norm. It is normative as opposed to merely (statistically) normal. But normative notions present a challenge for the philosophical program of placing complex concepts into a conception of nature, or "naturalizing" them as that project is usually known, especially given the most influential version of philosophical naturalism: reductionism. (In his book *Philosophical Naturalism,* David Papineau argues that its fundamental characteristic is "the thesis that all natural phenomena are, in a sense to be made precise, physical" [Papineau 1993, 1]. Hence, showing how concepts pick out real and natural features of the world involves, ultimately, reducing them to physical concepts.)

The reason that normativity presents a challenge to philosophical naturalism so understood is that, on an influential neo-Humean view, the natural world is not itself the source of normativity: thinking subjects are. As Hamlet says, on this view, "There is nothing either good or bad, but thinking makes it so." Thus, normative concepts cannot be thought of as describing the natural world but as reflecting human subjectiv-ity. This is clearest in cases where the normativity concerned, like Hamlet's line, takes the form of explicit value judgments.

Here is one such example in the philosophy of disorder. K. W. M. (Bill) Fulford defends an account of illness as an endogenously caused failure of ordinary doing (Ful-ford 1989). He argues against both Thomas Szasz, who contrasts mental and physical illness, and Robert Kendell, who assimilates them as value free, that mental illness and physical illness are *both* value terms (Szasz 1960). The idea that illness comprises an internally generated failure of ordinary doing explains its value-ladenness because the concept of *failure* itself suggests an ineliminable negative value judgment. But Fulford also argues that differences of opinion about the value judgments need not generally imply error because they do not answer to anything objective. Value judgments are projections of a subject's sentiments onto the world, and hence differences of opinions should be explored rather than corrected (e.g., Fulford 2004). Hence, the class of ill-nesses does not pick out anything objective. It is a reflection of both worldly facts but also subjective values about which there can be rational disagreement.

Fulford's account does not fit reductionist naturalism. Illness is not in that sense a "natural" concept but an alloy of worldly fact and human value with the latter under-pinning the prima facie normative element of illness. To naturalize illness—at least in accord with the dominant reductionist reading of that term—would require some way to account for the normative dimension in value-free and naturalistic terms. That pos-sibility is the subject matter of this chapter. To investigate its prospects, I will discuss Jerome Wakefield's influential harmful dysfunction model of disorder.

I. Wakefield's Harmful Dysfunction Model

To be clear from the start: Wakefield does *not* attempt to provide a value-free analysis of illness or disease or disorder (unlike others such as Christopher Boorse [1975] and Robert Kendell [1975], who do). (Note that although, perhaps influenced by Boorse, Wakefield talks of "disorder" rather than "illness" or "disease," he does not suggest any firm distinctions between them; he comments, "Some writers draw distinctions among *disorder, disease,* and *illness. Disorder* is perhaps the broader term because it cov-ers traumatic injuries as well as disease/illness. I ignore these differences" [Wakefield 1992, 374]. I will follow his lead.) But he suggests that disorder can be analyzed as a conjunction of one specific value and a value-free medical science core.

On his account, the normative dimension is divided between two elements. It fea-tures in the value "harm," which forms one conjunct and helps encode the practi-cal aims of medicine to intervene in only particular cases, the harmful ones. But it is also present in the concept of a dysfunction, which turns out to be "anchored in evolutionary theory" (Wakefield 1999, 465). The resulting "harmful dysfunction analysis" contrasts with Fulford's analysis in that, in the latter, facts and values mingle "all the way down." By contrast, Wakefield's approach aims to characterize a purely descriptive *core* for medical science using the idea of biological functions. In other words, the normative component of any illness is divided into an irreducibly value-laden element of harm and into a deviation from a biological function, which is then reduced to, or naturalized via, descriptive biological theory. The class of biological dysfunctions is thus a natural class even if the broader class of disorder is not. The focus here is that narrow class.

The challenge of giving a descriptive, nonnormative, or nonevaluative account of function to explain this core element of disorder goes hand in hand with giving an account of *failure* of function. Only if an account can be given of what a *divergence* of the behavior of a system from its function comprises has the notion of a function that could be successfully *or* unsuccessfully executed been substantiated. But if such an account of divergence of function can be given in value-free, descriptive terms, then it would ipso facto successfully account for failure of function. Thus, it would be a mistake to assume that in characterizing disorder partly as a *failure* of function, Wakefield has already conceded the game to value theorists because "failure" is an evaluative concept as Fulford seems to suggest (Fulford 1999, 2000). If function and divergence from it can be analyzed in descriptive terms, then so can "failure" of function: it is any divergence from function. An apparently normative or evaluative concept would be reduced to a value-free descriptive analysis.

It may still seem that, in the case of function, a nonnormative descriptive account is a hopeless nonstarter precisely because the distinction between *success* and *failure* surely cannot be reduced to a purely factual or descriptive vocabulary. But just such descriptivist accounts of natural function have been proposed elsewhere as part of the wider legacy of Darwin. In the philosophy of language and thought, for example, Ruth Garrett Millikan proposes that the intentionality or "aboutness" of thoughts and beliefs can be naturalized using the notion of biological functions (see especially Millikan 1984). She argues that even conscious human purposes—paradigm instances of genuine teleology—are susceptible to this form of reductionist naturalism (Millikan 1998, 309).

Much has been written on the definition of function. Two broad approaches are perhaps most influential: the views of Cummins and Wright. Rachel Cooper summarizes their differences thus:

Of the best known positions, those who adopt Cummins-type views (Cummins 1975) claim that the function of a sub-system is whatever it normally currently does that contributes towards the goals of a larger system. On such an account the function of the heart is to pump blood around the body, as this is what hearts currently normally do that contributes to the organism surviving and reproducing. On the other hand, those who favour Wright-style approaches (Wright 1973) think that the function of a sub-system is fixed by its history. In the biological domain, the Wright-function of a sub-system is whatever it was naturally selected to do. (Cooper 2007, 30–31)

Elsewhere, Cooper (2002, 268) suggests other options and suggests that there are prima facie difficulties with all of them for the analysis of disorder or disease.

For the function of X to be Z, any of the following might be considered necessary:

1. X was originally selected because it does Z.
2. In the recent past, selection has been responsible for maintaining X because it does Z.
3. Currently, selection is responsible for maintaining X because it does Z.
4. At all times, X has been selected because it does Z.

It is difficult to choose between these options as each is associated with potential problems. One of the problems that Cooper highlights is that if one opts for the original selective advantages of some trait that, as a matter of fact, now also prima facie serves another function, then failure of that current prima facie function will not count as disease. But if recent history is taken to be key, then, because human societies and technologies now affect actual reproduction, traits that might seem prima facie to be dysfunctional but that are compensated for through human intervention cannot count as diseases. I will ignore these particular difficulties here.

Both Wakefield and Millikan favor a historical approach (like Wright's) connecting functions to actual evolutionary selective histories, and as will become clearer, this is most apt for the reductionist project in question. Roughly speaking, the biological or proper function of a particular trait of an organism is what explains the evolutionary success and survival value of that trait. (In fact, Millikan defines functions within an account of reproductively established families, but the details of her theory will not matter here.)

Crucially, for the purposes of capturing the prima facie normativity of disorder (Wakefield) and intentionality (Millikan), biological functions are distinct from dispositions. The biological function of a trait and its dispositions can diverge. Engineering limitations might cause the actual behavioral dispositions of a trait to diverge from the biological function it thus only partially exemplifies. Further, the divergences might themselves be life threatening and play no positive part in explaining the value of the trait. The best explanation of the survival of that organism and those like it cites the function that helped propagation or predator evasion, for example, and not those aspects of its behavioral dispositions that diverged unhelpfully from it.

This point is sometimes put by saying that what matters is not which traits or dispositions are selected but what function they are selected *for*. The distinction between "selection of" and "selection for" can be illustrated by the example of a child's toy

(Sober 1984). A box allows objects of different shapes to be posted into it through differently shaped slots in the lid. The round slot thus allows the insertion of balls, for example. It may be that the actual balls allowed through or "selected" in one case are all green. But they are selected *for* their round cross section and not their green color. Millikan stresses the fact that the biological function of a trait may be displayed in only a minority of actual cases. It is the function of sperm to fertilize an egg, but the great majority of sperm fails in this regard (Millikan 1984, 34). Since biological functions can diverge from mere dispositions, they have extra resources necessary for accounting for the idea of *failure* of function. The distinction between success and failure of a system, organism or organ can be defined by reference to its functioning in accord with its biological function.

Wakefield's work on disorder is in the same tradition: providing a reductionist account of a problematic concept by appeal to evolutionary theory. He offers an initially distinct, but eventually similar, account of natural functions. Drawing on essentialist accounts of natural kinds, such as water or gold, he suggests that natural functions likewise have an underlying essence. Thus, natural functions are defined as sharing whatever the initially unknown essential process is, which explains prototypical nonaccidental beneficial effects such as eyes seeing. This is a surprising claim given that what unites natural kinds such as gold or water are first-order physical properties. No first-order physical properties unite natural functions. But Wakefield goes on to invoke explanation and natural selection in a much more standard way:

> A natural function of a biological mechanism is an effect of the mechanism that explains the existence, maintenance or nature of the mechanism via the same essential process (whatever it is) by which prototypical nonaccidental beneficial effects…explain the mechanism which cause them.…It turns out that the process that explains the prototypical non-accidental benefits is natural selection acting to increase inclusive fitness of the organism. (Wakefield 1999, 471–472)

Thus, like Millikan, Wakefield relies on an account of natural function drawn from explanation within evolutionary theory to distinguish those dispositions that accord with a system's naturally selected function from those that do not.

However, despite this connection between the prima facie normativity of the concept of disorder and the normativity, albeit rooted in evolutionary history, of biological functions, there remains an ambiguity between two possible reductionist aims for such an account. In the next section, I will clarify this through a detour into the philosophy of thought or mental content. I will then argue, in the following section, that an objection derived from Wittgenstein's discussion of rules threatens one version but not the other. In the final section, I will consider which aim is appropriate to naturalizing mental disorder.

II.   What Kind of Reductionist Naturalism?

In this section, I will distinguish between two aims for reductionist naturalism that can be compared to two horns of the Euthyphro dilemma. But to make this more concrete, I will characterize the difference using the actual aims of two competing, but reductionist, approaches in the philosophy of content: those of Millikan, already mentioned, and of Jerry Fodor.

In the lengthy appendix to his book *Psychosemantics*, Jerry Fodor articulates a general argument for reductionism in the philosophy of content:

> I suppose that sooner or later the physicists will complete the catalogue they've been compiling of the ultimate and irreducible properties of things. When they do, the likes of *spin, charm* and *charge* will perhaps appear upon their list. But *aboutness* surely won't; intentionality simply doesn't go that deep. It's hard to see...how one can be a Realist about intentionality without also being, to some extent or other, a Reductionist. If the semantic and intentional are real properties of things, it must be in virtue of their identity with (or supervenience on?) properties that are *neither* intentional *nor* semantic. If aboutness is real, it must be really something else. (Fodor 1987, 97)

The promise of the program is that intentionality itself will be fitted into a conception of nature—or "naturalized"—by a reduction to properties that are not essentially or intrinsically intentional or semantic. Since the latter are supposed to constitute the former (through identity or supervenience), it is not that they are not intentional or semantic, but they are not essentially so. Thus, the concepts in the reduction base can be understood independently of grasp of the concepts to be understood, thus serving a project of philosophical naturalism.

The work of the rest of the book looks at first sight to be a contribution to this task through the articulation of what Fodor calls a "representational theory of mind." This comprises a "language of thought" (LOT) to explain the relationships between mental representations construed as internal vehicles of mental content combined with a version of a causal theory of reference (an asymmetric dependence theory) connecting those internal vehicles to the world.

But, on reflection, while, if successful, the representational theory of mind would be a step toward a reduction of intentionality, it is not that the actual aim of the representational theory of mind as set out in *Psychosemantics* is quite as radical as the argument in the appendix. Consider the argument that mental representations must have a structure to map the structure of mental contents.

> Practically everybody thinks that the *objects* of intentional states are in some way complex: for example, that what you believe when you believe that...P & Q is...something composite, whose elements are—as it might be—the proposition that P and the proposition that Q.

> But the (putative) complexity of the *intentional object* of a mental state does not, of course, entail the complexity of the mental state itself. It's here that LOT ventures beyond mere Intentional Realism…LOT claims that *mental states*—and not just their propositional objects—*typically have constituent structure.* (Fodor 1987, 136)

The aim of the account seems to be to explain how it is possible for thinkers to think thoughts with the right systematic relations to other thoughts. It *is* possible if there are inner vehicles of thoughts with an isomorphous structure to the structure of thought and, in turn, if the syntactic properties of those vehicles mirror their semantic relations and are suitably connected to their causal properties. Fodor attempts to show that it is not mysterious—that it is natural—that creatures like us can think the thoughts we can. If I may use the phrase the "space of reasons" to stand for the rational relations between thought contents and between them and the world, it seems that Fodor takes his question to be:

- Given the space of reasons, how is it possible for creatures like us to respond to it?

His answer is a piece of a priori engineering design. We must be creatures with an innate conceptual repertoire carried by a language of thought. This is still a form of reductionist naturalism. The fact that, medical limitations aside, humans can grasp a potential infinity of thoughts and chart the rational relations between them can seem puzzling and call for philosophical attention. The representational theory of mind is an attempt to make that less mysterious by showing how it would be possible for suitably engineered creatures to have those characteristics. But it is less radical than it might be because, within the main body of the text at least, it takes the conceptual connections themselves for granted.

Millikan, by contrast, aims to do something more ambitious with her evolutionary, or teleosemantic, theory of mental content. As summarized above, she deploys a tool that seems more promising than a causal theory of reference to account for mental content because it is itself an apparently normative notion: biological or proper function. A biological function is normative because it sets a standard against which the actual behavior or dispositions of a biological trait or subsystem can be compared. She deploys this idea not just aim to explain how possessing mental content is the proper function of some cognitive system. Rather, particular representational contents are supposed to be explained in this way. The contents carried by inner vehicles are specified via the proper functions of those vehicles: that for which they are selected. Hence, the selective advantages conferred must be characterizable in nonintentional terms. The meaning or content carried must drop out of the evolutionary theory rather than be presupposed in specifying the advantage.

The aim of this analysis is thus more ambitious than Fodor's project because Millikan aims to naturalize the structure of conceptual connections or "the space of reasons" itself. Assuming that logic charts the rational connections between contents, it is significant that Millikan claims that given a teleosemantic account, logic itself will become "the first of the natural sciences" (Millikan 1984, 11). So her key question is something like:

• Given our biological natures, how is it possible for creatures like us to respond to what we take to be the space of reasons, whatever it is?

The difference in actual ambition between Fodor and Millikan is akin to the Euthyphro dilemma. Given a suitable theology, the following biconditional would be true:

• For any act X: X is pious if and only if X is loved by the gods.

The dilemma stems from considering the "order of determination," in Crispin Wright's phrase, of this biconditional (Wright 1992). Is the pious loved by the gods because it is pious, or is it pious because it is loved by the gods? Fodor's and Millikan's projects take opposing views. In effect, Fodor adopts the first horn and derives a priori engineering constraints on the gods (or thinkers) given that we know that they are able to track piety (or the space of reasons), antecedently understood. Millikan, by contrast, adopts the second horn and aims to explain piety (or the space of reasons) by describing the engineering of the gods (or thinkers) in independent (of piety or the space of reasons) evolutionary terms.

This distinction matters to the force of an objection that can be raised against Millikan's program, which I will now summarize.

III.   A Wittgensteinian Objection to Millikan's Project

There is a familiar objection to Millikan's program based on Wittgenstein's rule following considerations. It is tempting to think that meaning or mental content needs some sort of vehicle such as sign or symbol. Any such sign can, however, be interpreted in an unlimited number of ways and thus needs to be coupled with the correct interpretation. This point is often emphasized by commentators by suggesting interpretations of even extended demonstrations by example of the meaning of words or of mathematical series that are consistent with the examples given but that deviate or are "bent" in some future application (e.g., Blackburn 1984). But if mental content is explained as a mental sign that stands in need of the correct interpretation, then the content of the interpretation will also need to be similarly underpinned. And this initiates a vicious infinite regress.

> "But how can a rule shew me what I have to do at *this* point? Whatever I do is, on some interpretation, in accord with the rule."—That is not what we ought to say, but rather: any interpretation still hangs in the air along with what it interprets, and cannot give it any support. Interpretations by themselves do not determine meaning. (Wittgenstein 1953, §198)

The same goes for accounting for understanding written or spoken signs or symbols. In the absence of any coherent account of a final interpretation that somehow blocks the regress, any account of mental content that depends on an interpretation faces a challenge.

Millikan's teleosemantic account of mental content is a form of interpretation-based theory. Past behavior is a set of signs to be interpreted. Like the interpretation of signs, such behavior is consistent with an unlimited number of possible functions or rules including both continuations that seem natural and logical and an unlimited number of other "bent" rules that deviate in unnatural ways. The normativity of a function implies that not every aspect of the behavior of a trait or subsystem needs to match the function: what the trait is for. A trait may fail to match the function for which it was selected. What ensures the determinacy of biological function—what selects just one of the possible rules—is a particular *explanation* of the persistence of trait over evolutionary time. If the potential rewards of a trait are sufficiently great, it may be that actual behavioral dispositions of previous instances of the trait only rarely match the function that explains the trait's persistence. Hence the potential gap between actual past performance and the appropriate functional explanation. But the lesson from the discussion of "bent" rules is that finite past behavior could be explained as exemplifying many different or "bent" functions, all of which would have been equally successful in the past but that would diverge in the future. (Note also that this worry is not merely a kind of Quinian marginal indeterminacy akin to the difference between rabbits and undetached rabbit parts. Competing bent rules might be utterly different in future applications. By what principle is just one selected? I will return to this thought at the end.)

Millikan considers and responds to this objection in "Truth Rules, Hoverflies, and the Kripke-Wittgenstein Paradox." Male hoverflies spend their time hovering and waiting for female hoverflies to pass by at which point they accelerate in pursuit. "The geometry of motion dictates that to intercept the female the male must make a turn that is 180° away from the target minus about 1/10 of the vector angular velocity (measured in degrees per second) of the target's image across his retina" (Millikan 1993, 219). Millikan calls this the "proximal hoverfly rule" and suggests that male hoverflies are genetically programmed to follow it. That is, they have some internal mechanism "of a kind that historically proliferated in part because it was responsible for producing conformity to the proximal hoverfly rule, hence for getting male and female hoverflies together" (Millikan 1993, 219). So the biological function of the mechanism is to follow that rule.

But the behavior of actual hoverflies may not accord with just that. One possibility is that hoverflies have some optical blind spots such that a female arriving in the blind spot of a male provokes no reaction. Such a possibility, however, would not be part of what explains the continued existence of the mechanism in the fly population. It would be noise rather than signal. The more worrying possibility is a rule that accords with all past successful fly-on-fly action but that diverges in the future. What in the evolutionary historical record could rule that out? Millikan dismisses such possibilities as follows:

> [The "bent" rule] is not a rule the hoverfly has a biological purpose to follow. For it is not because their behaviour coincided with that rule that the hoverfly's ancestors managed to catch females, and hence to proliferate. In saying that, I don't have any particular theory of the nature of explanation up my sleeve. But surely, on any reasonable account, a complexity that can simply be dropped from the explanans without affecting the tightness of the relation of explanans to explanandum is not a functioning part of the explanation. (Millikan 1993, 221)

This is rather a brisk response. A key element of it is that the bent rule contains a complexity that Millikan's preferred explanation lacks. Her explanation is simpler. But from what perspective is her explanation simpler?

In the case of trying to naturalize mental content, her explanans is the meaning or content of particular vehicles of content. But she cannot invoke our prior grasp of what such contents seem more natural—of what it would be natural to *mean*—since that is what is supposed to drop out of, rather than being presupposed by, her analysis. And, of course, the content of the proper function is not just a matter of looking to behavioral dispositions but selecting a function that best explains them. But without presupposing the pattern that meaning imposes, the pattern of the space of reasons, what other principle is there to say what makes for a simpler explanation?

Millikan's response would be legitimate for an attempt to answer the question I have suggested that Fodor attempts (despite his appendix) to answer:

- Given the space of reasons, how is it possible for creatures like us to respond to it?

Fodor's implicit question presupposes, rather than seeks to explain, the pattern of normative liaisons between mental contents. Answering that question, it is *not* illicit to deploy a notion of simplicity that presupposes a prior grasp of the space of reasons because that is not what the question seeks to answer. But Millikan's question is more ambitious, and hence it is illicit in attempting it to presuppose a notion of simplicity that is based on prior grasp of the space of reasons.

IV.   Biological Function and Illness, Disease, and Disorder

What, then, is the reductionist aim of appealing to biological functions in the philosophy of mental disorder? Two options can be articulated by translating from Fodor's and Millikan's questions in the philosophy of content. I suggested that Fodor's question was:

- Given the space of reasons, how is it possible for creatures like us to respond to it?

Translated into the context of naturalizing disorder gives something like:

- Given the concept of disorder, how is it possible for creatures like us to suffer it?

Unlike the parallel question in the philosophy of content, however, this question does not seem worth an a priori answer. I do not mean to presuppose an articulated theory of what is, and isn't, worth philosophical attention. But there seems no pressing need to articulate a general theory of a failure to meet a normative standard by contrast with the felt need in the parallel semantic case to articulate a general theory of how it might be possible to meet one. Thus, this question is not an appropriate way to model reductionism about the concept of mental disorder. What of the other option?

Millikan's question was:

- Given our biological natures, how is it possible for creatures like us to respond to what we take to be the space of reasons, whatever it is?

Translated into the philosophy of mental disorder gives a question something like:

- Given our biological natures, how is it possible for creatures like us to suffer what we take to be disorder, whatever it is?

Millikan's looks the better model question for the philosophy of medicine. It makes questioning the nature of the concept of illness itself central rather than something presupposed.

It may be objected, however, that this cannot apply to Wakefield's analysis of disorder as harmful dysfunction because he relies on an approach that he describes using the phrase "black box." The notion of a natural function is defined as sharing whatever the initially unknown essential process is that explains prototypical nonaccidental beneficial effects such as eyes seeing. It merely transpires—it comes as an a posteriori discovery—that the process that explains the prototypical nonaccidental benefits is natural selection acting to increase inclusive fitness of the organism. And hence, the objection might run, this cannot be used to shed light on what is meant by the kind of dysfunction that underpins—when conjoined with harm—the idea of a disorder.

That objection goes too quickly, however. Although it is true that Wakefield does not engage in traditional conceptual analysis to underpin his conception of function, and hence dysfunction, that fact does not rule out the use of the supposedly empirically derived conception to shed light on the nature of function itself. It does not imply that he has to restrict himself merely to the kind of a priori engineering that Fodor attempts.

Furthermore, there is positive reason to think that he does more. One of the virtues that Wakefield claims for his analysis is that it is able to hold contemporary psychiatric taxonomy to account. In his persuasive coauthored book (with Allan Horwitz) *The Loss of Sadness*, for example, he argues that depression is overdiagnosed because "normal sadness"—that is, sadness that is in accord with human emotional biological function—is mistaken for genuine, pathological depression (Horwitz and Wakefield 2007). But since, he argues, mental disorder presupposes an underlying biological dysfunction, however unpleasant grief is, for example, it cannot be a disorder or an illness providing it is serving its (presumed) biological function. Given that the analysis is used to explain the very idea of disorder (via the underlying notion of dysfunction), the form of reductionist naturalism belongs to the more radical second horn.

But if so, because it shares the task of naturalizing the normativity of pathology, Wittgenstein's objection is a serious objection. That is, a biological teleological account cannot rule out wildly divergent accounts of the functions in play, functions that explain the presence of traits. And if so, we need a better version of naturalism for the philosophy of disorder.

V. A Quinian Response?

My attempt to shed light on the nature of, and hence prospects for, reductionism in the philosophy of disorder has turned on an analogy between it and the philosophy of content and the prospects for reductionism about semantics. But it might be objected that there is a key disanalogy between the two cases.

Consider an argument often compared with Wittgenstein's discussion of rules and meaning: Quine's argument for the indeterminacy of translation (Quine 1960. (Since the relation between indeterminacy of translation, inscrutability of reference, and holophrastic indeterminacy is subject to interpretation and debate within Quine scholarship, a rough summary of one aspect of the argument will suffice.) Quine approaches the study of meaning via a particular methodological constraint.

> In psychology one may or may not be a behaviourist, but in linguistics one has no choice. Each of us learns his language by observing other people's verbal behaviour and having his own faltering verbal behaviour observed and reinforced and corrected by others....There is nothing in linguistic meaning, then, beyond what is to be gleaned from overt behaviour in overt circumstances. (Quine 1987, 5)

This reflects a commitment to the idea that facts about meaning are public and shareable. But Quine goes further in limiting the kind of facts available to fix the facts about meaning to those that fit a particular scientistic worldview. The project is constrained by connecting prompted ascent to sentences with environmental stimuli physicalistically described. These facts, however, underdetermine the translation of sentences. Since they are the only relevant facts, this implies that sentence translation is indeterminate.

With this argument in place, one might object that the comparison deployed so far between meaning and the concept of disorder is inappropriate. While Quinian indeterminacy is revisionary of our prephilosophical concept of meaning, the concept of disorder can more readily tolerate some such slack. So on the assumption that the Wittgensteinian argument outlined in previous sections sufficiently matches the Quinian argument just sketched, and on the assumption that some degree of indeterminacy is no threat to the medical concept of disorder, the claim that the project of reducing the concept of disorder to naturalistic terms introduces an element of indeterminacy is no threat to the project.

Such a response fails, however, because the supposed parallel between Wittgenstein and Quine is misleading. Quine accepts a degree of indeterminacy in his positive account of meaning. He thinks that the evidence that fixes meaning only goes so far. This is, of course, because Quine builds in an assumption that the evidence has to be physicalistically described. Against that background, meaning would be indeterministic. But what, aside from scientism, justifies that restriction?

Wittgenstein, by contrast, does not think that meaning is indeterministic. The contexts that play a role in constraining it are described in intentional terms. The apparent parallel just sketched between Quine and Wittgenstein is not part of the latter's positive account but rather a reductio ad absurdum of reductionism. More significant, however, is that Wittgenstein's negative argument does not deliver merely a domesticated indeterminacy but rather no shaping of content in the future at all and hence undermines the very possibility of radical reductionist naturalism in the case of disorder too.

Conclusion

I suggested that if the Wittgensteinian argument against the more radical reductionist aim is successful while there is no rational reason to pursue the more modest aim, then the philosophy of disorder needs a better conception of philosophical naturalism. Fortunately, there are other approaches that can still justifiably claim to be forms of philosophical naturalism.

One can, for example, sketch the broader context in which apparently puzzling concepts are used in such a way as to make their use clear. One example of this is the way that Daniel Dennett attempts to demystify the mental by describing the "intentional stance" within which mental properties are characterized (Dennett 1991). Dennett's aim is, by describing how the stance works and by suggesting that it is merely one of many possible stances for making sense of the world, to show how the properties so ascribed are perfectly natural even though they cannot be reduced to the properties deployed in other stances, such as the physical stance.

Dennett's approach is one version of naturalism without reductionism. It helps to highlight the key assumption behind Fodor's argument for reductionism quoted earlier in this chapter. The passage starts with an appeal to the shape of a future, completed physics. That serves as the benchmark of the really real and hence prompts the challenge for puzzling concepts. If they do not appear on the ultimate list, then either they mark an unreal property or they must be reducible to concepts on the list. The challenge, however, presupposes without justifying the assumption that the physicists' list is such a benchmark and that assumption can be contested.

John McDowell, for example, has suggested that nature is not restricted to what can be described using the vocabulary of the physical sciences. Criticizing a reductionist construal of naturalism, McDowell, for example, says,

> What is at work here is a conception of nature that can seem sheer common sense, though it was not always so; the conception I mean was made available only by a hard-won achievement of human thought at a specific time, the time of the rise of modern science. Modern science understands its subject matter in a way that threatens, at least, to leave it disenchanted.... The image marks a contrast between two kinds of intelligibility: the kind that is sought by (as we call it) natural science, and the kind we find in something when we place it in relation to other occupations of 'the logical space of reasons,' to repeat a suggestive phrase from Wilfrid Sellars. If we identify nature with what natural science aims to make comprehensible, we threaten, at least, to empty it of meaning. By way of compensation, so to speak, we see it as the home of a perhaps inexhaustible supply of intelligibility of the other kind, the kind we find in a phenomenon when we see it as governed by natural law. It was an achievement of modern thought when this second kind of intelligibility was clearly marked off from the first. (McDowell 1994, 70–71)

McDowell commends a different response to the prospects of a failure of reductionism. Rather than regarding this as impugning the reality of the properties or concepts concerned, it may merely show that reductionists have started with an impoverished conception of the real or of nature. Central to McDowell's picture is the possibility of undermining a dualism of normativity and nature. Nature itself may contain norms; it may be "fraught with ought" in Sellars's phrase. It is not restricted to what fits within the "realm of law" articulated by the physical sciences but also includes those emergent patterns and properties that have to be fitted within a different pattern of intelligibility: the "space of reasons." This phrase marks in McDowell's work (following Sellars) the rational pattern of intentional states (broadly construed to include ethical demands; it is thus comparable with but broader than Dennett's intentional patterns [Dennett 1991]). But an analogous conclusion could be drawn for other, nonintentional, concepts for which naturalists have also attempted philosophical reduction (e.g., necessity, causality). Again, the failure of an attempt at reduction in these cases need not undermine their reality.

McDowell's views are influenced by a reading of Aristotle's ethical views. He argues, elsewhere, that that both moral values and also secondary qualities form part of the fabric of the world (McDowell 1983). The suggestion is that there may be features of the world for which one needs a particular kind of mind, perhaps formed partly as the result of training, to detect, respond to, and even to conceptualize. Thus, one needs an appropriate moral education to understand, be sensitive, and resonate, to the demands that, say, kindness, makes on one in particular circumstances (McDowell 1979). But just because these are demands that can be understood only from such a perspective does not undermine their basic reality.

Applied to the concept of disorder, such a conception of philosophical naturalism suggests a different approach to the prima facie normativity of mental illness and disease from reducing it. By contrast with apportioning it either to the irreducibly normative value of harm or to functions anchored, descriptively, in evolutionary theory, a more relaxed conception of nature allows that the normativity may be both more complex but no less part of the natural world. This has an important consequence. A substantial theory of disorder such as Wakefield's forges a connection between it and dysfunction. On a reductionist interpretation, the latter concept has to be understood independently of, and hence shed independent light on, the former. That connection, however, may be informative even without the reductionism. Our grasp of disorder may contribute to our grasp of function and dysfunction and vice versa. And hence Wakefield's analysis of the difference between, for example, sadness and depression may remain suggestive and helpful even in a new philosophical setting.

Acknowledgments

This chapter was written while a fellow of the Institute for Advanced Study, University of Durham. My thanks both to the IAS, Durham, and the University of Central Lancashire for granting me research leave.

References

Blackburn, S. 1984. The individual strikes back. *Synthese* 58(3): 281–301.

Boorse, C. 1975. On the distinction between disease and illness. *Philosophy and Public Affairs* 5(1): 49–68.

Cooper, R. 2002. Disease. *Studies in History and Philosophy of Biological and Biomedical Sciences* 33(2): 263–282.

Cooper, R. 2007. *Psychiatry and Philosophy of Science.* Acumen.

Cummins, R. 1975. Functional analysis. *Journal of Philosophy* 72(20): 741–765.

Dennett, D. 1991. Real patterns. *Journal of Philosophy* 88(1): 27–51.

Fodor, J. A. 1987. *Psychosemantics.* MIT Press.

Fulford, K. W. M. 1989. *Moral Theory and Medical Practice.* Cambridge University Press.

Fulford, K. W. M. 1999. Nine variations and a coda on the theme of an evolutionary definition of dysfunction. *Journal of Abnormal Psychology* 108(3): 412–420.

Fulford, K. W. M. 2000. Teleology without tears. *Philosophy, Psychiatry, and Psychology* 7(1): 77–94.

Fulford, K. W. M. 2004. Ten principles of values-based medicine. In *The Philosophy of Psychiatry: A Companion,* J. Radden (ed.), 205–234. Oxford University Press.

Horwitz, A. V., and J. C. Wakefield. 2007. *The Loss of Sadness.* Oxford University Press.

Kendell, R. E. 1975. The concept of disease and its implications for psychiatry. *British Journal of Psychiatry* 127(4): 305–315.

McDowell, J. 1979. Virtue and reason. *The Monist* 62(3): 331–350.

McDowell, J. 1983. Aesthetic value, objectivity, and the fabric of the world. In *Pleasure Preference and Value,* E. Schaper (ed.), 1–16. Cambridge University Press.

McDowell, J. 1994. *Mind and World.* Harvard University Press.

Millikan, R. G. 1984. *Language, Thought and Other Biological Categories.* MIT Press.

Millikan, R. G. 1993. *White Queen Psychology.* MIT Press.

Millikan, R. G. 1998. In defence of proper functions. In *Nature's Purposes: Analyses of Function and Design in Biology,* C. Allen and G. Lauder (eds.), 295–312. MIT Press.

Papineau, D. 1993. *Philosophical Naturalism.* Blackwell.

Quine, W. V. O. 1960. *Word and Object.* MIT Press.

Quine, W. V. O. 1987. Indeterminacy of translation again. *Journal of Philosophy* 84(1): 5–10.

Sober, E. 1984. *The Nature of Selection.* MIT Press.

Szasz, T. 1960. The myth of mental illness. *American Psychologist* 15: 113–118.

Wakefield, J. C. 1992. The concept of mental disorder: On the boundary between biological facts and social values. *American Psychologist* 47(3): 373–388.

Wakefield, J. C. 1999. Mental disorder as a black box essentialist concept. *Journal of Abnormal Psychology* 108: 465–472.

Wittgenstein, L. 1953. *Philosophical Investigations.* Blackwell.

Wright, C. 1992. *Truth and Objectivity.* Harvard University Press.

Wright, L. 1973. Function. *Philosophical Review* 82(2): 139–168.

24   Is Indeterminacy of Biological Function an Objection to the Harmful Dysfunction Analysis? Reply to Tim Thornton

Jerome Wakefield

I thank Tim Thornton for his chapter exploring the possibility and limits of naturalism in my harmful dysfunction analysis (HDA) of medical, including mental, disorder. The HDA claims that "disorder" refers to "harmful dysfunction," where dysfunction is the failure of some feature to perform a natural function for which it is biologically designed by evolutionary processes and harm is judged in accordance with social values (First and Wakefield 2010, 2013; Spitzer, 1997, 1999; Wakefield 1992a, 1992b 1993, 1995, 1997a, 1997b, 1997c, 1997d, 1998, 1999a, 1999b, 2000a, 2000b, 2001, 2006, 2007, 2009, 2011, 2014, 2016a, 2016b; Wakefield and First 2003, 2012). I have long benefited from Tim Thornton's extensive work not only in philosophy of the mental health professions but also philosophy of science and mind as well, and he brings his sophisticated understanding of these multiple domains of philosophy to his chapter's exploration of the HDA's naturalist evolutionary analysis of "biological function."

At the beginning of his paper, Thornton astutely draws attention to a cardinal feature of the HDA. In opposition to value-based approaches such as Fulford's (1989) that see values as foundational and pervading every component of "disorder," the HDA distinguishes a purely naturalist necessary component of "disorder" from a value component. This allows for a naturalist value-free zone of assessment and debate over diagnostic validity, offering a partial escape from values in the sense that one can critique disorder claims evidentially and scientifically without always having to address values. Nonetheless, due to its value component, the HDA will never satisfy those who are engaged in a thoroughgoing philosophical naturalist project. Although in a profession like medicine, values may not be fully escapable in its foundational concepts, the HDA's two-component approach allows that values can sometimes be put aside in a purely naturalist assessment of diagnostic validity based on questioning the presence of evolutionary dysfunction. The general issue Thornton raises, by way of a discussion of Millikan's ambitious project to naturalize meaning in terms of biological function, is whether the HDA's naturalist "function" component can remain truly value free given potential Wittgenstein-inspired indeterminacy issues in the specification of functions.

Thornton lucidly addresses a challenge to the HDA's position on separate value and factual components posed by Fulford (1999). Fulford argued that the "dysfunction" component of the HDA is in fact normative because it requires the "failure" of a function, and "failure," he claimed, is irreducibly value laden. (Apparently for Fulford, the fact that the latest Brexit proposal "failed to pass" in Parliament or that an argument "fails to be valid" is a value judgment.) "Failure" is indeed often used to indicate lack of success in value-defined outcomes, but in the context of the HDA, "failure of function" is just a way of saying that a mechanism did not perform its biologically designed function. As Thornton observes, "If function and divergence from it can be analysed in descriptive terms then so can 'failure' of function: it is any divergence from function." Thus, in disputes over disorder status, there is at least a potential "place to stand" from which one can offer a factual/scientific/naturalist critique of a judgment that a condition is a disorder. In many instances, this is a much more potent tool of critique than clashing value judgments or radical antipsychiatric arguments that deny the obvious fact that there really are mental disorders.

A small point: Thornton mentions that Robert Kendell, perhaps the most respected psychiatrist other than Robert Spitzer on the topic of the concept of mental disorder, initially grappled with an all-factual account. He also flirted with the factual but hopeless "whatever psychiatrists treat" notion at one point. It is perhaps of some slight interest where his odyssey ended on this issue. In one of his last papers before his sudden death, he endorsed the HDA: "It also would be well worthwhile revising the basic *Diagnostic and Statistical Manual of Mental Disorders (DSM)* definition of mental disorder in light of Wakefield's (1992) cogent analysis of the concept.... Having struggled myself (Kendell 1975, 1986) to decide whether disease or disorder are better regarded as normative concepts based on value judgments or as value-free scientific terms, I am impressed by Wakefield's arguments that both elements are necessarily involved" (2002, 5).

Another small point: Thornton incorrectly suggests that my insistence on the term "disorder" comes from Boorse. However, it was in fact in opposition to Boorse's confusing use of "disease" that I adopted "disorder." "Disease" has a common meaning that excludes medical disorders such as injuries and poisonings—and which Boorse eventually abandoned. "Disorder" has actually been used for centuries for this reason.

I am not going to attempt in this reply to follow Thornton's fascinating journey through the contemporary philosophical landscape ranging from Millikan and Fodor to Wittgenstein and McDowell. Instead, I will provide just a few thoughts on some central issues raised by his observations.

Thornton points out some obvious parallels in the understanding of "function" between the work of Ruth Millikan on intentionality and my own on disorder. Because Millikan brilliantly uses biological function in an attempt to analyze mental content, and I use biological function to analyze medical disorder, and we both understand biological functions broadly speaking in terms of natural selection, there is certainly a degree of affinity between our analyses. He then suggests that Wittgensteinian (or perhaps Kripkensteinian) doubts about content determinacy—due to the possibility of many different ways of generalizing a rule into the future from past behaviors—might also apply to disorder attributions and thus pose a challenge to function determinacy. I agree that this is an interesting issue, although I am doubtful that it leads to any deep problems specifically for the HDA for reasons I will explain.

First, I guess it is worth stating for the record that while I agree with Millikan that the intuitive notion of "natural/biological function" has a natural-selective evolutionary essence and can be elaborated in evolutionary terms, I do not believe that Millikan's program to leverage that understanding of "function" into a naturalist account of intentionality can possibly work for reasons related to Thornton's discussion. Meaning and content cannot be reduced to natural-selective history due to familiar indeterminacy considerations, namely, intentionality is more fine-grained and determinate than evolutionary history. In this regard, it seems to me that, although Thornton dismisses mere Quinian "gavagai" arguments as not relevant in his analysis (he is focusing on Wittgensteinian rule-paradoxical real divergences between rules and their "bent" analogs, which unlike the Quinian cases do actually diverge at some point and are not always and necessarily co-referential), in fact the gavagai-type examples seem to me to be conclusive counterexamples to Millikan's attempt to theorize meaning/content as naturally selected functions. The problem (analogous to the problem Quine pointed to in trying to use behavior or neurobiology to identify meaning) is that determinacy of meaning cannot be matched by determinacy of function. Simply and Quinianly put, there is a difference in meaning between "the heart's function is to pump blood cells throughout the body" and "the heart's function is to pump undetached parts of blood cells throughout the body," but there is no way that any theory in which functions are determined by natural selection can account for that difference because functions selected to accomplish necessarily co-occurring effects cannot be distinguished by natural selection history. Or, to take a favorite example of Millikan's, when the bee does its communicational dance to the hive's denizens after finding honey, there is no natural selection story that is going to allow a discrimination between the meanings "honey-yielding flowers at location X" and "undetached parts of honey-yielding flowers at location X." In other words, when push comes to shove, Millikan's view of meaning falls to the same old Quinian argument against content reduction that felled behaviorist and neurobiological reductions of content. So, to me, one does not require the additional machinery of Wittgenstein's critique of meaning to refute Millikan's project. Moreover, while Thornton emphasizes certain differences between Fodor and Millikan, Fodor's various theories of content similarly collapse before the elegant Quinian indeterminacy critique of content turned around by Searle to be an antireductionist argument, and Fodor's explicit attempts to address the problem don't work (Wakefield

2003). And, in keeping with this failure, Millikan and Fodor both admit that they don't have anything to say about consciousness (Wakefield 2018).

Obviously, I don't conclude from all this that therefore there is no such thing as content. Rather, I conclude, with Searle, that Quine's indeterminacy argument reduces to absurdity the notion that third-person accounts like Millikan's and Fodor's encompass all the evidence there is for content. The problem, of course, is that consciousness has been left out, but that is a long story that cannot be further addressed here.

Thornton's subtle analysis leads him to confront a problem facing not just the HDA but the concepts of function, dysfunction, and disorder within both evolutionary theory and medicine, namely, the problem of indeterminacy of function. Given an actual evolutionary history, there will be many ways of translating that into a function statement depending on how broadly or narrowly one interprets the selective "rule" being followed.

Now, although various philosophical problems have complex interrelationships, I don't think one can solve all these large general problems at once when addressing a special area. I can't solve "grue" and "underdetermination" and "Kripkenstein" when elaborating the concept of "disorder." Rather, I work within some standard assumptive systems. I grant that if these broader issues fall a certain way and it turns out that there are no filters to neutralize them down the line when doing concrete things like medical diagnosis, then there might be problems for psychiatric disorder judgments and medical diagnosis more generally, but this seems very unlikely to me. Evolutionary theory is an enormously successful scientific explanatory system, and whatever issues of indeterminacy arise for its notion of function presumably cannot undo that success, although exactly how that works needs to be understood. The HDA's evolutionary interpretations of "function" and of the intuitive notion of "biological design" take place within that framework, and thus whatever indeterminacy occurs in evolutionary theory is likely to occur within medical theory as well, but also medical theory can rely on whatever disambiguation techniques are found in the parent theories. This stance is similar to a point I recall being made by Christopher Boorse in response to those who argue that all scientific concepts are ultimately value laden so that "disorder" cannot be purely factual. He explained that if such universal value-ladenness turns out to be the case, then that would be a general limit on his claims and that he is only claiming in his "naturalist" theory that the concept of "disorder" has no *special* value loading over and above whatever value loading, if any, turns out to be routinely true of, say, physics and biology generally. Similarly, I am claiming that *given evolutionary theory's determination of functions* (however potential indeterminacies are dealt with at that level), disorder can be defined with adequate determinacy from there. If the theory of medical pathology piggybacks on the evolutionary theory of function, then it can rely on indeterminacy disambiguation within that home scientific discipline, and the claim is only that medical diagnosis does not introduce a new and seriously problematic level of indeterminacy. I see nothing in Thornton's paper that suggests that disorder judgments do add indeterminacy problems over and above issues involved with "function" at the evolutionary theory level, but of course this impression could be proven wrong.

There are places to look for such indeterminacies. I would say with issues of trade-offs, side effects, pleiotropy, reactions to changing environments, balancing selection, and especially the precise scope of function versus dysfunction in terms of the breadth of performances that qualify as function versus dysfunction, issues of indeterminacy could arise. My inclination is to think that confident judgments of dysfunction and thus disorder would escape such problems by being failures of a clear core of function, but admittedly this intuition requires serious examination.

Thornton's exploration raises a series of profound questions that he does not attempt to answer and that I cannot undertake to answer here but that are well worthy of further analysis (I nibble at these questions in my replies to Garson and Lemoine in this volume). The questions might be put as follows: First, to what extent and in what ways is the concept of "natural function" as interpreted in evolutionary terms indeterminate? Second, how, if at all, are such indeterminacies resolved within evolutionary theorizing? Third, to what extent or in what ways, if any, do such indeterminacies yield corresponding indeterminacies in the concept of disorder that can impact meaningful real-world judgments of disorder versus nondisorder? Fourth, if our actual disorder and nondisorder judgments involve implicit resolutions of such indeterminacies, what is the logic or justification, if any, for how such indeterminacies are resolved, and in particular, does that resolution involve hidden normativist/value premises, thus building values into a deeper level of what appears on the surface to be a factual criterion? And fifth, if, as it appears, evolutionary theory is a highly successful scientific explanatory theory despite any such indeterminacies, is there any problem with the concept of disorder piggybacking on whatever function indeterminacy resolution process occurs in evolutionary theory to avoid independent function indeterminacy issues, or does it have a problem in moving from evolutionary function to dysfunction over and above whatever such issues occur within evolutionary theory itself?

References

First, M. B., and J. C. Wakefield. 2010. Defining 'mental disorder' in *DSM-V*. *Psychological Medicine* 40(11): 1779–1782.

First, M. B., and J. C. Wakefield. 2013. Diagnostic criteria as dysfunction indicators: Bridging the chasm between the definition of mental disorder and diagnostic criteria for specific disorders. *Canadian Journal of Psychiatry* 58(12): 663–669.

Fulford, K. W. M. 1989. *Moral Theory and Medical Practice*. Cambridge University Press.

Fulford, K. W. M. 1999. Nine variations and a coda on the theme of an evolutionary definition of dysfunction. *Journal of Abnormal Psychology* 108: 412–420.

Kendell, R. E. 2002. Five criteria for an improved taxonomy of mental disorders. In *Defining Psychopathology in the 21st Century*, J. E. Helzer and J. J. Hudziak (eds.), 3–18. American Psychiatric Publishing.

Spitzer, R. L. 1997. Brief comments from a psychiatric nosologist weary from his own attempts to define mental disorder: Why Ossorio's definition muddles and Wakefield's "harmful dysfunction" illuminates the issues. *Clinical Psychology: Science and Practice* 4(3): 259–261.

Spitzer, R. L. 1999. Harmful dysfunction and the *DSM* definition of mental disorder. *Journal of Abnormal Psychology* 108(3): 430–432.

Wakefield, J. C. 1992a. The concept of mental disorder: On the boundary between biological facts and social values. *American Psychologist* 47: 373–388.

Wakefield, J. C. 1992b. Disorder as harmful dysfunction: A conceptual critique of *DSM-III-R*'s definition of mental disorder. *Psychological Review* 99: 232–247.

Wakefield, J. C. 1993. Limits of operationalization: A critique of Spitzer and Endicott's (1978) proposed operational criteria of mental disorder. *Journal of Abnormal Psychology* 102: 160–172.

Wakefield, J. C. 1995. Dysfunction as a value-free concept: A reply to Sadler and Agich. *Philosophy, Psychiatry, and Psychology* 2: 233–46.

Wakefield, J. C. 1997a. Diagnosing *DSM-IV*, part 1: *DSM-IV* and the concept of mental disorder. *Behaviour Research and Therapy* 35: 633–650.

Wakefield, J. C. 1997b. Diagnosing *DSM-IV*, part 2: Eysenck (1986) and the essentialist fallacy. *Behaviour Research and Therapy*: 35: 651–666.

Wakefield, J. C. 1997c. Normal inability versus pathological disability: Why Ossorio's (1985) definition of mental disorder is not sufficient. *Clinical Psychology: Science and Practice* 4: 249–258.

Wakefield, J. C. 1997d. When is development disordered? Developmental psychopathology and the harmful dysfunction analysis of mental disorder. *Development and Psychopathology* 9: 269–290.

Wakefield, J. C. 1998. The DSM's theory-neutral nosology is scientifically progressive: Response to Follette and Houts. *Journal of Consulting and Clinical Psychology* 66: 846–852.

Wakefield, J. C. 1999a. Evolutionary versus prototype analyses of the concept of disorder. *Journal of Abnormal Psychology* 108: 374–399.

Wakefield, J. C. 1999b. Mental disorder as a black box essentialist concept. *Journal of Abnormal Psychology* 108: 465–472.

Wakefield, J. C. 2000a. Aristotle as sociobiologist: The "function of a human being" argument, black-box essentialism, and the concept of mental disorder. *Philosophy, Psychiatry, and Psychology* 7: 17–44.

Wakefield, J. C. 2000b. Spandrels, vestigial organs, and such: Reply to Murphy and Woolfolk's "The harmful dysfunction analysis of mental disorder." *Philosophy, Psychiatry, and Psychology* 7: 253–269.

Wakefield, J. C. 2001. Evolutionary history versus current causal role in the definition of disorder: Reply to McNally. *Behaviour Research and Therapy* 39: 347–366.

Wakefield, J. C. 2003. Fodor on inscrutability. *Mind and Language* 18: 524–537.

Wakefield, J. C. 2006. What makes a mental disorder mental? *Philosophy, Psychiatry, and Psychology* 13: 123–131.

Wakefield, J. C. 2007. The concept of mental disorder: Diagnostic implications of the harmful dysfunction analysis. *World Psychiatry* 6: 149–156.

Wakefield, J. C. 2009. Mental disorder and moral responsibility: Disorders of personhood as harmful dysfunctions, with special reference to alcoholism. *Philosophy, Psychiatry, and Psychology* 16: 91–99.

Wakefield, J. C. 2011. Darwin, functional explanation, and the philosophy of psychiatry. In *Maladapting Minds: Philosophy, Psychiatry, and Evolutionary Theory*, P. R. Andriaens and A. De Block (eds.), 143–172. Oxford University Press.

Wakefield, J. C. 2014. The biostatistical theory versus the harmful dysfunction analysis, part 1: Is part-dysfunction a sufficient condition for medical disorder? *Journal of Medicine and Philosophy* 39: 648–682.

Wakefield, J. C. 2016a. The concepts of biological function and dysfunction: Toward a conceptual foundation for evolutionary psychopathology. In *Handbook of Evolutionary Psychology*, D. Buss (ed.), 2nd ed., vol. 2, 988–1006. Oxford University Press.

Wakefield, J. C. 2016b. Diagnostic issues and controversies in DSM-5: Return of the false positives problem. *Annual Review of Clinical Psychology* 12: 105–132.

Wakefield, J. C. 2018. *Freud and Philosophy of Mind: Vol. 1. Reconstructing the Argument for Unconscious Mental States*. Palgrave Macmillan.

Wakefield, J. C., and M. B. First. 2003. Clarifying the distinction between disorder and nondisorder: Confronting the overdiagnosis ("false positives") problem in *DSM-V*. In *Advancing DSM: Dilemmas in Psychiatric Diagnosis*, K. A. Phillips, M. B. First, and H. A. Pincus (eds.), 23–56. American Psychiatric Press.

Wakefield, J. C., and M. B. First. 2012. Placing symptoms in context: The role of contextual criteria in reducing false positives in *DSM* diagnosis. *Comprehensive Psychiatry* 53: 130–139.

IV The Harmful Component

25 Harmless Dysfunctions and the Problem of Normal Variation

Andreas De Block and Jonathan Sholl

In one of his key publications on the harmful dysfunction analysis of mental disorder (HDA), Jerome Wakefield acknowledged that he has "explored the value element in disorder less thoroughly than the factual element. This is in part because the factual component poses more of a problem for inferences about disorder and in part because the nature of values is such that it requires separate consideration" (Wakefield 1992, 384). More than twenty years have passed since this remark, and yet a thorough consideration of the value component in Wakefield's HDA is still lacking. Quite a few contributions to this volume promise to change that situation, and ours is one of these. In this contribution, we will analyze the harm or value component and argue that Wakefield's dealing with it is so problematic that it undermines, at least indirectly, the viability of the HDA.

In the first section, we explore Wakefield's emphasis on the subjective nature of harm and his exclusive focus on social values. The second section is devoted to an analysis of Wakefield's examples of conditions that are dysfunctional but harmless (fused toes, albinism, reversal of the heart, dyslexia in illiterate societies, etc.). We argue that these examples are quite problematic because they do not exemplify what they are supposed to exemplify. In the third section, we show how these two problems are connected: Wakefield uses the harmfulness of a condition as an implicit criterion to distinguish normal variation from dysfunction. In doing so, he blurs the distinction between the harm component and the dysfunction component, even though this distinction is central to his HDA.

I. The Downsides of a Hybrid Concept of (Mental) Disorder

Wakefield's HDA is commonly referred to as the most influential hybrid account of mental and bodily disorder. This account is said to be hybrid because it builds upon the idea that scientific judgments need to be accompanied by value judgments to draw the line between health and disorder. The reasons for proposing such hybrid concepts are easy to understand. First, both pure value accounts and pure objectivist accounts cannot do the work that objectivists or normativists expect them to do. Second, there is some philosophically attractive kernel in each of these accounts. It is clear that according to Wakefield, the HDA avoids the problems of other nonhybrid accounts (including the pure value account), while preserving the real insights of these accounts (including the pure value account). Because disorder cannot be identified with dysfunction—which is, according to Wakefield, a purely factual component—we need a value component in order to have a full analysis of disorder.

One reason that the factual component does not suffice is because of culture-relative aspects of diagnosis. As Wakefield (1995, 244) himself writes, "I believe it is important to identify both the aspects of diagnosis that are culturally relative and the aspects that remain invariant under cultural transformations." Obviously, the universal aspects of diagnosis are covered by the dysfunction component, while the culturally relative aspects have to do with value. Wakefield contends that bodily/mental state S constitutes a disorder in some cultural environments, while the same bodily/mental state is correctly seen as a healthy, albeit possibly dysfunctional, state in other cultural environments. Dyslexia, for example, is a mental disorder in literate societies, but it is not a mental disorder in illiterate ones. While dyslexia might be a dysfunction in both societies, it is the value component that makes it a disorder in literate ones. So it seems that cultures can be wrong about the dysfunction component, but they cannot be wrong about the value component (Wakefield 2007, 155). "The nature of values themselves plays no role in my analysis," or so Wakefield has argued (Wakefield 1995, 243). Yet, it does seem that he subscribes to a particular view about the nature of values that are relevant for the value component of the HDA. First, these values are not absolute values, for the values are the culture-relative element in his HDA. Second, these values are social values. This is actually mentioned as the real insight of the "pure value account" of health and disorder: "The value account reveals an important truth: because disorders are negative conditions that justify social concern, social values are involved" (Wakefield 1992, 336). So disorders are harmful according to social norms and not individual norms (Wakefield 2005). We are, after all, a social animal and Wakefield seems to find it awkward to leave out the evaluative responses of others when making judgments concerning how an individual organism functions (Wakefield 1992). What this amounts to is exemplified again by dyslexia: "in a literate society, a person who does not value reading still has a dyslexic disorder if incapable of learning to read due to a brain dysfunction" (Wakefield 2005, 98). In short, Wakefield holds that a dysfunction can only be a disorder if it is considered to be "harmful" (*value relativism*) within a particular cultural framework (*social values*).

This view, however, harbors a lot of problems. Most important, one wonders why Wakefield claims that someone who doesn't value reading and writing at all should be considered disordered in a literate society. If the individual experiences no harm, why should she be considered disordered? Would Wakefield be willing to bite the bullet and say that homosexuality is a disorder in cultures that value heterosexuality—assuming of course that homosexuality is dysfunctional as is indeed often assumed by those who defend an etiological account of function (see, e.g., Levin 1984)? One way to avoid this conclusion is by making a distinction between the distress/harm that results directly from the dysfunctional state and distress/harm caused by the social disapproval of the consequences of this condition. For example, one could argue that the harm caused by dyslexia follows directly from the difficulty with reading that is intrinsically tied to dyslexia, whereas the harm caused by homosexuality/bestiality is caused by being ostracized by your peers, a consequence that is not intrinsically tied to bestiality or homosexuality. Yet, "intrinsicality" is a very difficult concept in general (Francescotti 1999; Witmer et al. 2005), and in this case, it is relatively easy to come up with examples that blur the distinction. The examples of dyslexia and homosexuality are, however, closer to each other than one may suspect. After all, dyslexia is harmful in culture A because it is intrinsically tied to not being able to read and because culture A values being able to read, whereas (exclusive) homosexuality is harmful in culture B because it is intrinsically tied to not being able to be attracted to individuals of the other biological sex and because culture B is a heteronormative culture.

This difficulty with social values explains why the *Diagnostic and Statistical Manual of Mental Disorders* (*DSM*) adopted a different position on the relevant values and emphasized the importance of what Wakefield would call individual values for psychiatric diagnoses. For example, systematic cross-dressing is not considered a mental disorder as long as it is "ego-syntonic." Only if it becomes ego-dystonic will it qualify as a mental disorder (Gert and Culver 2009).

Now, it certainly is conceivable to develop a version of the HDA that treats individual values as central, rather than social values. One of the reasons Wakefield has put forward to break with an objectivist account like Boorse's, and to include values in his account of (mental) disorder, is the distinction between "evolutionary harm" (lowered fertility, lowered longevity) and harm to an individual's well-being. And even though well-being for most members of our species does clearly depend on social factors, it seems reasonable to let the individual judge this, rather than letting the individual's well-being be judged by cultural standards. In the case discussed above, the fact that a society values reading seems insufficient to judge someone with dyslexia as being disordered since the individual may not value such a skill and therefore experiences no harm for lacking it. There could be various conditions that a society disvalues but that produce no harm in the individual who does not share the same values, partly because social norms are neither understood in the same way by everyone, nor are they universally accepted.

Yet, this "individual value" solution is not without its own problems, as those familiar with pure value accounts of disorder and health know (Reznek 1987; Fulford et al. 2005). First of all, the individual values probably all have—at least in part—a social origin. So chances are that if transvesticism is ego-dystonic, this is mainly due to the cultural norms of the transvesticist individual. That is why the American Psychiatric Association decided to remove ego-dystonic homosexuality from the *DSM III-R* in 1987, after having removed homosexuality as such already thirteen years earlier from the *DSM-III* (De Block and Adriaens 2013). In 1987, it was generally agreed upon that much—if not all—of the distress homosexual individuals experience has to do with their being stigmatized and discriminated against. Second, adopting individual values as the relevant values to make the distinction between health and disorder is confronted with the problem of anosognosia. Quite a few patients who suffer from severe mental and neurological disorders do not seem to consider their condition problematic, let alone disordered. Yet, few philosophers would argue that they are not disordered, just like few people would defend the view that comatose patients are healthy because they are unable to have value judgments about their condition (Sullivan 2003).

The value component of Wakefield's HDA may result in one advantage of his account over pure objectivist accounts like Boorse's: it embraces an "important truth" of the pure value account. But as we have seen in this first section, the problems or downsides of a pure value account do not seem to be convincingly solved by the HDA, nor is it easy to come up with straightforward modifications of the HDA that do away with these downsides. In the following section, we will explore why Wakefield thinks he needs the value component to take into account the normativist truth that "all disorders are undesirable and harmful" (Wakefield 1992, 376). Does this "fact" really show "that values are part of the concept of disorder" (Wakefield 1992, 376), as he himself is clearly convinced that it does? Or could it be that all dysfunctions are harmful and that therefore we only need a scientific judgment to establish whether or not a condition is disordered?

II. Fused Toes and Albinism

The kind of analysis of disorder that Wakefield proposes is an analysis of the concept "disorder" as it is used by the lay public and by professionals. It aims at analyzing uncontroversial judgments about which conditions are disorders. Examples of these uncontroversial judgments include the judgments that acute leukemia is a disorder and the judgment that schizophrenia is a disorder. If the HD analysis is correct, (1) all uncontroversial disorders—what Boorse (1977, 544) has called "the paradigm objects of medical concern"—are both harmful and dysfunctional, and (2) our intuitions about more controversial cases can change due to discoveries with regard to their harmfulness or their functionality. For example, the HDA "predicts that if what is now considered a disorder is shown to be a selected feature, then our intuitions would change and we would come to consider it a non-disorder, re-conceptualizing it as a normal variation—as has happened with fever" (Wakefield 2011, 152).

This prediction is interesting and raises a series of issues. For example, what would the consequences be for the HDA if it would be shown that schizophrenia—a paradigm object of psychiatric concern—is an adaptation, as some speculatively inclined evolutionary psychiatrists have already hypothesized (Stevens and Price 1996)? Another issue, and one that we will focus on here, has to do with the idea that each of the conjuncts "harmful" and "dysfunctional" is in separation from the other insufficient for a condition to be a disorder. So, if the HDA is correct, (1) some conditions must be both dysfunctional *and* harmless, and (2) our judgment that these conditions are not disorders must also be relatively uncontroversial. It is important to note that the HDA fails if all dysfunctional conditions are harmful or if there are harmless and dysfunctional conditions that are generally considered disorders.

Do we have examples of conditions that are (1) dysfunctional, (2) harmless, and (3) uncontroversially not disordered? Wakefield gives a few examples of physical conditions that are supposed to meet these criteria: fused toes, albinism, and dextrocardia[1] ("reversal of the heart"). We will argue that, contrary to what Wakefield contends, each of these examples does not meet at least one of these criteria.

Let's start with the fused toes. According to the *International Classification of Diseases* (*ICD-10*) of the World Health Organization, fused toes and other forms of syndactyly are disorders. Of course, you can always argue that the WHO is wrong here. But does it really seem reasonable to think that one can speak of an uncontroversial medical judgment if this judgment—"fused toes is not a disorder"—goes against the arguably most important health classification system that is published by the arguably most important international health and disease agency? Since all three criteria have to be met, this would be enough to dismiss fused toes as relevant support for Wakefield's HDA. But let us, for the sake and the pleasure of the argument, check whether the other two criteria are met. Is it really harmless? Suppose for a moment that we could choose to have fused toes or toes that are not webbed. What would most people choose, all else being equal? We think this is pretty much a no-brainer, at least in our culture. Fused toes are often surgically treated, and we assume that this is because they are seen as undesirable. Of course, most people would choose not to have fused toes because of aesthetic reasons and not for more "serious" reasons. Fused toes do not, for example, impair walking or running. But why should we leave concerns over bodily beauty and attractiveness out of the "harm" evaluation? We readily admit that the harm associated with fused toes is mild and that the large majority of individuals with fused toes can live happy lives, but mild harm is harm nonetheless. So *syndactyly* is generally seen as a disorder and as something (mildly) harmful, even though Wakefield contends the opposite. What about Wakefield's assumption or claim that syndactyly is a dysfunction? The problem here is not so much that there isn't any account of function and dysfunction available according to which syndactyly clearly qualifies as a dysfunction. The problem is that it is far from obvious that this condition is dysfunctional if one accepts Wakefield's etiological account of function. Do people with fused toes have fused toes because of a mechanism that was naturally selected because it generated toes that are not fused? There are evolutionary reasons why we have toes, and it is most probably the case that having many digits is an adaptation. It seems far from certain, however, that having five rather than four or six digits is an adaptation. Nobody seems to know for sure why we have five (or ten) toes. We do not think it is very likely that something in the environment of our species (or of species' ancestors) made having ten toes selectively advantageous. In our view, the best supported hypothesis we have right now is that there is a developmental constraint at work (Amundson 2005) that tends to lead to ten toes rather nine or eight. But the loosening of this constraint in individual cases is not—or at least not obviously—a failure of the naturally selected developmental mechanism (Alberch and Gale 1985; Tabin 1992; Galis et al. 2001).

The second example, albinism, is also a disorder according the *ICD-10* (code E70.3). So it is *certainly* not the kind of example that Wakefield needs to support the need for a value component. Still, it seems somewhat better suited than the fused toes example because everybody seems to agree that albinism in humans is (the result of) a dysfunction in the etiological sense, more precisely a dysfunctional absence of the melanin pigment. Yet, it seems very awkward to claim that this condition is harmless. First, the albino phenotype is so salient that individuals with albinism are often socially stigmatized (Maron 2013). This is the case, for example, in Tanzania, where it is believed that owning albino body parts can make one powerful or wealthy, especially if those parts come from children who screamed while their parts were harvested. Understandably, many parents don't send their albinistic kids to school because they fear for their lives, thus leading to an increased risk of poverty among albinistic people. Second, even if one would dismiss the stigmatization harm as irrelevant for the HDA, one could still point to the increased skin cancer risk of people with the oculocutaneous type of albinism. Individuals with albinism need more skin protection than others to avoid skin cancer (and sunburn). Of course, an increased risk for certain disorders is not a disorder itself. Smoking is not a disease, even though it increases your risk to develop all sorts of diseases. However, it seems to square with Wakefield's account of harm to call the increased risk of developing skin cancer a form of harm, for the same reasons that smoking is generally considered harmful (even though it does not seem to be a dysfunction). Third, both individuals with the oculocutaneous and the ocular type almost invariably suffer from (mild to serious) visual problems. If photophobia and astigmatism in nonalbinistic people are seen as diseases of the eye, then why should we not see them as harmful in individuals with albinism?

In the *ICD-10*, albinism and fused toes can be found alongside Wakefield's third example, dextrocardia (Boorse 2011). Probably, many people would disagree with dextrocardia being classified as a disease (e.g., Boorse 1977). But again, it is really hard to argue that this condition is an uncontroversial nondiseased condition, given its being listed as a disease in the *ICD-10*. *ICD-10* distinguishes many types of this "disease," and Wakefield is right that at least one type (*dextrocardia situs inversus*) is quite harmless. People with this condition tend to live as long and as healthily as people without it. With regard to the third criterion, Wakefield himself notes that "a lesion can be a harmless abnormality that is not a disorder, such as when the heart is positioned on the right side of the body but *retains functional integrity*" (Wakefield 1992, 375, emphasis added). So Wakefield himself explicitly acknowledges that in the harmless form of dextrocardia, the heart still does what it was selected for. In his view, the condition is dysfunctional, but the dysfunction can clearly not be a dysfunction of the heart. He is less explicit, though, on what constitutes the dysfunction here, but our guess is that Wakefield considers it to be the result of a dysfunctional development. But why would this development be dysfunctional? The embryonic development of all humans is to some degree the result of selection. However, the issue is whether this development was selected or whether it was not only selected but also selected *for*. If there occurred selection of this development, but not selection for this development, the absence (or the mirroring) of this developmental pattern does not seem to constitute a dysfunction in the etiological sense.

Sober's (1984) well-known distinction between selection of and selection for has often been used in the literature on etiological accounts of functions (see, e.g., Sterelny 1990; Shapiro 1992). It is generally agreed upon that the difference between a trait/property that is selected for and one that is selected can be established by counterfactual reasoning that tracks the causal role of the target of selection (that which is selected for) in the selection process. For example, the warmth of the polar bear's coat has been selected for, while there has only been selection of its weight, because the polar bear's coat would not have been selected if it would have been heavy but not warm, and the coat would have been selected if it had been warm but not heavy (Sober 1984). According to the etiological account of function, the coat of the polar bear would dysfunction if it failed to be warm but not if it failed to be heavy. Likewise, if people with a particular form of dextrocardia tend to live healthy lives, this is reason to believe that the human embryogenetic processes were not selected for generating a heart at the left (and the lungs at the right). In other words, the harmlessness of this condition suggests that this is not a dysfunction. We do not claim to know the eventual selectionist story about the normal position of heart and other thoracic organs, but we do have reasons to doubt that the present biological knowledge renders *dextrocardia situs inversus* an uncontroversial example of a dysfunctional condition.

Albinism, fused toes, and dextrocardia are all physical disorders. Maybe, the HDA is better suited to deal with psychiatric judgments than with other medical judgments. If true, this could entail that the uncontroversially nondisordered conditions that are dysfunctional but harmless should be looked for in the psychiatric literature. And indeed, Wakefield also points to some mental conditions that are dysfunctional and harmless and are generally not seen as disorders. For instance, a dyslectic condition in illiterate societies wouldn't be a disorder because it is a harmless dysfunction. Likewise, lack of male aggression in current Western societies would be more harmless than the high level of aggression of most males, even though these higher levels of aggression were selected for in our ancestral environment.

The first example—dyslectic conditions in illiterate societies—is highly problematic. After all, the dysfunctional nature of the dyslectic condition is far from established. Most evolutionary social scientists think reading, writing, and dyslexia have no prior history of selection: "The ability to read and write are by-products of adaptations for spoken language, enabled by their causal structure. Random evolutionary noise exists as well, for example, the gene variants that cause dyslexia" (Tooby and Cosmides 2005, 26). Because Wakefield's HDA entails that psychological structures without a selective history cannot genuinely dysfunction (Murphy 2006, 82), dyslexia is not to be thought of as a dysfunction. Of course, one need not take Tooby and Comsides's view of dyslexia for granted, but there is little reason to prefer an adaptationist account of reading and writing above their account. Tooby and Cosmides are renowned adaptationists (in the Gould-Lewontin sense), and it is telling that they offer the example of reading and writing to show that they are not "panadaptationist." In other words, if there would be a more plausible adaptationist story to tell about our capacity for reading and writing, adaptationists like Tooby and Cosmides would most likely endorse it.

The second example is probably the most convincing example Wakefield gives of a condition that meets the three criteria. Evolutionary psychiatrists have emphasized over and over again that the absence of a particular emotion and/or attitude can be as dysfunctional as having too much of that emotion or attitude. They argue that extreme jealousy is rightly seen as a mental disorder but that the evolutionary perspective helps us to see that it is equally pathological not to feel any jealousy after finding out that your beloved husband cheated on you with your best friend. So evolutionary psychiatrists would argue that even though this lack of jealousy is currently not seen as a mental disorder, it should be seen as a disorder. The case that Wakefield presents here is different. Whereas the absence of jealousy is still maladaptive in our current social environment and thus a "harmful dysfunction" (although perhaps less so than in the ancestral environment, due to, for instance, modern birth control methods), the absence of aggression is not maladaptive now, even though it is the result of a breakdown of a mechanism that is thought to be a full-fledged adaptation. In this case, the mismatch model of evolutionary medicine is turned on its head: there are lucky individuals who would suffer from a disorder if they would live in the environment of evolutionary adaptedness, but they live happy and good lives because they are lucky enough to find themselves in a world where lack of aggression is highly valued and where the "typically male aggression" is punished severely enough to make it maladaptive. A benign environment makes all the difference here. We fully agree with

Wakefield that this condition is harmless—it's even beneficial—and that most laypeople and medical professionals would not see this as a disorder. It is less clear, however, whether this lack of aggression is really dysfunctional. Conditions like this "lack of aggression" are often used to counter the etiological account of function. For instance, McLaughlin critiques Wright's etiological account of function in the following way:

> At its first appearance, a beneficial trait in an organism doesn't have the proper etiology and thus cannot, according to Wright, be said to have a function—although a few generations later it will have acquired one: Organismic mutations are paradigmatically accidental in this sense. But that only disqualifies an organ from functionhood for the first—or the first few—generations. This is a problem that Wright shares with all the other etiological analyses. (McLaughlin 2001, 101)

While Wakefield would be likely to argue that those individuals without aggression are simply lucky accidents until this trait will have been selected,[2] the problem is that the only convincing example that he gives of a harmless dysfunction constitutes a classic counterexample to the natural selection account of function he considers crucial for his HDA.

Wakefield develops this example primarily as an example of a breakdown of mechanisms that usually result in highly aggressive responses, thereby suggesting that even reduced levels of aggression (and not just the total lack of aggression) would be dysfunctional: "For example, high levels of male aggression might have been useful under primitive conditions, but in present day circumstances such aggressive responses might be harmful. Consequently, even if a disposition to highly aggressive responses is the natural function of some mechanism, the loss of that function might not now be considered a disorder" (Wakefield 1992, 384).

In this example, mild aggression is a dysfunction in current societies and not just an example of normal variation (of aggression or of the underlying psychological mechanisms). Interestingly, as we will see in the next section, this is one of the very few places where he does not seem to use—implicitly—a harm judgment (or a related value judgment) to distinguish normal variation from dysfunction. The fact that this is so unusual could indicate that it is very difficult—and maybe even impracticable—to distinguish between suboptimal normal variation and dysfunction without using value judgments, even though Wakefield is trying to say the inverse.

III.   Normal Variation and Harmless Dysfunctions

One of the supposed benefits of the HDA is that it helps to distinguish harmful misfortunes and what are commonly considered to be true disorders (e.g., being illiterate due to circumstances vs. due to a reading disorder or being short vs. having a height disorder). With the former set of conditions, there is harm to the individual and yet there is no disorder, precisely because there is no underlying or accompanying dysfunction.

One interesting consequence of this is that in such instances, "no matter how harmful these conditions may be, they are part of the way we are biologically designed" (Wakefield 2010, 343). Such a claim, however, does not seem to capture what is at stake when looking at how a large majority of health conditions fall along a continuum. This problem should become apparent by looking at the following examples.

It has been argued that the nausea and vomiting experienced by many pregnant women is likely an evolved trait that protects the developing fetus against toxins, implying that while such symptoms are harmful for the mother, they need not indicate a disorder (Nesse and Williams 1994). Being able to determine, however, at what point variations in the intensity and duration of such symptoms shade into hyperemesis gravidarum, or severe morning sickness, which occurs in 0.3% to 2% of pregnant women (Goodwin 2008), is rather difficult. While Wakefield clearly accepts this latter condition to be a disorder (Wakefield 1999, 392), what seems implicit in his account is that because there is normal variation in this naturally selected function, it is actually only when such variation becomes harmful for the individual that it will be considered unhealthy. In making his argument, Wakefield does not refer to the lowered fitness of women suffering from hyperemesis gravidarum. The fact that he considers it disordered (and thus also dysfunctional) is not because he knows that pregnant women with severe morning sickness have on average lower fitness than pregnant women with mild morning sickness but because he implicitly uses harm to distinguish normal variants from dysfunctional ones. This also seems to square with most people's intuitions: if there are polymorphous traits that are equally well functioning (and with equally high fitness values), the trait that confers substantial harm would probably be seen as a disordered trait.

As Lilienfeld and Marino (1995) have argued, Wakefield's analysis needs to address the problem of normal variation. Natural selection is a process that filters out rather extreme forms, but while the resulting traits fixate within a population, there still remains much variation. In some cases, the remaining variants do not differ in fitness. Blood types are a good example of this, and this might also be true for severe and mild morning sickness. The existence of normal variation is especially interesting for medicine because not all suboptimal variation is judged as disordered. According to Wakefield's etiological approach, there is only a dysfunction when a trait within the variation that has been selected for breaks down, having detrimental effects on individual fitness. However, variation in suboptimal traits suggests that not all fitness reductions will be considered disordered, and this needs to be explained.

One example of this problem could be seen in the variation of heart rate–related conditions. The extreme of heart failure is a clear example of where the heart is failing to perform its naturally selected function of pumping blood, resulting in the death of the organism, and is thus disordered. The conclusion that death is unhealthy is rather trivial, though. Wakefield's HDA should also be able to capture diseases that are not the result of such drastic breakdowns. For example, within any given population, there will be variations in the level at which hearts perform this function, many of which will be suboptimal, as in the case of hypotension. The main question for Wakefield now becomes when hypotension becomes a dysfunction. Can the cutoff between suboptimal hypotension and dysfunctional hypotension be made without reference to the harm it causes? After all, what will constitute hypotension in any given case will differ between individuals, and while it is potentially harmful to the individual, hypotension is not in itself a disorder. It seems uncontroversial to argue, however, that severe forms of it are. Since the line between healthy and pathological hypotension is unclear (see also Schwartz 2007), in part because it is unclear when it would have negative effects on fitness, he seems caught in the trap of either considering all suboptimal variation as dysfunctional, since they are all fitness reducing (compared to the optimal heart rate), or using harm to determine when the variation should be considered a dysfunction. If Wakefield would opt for the first alternative—all suboptimal variation is dysfunctional—the value judgment is really all that matters for most diseases since most variants of a trait in a population are suboptimal. Furthermore, this would entail that Wakefield's use of "dysfunction" parts from how the concept is used in biology, where not all suboptimal variation is considered dysfunctional. If he opts for the second alternative—harm makes the difference between suboptimal and dysfunctional variants—he would blur the distinction between the harm component and the dysfunction component, a distinction that is absolutely basic for his hybrid account of disorder.

Another example of this problem arises when trying to distinguish shortness from height disorders (Wakefield 1999, 2010). When is normal variation in height to be considered a dysfunction? For Wakefield, there is a clear and commonly accepted divide between those unlucky individuals who are short, and who may experience some harm because of it, and those who are short because there is a hormone deficiency causing their diminished stature (1999, 379). He argues that where this line will be drawn will be a matter of convention and falls outside of conceptual analysis. This is an odd claim since no one disagrees with the fact that there is a difference between being short and having a hormone deficiency. The fruitfulness of such an analysis, however, stands or falls not on the extremes but precisely on these borderline "fuzzy" cases where a decision is needed. At the extreme end of normal variations in shortness, there is clear harm to the individual (according to social values), as witnessed in the frequent complaints and social stigmas attached to being short. Moreover, it is possible that this social harm could be linked to some form of evolutionary harm (and hence dysfunction) in the sense that average-height males have higher reproductive success than shorter and taller males (Stulp et al. 2012). As with the example of hypotension, would he then argue that all suboptimal deviations are dysfunctional? While Wakefield will likely cling to the argument that no matter how harmful being short is, without an underlying dysfunction there is no disorder, it seems reasonable to argue that extreme cases of shortness, like severe hypotension, cause enough harm/distress to render the individual dysfunctional. In other words, the line between suboptimal height and a dysfunction will be drawn precisely where the individual is sufficiently harmed due to their height. At this point, extreme shortness is just as much a disorder as having a hormone deficiency, even if there will obviously be a different prescription for the latter.

This problem of borderline cases is not an appeal to rare medical conditions but seems to plague all disorders that are a matter of degree (e.g., those with the prefix hyper- or hypo-, or those with dys-).[3] As such, Wakefield struggles to account for how the line is drawn between suboptimal variation and disorder within a large suite of common conditions. Is Wakefield led to conclude, then, that suboptimal functioning of the corpus callosum that produces a mild inability to read, or suboptimal developmental variations leading to mild abasia, or suboptimal hepatic regulation of cholesterol engendering mild hypercholesterolemia, or suboptimal loss-coping mechanisms producing mild intense sadness are all considered dysfunctional? If he does not wish to make such a judgment, then what might make Wakefield's account "unworkable," as Lilienfeld and Marino (1995) suggest, is that in order to work, it must assume precisely the opposite of what it claims: the suboptimal is considered dysfunctional when it is harmful.

We have seen, two different problems arising from normal variation. The first, which we explored through variations in morning sickness, suggests that fitness can be held equal across variations, and yet it is reasonable to consider some variations to be disorders precisely because they are harmful to the individual. The second, which we saw in terms of suboptimal variations, suggests that if there will be variations in fitness, and thus the attribution of a dysfunction, this attribution will most likely occur at that point where the variation is sufficiently harmful, in relation to individual or social values. In both cases, the line between dysfunction and harm is blurred. At the limits of the normal range of variation, which is precisely where medical judgment is needed and thus where conceptual analysis is put to the test, Wakefield smuggles the harm component into his account of dysfunction. As we have seen, this is the underlying problem that gets Wakefield into trouble when trying to provide uncontroversial examples of harmless dysfunctions, such as albinism or fused toes. If having fused toes is considered a suboptimal trait, then the point at which it would become a dysfunction is when it would pose enough harm to the individual. It is because he has not adequately accounted for the consequences that the problem of normal variation poses that his account cannot do what it set out to do.[4] In responding to a similar remark made by Murphy and Woolfolk (2000a) that there is a continuum in nature regarding the intensities and varieties of conditions, Wakefield argues that he is concerned with explaining what occurs outside of such ranges in the clear-cut cases (i.e., explaining the *intuition* that something is a disorder). The way in which he states this appeal to intuition is rather telling: "Our intuitions tend to attribute dysfunction and disorder in extreme cases where the behavior does not appear to be a useful strategy by any stretch of the imagination but rather seems *to devastate the individual's social functioning and interfere with other designed functions*" (Wakefield 2000, 260, emphasis added). In other words, the reason we seem to intuit that there is a *dysfunction*, let alone a disorder, is because as one moves into such an extreme, there is clearly harm to the individual. In other words, we also seem to have the "intuition" that conditions that exist on a continuum are only actually pathological if they are harmful to the individual. Prior to that, they are simply functional anomalies. It seems possible to have the intuition, then, that in such borderline cases, some levels of harm are sufficient to render someone disordered. At this point, the usual response of harm without dysfunction simply does not hold water.

As such, not even an appeal to intuitions seems sufficient to prop up the HDA. In the end, Wakefield only seems to describe the obvious or what is commonly accepted. He acknowledges that normal variations and fuzzy boundaries exist but claims that boundaries are not what conceptual analysis is meant to clarify. But if not, then the concepts seem redundant to medical judgments, and he seems to be doing nothing more than trying to find scientific support for some "folk psychiatry." As Murphy and Woolfolk write, "It is precisely the disagreements and divergent usages that provide the most information about the way the concept is used in the various theories that employ it" (2000b, 289). One would think that putting a concept to the test by appealing to those tough borderline cases would be yet one more chance to strengthen the HDA, but the fact that Wakefield avoids doing so seems to reveal a fundamental dysfunction at the heart of his endeavor.

Notes

1. These examples seem to come from Kendell (1975), who himself seems to take them as emblematic. Interestingly, roughly the same set of conditions (alongside hemophilia and color blindness), likely finding its source in the work of Geoffroy Saint-Hilaire, has been discussed quite some time ago by the philosopher of medicine, Georges Canguilhem (1991, 2008), suggesting that they are prototypical examples of where medical judgments differ. In the case of Canguilhem, he suggests that it is up to the individual to judge whether such conditions are mere anomalies or diseases.

2. In fact, Wakefield makes this argument by suggesting that if there would be a genetic mutation for blue eyes that is also protective of a disease, it could only be said to have this function after having been selected (2001, 357). Until that point, it would simply be a mutation with accidentally beneficial effects.

3. Murphy (2001) provides the example of dysthymia to suggest that there could be normally functioning mechanisms that are still deemed disordered, in this case due to having received deviant information.

4. The fact that one can more easily find examples of harmful conditions that are not dysfunctional has to do with one of the central tenets of error management theory (and evolutionary theory in general): type I errors (false positives) are less fitness undermining than false negatives.

References

Alberch, P., and E. A. Gale. 1985. A developmental analysis of an evolutionary trend: Digital reduction in amphibians. *Evolution* 39(1): 8–23.

Amundson, R. 2005. *The Changing Role of the Embryo in Evolutionary Thought: Roots of Evo-Devo.* Cambridge University Press.

Boorse, C. 1977. Health as a theoretical concept. *Philosophy of Science* 44(4): 542–573.

Boorse, C. 2011. Concepts of health and disease. In *Handbook of the Philosophy of Science Volume 16: Philosophy of Medicine,* F. Gifford (ed.), 13–64. Elsevier.

Canguilhem, G. 1991. *The Normal and the Pathological.* Trans. C. R. Fawcett and R. S. Cohen. Zone Books.

Canguilhem, G. 2008. *Knowledge of Life.* Trans. S. Geroulanos and D. Ginsberg. Fordham University Press.

De Block, A., and P. Adriaens. 2013. Pathologizing sexual deviance: A history. *Journal of Sex Research* 50(3–4): 276–298.

Francescotti, R. 1999. How to define intrinsic properties. *Noûs* 33(4): 590–609.

Fulford, K. W. M., M. Broome, G. Stanghellini, and T. Horton. 2005. Looking with both eyes open: Fact *and* value in psychiatric diagnosis? *World Psychiatry* 4(2): 78–86.

Galis, F., J. J. M. van Alphen, and J. A. J. Metz. 2001. Why five fingers? Evolutionary constraints on digit numbers. *Trends in Ecology and Evolution* 16(11): 637–646.

Gert, B., and G. Culver. 2009. Sex, immorality, and mental disorders. *Journal of Medicine and Philosophy* 34(5): 487–495.

Goodwin, T. M. 2008. Hyperemesis gravidarum. *Obstetrics and Gynecology Clinics of North America* 35(3): 401–417.

Kendall, R. E. 1975. The concept of disease and its implications for psychiatry. *British Journal of Psychiatry* 127: 305–315.

Levin, M. 1984. Why homosexuality is abnormal. *The Monist* 67(2): 251–283.

Lilienfeld, S. O., and L. Marino. 1995. Mental disorder as a Roschian concept: A critique of Wakefield's "harmful dysfunction" analysis. *Journal of Abnormal Psychology* 104(3): 411–420.

Maron, D. F. 2013. Witchcraft trade, skin cancer pose serious threats to albinos in Tanzania. *Scientific American,* October 11. http://www.scientificamerican.com/article.cfm?id=witchcraft-trade -skin.

McLaughlin, P. 2001. *What Functions Explain: Functional Explanation and Self-Reproducing Systems.* Cambridge University Press.

Murphy, D. 2001. Hacking's reconciliation: Putting the biological and sociological together in the explanation of mental illness. *Philosophy of the Social Sciences* 31(2): 139–162.

Murphy, D. 2006. *Psychiatry in the Scientific Image.* MIT Press.

Murphy, D., and R. L. Woolfolk. 2000a. The harmful dysfunction analysis of mental disorder. *Philosophy, Psychiatry, & Psychology* 7(4): 241–252.

Murphy, D., and R. L. Woolfolk. 2000b. Conceptual analysis versus scientific understanding: An assessment of Wakefield's folk psychiatry. *Philosophy, Psychiatry, and Psychology* 7(4): 271–293.

Nesse, R., and G. C. Williams. 1994. *Why We Get Sick: The New Science of Darwinian Medicine.* Vintage.

Reznek, L. 1987. *The Nature of Disease.* Routledge & Kegan Paul.

Schwartz, P. H. 2007. Defining dysfunction: Natural selection, design, and drawing a line. *Philosophy of Science* 74: 364–385.

Shapiro, L. A. 1992. Darwin and disjunction: Optimal foraging theory and univocal assignments of content. *Proceedings of the Philosophy of Science Association* 1: 469–480.

Sober, E. 1984. *The Nature of Selection.* MIT Press.

Sterelny, K. 1990. *The Representational Theory of Mind: An Introduction.* Blackwell.

Stevens, A., and J. Price. 1996. *Evolutionary Psychiatry: A New Beginning.* Routledge.

Stulp, G., T. V. Pollet, Verhulst, S., and A. P. Buunk. 2012. A curvilinear effect of height on reproductive success in human males. *Behavioral Ecology and Sociobiology* 66(3): 375–384.

Sullivan, M. 2003. The new subjective medicine: Taking the patient's point of view on health care and health. *Social Science & Medicine* 56: 1595–1604.

Tabin, C. J. 1992. Why we have (only) five fingers per hand: Hox genes and the evolution of paired limbs. *Development* 116: 289–296.

Tooby, J., and L. Cosmides. 2005. Conceptual foundations of evolutionary psychiatry. In *The Handbook of Evolutionary Psychiatry,* D. Buss (ed.), 5–67. John Wiley & Sons.

Wakefield, J. C. 1992. The concept of mental disorder: On the boundary between biological facts and social values. *American Psychologist* 47(3): 373–388.

Wakefield, J. C. 1995. Dysfunction as a value-free concept: A reply to Sadler and Agich. *Philosophy, Psychiatry, and Psychology* 2(3): 233–246.

Wakefield, J. C. 1999. Evolutionary versus prototype analyses of the concept of disorder. *Journal of Abnormal Psychology* 108: 374–399.

Wakefield, J. C. 2000. Spandrels, vestigial organs, and such: Reply to Murphy and Woolfolk's "The harmful dysfunction analysis of mental disorder." *Philosophy, Psychiatry, and Psychology* 7(4): 253–269.

Wakefield, J. C. 2001. Evolutionary history versus current causal role in the definition of disorder: Reply to McNally. *Behavior Research and Therapy* 39: 347–366.

Wakefield, J. C. 2005. On winking at the facts, and losing one's hare: Value pluralism and the harmful dysfunction analysis. *World Psychiatry* 4(2): 88–89.

Wakefield, J. C. 2007. The concept of mental disorder: Diagnostic implications of the harmful dysfunction analysis. *World Psychiatry* 6(3): 149–156.

Wakefield, J. C. 2010. Misdiagnosing normality: Psychiatry's failure to address the problem of false positive diagnoses of mental disorder in a changing professional environment. *Journal of Mental Health* 19(4): 337–351.

Wakefield, J. C. 2011. Darwin, functional explanation, and the philosophy of psychiatry. In *Maladapting Minds: Philosophy, Psychiatry, and Evolutionary Theory*, P. R. Adriaens and A. De Block (eds.), 43–172. Oxford University Press.

Witmer, D. G., W. Butchard, and K. Trogdon. 2005. Intrinsicality without naturalness. *Philosophy and Phenomenological Research* 70(2): 326–350.

26   Can the Harmful Dysfunction Analysis Distinguish Problematic Normal Variation from Disorder? Reply to Andreas De Block and Jonathan Sholl

Jerome Wakefield

I thank Andreas De Block and Jonathan Sholl for their fresh and energetic attempt to rethink the relationship between the harm and dysfunction components of the harmful dysfunction analysis (HDA) of medical, including mental, disorder. The HDA claims that "disorder" refers to "harmful dysfunction," where dysfunction is the failure of some feature to perform a natural function for which it is biologically designed by evolutionary processes and harm is judged in accordance with social values (First and Wakefield 2010, 2013; Spitzer 1997, 1999; Wakefield 1992a, 1992b, 1993, 1995, 1997a, 1997b, 1997c, 1997d, 1998, 1999a, 1999b, 2000a, 2000b, 2001, 2006, 2007, 2009, 2011, 2014, 2016a, 2016b; Wakefield and First 2003, 2012).

De Block and Sholl grapple with one of the most challenging problems for any account of mental disorder, namely, the differentiation of disorder from normal variation. If I understand De Block's position correctly from this and other (De Block 2008) papers, he focuses on the organism-environment interactive aspect of evolutionary theory and holds that "dysfunction" is just a way of describing a harmful interaction between the organism's nature and the current environment. On this view, dysfunction encompasses harm, so disorder can be understood simply as dysfunction: "the concept of mental disorder is identical to the concept of mental dysfunction....It is...redundant to conceptualize mental disorders as 'harmful dysfunctions', and not simply as 'mental dysfunctions'" (2008, 338). If this is (or was) his view, then he is using "dysfunction" and "disorder" in a way that equates them with current harm, and that would pathologize an enormous range of mismatches between individual natures and social demands. I believe that this approach confuses the technical biological meaning of dysfunction as failure of biologically designed function with the colloquial meaning of dysfunction as simply any negative interaction or performance (e.g., "I'm in a dysfunctional marriage"; "The congress is dysfunctional"). Consequently, this approach collapses the distinction between disorder and social deviance, undermining the ability to respond to antipsychiatric critiques and losing the value of a clarified concept of disorder.

De Block and Sholl's analysis in their chapter leads them to conclude that the HDA's harm criterion harbors problems "so problematic that it undermines, at least indirectly, the viability of the HDA." The problem, they argue, is that there is no genuine distinction between harm and dysfunction judgments. That is, dysfunction judgments are just harm judgments to begin with, so the HDA's essential contribution of separating those two components of disorder judgments turns out to be illusory. This is a projection onto the HDA of De Block's prior view, but their several resourceful arguments for this position lead to no such conclusion. I cannot address every one of the objections but have selected a few that I consider most important and will answer those in depth.

Dyslexia, Homosexuality, and Social versus Individual Values

Like Cooper and Forest in this volume, De Block and Sholl find fault with my claim that the evaluation of harm must be sensitive to social values. Specifically, they challenge my example that "in a literate society, a person who does not value reading still has a dyslexic disorder if incapable of learning to read due to a brain dysfunction" (Wakefield 2005, 98), asking, "why Wakefield claims that someone who doesn't value reading and writing at all should be considered disordered even in a literate society. If the individual experiences no harm, why should she be considered disordered?"

There are two answers to the question of why the HDA attributes disorder to such an individual. The first answer is simply that that's the way diagnosis works. The HDA is primarily an explanatory/descriptive account of the conceptual underpinnings of lay and professional disorder judgments. Medical disorder judgments of dyslexia are made without reference to the patient's personal values regarding reading, and an adequate analysis should explain that fact.

The more basic explanation, however, is that, contrary to De Block and Sholl's narrow characterization, the dyslexic individual *is* harmed in the diagnosis-relevant sense, whatever her personal values. Harm is not exhausted by whether, at the time of diagnostic assessment, the patient values a certain capacity or feels harmed by its lack. It is of course difficult to know how to interpret such disclaimers, but the issue is much deeper than that. In a society as dependent on reading as ours, with multiple opportunities and resources from occupational to recreational activities dependent on the ability, someone incapable of learning to read and thus incapable of accessing such resources is considered to be harmed *pro tanto* even if she claims not to value reading. She is no more unharmed just because of her disclaimer than someone without legs who says they don't care about walking. The harm lies in the objective loss of the capacity to access the social practices, institutions, and resources of the society within which she lives, whether or not at a certain time she would wish to exercise such capacities if she possessed them.

De Block and Sholl follow the same path trod by Cooper in her essay in this volume and assert that "it certainly is conceivable to develop a version of the HDA that treats individual values as central, rather than social values," and that "it seems reasonable to let the individual judge this, rather than letting the individual's well-being be judged by cultural standards." This can seem reasonable only if one does not actually think through the consequences. De Block and Sholl themselves acknowledge some of the serious problems with an "individual values" approach to harm and diagnosis: most individual values in the end are socially shaped, and many individuals with even the most severe and disabling cases of mental disorder deny that they are disordered. However, again, the problems run deeper than these issues. Although valuable for deciding among treatment options, the "individual harm" approach would make a hash of diagnosis for a variety of reasons. For starters, people's values change over time and sometimes within a short span. Moreover, there often is denial of caring about some impaired capacity as a self-protective strategy, and there are conflicts between first- and second-order desires regarding a capacity. A physician's job in diagnosis is not to psychoanalyze the patient and decide what the patient *really* wants or to discern whether the patient might change their mind the next day or ten years hence and more generally what the patient might want in the future. All of that may enter into consideration of whether and how to treat, but not into diagnosis. Contrary to the individual harm view, the patient's cultivation of a neutral attitude about the loss of a socially important capacity does not negate the harm or block a disorder judgment.

De Block and Sholl suggest that, by parity of reasoning with the dyslexia example, the social values view of harm could repathologize homosexuality: "Would Wakefield be willing to bite the bullet and say that homosexuality is a disorder in cultures that value heterosexuality—assuming of course that homosexuality is dysfunctional?" The assumption that homosexuality is due to a dysfunction takes this thought experiment beyond current consensus scientific judgments. However, granting the premise of a dysfunction as the cause of some forms of homosexuality, the standard answer to this sort of comparison is to distinguish between the direct harm of, for example, being unable to read and the indirect harm of, for example, being treated poorly by others as a result of sexual preference. Indirect harm, it is commonly held, does not warrant a disorder attribution, regardless of dysfunction.

De Block and Sholl are aware of this traditional answer in terms of direct versus indirect harm and they challenge it. They argue that there is more parity between the cases of dyslexia and homosexuality than the "direct versus indirect harm" response allows: "After all, dyslexia is harmful in culture A because it is intrinsically tied to not being able to read and because culture A values being able to read, whereas (exclusive) homosexuality is harmful in culture B because it is intrinsically tied to not being able to be attracted to individuals of the other biological sex and because culture B is a heteronormative culture." This analogy does not hold up upon examination. The reason that the harm from dyslexia is considered direct in culture A is not simply because "culture A values being able to read" but because reading is crucial to accessing the educational, occupational, recreational, and informational resources of (our) culture

A. Unlike homosexuality, dyslexia has harmful effects that are not only or primarily due to social disapproval of individuals who do not read but are the direct result of the inability to read because access to occupations, resources, and other opportunities is tied to the ability to read. As Spitzer came to see after a momentous clandestine meeting with closeted homosexual leaders in psychiatry—many of whom, he observed, were occupationally successful, socially engaged, enduringly attached in loving relationships, and personally happy—there is no such direct substantial harm independent of the attitudes of others in homosexuality. De Block and Sholl's facile analogy between dyslexia and homosexuality does not hold water.

Does the *DSM*'s "Clinical Significance Criterion" Require Individual-Perceived Harm?

De Block and Sholl claim that, contrary to the HDA's "social values" approach to harm, the *Diagnostic and Statistical Manual of Mental Disorders* (*DSM*) adopts an "individual values" approach, and they cite as evidence the "clinical significance criterion" (CSC) that was added to the diagnostic criteria for most categories of disorder in *DSM-IV* (1994). The CSC typically requires that, to be a disorder, the symptoms must "cause clinically significant distress or impairment in social, occupational, or other important areas of functioning." (The CSC is also cited by Cooper in her chapter in this volume as a device to ensure harm; for a critique of the CSC, see Spitzer and Wakefield 1999.)

In their discussion of the CSC, De Block and Sholl confuse two importantly different notions: whether *harm occurs to the individual* versus whether there is harm *as judged according to the individual's own values*. The latter idea is not found in the CSC, which requires socially defined harms that may or may not be harms from the individual's own perspective.

It is true that the individual's distress is one form of harm specified in the CSC, and in some *DSM-5* categories, such as some sexual dysfunctions, the individual's distress is a necessary condition for diagnosis. One assumes that patients disvalue distress, but perhaps this does not apply to everyone. However, the *DSM* distress criterion applies to all those who are distressed, whether they care about being distressed or not. It is based on our fundamental cultural agreement that distress is undesirable, which in turn is based on the virtually universal desire to end distress. If Nietzsche walked into a modern New York psychiatrist's office insisting that "What doesn't kill me makes me stronger" (1888/2005) and that he was therefore glad to experience distress from his condition, that would not block his *DSM* diagnosis based partly on distress. However, treatment planning for Nietzsche might be another matter.

The point is even clearer with regard to the CSC's role impairment clause. Social roles are socially defined, and thus impairment in important social roles is socially defined. The nature of child-caring, socializing, and work varies from culture to culture, and if the individual's symptoms make the individual incapable of caring adequately for children, working effectively, or attending to social interactions in socially defined ways, disorder is diagnosable, whether or not the patient values adequate parenting or work performance or social interaction as culturally defined. Again, of course, whether or how the clinician intervenes in partnership with the patient will depend strongly on the patient's values and attitudes. I conclude that, the *DSM*'s CSC notwithstanding, De Block and Sholl's attempt to relativize the harm component to the individual's values fails to make any headway.

What If We Discovered That a Paradigmatic Disorder Was Naturally Selected?

A perennial objection to the HDA is that evolutionary dysfunction can't be necessary for disorder because it is conceivable that we could discover that a disorder was in fact naturally selected. This led me to make a risky, bold, novel HDA prediction: "if what is now considered a disorder is shown to be a selected feature, then our intuitions would change and we would come to consider it a nondisorder, reconceptualizing it as a normal variation—as has happened with fever" (Wakefield 2011, 152). De Block and Sholl challenge this answer, asking, "What would the consequences be for the HDA if it would be shown that schizophrenia—a paradigm object of psychiatric concern—is an adaptation, as some speculatively inclined evolutionary psychiatrists have already hypothesized (Stevens and Price 1996)?"

The answer to De Block and Sholl's question is that, if schizophrenia turned out to be an adaptation that was a normal variation of biologically designed humanity that modern societies have rendered disadvantageous, it would remain a problem in modern societies but it would no longer be understood as a medical/mental disorder. There is evidence for this claim: in those instances in which theorists, ranging from R. D. Laing and some family dynamics theorists to some behaviorists, have come to the conclusion that schizophrenia is a nondysfunction reaction to an abnormal situation, they have also held that it is not a disorder (see my reply to Garson in this volume for further comments and references on this point). Indeed, there is recent additional striking support for my prediction. Moderate forms of psychopathy—which are equally "a paradigm object of psychiatric concern"—have recently come to be understood by some researchers as likely adaptations, and those researchers consequently have come to recategorize psychopathy as nondisorder (for a detailed discussion of the psychopathy example, see my reply to Cooper in this volume).

A common mistake is to confuse various evolutionary explanations of the persistence of a condition with explanations specifically in terms of natural selection of the condition; it is only the latter that establish a function and thus provide the basis for attribution of a dysfunction when failure occurs. De Block and Sholl's comments on schizophrenia, drawing on Stevens and Price's (1996) "group splitting hypothesis," illustrate this sort of confusion. Stevens and Price speculate that in the environment of human evolutionary adaptation, the challenging but necessary process of splitting a new group off from a primary group that has grown too large may have been facilitated by the presence of charismatic leaders who could inspire a subgroup of the community to follow him or her under the influence of a new belief system. Such a leader might have been advantaged by some schizotypal traits (e.g., "religious themes," "use of neologisms," "mood changes," "delusions and hallucinations" [151]), which carry a genetic load on a spectrum with schizophrenia. De Block and Sholl use this hypothesis as an example of evolutionary explanations for clear disorders.

However, a close reading of Stevens and Price indicates that they do not claim that schizophrenia itself in its full clinical form was specifically selected for. Rather, they argue that "certain schizotypal features on the schizophrenia spectrum can under specific conditions and in certain levels be advantageous" and that "the predisposition to schizophrenia" may be "inherited in a graded fashion" that has "a counterpart in the behavior of normal individuals" (145). Indeed, current clinical descriptions of schizophrenia include negative symptoms that often imply lack of ability to manage positive symptoms and inclination to social withdrawal, directly in tension with what the hypothesized charismatic group leaders would require. So, Stevens and Price are not at all hypothesizing selection for the clinical condition of schizophrenia as we know it. Rather, analogous to "heterozygote advantage" in such conditions as sickle cell trait, Stevens and Price hypothesize selection for certain genes that may be advantageous in themselves but, when they occur in specific combinations or numbers, yield the nonselected and strictly disadvantageous pathology of schizophrenia. De Block and Sholl's suggestion that there exist credible arguments for the selection for schizophrenia confuses selection for preconditions or risk factors for a disorder with selection for the disorder itself.

Past Examples of Harmless Dysfunctions That Are Not Considered Disorders

De Block and Sholl expend most of their paper arguing in a variety of ways that I am wrong to claim that dysfunctions can be identified independently of harm. They thus expend considerable effort disputing the HDA's "idea that each of the conjuncts 'harmful' and 'dysfunctional' is in separation from the other insufficient for a condition to be a disorder." For me, a fundamental task of an analysis of mental disorder—indeed, a transcendental sine qua non of a successful analysis in response to the antipsychiatric challenge—is to distinguish problematic normal variation (harmful nondysfunction) from disorder (harmful dysfunction). If the only way to tell that there is dysfunction is via harmfulness, this implies, according to De Block and Sholl's argument, that the HDA cannot in fact distinguish between harmful normal variation and disorder and thus fails in its goals. De Block and Sholl frame the issue as follows: "So, if the HDA is correct, (1) some conditions must be both dysfunctional *and* harmless, and (2) our judgment that these conditions are not disorders must also be relatively uncontroversial." They thus challenge me to describe "examples of conditions that are (1) dysfunctional, (2) harmless, and (3) uncontroversially not disordered."

De Block and Sholl's initial attack on the possibility of separating dysfunction from harm is to argue that none of the examples I have presented of harmless dysfunctions that are nondisorders really are such. They pose objections to each of the three examples of harmless dysfunctions—fused toes, albinism, and reversal of heart position—that I presented in my 1992 paper on the HDA, which I borrowed from Robert Kendell's (1975) paper on the concept of disorder, as well as my own later example of dyslexia in a preliterate culture, claiming each one is either nondysfunction or harmful or/and a disorder. I will not quibble at length about these past examples; I have revisited the literature on each of them and stand by these examples. Before turning to some fresh examples, I offer the following brief comments.

In claiming that the above conditions are judged disorders, De Block and Sholl rely heavily on the fact that fused toes, albinism, and situs inversus all have disorder codes in the *International Classification of Diseases* (*ICD-10*). However, some conditions are listed within disorder categories of *ICD-10* because of the need for codes for reimbursement due to associated conditions even when the specific condition itself is clearly a nondisorder. For example, the *ICD-10*'s "O-codes" in chapter XV include disorders related to "pregnancy, childbirth, and the puerperium" but also include such nondisordered conditions as "O80. Single spontaneous delivery" that explicitly states that it "includes delivery in a completely normal case," as well as "O80.0. Spontaneous vertex delivery" (i.e., a completely normal unaided head-first delivery) and "O04.9. Medical abortion, complete without complication." All of my examples of harmless dysfunctions have complicated versions in which medical intervention is necessary, justifying the codes. Indeed, De Block and Sholl themselves report Canguilhem's statement that some of these same conditions are "prototypical examples of where medical judgments differ," suggesting that their status as disorders is more dubious than De Block and Sholl suggest.

De Block and Sholl's discussion of my "dyslexia in a preliterate culture" example reveals a basic misunderstanding of the HDA that may explain some of their puzzling responses to the other examples. There is a theory that dyslexia is caused by a minor dysfunction of the corpus callosum that interferes with the individual's ability to transfer information across brain hemispheres at the extremely high rates uniquely demanded by reading, and this dysfunction has no other effects. I argue that if this is so, then someone with that dysfunction who lived 50,000 years ago in a preliterate society would not have a medical disorder because there is no conceivable harm. This illustrates a dysfunction without harm, the very thing that De Block and Sholl deny exists. In response, they say that this example is highly problematic because "the dysfunctional nature of the dyslectic condition is far from established. Most evolutionary social scientists think reading, writing, and dyslexia have no prior history of selection."

However, as I have repeatedly explained in various publications, of course reading is not a naturally selected capacity but rather an invention that exploits the capacities of various brain mechanisms that evolved for other reasons. The failure to be able to learn to read is the *harm* in dyslexia, and harm cannot be defined in evolutionary terms. Dyslexia is supposed to be diagnosed only when the clinician infers the existence of a neurological dysfunction of an as yet unknown nature that is causing that harm.

De Block and Sholl make two basic errors here. First, they think that the HDA implies that the disorder's harm itself must be a failure of a naturally selected function, but the HDA only requires that the harm be caused by *some* dysfunction that has the harm as an effect, not that the harm itself be the failure of the function. Second, in saying that the cause of dyslexia in a neurological dysfunction is far from established, they confuse conceptual analysis of the meaning of "disorder" with scientific discovery about causes of disorder. The issue for conceptual analysis is not whether dyslexia is in fact caused by a dysfunction but whether nosologists and clinicians tend to classify lack of ability to read as due to a disorder of dyslexia when and only when they believe that it is due to a neurological dysfunction. A careful reading of the literature of dyslexia diagnosis indicates that this is precisely what they do, and that diagnosis proceeds by first eliminating all other plausible explanations of the reading problem as well as looking for symptoms distinctive of neurological dysfunction. Once these points are understood, the dyslexia example does provide a clean separation of dysfunction and harm.

New Examples of Clear Cases of Harmless Dysfunctions Not Considered Disorders

Rather than further disputing mostly borrowed past illustrations of nondisorder harmless dysfunctions, I present here four fresh examples (for further examples, see Wakefield 2014).

First, then, there are many examples of dysfunctions in which a genetic mutation alters biologically designed functioning and thus constitutes an evolutionary dysfunction in the HDA's sense, but rather than causing harm, the result fits better with our modern social environment than the original version of the gene that was naturally selected in the EEA and so the dysfunction is beneficial. A fanciful example I provided in the past was of a dysfunction that reduced naturally high levels of male aggression to a level more in keeping with what is demanded by modern social environments. In this case, I argued, there is a dysfunction that causes no harm, and consequently no one would consider this individual disordered. De Block and Sholl respond, "We fully agree with Wakefield that this condition is harmless—it's even beneficial—and that most laypeople and medical professionals would not see this as a disorder." They object that "it is less clear, however, whether this lack of aggression is really dysfunctional," but that objection is based on their own idiosyncratic approach to dysfunction, and per hypothesis, there is a dysfunction in the HDA's evolutionary sense.

There are limits to such hypothetical examples, but fortunately, there are many real examples that share a similar structure to the aggression-reducing example. Consider, for example, apolipoprotein C-III (C-III), a lipid that plays a role in the production of triglycerides. Due to various dietary and stress factors in a modern environment, high normal-variation triglycerides significantly increase the risk of heart attack. A small number of individuals are born with a knockout loss-of-function mutation of the C-III gene on one DNA strand that stops that gene from producing any C-III, leaving the individual with much lower than the naturally selected level of C-III and thus a lower level of triglycerides (Norata et al. 2015; Jørgensen et al. 2014; TG and HDL Working Group 2014). In a modern environment, this lowered level of triglycerides turns out to be protective against cardiovascular disease and early death. In other words, modern social environments make high but normal-variant levels of triglycerides harmful, so a mutation that makes one C-III gene dysfunctional, thereby lowering C-III levels and consequently lowering triglycerides below the naturally selected level, turns out to be beneficial without any apparent cost. This, then, is a real example of a harmless dysfunction analogous to the aggression example.

Second, I have a little red dot on my abdomen. Technically, it is a benign angioma. It is known that it is due to a dysfunction in the mechanisms that cause capillaries to smoothly connect to each other during development, so that this particular capillary grew in another direction and connected with the skin instead. Despite its ominous classification as a neoplasm due to the abnormal cell growth, it is entirely harmless both physically and, because it is on a part of my body that is almost always covered, socially and aesthetically as well. Consequently, no one would seriously consider it a medical disorder; it is a harmless anomaly. My benign angioma is a clear case of a harmless dysfunction that is not a medical disorder.

My third example illustrates the fact that by far the vast majority of dysfunctions are harmless nondisorders. Mutations that cause dysfunctions of specific genetic loci are occurring all the time in the cells of one's body. Indeed, the somewhat frightening reality is that, as the title of a science article in *The Atlantic* put it, "Your Body Acquires Trillions of New Mutations Every Day" (Zhang 2018). When you walk out into the sun with exposed skin, you acquire literally millions of mutations within a short period that cause genes to stop being able to perform their natural functions, and many of these mutations are potential contributors to cancer if reparative mechanisms don't fix them and just the right (or wrong) other mutations should occur in the same cells. Yet, in themselves, they are not harmful, and so physicians and researchers consider the skin to be normal (articles on these genetic mutations often specify that the skin is normal) despite it being filled with such mutations that actually are known to vie with one another for skin space. The constant stream of trillions of harmless mutations that occur to the skin and to the insides of the body are clear cases of harmless dysfunctions that are not considered disorders.

My fourth domain of examples offers a made-to-order historical test case for the HDA's thesis that harmless dysfunctions are not considered disorders as against De Block and Sholl's contrary position. As virology and bacteriology have progressed using recently developed tools for genetic analysis, it has been discovered that many viruses and bacteria can chronically infect individuals without causing any symptoms or other harm; they are known as "commensal" infectious agents that benefit without harming the host. The reaction of the microbiology community has been crystal clear: these harmless infections, though they do involve cellular-level dysfunctions such as viral exploitation of cellular genetic machinery for reproduction, are not diseases or disorders as long as they are harmless. For example, the Epstein-Barr virus, which exists in roughly 90% of the world's population without resulting in disease, also under certain circumstances causes mononucleosis. It is only when Epstein-Barr gives rise to harmful symptoms—which tends to occur with exposure during adolescence and young adulthood—that it is classified as the disease of mononucleosis: "Epstein-Barr virus (EBV) was initially found to infect most healthy laboratory staff with no apparent disease" (Griffiths 1999, 74). A similar differentiation is for the bacterium *Streptococcus pneumoniae*, which has been recognized as a major cause of pneumonia since the nineteenth century, yet the dysfunction that consists of infection with this bacterium does not always constitute a disorder because the vast majority of infections occur harmlessly in the nose and sinuses and the bacterium only becomes problematic under special circumstances, when it migrates to the lungs and becomes more virulent (Vu and Kaiser 2017). Infection with the bacterium is not described in the literature as a disease, disorder, pathology, or pathogenic, and individuals are described as "healthy" and "normal" when it harmlessly resides in the nasal passages. This changes to the language of disease and sickness when the virus becomes harmful: "Bacteria are all around—and inside—us. Some are harmless, some are beneficial and some, of course, cause disease....The common bacterium *Streptococcus pneumoniae*...dwells harmlessly in people's nasal passages. Every so often, however, when *S. pneumoniae* senses danger, it disperses...making us sick" (Braun 2013, 2–3). Harmless viral and bacterial infections are a clear and very widespread instance of harmless dysfunctions that are not considered medical disorders. I conclude from these examples that De Block and Sholl's bold claim that there are no harmless dysfunctions that are considered nondisorders is amply falsified and any general claim that dysfunction cannot be distinguished from harm disproven.

Why Do We Classify Morning Sickness as Normal and Hyperemesis Gravidarum as a Disorder?

I now turn to the final section of De Block and Sholl's paper, in which they challenge the HDA's ability to distinguish problematic normal variation (misfortune) from harmful dysfunction (disorder) within two specific domains—conditions in which normal and disordered variants fall along a symptom-severity dimension and suboptimal conditions. They argue that the purported ability of the HDA to explain the difference between harmful normal conditions and harmful disordered conditions fails to materialize in these domains because the question of whether a dysfunction is causing the harm is not answerable independently of the harm judgment. I believe that the suboptimality argument is based on a confusion of optimality with biological design and will leave it aside here to focus on the dimensionality argument. Dimensional approaches to diagnosis are quite popular at the moment, and the view that a dimensional symptom-severity psychometric structure can somehow preempt a categorical HDA-driven disorder attribution has become widespread in psychiatric nosology, expressed in proposals to reconstruct diagnosis in dimensional terms (Kotov et al. 2017; Krueger et al. 2018). This approach finds culminating expression in Robert Plomin's (2003, 2018) dramatic claim that from a genetic perspective, "there are no disorders, only dimensions," and so warrants close examination.

De Block and Sholl argue that when symptoms generated by some mechanism fall along a dimensional severity continuum from none to severe, the HDA cannot distinguish where on the dimension to draw the distinction between dysfunction and nondysfunction and thus between disorder and nondisorder because of a lack of independent evidence. Consequently, the severity cut-point for drawing the HDA's supposed distinction between dysfunction-caused and nondysfunction-caused symptoms must be based simply on whether the symptoms are harmful, undercutting the distinction that is at the HDA's core. To assess these claims, I take an in-depth look at De Block and Sholl's primary example, the distinction between normal-range "morning sickness," which is medically labeled "nausea and vomiting of pregnancy" (NVP) and is not literally considered to be a sickness or disorder in the medical pathological sense, and the severe form of such symptoms in which there is extreme nausea and vomiting during pregnancy, which is considered a disorder and labeled "hyperemesis gravidarum" (HG).

De Block and Sholl's argument that the dimensionality of these symptoms poses a problem for the HDA goes as follows:

> It has been argued that the nausea and vomiting experienced by many pregnant women is likely an evolved trait that protects the developing fetus against toxins, implying that while such symptoms are harmful for the mother, they need not indicate a disorder. Being able to determine, however, at what point variations in the intensity and duration of such symptoms shade into hyperemesis gravidarum, or severe morning sickness...is rather difficult. While Wakefield clearly accepts this latter condition to be a disorder, what seems implicit in his account is that because there is normal variation in this naturally selected function, it is actually only when such variation becomes harmful for the individual that it will be considered unhealthy. In making his argument, Wakefield does not refer to the lowered fitness of women

suffering from hyperemesis gravidarum. The fact that he considers it disordered (and thus also dysfunctional) is not because he knows that pregnant women with severe morning sickness have on average lower fitness than pregnant women with mild morning sickness but because he implicitly uses harm to distinguish normal variants from dysfunctional ones. This also seems to square with most people's intuitions: if there are polymorphous traits that are equally well functioning (and with equally high fitness values), the trait that confers substantial harm would probably be seen as a disordered trait. (De Block and Sholl, this volume)

The basic idea of De Block and Sholl's argument is that nausea and vomiting during pregnancy, according to current theory, is likely a naturally selected protective mechanism, but this selected mechanism manifests in different levels of severity of the symptoms, forming a polymorphous set of reactions that lie on a continuous dimension from mild to very severe. Given that all the points on this dimension are equally expressions of the same naturally selected mechanism and thus presumably represent roughly equal fitness in the EEA and do not represent evolutionary dysfunctions ("In some cases, the remaining variants do not differ in fitness. Blood types are a good example of this, and this might also be true for severe and mild morning sickness"), the only basis for medicine dividing the dimension into normal-range versus disordered levels of symptoms must be harm: "If there are polymorphous traits that are equally well functioning (and with equally high fitness values), the trait that confers substantial harm would probably be seen as a disordered trait." Thus, the basis for so dividing the dimension—and the only real meaning of "dysfunction" if the term is applied to HG—must lie in the greater harm that occurs at the higher end of the dimension rather than in any inferred literal evolutionary dysfunction: "What seems implicit in his account is that because there is normal variation in this naturally selected function, it is actually only when such variation becomes harmful for the individual that it will be considered unhealthy." Thus, De Block and Sholl conclude, "We have seen, then, two different problems arising from normal variation. The first, which we explored through variations in morning sickness, suggests that fitness can be held equal across variations, and yet it is reasonable to consider some variations to be disorders precisely because they are harmful to the individual."

Before proceeding, there is one objection posed by De Block and Sholl that needs to be addressed to clarify the nature of the argument. They observe that in accepting that HG is a disorder, I "did not refer to the lowered fitness of women suffering from hyperemesis gravidarum." Consequently, they argue, my judgment that it is a disorder caused by a dysfunction is based not on lower EEA fitness "but because he implicitly uses harm to distinguish normal variants from dysfunctional ones." There are two problems with this objection. First, we have no data on the actual fitness effects of HG or NVP in the EEA, and knowing HG's fitness effects in our current environment does not help because there are widely available modern medical interventions, such as intravenous feeding, that have radically reduced HG's dangers and fitness disadvantages.

Anyway, disorder judgments generally do not involve explicit fitness estimates but implicit judgments about biological design and its failures based on circumstantial evidence. Second, the fact that De Block and Sholl pose my failure to cite fitness data as a criticism of the HDA shows that they misunderstand the difference between testing the substantive scientific hypothesis that HG is a disorder, for which EEA fitness data would conceivably be helpful, versus testing the HDA's conceptual analytic hypothesis that *HG is judged to be a disorder because it is judged to be a harmful failure of biological design*. For the latter purpose of evaluating the HDA—which I assume is De Block and Sholl's purpose—EEA fitness data are irrelevant. Instead, one has to examine what people say and believe about HG and NVP, a task undertaken in the analysis below.

To be capable of supporting De Block and Sholl's dimensional argument, their NVP/HG example must satisfy their argument's dimensional presuppositions. Those presuppositions are as follows: (1) certain kinds of harmful symptoms are considered to fall on a single dimensional continuum from lack of harmful symptoms to severely harmful symptoms of the same kind, (2) part of the dimension is considered normal, (3) the rest of the dimension is considered disordered, and (4) there is no established nonarbitrary dividing line between the two along the common dimension of harm. With these four dimensional presuppositions in the background, they then go on to claim that all the points along the dimension, being commonly generated by a naturally selected mechanism, must be considered equally naturally selected, and yet some are considered disordered and some not, thus contradicting the HD analysis.

The four background presuppositions are fully satisfied by De Block and Sholl's NVP/HG example. First, HG's symptoms are consistently described as a severe or extreme form of NVP (e.g., Fejzo et al. 2018, 2; Holmgren et al. 2018, 1; National Organization for Rare Disorders 2015; McParlin et al. 2016, 1392) and as at the "extreme end of the pregnancy sickness spectrum" (Pregnancy Sickness Support 2019), locating the condition on the same symptom-severity dimension with common NVP. Second, NVP is described not only as common but as "a normal part of a healthy pregnancy" (Ben-Joseph 2014) and generally as "normal" (Holmgren et al. 2018, 1; UK National Health Service 2016; WebMD Medical Reference 2019, 1, 2; Wood et al. 2013, 100). Third, in contrast to milder NVP, HG is consistently considered a "disorder" (Dean et al. 2018; National Organization for Rare Disorders 2015) or "disease" (Fejzo 2018, 2; London et al. 2017, 161). Indeed, once Antoine Dubois, obstetrician to Napoleon Bonaparte's second wife Empress Marie Louise, described the syndrome of "pernicious vomiting of pregnancy" to the French Academy of Medicine in 1852, a flourishing literature arose speculating on the pathogenesis of the disorder, with etiological theories ranging from "irritation of the vomiting reflex from the stretching of the uterine fibers" and "irritation of the cervix" to "toxinemia" (London et al. 2017, 162). Fourth, as De Block and Sholl suggest, and as is indicated in the common assertion that HG is a severe form of NVP, the consensus has been that there is no apparent natural dividing line on the continuum of symptom expressions between HG and NVP: "Many researchers believe that NVP should be regarded as a continuum of symptoms that may impact an affected woman's physical, mental and social well-being to varying degrees. Hyperemesis gravidarum represents the severe end of the continuum. No specific line exists that separates hyperemesis gravidarum from NVP" (National Organization for Rare Disorders 2015). Thus, this is precisely the kind of example that should support De Block and Sholl's case and reveal a problem for the HDA, if their analysis is correct. The question is whether they are correct in their assumption that, under these conditions, those distinguishing HG as a disorder do not see it as due to a dysfunction that represents a breakdown in biological design.

Before tackling whether the HDA works to explain the NVP/HG distinction, it is worth noting that De Block and Sholl's assertion that the division between NVP and HG is based sheerly on harm, were it to be formulated as an alternative account of the distinction, would fail to be explanatory of where even roughly on the symptom-severity dimension the line is generally drawn between HG and NVP. Moderate to severe non-HG NVP is itself quite unpleasant and somewhat impairing and thus significantly harmful: "[NVP's] impact on women's lives is not necessarily minimal. For some women, the implications of NVP are substantial with multi-faceted effects, hindering their ability to maintain usual life activities, and particularly their ability to work" (Wood et al. 2013, 100). Surely if not occurring during pregnancy, NVP-level harm would be considered indicative of possible disorder. Nor can the dividing line reflect when NVP is harmful enough to justify treatment, for "as many as 18% of pregnant women take medication to treat this condition" (Fejzo et al. 2018, 2). Yet, even when treated, NVP is not considered a disorder any more than pain during childbirth, for which most women are treated. If one simply asserts that it is greater harmfulness along the severity dimension that warrants the disorder/nondisorder division, one runs into the problem that moderate to strong NVP is of relatively greater severity than mild or no NVP along the very same dimension of harmfulness, and so according to this account should be labeled a disorder, but it is not. Nor does such a symptom-gradient account work elsewhere; for example, severe major depression is much more harmful than mild major depression, yet the entire dimension is considered disorder territory, whereas severe (normal) grief is much more painful than mild grief, yet the entire dimension is considered nondisordered. Of course, many physical disorders as well occur with varying degrees of harm from very modest to extremely severe symptoms, with the entire dimension considered disordered.

Harmfulness itself thus fails to explain the location of the fuzzy division between HG disorder and NVP nondisorder. This failure presents a seeming paradox because, as De Block and Sholl emphasize, prior to recent developments (to be described shortly), the harmful symptoms were all the evidence we possessed in regard to HG and NVP. So, why is the harm of HG seen as indicative of disorder, whereas the harm of NVP is not?

The way out of this conundrum is that what De Block and Sholl singly label "harm" consists of symptoms with many aspects other than their harmfulness and so additional explanatory variables beyond sheer severity of harm can yield the divergent dysfunction versus nondysfunction attributions. Although dysfunction and harm are conceptually distinct components of HDA disorders, the same set of symptoms may be evidentially relevant to both, manifesting harmfulness in certain features and manifesting a likely failure of biological design in other features. Moreover, a smooth dimensional distribution of harmful symptoms can be generated by multiple underlying etiologies. I will argue that a careful reading of the literature reveals that a belief in multiple etiologies and multiple fitness levels underlies the NVP/HG distinction. Thus, what De Block and Sholl singly label "harm" does double duty, playing two distinct roles based on different properties of the symptoms with different explanatory pathways.

What is this difference in features over and above sheer severity of nausea and vomiting that suggests different fitness values? In one sense, HG is literally a severe form of NVP along the NVP symptom dimension because it consists of continuous, intractable, extreme nausea and vomiting. However, as a result of the extreme severity of NVP-type symptoms, HG is also harmful to both maternal and fetal health in ways that experts distinguish as quite different from what happens in standard NVP and that transcend the nausea and vomiting themselves as clinical issues. For one thing, women with NVP can continue to gain weight consistent with healthy pregnancy and remain adequately hydrated, whereas women with HG can lose substantial amounts of weight while pregnant and can become dangerously dehydrated or malnourished (National Organization for Rare Disorders 2015; Dulay 2017). Women with HG can experience ketonuria, nutritional deficiencies, muscle wasting, electrolyte disturbances, tachycardia, Wernicke's encephalopathy, renal failure, liver function abnormalities, and esophageal rupture, whereas women with NVP experience none of these. Intravenous fluids and sometimes feeding tubes are often necessary to bring HG under control, with HG the second leading cause of hospitalization during pregnancy (e.g., Dean et al. 2018; Fejzo et al. 2016; Fejzo et al. 2018, 1–2; McParlin et al. 2016, 1392; Walker and Thompson 2018, 2698). Dr. Amos Grunebaum, then director of obstetrics at New York Presbyterian/Weill Cornell Medical Center, distinguished HG from NVP as follows: "Unlike simple nausea and vomiting that accompanies many pregnancies, hyperemesis gravidarum is a medical emergency that usually requires hospitalization....If not treated properly with intravenous fluids and sometimes also intravenous nutrition, it can be life-threatening to pregnant women and their fetuses" (as quoted in Flam 2014, 3).

Walker and Thomas (2018) observe, "Interestingly, an absence of NVP is associated with a higher risk of miscarriage, whereas having HG is associated with poor fetal outcomes ranging from preterm birth and neurodevelopmental delay" (2698; see also Fejzo et al. 2018, 2). This divergence between NVP and HG is of particular interest because the reduction of miscarriage is the only established offsetting benefit of NVP that provides some support for the theory that it is a naturally selected defense against substances toxic to the fetus rather than just an unpleasant side effect of hormonal changes. The fact that HG's effect on the fetus's prospects is instead negative in multiple ways removes the only known rationale for a "naturally selected defense" theory of HG that makes it as fit as NVP.

As Grunebaum notes, aside from the great variety of other potentially serious medical problems that could place the mother's health and the pregnancy at risk, HG's potential harms include the substantial risk of death to the mother and the fetus, placing it in a discontinuous class of basic threats to fitness not comparable even dimensionally to NVP's benign nausea-and-vomiting profile. This was especially true in the EEA and historically before modern medical interventions (National Organization for Rare Disorders 2015) but to some extent remains so today. For example, in their history of HG, London et al. (2017) note that "reports of maternal death from symptoms that now appear attributed to hyperemesis date as far back as religious documentation" (162). Fejzo et al. (2016), in their aptly titled article, "Why Are Women Still Dying from Nausea and Vomiting of Pregnancy?" state, "Until the 1950's, maternal deaths were commonly associated with hyperemesis gravidarum (HG). Although maternal mortality secondary to HG has since decreased, 6 deaths were reported recently in the literature" (1).

Perhaps the most famous case of a death from HG is that of the author Charlotte Bronte in 1855. Drife (2012), noting that "newly married and pregnant at 38, [Bronte] soon began vomiting," observes that "today her hyperemesis would be treated with a routine drip," but "When I was a student, ... our textbooks pointed out that hyperemesis can lead to liver failure and it may be necessary to terminate the pregnancy" (51). Before intravenous feeding and hydration, termination was the only available solution for unremitting HG to avoid maternal death. Drife quotes the reaction to Bronte's death expressed in a letter written by her friend, Elizabeth Gaskell, who did not know about Bronte's condition until after her death: "A wren would have starved on what she ate during those last six weeks. How I wish I had known! I do fancy that if I had come, I could have induced her,—even though they had all felt angry with me at first,—to do what was absolutely necessary, for her very life. Poor poor creature" (Gaskell as quoted in Drife 2012, 51). Gaskell's letter reveals that it was understood at the time that HG is potentially fatal and that the only reliable way to stop HG was to terminate the pregnancy. Despite medical progress, termination of pregnancy is still often the selected intervention to address unremitting HG that does not respond to standard antiemetics and threatens the mother (Boelig et al. 2018; London 2017; Dulay 2017). This choice remains common enough that Al-Ozairi et al.'s (2009) study of the use of high-dose steroids to suppress unremitting HG is explicitly posed as a challenge to the standard practice of pregnancy termination.

In sum, although severity of nausea and vomiting may form a continuous dimension, there is a crucial inflection point in the nature of the outcomes and side effects of the dimensional harm at roughly around where the distinction is drawn between normal NVP and disordered HG. This inflection point between NVP and HG, although located with somewhat arbitrary precision in modern diagnostic systems (e.g., >5 lbs. of lost weight), reflects judgments on the question of function versus dysfunction. A condition that under EEA circumstances seriously threatened the life of the mother and the fetus without any plausible offsetting benefit is a prima facie failure of biological design. It is this inference that draws observers to the conclusion that there must be a dysfunction underlying HG and that the broader morning sickness adaptation or side effect has gone terribly wrong.

If the HDA analysis is correct, then, rather than simply accepting NVP-HG as a seamless severity dimension, the natural logic of nosology should lead researchers to explore potential differential underlying factors explaining the superficial symptom-severity differences and the inflection point at which they shift that might allow for the identification of a causal differentiation between the domain of intuitive dysfunction versus normal variation along the NVP symptom dimension, with the variables uncovered justifying the disorder attribution. The scientific attempt to isolate the etiology of the symptoms and specifically to identify a dysfunction—the abnormality that causes the harm—is exactly what recent research has begun to accomplish:

> A new study has identified two genes associated with hyperemesis gravidarum, whose cause has not been determined in previous studies. The genes, known as GDF15 and IGFBP7, are both involved in the development of the placenta and play important roles in early pregnancy and appetite regulation.... For this study, the team compared the variation in DNA from pregnant women with no nausea and vomiting to those with hyperemesis gravidarum to see what the differences were between the two groups. DNA variation around the genes GDF15 and IGFBP7 was associated with hyperemesis gravidarum. The findings were then confirmed in an independent study of women with hyperemesis gravidarum. In a separate follow-up study, researchers then proved the proteins GDF15 and IGFBP7 are abnormally high in women with hyperemesis gravidarum. (University of California–Los Angeles Health Sciences 2018)

In fact, as the authors' comments indicate, the study's results suggest more than just a correlation between the identified genetic mutations and disorder:

> The association between this gene and HG is of particular importance because it highlights the possibility of a pathway involved in the etiology of the condition. GDF15...increases significantly in the first two trimesters. GDF15 is believed to suppress production of proinflammatory cytokines in order to facilitate placentation and maintain pregnancy. In addition to its role in pregnancy, GDF15 has been shown to be a regulator of physiological body weight and appetite via activation of neurons in the hypothalamus and area postrema (vomiting center) of the brainstem. It is also notable that abnormal overproduction of GDF15 in cancer was recently found to be the key driver of cancer anorexia and cachexia which, like HG, exhibits symptoms

of chronic nausea and weight loss. Of particular clinical interest, inhibition of GDF15 restored appetite and weight gain in a mouse model of cancer cachexia, suggesting a therapeutic strategy that may be applicable to patients with HG, if GDF15 proves to be the implicated gene. (Fejzo et al. 2018, 6)

But, how do we know that "abnormally high" (presumably in the statistical sense) proteins generated by specific variations at certain genetic loci reveal dysfunctions rather than normal variations? Here a web of circumstantial evidence generated by further studies to establish causality, in particular by Fejzo et al. (2019), is helpful. In particular, there is no evidence of a continuous distribution of effects. The critical findings for present purposes were, first, that "the serum concentrations of GDF15 and IGFBP7 were significantly increased … in women hospitalized for HG compared to women with NVP" and, in the case of GDF15, also compared to women with no NVP, the levels in the women with HG subsided to baseline when the HG itself subsided late in the pregnancy, but—most strikingly—"there was no difference in serum GDF15 or IGFBP7 levels in patients with NVP compared to NO NVP" (Fejzo et al. 2019, 385). These findings suggest that the variations in genetic loci are not continuously distributed (which in any event is misleading because genes are discrete by nature) in parallel to levels of NVP from none through severe NVP and HG, but rather that HG is caused by distinctive pathogenic variants of GDF15 that interact with the changes during pregnancy to cause HG—in other words, a likely dysfunction. Furthermore, the two loci are "both known to be involved in placentation, appetite, and cachexia" (cachexia is the distinctive loss of appetite and wasting of the body that occurs in some forms of cancer and some other chronic diseases), providing an additional pathological mechanism for generating part of the NVP-like symptom dimension, in addition to mechanisms naturally selected to generate NVP. The link to cachexia as a disorder of appetite is revealing; these are structures that normally regulate body weight and appetite but are known to be capable of going horribly wrong under some circumstances. These studies in which specific variants at genetic loci create abnormally high levels of a protein tied to pathological appetitive changes verify the initial suspicion that the difference between HG and NVP is not merely a quantitative difference in symptom severity but also a qualitative difference in type of underlying causation, with the implicit assumption that it is a dysfunction.

Contrary to De Block and Sholl's suggestion that these differences are not formulated in terms of implications for biological design and fitness in the EEA, these days, the implicit intuition about biological design is translated by researchers into explicit evolutionary talk. As noted, given HG's extreme symptoms and their effects, and extrapolating into earlier time periods, there is a strong prima facie presumption that the impact of this condition on fitness in the EEA was substantial and negative, and this always leads to the puzzle of why the risk factors were preserved. HG researchers have made this puzzle explicit and portrayed the condition as an evolutionary anomaly beyond any plausible biologically designed limits, so that something has gone wrong with the way pregnancy is biologically designed to occur: "The cause of hyperemesis gravidarum is currently unknown and the rationale for maintenance of genes that predispose to dehydration and malnutrition in pregnancy remains an evolutionary enigma. One would think that a condition that commonly resulted in maternal and fetal death before the introduction of intra venous fluids in the 1950s would have been strongly selected against in nature" (National Organization for Rare Disorders 2015). As etiological research yields some understanding, researchers attempt to address that initial puzzle: "Finally, the findings herein suggest an answer to an age-old paradox. HG can lead to prolonged dehydration and undernutrition, which can be detrimental to maternal and fetal health and can decrease reproductive fitness. The dual roles of GDF15 and IGFBP7 in maintaining pregnancy and in increasing the risk of HG may provide a molecular explanation for why NVP still exists in nature" (Fezjo et al. 2018, 6). Thus, De Block and Sholl's crucial premise that all points along the NVP-HG dimension are considered to have equal fitness fails, and their argument dissolves.

In sum, there is no need to rely entirely on the nausea-and-vomiting harm dimension alone to explain why HG has been considered a disorder and NVP has been considered within normal range. A dimension of harm may run continuously atop multiple deeper etiological mechanisms, so the continuity need not reflect a single continuous causal or etiological process. Based on additional qualitative features, two different parts of a continuous dimension can be understood to result from naturally selected mechanisms and from dysfunctions, respectively. The thinking of leading HG researchers and clinicians confirms that this is how the NVP/HG distinction is understood. Thus, De Block and Sholl's claim that it is simply the degree of harm on the symptom-severity dimension alone that determines their disorder judgments is disconfirmed. The HDA's claim that judgments distinguishing NVP normality from HG disorder presuppose inferences regarding biological design and dysfunction that are not reducible to sheer degree of harm along the NVP dimension is confirmed. De Block and Sholl's crucial premise—that those (including myself) who accept the division of the NVP dimension into normal suffering and disorder implicitly also accept that there is no difference between the two in their biological design status—is falsified. Despite sharing a symptom dimension, NVP is presumed to be naturally selected, whereas HG is presumed to be due to an inferred underlying dysfunction. Research investigations following out the HDA conceptual path are revealing valuable new truths about these conditions.

The Example of Premenstrual Dysphoric Disorder

The analysis above shows how the distinction between NVP as normal variation and HG as disorder depends on more than just a dimensional assessment of harm. It relies as well on an intuition about, and ultimately research into, underlying dysfunction. To illustrate that the analysis can also shed light on how disorder is distinguished from nondisorder in dimensional psychological conditions, I very briefly and schematically present the example of premenstrual dysphoric disorder (PMDD), a condition that was previously listed in *DSM-IV*'s Appendix B of "Criteria sets … provided for further study" but was moved into the main part of the manual as a stand-alone criterial disorder category in *DSM-5*'s depressive disorders chapter.

A panel of experts appointed by the *DSM-5* Mood Disorders Work Group concluded that there was sufficient empirical evidence to support such a move (Epperson, 2013; Epperson et al., 2012). PMDD is defined as the extreme along the dimension of symptom severity of common premenstrual syndrome (PMS) psychological symptoms that most women experience to some degree. According to statistical views of disorder, simply being the extreme of the dimension should have been sufficient to allow consensus classification of PMDD as a disorder, but that was not the case. Although the condition's level of impairment and distress had convinced the FDA to approve PMDD as an indication for antidepressant medication, worries were expressed about the dimensionality issue (Food and Drug Administration 1999). The problem was that many feminist and psychiatric critics believed that PMDD was just an extreme level of a normal-range female issue and were concerned that its invalid pathologization might lead to broader pathologization of women working its way down the severity dimension (Vargas-Cooper 2012). The skepticism that there was any dysfunction involved in PMDD was supported by the negative results of studies examining whether women with PMDD had abnormal levels of menstruation-related hormones, a favored theory of the nature of the dysfunction.

So, what convinced the *DSM-5* panel to recommend a change of PMDD to full disorder status? It was not evidence of greater symptom severity or being at the extreme of the dimension, which was already established by definition. Rather, it was emerging evidence that bore on the question of whether the greater severity of PMDD symptoms likely involves a distinctive dysfunction. Two points in particular stand out. First, the surprising discovery of the rapid efficacy of selective serotonin reuptake inhibitors when taken only during PMDD symptomatic periods, which is unlike the usual delayed and gradual impact of such drugs on other depressive disorders, suggested a distinctive condition responsive to medication. Second, and most impressively, was the pronounced symptomatic response in hormonal add-back studies only in those with a PMDD history and not for others with PMS, thus offering evidence of a latent categorical distinction between PMDD and PMS. Given that differences in hormone levels had not been found between those women with PMS versus PMDD, researchers turned to the question of whether there might be a different reaction to similar hormonal levels. In these studies, women with and without PMDD histories were administered agonists that rid the bloodstream of relevant circulating hormones such as progesterone, and then from these no-hormone base levels the hormone is gradually added back into the bloodstream, simulating the normally changing amount of hormone during the menstrual cycle. These studies (e.g., Baller et al., 2013; Schmidt et al., 1998) demonstrated a marked difference in the type of behavioral and brain reactivity to hormone fluctuation in women with PMDD versus controls, revealing what appears to be a qualitative difference hidden within the severity dimension.

This finding of different reactions to hormone fluctuations helped resolve the *DSM-5* debate, but it did not end the search for a more definitive identification of a presumptive dysfunction cut-point that could define the PMDD category. As in the HG example, later research went further and examined whether the greater reactivity to hormone variation by women with PMDD versus controls is mediated by specific genetic mutations (Dubey et al., 2017), with follow-up replicative genetic studies in nonhuman models of PMDD (e.g., Marrocco et al. 2020). This research revealed both overexpression of some genes and underexpression of others in women with PMDD versus controls, with divergent genetic responses in PMDD and control subjects (Physician's Briefing, 2017). Despite the uncertainties of this research program, the point is that the aspiration is clearly to verify that there is some underlying dysfunction that explains the intuition that PMDD is a disorder whereas milder PMS conditions are not. The issue with regard to establishing the disorder status of PMDD is not just its relative severity along a harm dimension, which is apparent, but whether the processes generating those heightened levels of severity consist of identifiable dysfunctions.

Harm Is Not the Only Dimension in Judging Disorder

Our consideration of De Block and Sholl's "dimensionality" argument reinforces the HDA's basic point that judgments of disorder depend on two dimensions, not one. It is true that if, like De Block and Sholl, one focuses on symptoms as harms, then it is tempting to arrange disorders along a symptom severity scale. In fact, the *DSM-5* Task Force planned to do this with all major disorders as part of their diagnostic criteria and actually formulated such scales. One of the task force chairs suggested that empirical research might eventually refine where along the severity dimension was the optimal cut-point for drawing the nondisorder versus disorder distinction (Greenberg 2011). The whole approach was eventually abandoned as without adequate empirical warrant for the scales. (Also, a pragmatic consideration intervened; once such severity measures were part of diagnosis, insurance companies might not wait for psychiatric research and might establish their own cut-points for insurance coverage, as they had with requiring certain levels of disability for admission to inpatient treatment.)

From the HDA perspective, the idea made no sense. Symptom severity is one dimension, and dysfunction is another, and neither by itself determines disorder. Thus, there is not necessarily a cut-point anywhere on the symptom severity dimension that is the proper cut-point between disorder and nondisorder. The dysfunction judgment always goes beyond sheer harm per se to consider the kind of harm in the light of what seem plausible hypotheses about biological design.

References

Al-Ozairi, E., J. J. S. Waugh, and R. Taylor. 2009. Termination is not the treatment of choice for severe hyperemesis gravidarum: Successful management using prednisolone. *Obstetric Medicine* 2: 34–37.

Baller, E. B., S.-M. Wei, P. D. Kohn, D. R. Rubinow, G. Alarcón, P. J. Schmidt, and K. F. Berman. 2013. Abnormalities of dorsolateral prefrontal function in women with premenstrual dysphoric disorder: A multimodal neuroimaging study. *American Journal of Psychiatry* 170: 305–314.

Ben-Joseph, E. P. 2014. Severe morning sickness (hyperemesis gravidarum). *Kidshealth: For Parents*. https://kidshealth.org/en/parents/hyperemesis-gravidarum.html.

Boelig, R. C., S. J. Barton, G. Saccone, A. J. Kelly, S. J. Edwards, and V. Berghella. 2018. Interventions for treating hyperemesis gravidarum: A Cochrane systematic review and meta-analysis. *Journal of Maternal-Fetal & Neonatal Medicine* 31(18): 2492–2505.

Dean, C. R., K. Bannigan, and J. Marsden. 2018. Reviewing the effect of hyperemesis gravidarum on women's lives and mental health. *British Journal of Midwifery* 26(2): 109–119.

De Block, A. 2008. Why mental disorders are just mental dysfunctions (and nothing more): Some Darwinian arguments. *Studies in History and Philosophy of Biological and Biomedical Sciences* 39: 338–346.

Drife, J. O. 2012. Saving Charlotte Brontë. *British Medical Journal* 344(7841): 51.

Dubey, N., J. F. Hoffman, K. Schuebel, Q. Yuan, P. E. Martinez, L. K. Nieman, et al. 2017. The ESC/E(Z) complex, an effector of response to ovarian steroids, manifests an intrinsic difference in cells from women with premenstrual dysphoric disorder. *Molecular Psychiatry* 22(8): 1172–1184.

Dulay, A. T. 2017. Hyperemesis gravidarum. *Merck Manual*. https://www.merckmanuals.com /professional/gynecology-and-obstetrics/abnormalities-of-pregnancy/hyperemesis-gravidarum.

Epperson, C. N. 2013. Premenstrual dysphoric disorder and the brain. *American Journal of Psychiatry* 170: 248–252.

Epperson, C. N., M. Steiner, S. A. Hartlage, E. Eriksson, P. J. Schmidt, I. Jones, et al. 2012. Premenstrual dysphoric disorder: Evidence for a new category for *DSM-5*. *American Journal of Psychiatry* 169: 465–475.

Fayed, L. 2018. Neoplasm types and factors that cause them. *VeryWell Health,* December 15. https://www.verywellhealth.com/what-is-a-neoplasm-513708.

Fejzo, M. S., P. A. Fasching, M. O. Schneider, J. Schwitulla, M. W. Beckmann, E. Schwenke, K. W. MacGibbon, and P. M. Mullin. 2019. Analysis of GDF15 and IGFBP7 in hyperemesis gravidarum support causality. *Geburtshilfe und Frauenheilkunde* 79(4): 382–388.

Fejzo, M. S., K. MacGibbon, and P. M. Mullin. 2016. Why are women still dying from nausea and vomiting of pregnancy. *Gynecology & Obstetrics Case Report* 2(2): 1–4.

Fejzo, M. S., O. V. Sazonova, J. F. Sathirapongasuti, I. B. Hallgrímsdóttir, 23andMe Research Team, V. Vacic, et al. 2018. Placenta and appetite genes GDF15 and IGFBP7 associated with hyperemesis gravidarum. *Nature Communications* 9: 1–9.

First, M. B., and J. C. Wakefield. 2010. Defining 'mental disorder' in *DSM-V*. *Psychological Medicine* 40(11): 1779–1782.

First, M. B., and J. C. Wakefield. 2013. Diagnostic criteria as dysfunction indicators: Bridging the chasm between the definition of mental disorder and diagnostic criteria for specific disorders. *Canadian Journal of Psychiatry* 58(12): 663–669.

Flam, L. 2014. What is hyperemesis gravidarum? The rare pregnancy complication making Duchess Kate sick. *Today,* September 8. https://www.today.com/parents/hyperemesis-gravidarum-why -its-worst-royal-or-not-1D80133997.

Food and Drug Administration. 1999. Minutes of the meeting of the Psychopharmacologic Drugs Advisory Committee of the Food and Drug Administration Center for Drug Evaluation and Research, Hearing on NDA 18–936(S), Prozac (fluoxetine hydrochloride), Ely Lilly and Company, indicated for the treatment of premenstrual dysphoric disorder. FDA.

Holmgren, C., D. Olsen, and L. Sittig. 2018. Management of nausea and vomiting of pregnancy (NVP) and hyperemesis gravidarum. *Intermountain Healthcare: Care Process Model.* intermountain-physician.org/clinicalprograms.

Jørgensen, A. B., R. Frikke-Schmidt, B. G. Nordenstgaard, and A. Tybjærg-Hansen. 2014. Loss-of-function mutations in *APOC3* and risk of ischemic vascular disease. *New England Journal of Medicine* 371(1): 32–41.

Lilienfeld, S. O., and L. Marino. 1995. Mental disorder as a Roschian concept: A critique of Wakefield's "harmful dysfunction" analysis. *Journal of Abnormal Psychology* 104: 411–420.

Lilienfeld, S. O., and L. Marino. 1999. Essentialism revisited: Evolutionary theory and the concept of mental disorder. *Journal of Abnormal Psychology* 108: 400–411.

London, V., S. Grube, D. M. Sherer, and O. Abulafia. 2017. Hyperemesis gravidarum: A review of recent literature. *Pharmacology* 100(3–4): 161–171.

Marrocco, J., N. R. Einhorn, G. H. Petty, H. Li, N. Dubey, J. Hoffman, et al. 2020. Epigenetic intersection of BDNF Val66Met genotype with premenstrual dysphoric disorder transcriptome in cross-species model of estradiol add-back. *Molecular Psychiatry* 25(3): 572–583.

McParlin, C., A. O'Donnell, S. C. Robson, F. Beyer, E. Moloney, A. Bryant, et al. 2016. Treatments for hyperemesis gravidarum and nausea and vomiting in pregnancy: A systematic review. *Journal of the American Medical Association* 316(13): 1392–1401.

National Institute of Mental Health. 2017. Sex hormone-sensitive gene complex linked to premenstrual mood disorder [Press release]. https://www.nimh.nih.gov/news/science-news/2017/sex -hormone-sensitive-gene-complex-linked-to-premenstrual-mood-disorder.shtml.

National Organization for Rare Disorders. 2015. Hyperemesis gravidarum. *Rare Disease Database.* https://rarediseases.org/rare-diseases/hyperemesis-gravidarum/.

Nietzsche, F. 1888/2005. *Twilight of the Idols.* In *The Anti-Christ, Ecce Homo, Twilight of the Idols and Other Writings,* A. Ridley and J. Norman (eds.) and J. Norman (trans.), 155–229. Cambridge University Press.

Norata, G. D., S. Tsimikas, A. Pirillo, and A. L. Catapano. 2015. Apolipoprotein C-II: From pathophysiology to pharmacology. *Trends in Pharmacological Sciences* 36(10): 675–689.

Physician's Briefing. 2017. Sex hormone-sensitive gene complex implicated in PMDD. https://www.physiciansbriefing.com/obgyn-women-s-health-11/genetics-news-334/sex-hormone-sensitive-gene-complex-implicated-in-pmdd-718359.html.

Plomin, R. 2003. Genes and behavior: Cognitive abilities and disabilities in normal populations. In *Disorders of Brain and Mind,* M. Ron and T. Robbins (eds.), 3–29. Vol. 2. Cambridge University Press.

Plomin, R. 2018. *Blueprint: How DNA Makes us Who We Are.* MIT Press.

Pregnancy Sickness Support. 2019. What is hyperemesis gravidarum? https://www.pregnancysicknesssupport.org.uk/what-is-hyperemesis-gravidarum/.

Schmidt, P. J., L. K. Nieman, M. A. Danaceau, L. F. Adams, and D. R. Rubinow. 1998. Differential behavioral effects of gonadal steroids in women with and in those without premenstrual syndrome. *New England Journal of Medicine* 338: 209–216.

Spitzer, R. L. 1997. Brief comments from a psychiatric nosologist weary from his own attempts to define mental disorder: Why Ossorio's definition muddles and Wakefield's "harmful dysfunction" illuminates the issues. *Clinical Psychology: Science and Practice* 4(3): 259–261.

Spitzer, R. L. 1999. Harmful dysfunction and the *DSM* definition of mental disorder. *Journal of Abnormal Psychology* 108(3): 430–432.

TG and HDL Working Group. 2014. Loss-of-function mutations in *APOC3,* triglycerides, and coronary disease. *New England Journal of Medicine* 37(1): 22–31.

UK National Health Service. 2016. Your pregnancy and baby guide: Severe vomiting in pregnancy. https://www.nhs.uk/conditions/pregnancy-and-baby/severe-vomiting-in-pregnancy-hyperemesis-gravidarum/.

University of California–Los Angeles Health Sciences. 2018. Two genes likely play key role in extreme nausea and vomiting during pregnancy. *Science Daily,* March 21. https://www.sciencedaily.com/releases/2018/03/180321090849.htm.

Vargas-Cooper, N. 2012. The billion dollar battle over premenstrual disorder. *Salon.* https://www.salon.com/2012/02/26/the_billion_dollar_battle_over_premenstrual_disorder/.

Wakefield, J. C. 1992a. The concept of mental disorder: On the boundary between biological facts and social values. *American Psychologist* 47: 373–388.

Wakefield, J. C. 1992b. Disorder as harmful dysfunction: A conceptual critique of *DSM-III-R*'s definition of mental disorder. *Psychological Review* 99: 232–247.

Wakefield, J. C. 1993. Limits of operationalization: A critique of Spitzer and Endicott's (1978) proposed operational criteria of mental disorder. *Journal of Abnormal Psychology* 102: 160–172.

Wakefield, J. C. 1995. Dysfunction as a value-free concept: A reply to Sadler and Agich. *Philosophy, Psychiatry, and Psychology* 2: 233–46.

Wakefield, J. C. 1997a. Diagnosing *DSM-IV*, part 1: *DSM-IV* and the concept of mental disorder. *Behaviour Research and Therapy* 35: 633–650.

Wakefield, J. C. 1997b. Diagnosing *DSM-IV*, part 2: Eysenck (1986) and the essentialist fallacy. *Behaviour Research and Therapy*: 35: 651–666.

Wakefield, J. C. 1997c. Normal inability versus pathological disability: Why Ossorio's (1985) definition of mental disorder is not sufficient. *Clinical Psychology: Science and Practice* 4: 249–258.

Wakefield, J. C. 1997d. When is development disordered? Developmental psychopathology and the harmful dysfunction analysis of mental disorder. *Development and Psychopathology* 9: 269–290.

Wakefield, J. C. 1998. The *DSM*'s theory-neutral nosology is scientifically progressive: Response to Follette and Houts. *Journal of Consulting and Clinical Psychology* 66: 846–852.

Wakefield, J. C. 1999a. Evolutionary versus prototype analyses of the concept of disorder. *Journal of Abnormal Psychology* 108: 374–399.

Wakefield, J. C. 1999b. Mental disorder as a black-box essentialist concept. *Journal of Abnormal Psychology* 108: 465–472.

Wakefield, J. C. 2000a. Aristotle as sociobiologist: The "function of a human being" argument, black box essentialism, and the concept of mental disorder. *Philosophy, Psychiatry, and Psychology* 7: 17–44.

Wakefield, J. C. 2000b. Spandrels, vestigial organs, and such: Reply to Murphy and Woolfolk's "The harmful dysfunction analysis of mental disorder." *Philosophy, Psychiatry, and Psychology* 7: 253–269.

Wakefield, J. C. 2001. Evolutionary history versus current causal role in the definition of disorder: Reply to McNally. *Behaviour Research and Therapy* 39: 347–366.

Wakefield, J. C. 2006. What makes a mental disorder mental? *Philosophy, Psychiatry, and Psychology* 13: 123–131.

Wakefield, J. C. 2007. The concept of mental disorder: Diagnostic implications of the harmful dysfunction analysis. *World Psychiatry* 6: 149–156.

Wakefield, J. C. 2009. Mental disorder and moral responsibility: Disorders of personhood as harmful dysfunctions, with special reference to alcoholism. *Philosophy, Psychiatry, and Psychology* 16: 91–99.

Wakefield, J. C. 2011. Darwin, functional explanation, and the philosophy of psychiatry. In *Maladapting Minds: Philosophy, Psychiatry, and Evolutionary Theory,* P. R. Andriaens and A. De Block (eds.), 143–172. Oxford University Press.

Wakefield, J. C. 2012. Are you as smart as a 4th grader? Why the prototype-similarity approach to diagnosis is a step backward for a scientific psychiatry. *World Psychiatry* 11(1): 27–28.

Wakefield, J. C. 2014. The biostatistical theory versus the harmful dysfunction analysis, part 1: Is part-dysfunction a sufficient condition for medical disorder? *Journal of Medicine and Philosophy* 39: 648–682.

Wakefield, J. C. 2016a. The concepts of biological function and dysfunction: Toward a conceptual foundation for evolutionary psychopathology. In *Handbook of Evolutionary Psychology,* D. Buss (ed.), 2nd ed., vol. 2, 988–1006. Oxford University Press.

Wakefield, J. C. 2016b. Diagnostic issues and controversies in *DSM-5*: Return of the false positives problem. *Annual Review of Clinical Psychology* 12: 105–132.

Wakefield, J. C., and M. B. First. 2003. Clarifying the distinction between disorder and nondisorder: Confronting the overdiagnosis ("false positives") problem in *DSM-V*. In *Advancing DSM: Dilemmas in Psychiatric Diagnosis,* K. A. Phillips, M. B. First, and H. A. Pincus (eds.), 23–56. American Psychiatric Press.

Wakefield, J. C., and M. B. First. 2012. Placing symptoms in context: The role of contextual criteria in reducing false positives in *DSM* diagnosis. *Comprehensive Psychiatry* 53: 130–139.

WebMD Medical Reference. 2019. Common pregnancy pains and their causes. *WebMD*. https://www.webmd.com/baby/guide/pregnancy-discomforts-causes#1.

Wood, H., L. V. McKellar, and M. Lightbody. 2013. Nausea and vomiting in pregnancy: Blooming or bloomin' awful? A review of the literature. *Women and Birth* 26(2): 100–104.

Zachar, P., and K. S. Kendler. 2014. A *Diagnostic and Statistical Manual of Mental Disorders* history of premenstrual dysphoric disorder. *Journal of Nervous and Mental Disease* 202(4): 346–352.

Zhang, S. 2018. Your body acquires trillions of new mutations every day: And its somehow fine? *The Atlantic,* May 7. https://www.theatlantic.com/science/archive/2018/05/your-body-acquires-trillions-of-new-mutations-every-day/559472/.

27 On Harm

Rachel Cooper

Jerome Wakefield holds that disorders are harmful dysfunctions. Although the harmful element is an essential component of his account, Wakefield has said comparatively little about it and has concentrated on fleshing out the dysfunction part of his account. One of the key aims of Wakefield's project has been to use his account of disorder to weed out "false positives." In such applications, Wakefield has tended to use the dysfunction part of his account to do the work. Thus, he has argued that normal misery and much misbehavior by young people are not disorders because there are no dysfunctions (Horwitz and Wakefield 2007; Wakefield et al. 2002).

This chapter takes as its starting point that Wakefield is correct in thinking that disorders must be harmful and examines what it means to say a condition is harmful. In his best-known work, Wakefield argues that disorders are harmful dysfunctions where "harmful is a value-term based on social norms" (1992a, 373). I will argue that an account of harm as whatever is disvalued by a society should be rejected. This is because whole societies can be wrong in how they evaluate a condition. Determining the correct account of harm is very difficult, but I argue that on all plausible accounts, it will be possible to argue that a condition should not be considered a disorder because it is not harmful. Thus, when properly understood, the harm component of Wakefield's account can also be used to provide a barrier against medicalization. I finish by considering how the idea that disorders are necessarily harmful has a crucial role to play in ensuring that classifications of disorders, such as the influential *Diagnostic and Statistical Manual of Mental Disorders* (*DSM*), do not medicalize normal oddities.

I. Wakefield's Struggle with an Account of Harm

In his 1992 paper "The Concept of Mental Disorder: On the Boundary between Biological Facts and Social Values," Wakefield sees the claim that disorders are harmful to be an essential part of his account. The criterion that disorders must cause harm allows Wakefield to say that certain conditions that may well be evolutionarily dysfunctional, but that cause no harm, do not count as disorders. In his paper, Wakefield offers fused toes and slow aging as possible examples (1992a, 384). More influentially, although it is a case little discussed by Wakefield himself, the harm element of Wakefield's account also enables the claim that homosexuality is not a disorder; it may be an evolutionary dysfunction, but insofar as it is not harmful, it is not a disorder.

Wakefield (1992a) tells us that "harmful is a value-term based on social norms" (373), a disorder is a dysfunction that "impinges on the person's well-being as determined by social values and meanings" (373), and harmful is "a value term referring to the consequences that occur to the person because of the dysfunction and are deemed negative by sociocultural standards" (374). Wakefield doesn't tell us much about why he thinks that whether a condition is harmful should be determined by social norms. One gets the impression that to him, it seems obvious that this is the only way in which harm might be defined. In the course of this chapter, I will show that there are actually numerous possible accounts of harm (or the flipside of the good life). Figuring out what harms an individual, or what comes to the same thing—what the good life is for an individual—is very difficult. This is not an issue that I will be able to resolve here. On one point I am sure, however, and that is that saying that harm is determined by one's society will not do.

The problem with holding that any condition that a society values is valuable is that this claim has profoundly counterintuitive consequences. There are cases where it is extremely plausible that a cultural group can be mistaken about what is valuable. Take the case of "pro-ana" groups, which are groups that promote the idea that anorexia is a good thing. Pro-ana groups are generally web based. On their sites, you can access chat rooms in which people swap diet tips, compare body statistics, and support each other during fasts. There are also galleries of "thinspiration" images, which are photos of very thin people looking beautiful. The members of pro-ana groups celebrate an aesthetics of extreme thinness, they admire the control that is required to limit food intake, and they delight in the euphoric experiences that can be produced by fasting.

On Wakefield's account, it looks like one is forced to say that as a cultural group values anorexia, there is no harm in being anorexic. Maybe Wakefield would avoid this by claiming that anorexics merely form a subculture rather than a full-blown culture— perhaps on the basis that those who celebrate anorexia are few and far between and meet virtually rather than in person. However, this response is not robust to slightly different circumstances. Suppose that the members of pro-ana groups get fed up with members of the dominant culture interfering in their chosen lifestyle. They purchase a small island and set up their own community. Anorexia becomes fashionable, and the numbers of the island swell. At some point, the pro-ana group will form a culture that is just as surely a culture as any other. Nevertheless, and even though the pro-ana community thinks that anorexia is a good thing, I suggest that the group is wrong. Anorexia is not a good because people with anorexia become obsessed with food-related issues (and having a life that revolves around this is an impoverished life) and risk death. Whatever their beliefs, anorexia remains a disorder because it remains harmful.

In a 2013 commentary, Wakefield shows sensitivity to this sort of case and starts to move away from the view that initial social judgments alone determine harm. Infamously, slaves who had a tendency to run away were at one time considered by some to be disordered. In earlier work, Wakefield had used the dysfunction component of his account to argue that the view that these slaves had a disorder was a mistake; they were not disordered because they did not have a dysfunction (2002, 150). Now, Wakefield considers the possibility that runaway behavior might in fact have been caused by some minor brain dysfunction that rendered certain individuals less able to adapt to oppressive environments (thus satisfying the "dysfunction" criterion). Given that the slave-owning society disvalued runaway behavior, on his original account, Wakefield would be forced to claim that the slaves were in fact disordered. The example now prompts Wakefield to concede that "to this extent, my (1992) claim that harm is judged by social values was overly simplistic" (2013, 1). He suggests, "The HD 'harm' component, being normative, reflects deliberation about broader normative commitments, not just immediate social reactions" (2013, 2). This idea goes in the right direction, but Wakefield does not expand on it. One of the main aims of section III is to consider in greater detail how we might reflect on our initial gut reactions regarding harmfulness and improve upon them. First, however, we need to consider further accounts of harm. Given that it is highly plausible that whole cultures can be mistaken in their assessment of harm, and insofar as Wakefield's initial account of harm struggles to allow for this possibility, we must look for a different account of harm.

II. Starting Again—How to Assess Harm?

Wakefield has struggled to provide an acceptable account of harm, but in this, he has the comfort of good company. The depth of the difficulty can be seen once it is appreciated that the flipside of deciding whether a condition causes harm is deciding what sorts of conditions are good for an individual. Figuring out what makes up the "good life" is, of course, one of the most long-standing and contentious of philosophical questions. Although various accounts of the good for an individual have been proposed, all are problematic (for an in-depth overview, see Griffin 1986). In this chapter, I will not be able to determine the correct account of the good life. My aims are more modest. I will briefly review a range of options and show the problems that they face. I will then move on to show how, even though we lack an acceptable account of the good life, some progress may yet be made in considering whether particular specific conditions are harmful.

The problems that emerge in seeking to develop an account of the good life can best be understood via thinking of the possible ways of determining what is good for an individual as varying along a scale. At one end of the scale, one might rely on asking actual people what they want (the "subjective," or "desire," approach). At the other end of the scale, one might appeal to ideal standards of human flourishing (the "objective," or "Aristotelian," approach). Between these extremes lie methods that claim that something is good for an individual if that individual would judge it to be good in ideal circumstances, for example, if he or she were calmer, wiser, and better informed than in reality.

Wakefield's suggestion that harm might be judged on the basis of the judgments of the social group is an account that relies on the judgments of actual people. I have suggested that Wakefield's account runs into difficulties because actual communities can be mistaken in their assessments of harm. This is a basic problem that afflicts all those accounts of the good life that rely of the judgments of actual people (whether individually or in groups). The key difficulty is that people often do not know what is in their own best interest or in the best interest of others. People make mistakes for a multitude of reasons. It is an unfortunate fact that humans are quite commonly ignorant, self-deceived, short-sighted, biased, deluded, and foolish.

The fact that actual humans make mistakes makes accounts of the good life that rely on more abstract notions of the good seem attractive. Various neo-Aristotelian accounts have recently become popular. On some accounts, the character of the human good life can be thought of as being analogous to the good life for a species of plant or animal (e.g., Hursthouse 1999). For example, it is a natural fact about gerbils that they are social burrowing creatures who are thus happiest living in company and with something they can dig. Similarly, cheetahs are naturally such that they like to roam long distances and are solitary. The neo-Aristotelian may suggest that humans are creatures that are naturally such that they need friends and intellectual stimulation. Regardless of what any individual claims, such things are good for humans. Such views take on a certain amount of plausibility when one bears in mind that it is commonplace for individuals to come to take pleasure in certain activities even when they initially had to be coerced into them. It seems empirically plausible, for example, that exercise improves mood even in those who claim to enjoy being couch potatoes, because humans are animals that benefit from exercise.

The difficulty with neo-Aristotelian accounts is that it is unclear exactly what grounds the notion that certain ways of living are good for certain types of creatures. The risk is that the neo-Aristotelian either comes to lean too much on biology or else ends up making claims that are ultimately ungrounded. Relying on biology becomes problematic because it is highly implausible that the good human life is identical with that which is evolutionarily most successful. Evolutionary success is dependent on acting to ensure that one's genes spread, but plausibly, the good life cannot be reduced to this (consider that Genghis Khan is postulated to be an exceptional evolutionary success but surely doesn't represent a role model [Zerjal et al. 2003]). Turn away from biology, however, and it becomes unclear what there is that might ground the claim that certain ways of living are good for humans quite apart from what anyone thinks. Appeals to "ideal standards of human flourishing" seem disturbingly abstract. It is not clear how the ideal standards are fixed, nor is it clear how we can find out about them.

Middling positions that appeal to the idealized judgments of humans also face problems. If there is only a bit of idealization, then mistakes can still be made. Suppose, for example, that we say that it is only the well-considered judgments of actual communities that should be considered in judging harm. The problem is that history shows that quite frequently, whole communities have reflected long and hard and have still reached the wrong conclusions. Consider, for example, all those traditional patriarchal societies that have had their best (male) minds thinking about the role of women for decades or even centuries; even after much thought, many still maintain that women are less worthy of respect than men. Oftentimes, actual deliberative processes misfire. Sometimes the fault lies with the individuals involved. For example, those who are very clever may still be self-deceived. Sometimes the deliberative forum lacks the sorts of social and cultural support required to move debate forward (e.g., a forum may be too deferential to authority or exclude those who could challenge prevailing beliefs). If we rely on idealization in our account of harm, we will need quite a bit of idealization if we are to rule out the possibility of mistakes being made. The problem is that the more idealization we have, the less grounded our account becomes. If I say, for example, that harm is to be judged by fully informed, unbiased, clever, and virtuous humans in a forum that involves all appropriate participants and is organized to promote progressive discussion, then I'm moving very far from the actual debates of actual humans. How I am to judge what such ideal agents would decide?

Here I will not resolve the problem of how to determine the nature of the good life or of harm. Luckily, we will be able to make some progress when it comes to evaluating the harmfulness of particular conditions even in the absence of an overarching account. Whatever account of the good we adopt, it is clear that rather than relying on gut reactions to determine whether a condition is harmful, we should require at least some reflection. This on its own will be enough to give the idea that disorders are harmful some critical bite. In the next section, I will show how we can use the claim that disorders are harmful to determine whether certain conditions should be considered disorders.

III. Making Progress

Suppose we accept that disorders must cause harm and set out to consider whether some particular condition causes harm. How should we proceed? I have argued that no fully satisfactory account of the good life exists. Luckily, however, seeking to establish whether some particular condition is harmful is often much easier than seeking to produce some abstract account of harm in general. I will discuss three methods for thinking about harm. These methods are intended to be illustrative rather than comprehensive. Together, they show how the idea that disorders are harmful can do critical work. The legitimacy of each method should be uncontroversial, and yet each can be used to argue that particular conditions should not be medicalized.

3.1 Method 1: Think!

When it comes to judging specific conditions, quite often simply posing the question, "Does this condition cause any harm?" is sufficient to unearth conditions that have wrongly been classified as disorders. Wakefield (2002) discusses the example of childhood disorder of atypical stereotyped movement disorder, which was included in *DSM-III* (the third edition of one of the main classifications of mental disorders). Many children with severe developmental disorders engage in repetitive movements—rocking, repetitive hand movements, head banging, and so on. Some otherwise normal children also engage in such actions, for example, rocking before they go to sleep. The movements are voluntary and are often experienced as comforting. Under the *DSM-III*, all children engaging in these sorts of repetitive movements could be diagnosed. Wakefield thinks it likely that such repetitive movements may well be associated with some sort of brain dysfunction (even in the children who are otherwise normal). Yet, he points out that given that the movements themselves generally cause no harm (except in cases where, for example, a child head bangs walls), there is no good reason to consider the child to have a disorder. In this example, simply asking whether there is any harm in a child rocking can be sufficient to rule out the fallacious diagnoses.

Medical thought has on occasion displayed a tendency to elide the distinctions between a state being unusual, it being a dysfunction, and it being a disorder. Amundson (2000) discusses the ways in which medics have all too often viewed infants born with unusual genitals, extra fingers, or webbed toes to be disordered simply in virtue of their difference. Against such a climate of thought, merely stopping to question whether a condition causes any harm can in itself act as a buffer against unnecessary medicalization.

3.2 Method 2: Breaking Down Claimed Costs and Benefits

There are numerous conditions where we may be unsure whether they should count as disorders because we are unsure whether they are harmful. Consider Asperger's syndrome, asexuality, Deafness, and hearing voices. In such complex cases, I suggest we can adopt the following strategy: we should go through potential alleged benefits and disadvantages of having the condition one by one and see if they survive scrutiny.

In detail, we start by asking those who think a condition is a good thing why they think it is a good thing, and those who think it is a bad thing why it is a bad thing. We can expect the responses to involve a mixture of factual and value-based claims. For example, someone with bipolar disorder may claim that an advantage of the condition is that during manic phases, they create great art. This claim is partly amenable to empirical investigation—do they paint more during manic phases? Are those paintings they produce then judged among their best? Partly, the claims depend on basic intuitions about values that may not be amenable to empirical evidence. Is it a good thing to produce art? And if so, how does this good rank against others? Is the production of great art worth producing even if its production involves creating distress in the artist, for example? In considering what sorts of things are good, we should start by making use of our commonplace intuitions. These intuitions are a starting point that in some cases will themselves be subject to critical revision. In seeking to evaluate claims that some condition is good, my suggestion is that we should break down the justification as much as we can and see whether the justification survives rational scrutiny.

In my 2007 paper "Can It Be a Good Thing to Be Deaf?" I employ this method in thinking through whether it can be a good thing to be Deaf. While being Deaf is not a mental disorder, the case serves to demonstrate the methodology and is useful because it has been subject to much discussion. The issue around Deafness is that some Deaf people claim that Deafness is not pathological but is rather a way of living.[1] This is because they think it is a good thing to be Deaf. Primarily, they have in mind people who have been Deaf from birth and use sign language, rather than those who have become deaf in later life. In considering whether it is true that it can be good to be Deaf, we need first to compile a list of the differences between Deaf and hearing people. Most notably, hearing and Deaf people differ in the sensations that they experience and in the languages that they typically employ. Once we have a list of the differences, we need to consider the benefits and costs that can be expected to flow from each difference. Thus, we should consider, for example, whether sign language is as good as spoken language. Those who argue for the benefits of sign languages make many claims that can be subjected to empirical test. For example, it is claimed that sign languages are often better able to convey information about the spatial location of objects. Whether this is true can be tested. Whether a difference should be considered a benefit or cost can be subjected to commonplace intuitions. In judging a language, for example, all things being equal, a language that can convey complex information easily is better than one that cannot. Or, consider the fact that Deaf people have different sensations than hearing people. Sensations provide us with pleasure and are a source of information. Deaf people miss out on sound sensations, but they may develop some enhancement in other sensations (e.g., better peripheral vision, being more attentive of vibrations). Again, the extent to which Deaf people do have different sensations can be tested. Once all the differences between Deaf and hearing people have been considered, a final summing of costs and benefits can be attempted. In the case of Deafness, I argue that the final summing is uncertain. Many factors are context dependent (using sign language is only practical where others sign) or depend on personal taste (some people get more pleasure listening to music than others). Thus, whether it is good to be Deaf will probably vary between different Deaf people.

It should not be considered a problem that the application of my method yields an unclear conclusion. Knowing that it is unclear whether it can be good to be Deaf is itself useful. Uncertainty in itself has policy implications. In this case, it means that any justifications for interfering in cases where parents choose to bring up their child as either Deaf or as hearing are weak. There is, for example, thin justification for removing a Deaf child who is happy in a Deaf community and whose parents refuse cochlear implants.

Our commonplace intuitions about goods and harms can enable judgments as to whether some condition is harmful. But it's also the case that the experiences of those with various types of medical condition can help inform our notion of the good life. For example, we may start by assuming that it is bad not to be able to talk. We have a tacit assumption that all languages are verbal. Then we learn about sign languages. We revise our initial assumption. Rather than saying that it is bad not to be able to talk, we say it is bad not to be able to communicate. The experiences of those who are physically and psychologically different can also inform us of goods that we might otherwise overlook. Consider the unease produced by feelings of derealization. These may prompt us to consider "feeling at home in the world" to be an important good, although if we had never come across accounts of derealization, this good would never have become salient to us.

3.3 Method 3: Considerations of Consistency

In some cases, considerations of consistency can prompt us to revise our initial judgments as to whether a condition can be considered harmful. Let us compare two cases:

First let us consider someone who has no interest in sex. Asexuality has at times been considered a disorder, but many asexual people do not consider themselves to have a problem. The Asexuality Visibility and Education Network (AVEN) provides web forums for people who identify as asexual. The forum asserts, "We here at AVEN get along just fine without sex" (http://www.asexuality.org/home/), and many of those posting on the forum seem pretty content. Many asexual people do not consider it a disadvantage not to desire sex. They may not have a sexual relationship but have more time for friends, and they claim that nonsexual adult relationships can be as rewarding as sexual ones. Suppose the claim that it is perfectly okay to be asexual strikes me as reasonable.

Now consider a different case, someone whose sexual desires exclusively revolve around solitary activities with shoes. The interests of those with shoe fetishes can vary in ways that can significantly affect their likelihood of living a good life (see, e.g., the case studies in Krafft-Ebing 1965). Some fetishes involve partners (the shoes need to be worn by someone); some just involve shoes. Some forms of shoe fetishism involve masochistic interests (being walked on, licking dirty shoes, etc.); some do not. In this case, I want to consider someone whose sexual interests revolve around masturbating with shoes that are bought from shops (as opposed to, for example, stolen).

Now suppose that having listened to the advocates of asexuality, I find it plausible that not having a sexual adult relationship is no loss. Fair enough, I think, the asexual person will have no adult sexual relationship, but this will be made up for by them having increased opportunities for forming friendships instead. But, then suppose that I listen to the shoe fetishist. He explains that he has an advantage in that his sexual desires are easily satisfied. Given that buying shoes is much easier than wooing women, he finds that he has more time to spend on other activities and on nonsexual friendships than do many of his conventionally heterosexual peers. He does not feel the lack of a sexual adult relationship. Suppose that in this case I find myself less convinced. As a good liberal, I assert that I make no judgment about how people get their kicks. So long as no nonconsenting partners are involved, I claim to judge all sexual pleasures equal. I claim that it's not that I find the shoe fetishist's pleasures ridiculous or disgusting but that I worry that in missing out on an adult sexual relationship, he misses out on something important.

Now, when I consider my responses to these two cases together, I notice that there is a tension. I must be consistent in my thinking as to whether an adult sexual relationship is an essential component of a good human life or not. If it's fine for an asexual person to have friendships instead, then this should also be the case for the shoe fetishist. Considerations of consistency can thus force the revision of initial judgments.

Through considering these cases, I have shown how we may make progress in deciding whether specific conditions cause harm and should be considered disorders or not. This enables the claim that disorders are necessarily harmful to have critical bite—that is, it will be possible to use it to argue that in certain cases, we have made a mistake. In some cases, we can use the claim that disorders are necessarily harmful to show that some condition that we currently consider a disorder should not be considered a disorder. What's more, we don't need to wait to establish a correct account of harm for such projects to get under way.

IV. Loose Ends

I have shown how we might use the idea that disorders are harmful in critical projects. In this final section, I address some loose ends.

4.1 Individualization

As the examples we have considered show, many conditions are such that they cause harm to some people but not others. Different people have different interests, abilities, and needs and live in different environments. Thus, the impact of Deafness varies from person to person. Using sign is easier for someone who lives among signers; some people like listening to music more than others. The same condition can have very different effects on different people. Consider Tourette's; some tics are rude (breast touching, racist shouts) or hurt (hitting), and others are subtle (standing on one's toes).

   That harm will vary from individual to individual presents us with a choice. We might say that a condition that is generally harmful within a particular society should be considered a disorder in the case of everyone who has that condition, even if a particular individual is not harmed. Thus, as schizophrenia is generally harmful, it will count as a disorder even in those individuals who only hear encouraging voices. Alternatively, we can say that whether a condition is a disorder will vary from person to person. Thus, schizophrenia is a disorder in those people that it harms and a mere difference in those individuals who it does not harm. In his writings, Wakefield seems to suggest that he adopts the first society-wide option (although he discusses harm so little that this is somewhat unclear). When Wakefield discusses how the harm criterion means that the same conditions can be a disorder in some contexts but not others, he considers dyslexia, which causes harm in literate societies but not in societies that do not use writing (2002, 151). If Wakefield's view is that a condition counts as a disorder for everyone in a particular society if it harms most people in a society, this is a mistake. It is better to claim that a disorder must be harmful for the particular individual who has it. This is for two reasons: the first ties in with the justification for having a criterion that disorders must cause harm at all. Wakefield (1992b) considers why we should require that disorders be harmful. He argues that attributions of disorder involve a value component because disorder is in certain respects a practical concept that is supposed to pick out only conditions that are undesirable and grounds for social concern, and there is no purely scientific nonevaluative account that captures such notions (Wakefield 1992b, 237). Such considerations suggest that we should consider whether a condition causes harm and will thus count as a disorder at the individual level, as only those individuals who are harmed are in need of help.

   Second, judging whether a condition harms a particular individual is far easier than seeking to work out whether a condition causes harm for most people within a society who have it. Figuring out what counts as a "society" is tricky. In multicultural countries, "societies" are hard to delimit. Even once one has decided on the relevant grouping of people, figuring out whether most of them are harmed by a condition or not would require complex surveys. Asking whether a particular individual is harmed by their condition is easier because the individual can be easily identified and their context can be known.

   On the downside, some worry that saying that the same condition should be considered a disorder for some individuals but not others will cause problems for certain types of research. Epidemiologists would prefer to be able to count cases of a particular disorder without having to worry about the life situations, hopes, and interests of each individual. The way to get around this worry is to slightly reconceptualize the work of medical researchers and epidemiologists. Rather than characterizing this research as investigating disorders per se, we can think of it as investigating those conditions that are of interest because they often cause harm and are therefore often disorders. This allows researchers to employ criteria that pick out subject populations without regard to whether or not the particular individuals experience harm.

4.2 Harm to Whom?

Must a disorder cause harm to the individual who has it, or is harm to others sometimes sufficient? Examples of conditions that might be thought disorders because of the harm they cause to other people are the personality disorders and paraphilias (sexual perversions). Generally, Wakefield says that the harm must be to the patient, but on occasion, he wavers (e.g., 2002, 148), and this is a matter on which we need to be clear.

I suggest that we should claim that disorders must be bad for the patient. This stance is linked to the solution to another problem; how can we distinguish between disorders and normal criminal or antisocial behavior that harms others? The difficulty is that not all of those who harm others suffer from disorders. Everyone sometimes does things that are naughty, cruel, or selfish, and some people do bad things quite often. We need to be able to say what distinguishes disordered people from those who are simply criminal or antisocial.

The most plausible distinction is that normal badness is voluntary, while behavior that is symptomatic of a disorder is not under normal voluntary control. The distinction is not completely clear-cut, but the extremes of voluntary and involuntary behavior are clearly distinct. The normal criminal may get into fights for fun and manipulate others for cash. He may plan his misdeeds and boast of them afterward. He moderates his actions in a rational way; he picks fights only with those who are weaker and only when there is no CCTV. The criminal's actions are planned, motivated, and controlled; they are fully voluntary.

Consider in contrast this description of behavior performed during dissociative flashbacks associated with posttraumatic stress disorder. This is described as "unpremeditated and sudden and uncharacteristic of the individual. ... Furthermore, there does not appear to be an alternate motive. Most individuals experience amnesia for the episode and are unaware of the specific ways they have repeated or re-enacted war experiences" (Frierson 2013, 83).

Plausibly, the difference between behavior that is indicative of normal bad behavior and disorder is that the former is voluntary, while the latter is in some way involuntary. Plausibly, it is also the case that not having normal control over one's behavior is a bad thing. If so, all those behaviors that harm others and that are also indicative of disorder will simultaneously be bad for the patient.

To illustrate how the idea that disorders must harm the patient and not just others might be applied in practice, let's consider pedophilia. Pedophiles may all be sexually attracted to children but differ in their behavior. Some find their desires repugnant and struggle against them; they may avoid the company of children and never act on their desires. In this sort of case, the pedophile is harmed by his condition; he finds himself with desires that cause him distress. Other pedophiles do not control themselves; they groom and abuse boys and girls. Possibly some abusive pedophiles would prefer not to abuse children but have unusually strong desires that they cannot resist. Given that it is bad not to be able to control oneself, such individuals are again harmed by their condition. But what of the individual who finds himself sexually attracted to children and acts on these desires without compunction? Does pedophilia harm this individual, or does it just harm others? This is a tricky question and depends on the account of good that one adopts. Some of those who adopt Aristotelian accounts will claim that the pedophile is harmed by his condition even if he claims to be quite happy. They can claim that the good human life is one that involves sexual relations only with other consenting adults. From this standpoint, the pedophile fails to flourish regardless of his claims. Some other accounts of the good life do not permit such a line to be taken. On desire-satisfaction accounts, the active pedophile who does not struggle against his desires is doing just fine. He has desires, and these desires are met. From such a standpoint, this pedophile harms others but is not himself harmed. If, as I suggest, one claims that behavior characteristic of disorders must be involuntary and that disorders have to harm the patient, then one is forced to say that the active and unrepentant pedophile should be considered bad rather than disordered. I think this is an acceptable line to take.

Of course, many of the disorders treated by psychiatrists are puzzling precisely because the behaviors associated with them seem to fall somewhere between those that are under normal voluntary control and those that are completely involuntary. In such cases, I suggest that it is simply unclear whether the condition should be considered a disorder or a moral failing.

4.3   Harm in Practice: The *DSM-5*

The importance of the idea that disorders are necessarily harmful is brought out if we consider the consequences for medical classification. The *DSM* is a classification of mental disorders that is published by the American Psychiatric Association and used by those many of those researching and treating mental disorders around the world. The *DSM* has long conceived of harm as being an essential element of disorder. This viewpoint came to be widely adopted in psychiatry following debates about the status of homosexuality in the late 1960s and 1970s. A consensus developed that although homosexuality might turn out to be some sort of evolutionary dysfunction insofar as it is not harmful, it should not be considered a disorder. The definition of disorder included in editions of the *DSM* in use from 1987 to 2013 states that

> each of the mental disorders is conceptualized as a clinically significant behavioral or psychological syndrome or pattern that occurs in a person and that is associated with present distress (a painful symptom) or disability (impairment in one or more important areas of functioning) or with significantly increased risk of suffering death, pain, disability, or an important loss of freedom. (American Psychiatric Association 1987, xxii; 1994, xxi)

However, in the latest edition, the *DSM-5*, published in May 2013, the role of harm has been downgraded. The new definition states only that

> mental disorders are *usually* associated with significant distress or disability in social, occupational, or other important activities. (American Psychiatric Association 2013, 20, emphasis added)

The *DSM-5* is a product of much work by many committees. The new *DSM-5* definition was a compromise between advocates of the view that disorders must necessarily be harmful and advocates of a quite different tradition, which considers "disorder" to be a value-free term. Among the committees involved in revising the *DSM*, the Impairment and Disability Assessment Study Group drafted a completely value-free definition of disorder that sought to bring the *DSM* into line with the view implicit in the *International Classification of Diseases* (*ICD*), published by the World Health Organization (WHO).[2] In the *ICD* system, disorder and disability are thought of as being quite distinct, and the WHO publishes a distinct classification, *The International Classification of Functioning, Disability and Health*, which supplies codes for disability. The thinking here will already be familiar to those who have had some exposure to disability studies, where the social model of disability conceptualizes impairment and disability separately; impairment refers to the biological difference (e.g., having no legs), and disability refers to problems in everyday living that are conceived of as arising from the social response to the impairment (e.g., a lack of ramps for wheelchairs). In the eyes of the Impairment and Disability Assessment Study Group, someone who, say, hears voices but is not bothered by them and has a good life should be said to have schizophrenia (supposing that criteria for duration, etc. are met) but not to be impaired or to necessarily need treatment. The value-free definition of disorder proposed by the Impairment and Disability Assessment Study Group was not adopted, but the downgrading of the role of harm in the *DSM* definition of disorder (from definitional to merely characteristic) is a legacy of the actions of this group.

So far, in practice, the altered *DSM* definition of disorder will have had little impact on the actual contents of the classification. The definition was developed far too late in the revisionary process to have influenced decisions about the contents the classification. Looking to the future, however, the change to the definition included in the *DSM* should be a real concern for those who think that disorders are necessarily harmful. Currently, it remains the case that many of the individual sets of diagnostic criteria included in the *DSM* include a requirement that the particular disorder can only be diagnosed if it produces harm. The exact wording varies but generally requires that "the disturbance causes clinically significant distress or impairment in social, occupational, or important areas of functioning" (American Psychiatric Association 2013, 21). The *DSM-IV* had many similar criteria, and these have generally been maintained in the *DSM-5*. The difference is that, with the change in the definition of mental disorder, there is no longer a robust rationale for the inclusion of the harm-related criterion in the individual sets of diagnostic criteria. Previously, this criterion was included as a reminder to clinicians that the diagnosis should only be made if harm was caused because the definition of disorder required harm (i.e., the rationale was conceptual). With the change in the definition, there is nothing to guard against some future edition of the *DSM* deciding to ditch the idea that disorders have to cause harm altogether. The change to the definition of disorder included in the *DSM* means that the notion that disorders necessarily cause harm is under threat. This should be cause for concern because the criterion that requires that disorders cause harm is crucial to prevent some of those who are merely different from being diagnosed. In many cases, unwarranted medicalization can only be prevented by appealing to the harm part of the harmful dysfunction account.

Notes

1. In these debates, "Deaf" with a capital "D" is used to refer to people who culturally identify as Deaf people (they tend to have been Deaf from birth and sign), while "deaf" with a little "d" refers to all those who cannot hear.

2. This definition and the rationale for its development were available on an American Psychiatric Association website while the *DSM-5* was being developed but has been removed since its publication.

References

American Psychiatric Association. 1987. *Diagnostic and Statistical Manual of Mental Disorders*. 3rd ed. revised. American Psychiatric Association.

American Psychiatric Association. 1994. *Diagnostic and Statistical Manual of Mental Disorders*. 4th ed. American Psychiatric Association.

American Psychiatric Association. 2013. *Diagnostic and Statistical Manual of Mental Disorders*. 5th ed. American Psychiatric Association.

Amundson, R. 2000. Against normal function. *Studies in History and Philosophy of Biological and Biomedical Sciences* 31(1): 33–53.

Cooper, R. 2007. Can it be a good thing to be deaf? *Journal of Medicine and Philosophy* 32: 563–583.

Frierson, R. 2013. Combat-related posttraumatic stress disorder and criminal responsibility determinations in the post-Iraq era: A review and case report. *Journal of the American Academy of Psychiatry and the Law* 41(1): 79–84.

Griffin, J. 1986. *Well-Being*. Clarendon.

Horwitz, A., and J. C. Wakefield. 2007. *The Loss of Sadness: How Psychiatry Transformed Normal Sorrow into Depressive Disorder*. Oxford University Press.

Hursthouse, R. 1999. *On Virtue Ethics*. Oxford University Press.

Krafft-Ebing, R. 1965. *Psychopathia Sexualis*. Trans. from the twelfth German edition by Franklin Klaf. Stein and Day.

Wakefield, J. C. 1992a. The concept of mental disorder: On the boundary between biological facts and social values. *American Psychologist* 47(3): 373–388.

Wakefield, J. C. 1992b. Disorder as harmful dysfunction: A conceptual critique of *DSM-III-R*'s definition of mental disorder. *Psychological Review* 99(2): 232–247.

Wakefield, J. C. 2002. Values and the validity of diagnostic criteria: Disvalued versus disordered conditions of childhood and adolescence. In *Descriptions and Prescriptions: Values, Mental Disorders, and the D.S.M.s*, J. Sadler (ed.), 148–164. John Hopkins University Press.

Wakefield, J. C. 2013. Addiction, the concept of disorder, and pathways to harm: Comment on Levy. *Frontiers in Psychiatry* 4: 34.

Wakefield, J. C., K. Pottick, and S. Kirk. 2002. Should the D.S.M.-IV diagnostic criteria for conduct disorder consider social context? *American Journal of Psychiatry* 159(3): 380–386.

Zerjal, T., Y. Xue, G. Bertorelle, R. S. Wells, W. Bao, S. Zhu, R. Qamar, Q. Ayub, A. Mohyuddin, S. Fu, P. Li, N. Yuldasheva, R. Ruzibakiev, J. Xu, Q. Shu, R. Du, H. Yang, M. E. Hurles, E. Robinson, T. Gerelsaikhan, B. Dashnyam, S. Qasim Mehdi, and C. Tyler-Smith. 2003. The genetic legacy of the Mongols. *American Journal of Human Genetics* 72(3): 717–721.

28 Must Social Values Play a Role in the Harm Component of the Harmful Dysfunction Analysis? Reply to Rachel Cooper

Jerome Wakefield

Rachel Cooper is one of our field's most productive and insightful thinkers, and I have learned much from her. I thank Cooper for her critique of the "social" aspect of the harm component of my harmful dysfunction analysis (HDA) of medical, including mental, disorder. The HDA claims that "disorder" refers to "harmful dysfunction," where dysfunction is the failure of some feature to perform a natural function for which it is biologically designed by evolutionary processes and harm is judged in accordance with social values (First and Wakefield 2010, 2013; Spitzer 1997, 1999; Wakefield 1992a, 1992b, 1993, 1995, 1997a, 1997b, 1997c, 1997d, 1998, 1999a, 1999b, 2000a, 2000b, 2001, 2006, 2007, 2009, 2011, 2014, 2016a, 2016b; Wakefield and First 2003, 2012).

Cooper accepts the HDA's claim that harm is a necessary requirement for disorder ("Wakefield is correct in thinking that disorders must be harmful") and undertakes to examine "what it means to say a condition is harmful," particularly objecting to my claim that harm must be understood in terms of social values. Cooper hopes to deploy a culturally transcendent harm criterion to prevent misdiagnosis ("when properly understood, the harm component of Wakefield's account can also be used to provide a barrier against medicalization"). Her critique is part of a recent surge of interest in the nature of the HDA's harm component (e.g., Feit 2017; Limbaugh 2019; Muckler and Taylor 2020; Powell and Scarffe 2019), and I thank her for pushing that discussion further. In the course of considering harm, she also proposes an analysis of "disorder" based on the involuntariness of action, which I address.

Cooper's chapter focuses on the HDA's harm component, but elsewhere Cooper (2007b) critiques the HDA's dysfunction component and disputes the HDA's claim that disorder requires evolutionary dysfunction. That critique is cited by other critics in this volume, including Leen De Vreese, who cites Cooper's discussion as a justification for considering the HDA to be refuted. Consequently, in a supplementary reply, I respond to Cooper's objections to the HDA's evolutionary perspective on dysfunction.

As Cooper observes, with a few recent exceptions (Wakefield 2013; Wakefield and Conrad 2019; Wakefield and First 2013), I have written relatively little about the HDA's harm component other than to defend the necessity of a harm criterion against pure naturalist accounts (Wakefield 2014). One reason for this emphasis is that the HDA is intended partly as a response to antipsychiatric claims that mental disorder judgments are nothing but social value judgments, so I have focused on explaining how disorder judgments go beyond social value judgments via the dysfunction criterion, yielding some degree of scientific objectivity and locating them within a legitimate medical domain that is partly factually anchored. Cooper observes as well that my focus on dysfunction was motivated by my specific interest in false-positive diagnosis, which was the problem at the heart of the antipsychiatric critique, because the most egregious false-positive abuses of psychiatric diagnosis have generally been due to failures to observe the dysfunction requirement. Moreover, the analysis of function and dysfunction has broader implications for philosophy of biology, philosophy of science, philosophy of mind, and the human sciences.

A further and more negative reason for focusing more on dysfunction than harm is that it seemed to me that something useful and relatively incisive can be said about dysfunction, whereas this is less clear for the harm component. Serious exploration of the harm component quickly leads one to confront profound disputes in value theory that are notoriously intractable and unlikely to be advanced by evidence of intuitions about disorder versus nondisorder. Indeed, one might wonder if harm is so contestable that it is best left imprecise within the HDA for the time being. We shall see that Cooper's contribution strongly underscores these doubts about attempting to be precise about harm.

Mea Culpa!

Before addressing the specifics of the harm criterion, I start with some general reorienting comments about the nature and limits of my "social values" qualifier to the harm criterion. I stoked controversy from several quarters by stating that harm is evaluated relative to social values. Some psychiatrists saw the reference to social values as introducing an unwanted element of cultural relativity into disorder diagnosis. Some philosophers saw it as a threat to a larger naturalist program. Other philosophers were concerned that I was embracing a naive cultural relativism that conflicts with the aspirations of some metaethicists to establish the transcultural objectivity of value judgments.

It has become obvious that I was not sufficiently clear or careful regarding the "social values" aspect when I formulated the HDA, and as Cooper notes, I (Wakefield 2013) recently attempted to clarify my intentions and present a broadened vision of harm in the context of social values. It apparently seemed to many readers that I was saying that actual social attitudes, opinions, and judgments at a given time are final arbiters of harm for medical purposes. That's absurd, of course. What is thought to be harmful may not really be harmful upon reflection when one takes into account a culture's overall moral vision, its changing circumstances, and basic human aspirations that infuse all social value systems. Social values in the sense I intended are not initial superficial subjective reactions but value claims that have been subjected to a dialectic that goes deeper than immediate reactions or consensus to explore which of a culture's many often-conflicting value commitments are its most basic values, which serve long-run interests of justice, which might be reactions that rationalize power relations, and so on. I thus agree with Cooper's three methods for challenging initial value judgments (see below) and more; social values include what can emerge from such a process.

When I claimed that social values provide an essential filter for judgments of medical harm, I did not mean to assert absurdities such as that "whatever is disvalued by a society should be rejected" or that "any condition that a society values is valuable"—views that Cooper targets for criticism as my views. The reference to social values was intended not as a relativist metaethical statement or an absolute constraint—harm is harm, and if it can be shown that there is diagnostically relevant harm that transcends social value systems, then I accept that that can qualify as HDA harm—but rather as a qualifier to explain features of actual medical diagnostic practice, detailed below.

I want to emphasize that the social values guideline went beyond strict conceptual analysis of the general concept of disorder and should be understood analogously to the HDA's commitment to the selected effects reading of dysfunction (see Lemoine and my response in this volume) as a theoretical codicil to the conceptual analysis. Bluntly put, disorder is harmful dysfunction, period, however harm can be established. Nonhuman nonsocial organisms, for instance, can have disorders because they can have harmful dysfunctions without reference to social values. However, my discussions focus on the human case, and in my view, the best available understanding of "harm" in the human case is through the prism of social values, for reasons provided below. Humans are social animals whose values and judgments of harm—and actual harms—are to a large extent mediated by, and vary with, social context. Of course, there are harm judgments that are virtually universal, but such universal values are expressed as well through cultural value systems, even if only latently, and so are encompassed within a broad social values perspective. But, the social values addendum is not strictly part of the concept of disorder, and an alternative theory of human harm would be possible.

Cooper is particularly concerned that my "social" approach anchors judgments of medical harm in the judgments of fallible "actual people"—think here of an earlier homogeneously homophobic America—who can err about what is harmful: "Wakefield's suggestion that harm might be judged on the basis of the judgments of the social group is an account that relies on the judgments of actual people. I have suggested that Wakefield's account runs into difficulties because actual communities can be mistaken in their assessments of harm.…The key difficulty is that people often do not know what is in their own best interest or in the best interest of others."

There are two ways to respond to this concern and "correct" what are seen as a culture's potential moral errors. One is to seek a realm of culture-transcendent moral values that override cultural values; this appears to be Cooper's solution, but it raises challenging epistemological and metaethical questions that are, as we shall see, quite difficult to answer. The other is to seek redress in the potential for moral change that exists within the resources and complexities of any actual human culture's value system; Cooper inadvertently seems to take this route as well, in her proposed methods for correction of faulty harm judgments (see below). Until the viability of the transcendent route is proven, the value-system approach seems to me to make the most practical sense. The process of self-interrogation of a culture's values in the domain of medically relevant harm is well illustrated by the remarkable reading of our culture's deeper values by Robert Spitzer and the consequent revolution in attitudes toward gay marriage and homosexual civil rights partly triggered by depathologization. No simple reduction of a social value system to a poll of the people in a society can explain such dynamic phenomena, nor can it best be explained by appeal to a transcendent value universe, for all the value issues Spitzer raised lie squarely within the complexities of our society's social value system.

Consistent with such an approach, a close examination of what I said in my papers reveals that my references to social values are not people's opinions or feelings or the "judgments of actual people" but are consistently to a more abstract level of "social norms" and "sociocultural standards" that allows for conflict and dialectic. As Cooper documents, in my original HDA publication, I indicated that harm is "based on social norms" (1992a, 373), "determined by social values and meanings" (373), and "deemed negative by sociocultural standards" (374). Fifteen years later, in a presentation of the HDA to a psychiatric audience, I (Wakefield 2007) said that harm "is judged negative by sociocultural standards" (149) and is judged "according to social values" (150). These references are not to the reactions of specific actual people but to more abstract entities that are complex and have various conflicting currents and levels that dynamically interact and evolve. Although supervenient on an ongoing meaning system of a culturally coherent collective of individuals, a system of values has structures and potentials that do not necessarily map on to any superficial reading of what people think or feel at a given time. As to my openness to any form of harm that can be defended, I stated that harm "is construed broadly here to include all negative conditions" (2007, 151).

The concept of disorder evolved in a world in which cultural values in relatively homogeneous societies may have seemed like ultimate objective values; indeed, societies sometimes support their value systems by erroneously seeing local values as objective universal truths, just as they support their values by elevating values into features of human nature and deviance into dysfunction and disorder. Such objectification of cultural values can lead to the devaluation of alternative ways of life and the oppressive deployment of medical power in the name of some supposed universal (e.g., see Powell and Scarffe 2019). Cooper is focused on addressing this danger in her attempt to go beyond cultural values and postulate an objective way of evaluating a condition's harmfulness in making a diagnosis. However, her solution is open to the same danger of reification of local values into transcendent truths as is the problem it is meant to solve.

There is nothing sacred about the precise way I formulated the harm criterion. I am open to rethinking and amending it if an alternative approach can be cogently elaborated and defended so that it is not an arbitrary imposition that is simply an expression of Western triumphalism (for discussion of some of the inevitable dangers of such an attempt, see Wakefield and Conrad 2019). I argue below that Cooper fails to provide any such rationale. For now, I tend to see such hypothesized transcendent value considerations as latent or implicit strands in virtually every human community's social value system rather than something standing outside of and in addition to social values.

Why Social Values?

All that said, why, then, did I feel it useful to specify that diagnostic harm reflects social values? One tactical motive was to prevent the possible misunderstanding that the harm is also, like dysfunction, related to evolutionary theory and represents a lowering of fitness. The evolutionary view of harm has been expressed in the literature and is easily confused with the HDA, and I disputed it in my original HDA paper (Wakefield 1992a). Without clarity on this point, the disorder status of conditions that cause sheerly socially anchored harms, such as dyslexia (reading disorder), is more difficult to address. Dyslexia has been a much-discussed controversial example deployed by critics of the HDA from the outset because its harm seems distant from evolutionary considerations and it does not involve alteration in fitness so far as we know, and the "social values" addendum makes clear how dyslexia can be harmful in the relevant way.

However, the primary motivation for the social values addendum was a theoretical-explanatory consideration. Whether a condition is a disorder is not determined by how the diagnosed individual subjectively happens to feel about the condition's effects but by more "objective" standards determined by the culture's value system. Thus, for example, infertility at prime childbearing age is a disorder even if a patient has decided not to have children because ability to reproduce is generally considered a valuable capability in our society and deprivation of this ability is considered a prima facie harm irrespective of benefits that might accrue. Harm is also not determined by the idiosyncratic values of the physician. Medicine in our time is a socially sanctioned activity that carries with it the obligation to alleviate harm as it is understood by the society at large. Of course, in medicine, as in all professions, there are occasional conflictual situations in which supererogatory moral commitments override such standard understandings.

The "social values" qualifier also captures the inevitable degree of social relativity present in disorder status. If a failure of function has no impact on anything valued by a specific culture, it is not a disorder for that culture but merely a harmless dysfunction or anomaly. The HDA allows for an appropriate degree of such cultural relativity. The HDA of course severely limits value-based cultural relativism of disorder because of the factual dysfunction requirement that is in principle independent of social values. The factual dysfunction requirement prevents disorder from being manufactured from the whole cloth of cultural values. But, equally, the social values anchoring of harm prevents disorder from being manufactured from dysfunction within a culture in which the dysfunction is not harmful.

For example, assume that the theory is true that dyslexia is caused by a minor malfunction of the corpus collosum linking the two brain hemispheres, such that the dysfunction limits the rate of information transfer from one hemisphere to the other, and it is then difficult to learn to read due to the unique and extraordinary cross-brain-hemispheric information integration demanded by our reading, but the dysfunction has no other negative effects. Because in our culture, reading is a highly valued practice, this dysfunction is harmful and thus a medical disorder. However, the same dysfunction in a preliterate society that existed 1,000 years before reading was invented, or in a postliterate society 1,000 years from now in which reading is obsolete, would not be considered a medical disorder but rather a harmless anomaly. Variations in values from society to society also enter into harm judgments when there may be agreement on broader values but disagreement on the details of how those values are realized. It seems to me that some degree of such cultural relativity of disorder cannot be avoided.

Social context must enter into the medical evaluation of harm because it is possible for different cultures to have different fundamental values that yield differences in what is harmful, and yet both societies are morally acceptable. Consequently, what is harmful dysfunction in one society can be a harmless anomaly in another society. To take a well-known example, there are fundamental differences between cultures in the attitude toward the balance between personal striving and individual autonomy, on one hand, and group cohesiveness and subservience to group well-being, on the other. In a society focused on individual self-realization, a dysfunction that caused pronounced behavior fitting the group-above-self society's ideal of subservience to the group might be considered a disorder, but the same dysfunction would not be considered a disorder—and might actually be considered a desirable advantage—in the other society. To consider a more mundane example, there are many harmless "commensal" viruses that infect human beings with no harm, and they are not considered disorders. There is also a virus that causes a modest weight gain due to disruption of appetitive mechanisms and no other negative effects. In our society, we are very weight conscious in our aesthetics, and this virus would be considered a disorder. However, in other societies in which an ample figure is the ideal, this virus would not be considered a disorder but commensal.

Moreover, there are many universal human features that have culturally variable parameter settings so that the actual instantiations of these values differ across cultures.

What foods are acceptable to eat, what sexual activities are acceptable at what age and with whom, what emotions at what intensity and duration are acceptable and are proportional reactions to events (e.g., how much sadness or grief is appropriate and for how long given each kind of loss), and so on all vary enormously. This is not necessarily a matter of one society having better values than another and is comparable to different societies having different languages that instantiate the universal human capacity for language, so that whether an utterance is a grammatical sentence depends on the culture within which it is uttered. The social embedding of harm is indicated by the *Diagnostic and Statistical Manual of Mental Disorders*'s (*DSM*'s) emphasis on role impairment as a basic form of harm. Role impairment is a form of *pro tanto* harm across cultures, but cultures differ in their social roles and role expectations and thus will differ in whether specific inabilities represent role impairment. An inability to deal with certain bureaucratic social demands of a developed economy may be irrelevant in a simpler society in which individuals can go alone on long hunting trips for much of the year. Conversely, a dysfunction that causes an inability to engage in a simpler society's most important activities of hunting and gathering may be irrelevant in a developed society in which there are myriad occupations with varying required abilities from which to choose.

Anorexia Island

As we saw, Cooper's basic objection is that my "social values" approach to harm anchors harm in the judgments of fallible "actual people" who can err about what is harmful. Cooper at times appears to look to some other source of value that lies beyond the entire social value system, given that "people often do not know what is in their own best interest or in the best interest of others." If we interpret her in this way, then what we would need to make sense of Cooper's position is some account of the nature and epistemological accessibility of the culture-transcendent values that determine medically relevant harm within a culture. However, such a rationale is not on offer. Cooper oddly combines an unwavering confidence that the HDA is incorrect in specifying that harm is understood in terms of social values with a professed lack of any systematic rationale for judging harm in any other way, other than by her own intuitions. Cooper repeatedly asserts that she has no such account that would justify or explain the validity of her intuitions and suggests that no such account is in reach: "Figuring out what harms an individual, or what comes to the same thing—what the good life is for an individual—is very difficult. This is not an issue that I will be able to resolve here"; "Although various accounts of the good for an individual have been proposed, all are problematic"; "In this chapter, I will not be able to determine the correct account of the good life"; "Here I will not resolve the problem of how to determine the nature of the good life or of harm"; "I have argued that no fully satisfactory account of the good life exists." Having no theory of value transcendence, she still insists, "On one point

I am sure, however, and that is that saying that harm is determined by one's society will not do."

Nevertheless, Cooper is confident that the social values construal of harm is wrong, and she thinks that she has a knock-down counterargument: "There are cases where it is extremely plausible that a cultural group can be mistaken about what is valuable." That is, entire societies can be wrong about what is harmful, so social values cannot be the baseline for judging harm. In support of the claim that entire societies can be wrong about what is harmful, Cooper provides the following thought experiment in which a society adopts an anorexic-like aesthetic:

> There are cases where it is extremely plausible that a cultural group can be mistaken about what is valuable. Take the case of "pro-ana" groups, which are groups that promote the idea that anorexia is a good thing. Pro-ana groups are generally web based....Suppose that the members of pro-ana groups get fed up with members of the dominant culture interfering in their chosen lifestyle. They purchase a small island and set up their own community. Anorexia becomes fashionable, and the numbers of the island swell. At some point, the pro-ana group will form a culture that is just as surely a culture as any other.

I am not sure I agree that a special-purpose isolated group set up for people who already share a minority aesthetic that emerged in a larger culture is therefore a culture. But leave that issue aside. This seems on its face to be an example about harm and culture, not about medical judgment. The individuals on this imagined island think anorexic-level thinness is a desirable aesthetic ideal, but that does make them anorexic in the psychiatric sense because their behavior does not result from a dysfunction. It becomes relevant to the HDA if we imagine either that they are all suffering from dysfunctions and are truly anorexic and embrace their condition (much like, say, the hearing impaired have created a community that embraces their lack of hearing), or that in such an anorexia-positive society, an individual develops a dysfunction that causes anorexia. Let's proceed with the latter scenario, in which there is a dysfunctional individual whose dysfunction's effects match the culture's anorexic ideal. The question is: first, does this individual have a disorder and, second, do they have a disorder according to the HDA? Cooper's point is that such an individual would not be harmed as judged by cultural standards, and thus would not be judged to have a disorder by the HDA, when in fact the individual is harmed and does have a disorder.

I think the anorexic individual in the anorexic society would still have a disorder according to the HDA. To see why, we might first ask, how does Cooper know that the anorexic ideal that is highly valued in this culture is harmful in the case of the dysfunctional individual despite being valued? She explains, "Anorexia is not a good because people with anorexia become obsessed with food-related issues (and having a life that resolves around this is an impoverished life) and risk death. Whatever their beliefs, anorexia remains a disorder because it remains harmful."

Cooper's supposedly culture-transcendent judgment that there is harm is perfectly accessible to members of the anorexic society, but Cooper seems to run together the anorexic ideal with the described harms of being anorexic so as to suggest that the afflicted individuals don't judge there to be harm. However, like just about all other human beings, pro-ana individuals presumably understand that death is a bad thing and should be avoided if possible. They may, like mountain climbers and military officers, realize that their chosen ideal life entails a greater risk of physical weakness or death than they might otherwise have but accept the management of that risk as part of the pursuit of their ideal. They also understand that it is bad to lead an impoverished life, although whether they consider a life focused on sharing ideas with friends about dieting, food regulation, and the pursuit of bodily aesthetics (as occurs on the pro-ana websites) to be an impoverished life remains questionable; obsessed "foodies" or extreme-thinness-yields-longevity dieters seem to have related preoccupations that do not necessarily yield impoverished lives. Moreover, like virtually all human beings, the pro-ana people understand that a very large part of the good life is being a successful and admired member of one's society, which entails partaking of socially valued roles and aims. Those who fail to engage in these cultural practices may thereby lose out in multiple social domains and roles or fail to participate socially as well as they might, which is a basic *pro tanto* harm. On the other hand, those who have a dysfunction causing their anorexic pursuits do benefit from successful social engagement but suffer a variety of other harms easily recognized as direct *pro tanto* harms by the pro-ana members themselves, eventually possibly including, for example, such harms as pain, loss of mobility, fatigue, and, ironically, the inability to thus present one's desirable body to others in social interactions.

In sum, in ways that Cooper does not acknowledge, the pro-ana people have the resources within the values of their culture to engage in the very dialectic that Cooper is engaging in. They are capable based on their available value resources of arriving at a reasoned conclusion about the potential harmfulness of their pursuit of thinness, but they value it nonetheless. And, they are able to understand that any individual—whether everyone in the society or just a few individuals—who has a psychological dysfunction that causes the individual to pursue anorexic values is disadvantaged in not being as capable of managing the potential *pro tanto* harms that come with these pursuits. These *pro tanto* harms, which are separable from the anorexic ideal itself, are sufficient for satisfying the harm requirement for HDA disorder attribution.

All that said, I would not want to deny that there is a sense in which entire cultures can be wrong about what is harmful. I believe, however, that whatever universal values can come to the rescue of such a culture are already implicit in and excavatable from within a culture's value system. Moreover, it is simply a fallacy to reason from "social values can get medically relevant harm wrong" to "therefore, there must be a source entirely beyond social values for discovering medically relevant harm," just as it is a fallacy to reason from "perception of what is immediately around us can go wrong" to "therefore, there must be a source entirely beyond perception for discovering what is immediately around us," and a fallacy to reason from "the available evidence in support of a theory can mislead us" to "therefore, there must be a source entirely beyond the available evidence for discovering which theory it is justified to believe."

Cooper is sufficiently confident that her intuitions can override the value foundations of an imagined society devoted to the value of thinness that she does not stop to wonder whether her judgment could just be her own culturally anchored values being projected into the world, in much the same manner as in an earlier time, "objective" European values were seen as superior to the immoral and harmful practices of "primitive" cultures. Should we equally reject culturally accepted practices such as lip-stretching, tattoos, circumcision, and other potentially harmful bodily modifications that define entry into a community or are aesthetic ideals in cultures other than our own? Oddly enough, while a society supporting thinness doesn't make the grade for Cooper as an acceptable cultural value, elsewhere she (Cooper 2007a) is sympathetic to deaf mothers depriving their children of the cochlear implants that would give the children the lifelong ability to hear because the parents prefer the child to be a full part of the deaf subcommunity. This suggests a lack of parity of reasoning that may reflect a confusion of local views du jour with transcendent insight.

Three Methods for Challenging Initial Harm Judgments

Having claimed that a culture's judgments of harm can be fundamentally wrong, Cooper then offers her attempt at a solution to how to reach culturally transcendent values ("One of the main aims of section III is to consider in greater detail how we might reflect on our initial gut reactions regarding harmfulness and improve upon them"), namely, three methods for how to engage in extended reflection and challenge standard gut-reaction views on whether a condition is harmful. The three methods are as follows: *(1) Think: Does this condition really cause any harm? (2) Break down claimed costs and benefits and make a list. (3) Consider consistency across judgments.*

Cooper's methods for exploring harm are innocuous enough, but there are several problems. First, the "list" approach of method 2 reveals an important point on which Cooper goes astray, undermining several of the arguments in her paper. The harm component of the concept of disorder works in terms of *pro tanto* direct harms (except where there is a biological "trade-off" situation), whereas Cooper allows her guidelines to encompass all the possible harms and benefits that a condition may bring and aims to judge overall benefit versus harm. This diverges dramatically from the way "disorder" is used in medicine.

Medical judgments of disorder examine harm in a restricted, diagnostically relevant way that stays close to the immediate effects of the dysfunction and usually involves pretty basic harms. There are many larger considerations regarding whether a diagnosed disorder should be treated, but those larger considerations do not generally enter into the diagnostic judgment itself. In judging more generally whether a dysfunction is harmful outside of a diagnostic context, one can take into account all the negatives and positives that issue from the dysfunction and form an "on-balance" judgment of overall harm versus benefit. However, the harm component of medical diagnosis does not work this way, which is why a physician does not need to evaluate your overall life, consider your life plans, and discern your hidden desires to reach a diagnosis. The diagnostically relevant harm associated with dysfunctions is not a matter of on-balance overall net harm but of *pro tanto* harm that emerges relatively directly from the dysfunction. This has long been obvious from examples such as the fact that cowpox can prevent smallpox; cowpox is a disorder due to its direct harmful *pro tanto* symptoms even if it later saves you from dying of smallpox and is an overall benefit. Similarly, your broken arm is a disorder even if it earns you a fortune from insurance that outweighs in benefit any harm suffered from the broken arm itself. In judging whether or how to treat a condition, of course all potential benefits and harms can be taken into account, but when judging whether a condition is a disorder, only *pro tanto* harm is relevant. Cooper's discussions of disorders here and elsewhere include a wide-ranging identification of harms and benefits in a way that potentially runs afoul of the *pro tanto* nature of diagnostically relevant harm for disorder attribution. Cooper's recommendation to evaluate whether a condition is harmful by making a list of the condition's overall harms and benefits is not in any simple way applicable to attribution of disorder versus nondisorder, although it may serve other purposes such as deciding whether overall it is preferable to treat or leave a condition untreated, as in the case deafness (Cooper 2007a).

Schwartz (2007) makes a similar error in his critique of the HDA's harm component, arguing that a disorder, whatever harm it causes, might have a benefit as well that makes it overall beneficial and not harmful: "Making harm a necessary requirement opens the theory to counterexamples involving diseases that benefit their victims, such as flat feet keeping a young man out of the army or cowpox conferring immunity during a smallpox epidemic" (56). However, a dysfunction's direct *pro tanto* harms, not on-balance harms, are the diagnostically relevant harms, which is why *DSM* contains symptom lists, not vast questionnaires for evaluating a condition's possible overall impact on a person's life. Thus, if flat feet are due to a dysfunction and cause discomfort when walking or running or bearing weight, then there is a disorder, even if the condition has the indirect and on-balance beneficial effect of saving one's life by keeping one out of the army. Moreover, harm is not judged on an individual basis that depends on accidental facts like one's being evaluated for forced entry into the armed services. One would judge the harmfulness of flat feet in terms of the disposition to typical and direct harm from the condition itself.

Second, Cooper does not really demonstrate with her examples that the guidelines are likely to yield agreement on conclusions about harm, with the outcomes of the described explorations seeming quite uncertain. For example, as anyone who has used the method of making lists of pros and cons will know, her advice to make a list of harms and benefits (and leaving aside her embrace of all possible harms and benefits rather than *pro tanto* harms) may not help very much. This is because, although listing may usefully bring additional considerations into play, it offers little guidance when it comes to the main obstacle to decision making, namely, figuring out which choice provides an overall superior outcome given the incommensurability of many desired goods (or in this case, harms versus benefits). For example, responding to claims by some members of the deaf community, Cooper (2007a) engages in an extended consideration of whether, based on a listing of harms and benefits, deafness should be considered harmful: on one hand, one is unable to hear music, but on the other, one is part of a vibrant community, and so on. In the end, she is unable to make a firm judgment on whether deafness is a disorder given these diverse and difficult-to-compare harms and benefits ("I conclude that whether it is a good or bad thing to be deaf is hard to determine" [579]). Making a list did not really address the issue, which is the incommensurability and variability of various benefits and harms. In any event, as argued above, whether or not deafness is overall harmful and should be treated, it is *pro tanto* harmful and a disorder.

Finally, recall that Cooper's argument is that the value considerations in judging harm may transcend culture, and the motive for the guidelines for challenging one's immediate superficial value reactions is to enable one to transcend one's culturally anchored reactions. The problem is that there is nothing in her three guidelines for amplifying value considerations that offers any grounds for going beyond one's existing culturally anchored value assumptions, though they do helpfully promote an exploration of value implications in a potentially challenging and deeper manner. I would argue that this reveals the actual situation, namely, that we can engage in a value dialectic to get a deeper insight into the harmfulness of a condition and thereby challenge the immediate superficial standard cultural view, but that dialectic takes place within a broader value framework that is itself culturally anchored but at the same time may move the culture forward. Perhaps in putting forward these guidelines, this sort of within-social-values dialectic is all that Cooper had in mind, and if so, we are in agreement.

I believe the above perspective applies to what would thus far be the prototype for supposed culture transcendence, the value arguments put forward by Spitzer when confronting the diagnostic status of homosexuality in the context of the deeply anchored disvaluing of homosexuality in our culture. Rather than standing outside our culture and declaring superior moral knowledge as Cooper does in her pro-ana example, all of the considerations Spitzer brought forward with regard to homosexuality's harmlessness, ranging from lack of distress or role impairment to the lessening importance of childbearing in an overpopulated world and the primary importance of the ability to have loving adult relationships, were culturally anchored considerations. However, they were edgy and pushed the culture beyond immediate reactions to confront foundational value issues in a value dialectic that allowed values that were already existent in the culture—for example, equality and acceptance in certain respects—to newly extend to individuals and features they previously did not cover.

Cooper on the Concept of Mental Disorder

In the course of her argument regarding the nature of the harm required for disorder, Cooper offers her own analysis of the concept of mental disorder as an alternative to the HDA. Taking Cooper's statements literally, it might appear that she is proposing that involuntary behavior in general is pathological: "Plausibly the difference between behavior that is indicative of disorder and normal bad behavior is that the former is voluntary, while the latter is in some way involuntary" [*sic*: presumably "former" and "latter" are switched here—JW]; "behavior characteristic of disorders must be involuntary." However, any notion that involuntariness is somehow intrinsically pathological is implausible on its face because many involuntary reactions are perfectly normal, ranging from emotional reactions (e.g., inability to be calm in the face of an immediate danger; inability to focus on work when one is intensely in love; inability to be cheerful when one has just experienced a loss) and biologically or developmentally based limitations (inability to engage in deliberate action when one is asleep; inability to will oneself to fall sleep; involuntary sexual attraction and arousal) to constraints imposed by moral conscience in individuals of firm conviction (inability to hurt a child or betray a lover). One passage, however, hints at the more plausible proposal that involuntariness is disordered when it is a deviation from what is normally voluntary ("The most plausible distinction is that normal badness is voluntary, while behavior that is symptomatic of a disorder is not under normal voluntary control"). In accordance with this passage, I will more charitably interpret Cooper as proposing not that psychopathology is involuntariness of action per se but that it is rather involuntariness of actions that is usually or formerly or expectably—or "normally"—under voluntary control.

I thus take Cooper to be proposing that a condition is a mental disorder when and only when there is a lessening of voluntary control of behavior from former or expectable levels. The lessening of the scope of the individual's agency is claimed by Cooper to be intrinsically harmful, so distress or role impairment is not required for disorder, just lessening of voluntariness. Note that if there is a loss of normal voluntary control over action, that often constitutes a dysfunction, that is, a failure of some internal system to operate as biologically designed, as in compulsive disorders. If Cooper is correct that such losses of voluntariness are intrinsically harmful, then in those cases both dysfunction and harm would be present, and so that subset of the conditions that Cooper's criterion identifies as disorders would also be disorders under the HDA.

Cooper's emphasis on the voluntary versus involuntary distinction as defining of disorder is reminiscent of Widiger and Sankis's (2000) "maladaptive dyscontrol" account of mental disorder, as well as Bergner's (1997) account, in the course of his explicating a definition of disorder proposed by Ossorio (1985), according to which the essence of psychopathology is loss of ability to engage in deliberate action: "When we observe that persons cannot, to a significant degree, choose their actions—that is, when they seem to lack considerable control with respect to initiating or restraining these actions—we take this as grounds for the attribution of psychopathology" (Bergner 1997, 239).

Cooper's proposal fails for reasons similar to the problems that confronted these earlier proposals (Wakefield 1997). When action that is normally under voluntary control becomes involuntary, that sometimes constitutes a dysfunction and, if harmful, a disorder, but not all such reductions in voluntariness are dysfunctions, and so the proposal is overly inclusive. Moreover, by limiting disorders to dyscontrol of normally controlled behaviors, Cooper and these other authors narrow the range of relevant psychological dysfunctions to those that concern failures of agency, yet surely that is not the only way psychological functioning can go wrong. The HDA can make the discriminations necessary here, whereas Cooper's definition cannot.

So, first, it is plain that mental disorder does not in fact require as a necessary condition the movement of some psychological process from the domain of the voluntary to the domain of involuntary control. For one thing, there are many disorders that occur entirely within the domain of the involuntary, where both normal functioning and pathological failure are involuntary. For example, we do not normally have willful control over when we fall asleep, yet the inability to involuntarily fall asleep is a disorder. We do not normally have voluntary control over our feelings of sadness after a loss, yet there are malfunctions of involuntary sadness responses that are depressive disorders. Going all the way back to Augustine, it has been lamented that we normally lack voluntary control over whether or not we become sexually aroused, yet the involuntary inability for a male to have an erection under standardly arousing conditions is considered a disorder. We generally do not have voluntary control of what we perceptually experience when we look at the world around us, yet malfunctions of visual perception (i.e., visual hallucinations) indicate disorder. Contrary to Cooper's analysis, in these and many other cases, involuntary responses are considered disorders despite the fact that the relevant kinds of responses have not previously or normally been voluntary, so there is no change from voluntary to involuntary. Cooper's analysis thus provides no way to distinguish normal from pathological involuntary responses (i.e., responses that are normally not under voluntary control) and thus fails to explain the many disorder judgments about such conditions. These examples are all counterexamples to the necessity of Cooper's analysis.

In addition to pathologies of normally involuntary responses, another kind of counterexample to the necessity of Cooper's voluntary-to-involuntary analysis of mental disorder consists of voluntary reactions that are disorders. Indeed, sometimes increases in voluntariness can constitute a disorder. There are some internal mechanisms that are biologically designed to act involuntarily and some mechanisms designed to preclude or inhibit certain potential voluntary behaviors, and in those cases, an increase in voluntary control can reveal a dysfunction and, if harmful, a disorder. Consider a person completely in control of his or her emotions, so that the person experiences no involuntary, spontaneous sadness or joy or surprise or love. Or imagine someone who must voluntarily and deliberately select each word when speaking rather than this process occurring largely outside of voluntary awareness. The ability to voluntarily engage in certain behaviors, such as the ability to easily betray those closest to one, to harm other people terribly without suffering involuntary guilt and without involuntary empathy, the ability to act without a sense of integrity limiting one's behavior, and so on, would all be considered health under Cooper's definition because they increase the domain of voluntary psychological action from the normal level. However, these conditions are more likely to be considered pathologies by experts and laypersons alike, just as the broadening of voluntary control in normally automatic physiological functions such as adjustment of heart rate to exercise, the adjustment of pupil dilation to the level of ambient light, and the adjustment of visual perception to indicate size and distance of objects from complex cues would be considered potential pathologies.

Cooper's theory of disorder as transformation of voluntary control to involuntary action does not work as a necessary condition even for some of the very sorts of cases that she cites, such as personality disorders and paraphilias. Both of these kinds of disorders involve behavior that need be no less voluntary than their normal counterparts. The problem is often not the voluntariness but the nature of the desires and perceptions on which the voluntary choice is based. Personality disorders involve voluntary actions within the distorted lens of the personality disorder, but in response to the distortions of that lens, the actions can be just as voluntary as the normal-range individual's actions are voluntary within the lens of a normal-range personality formation. Indeed, sometimes personality disorders open areas of potential action that the normal individual's meaning system would not allow. Although it is true, as Cooper argues, that "we need to be able to say what distinguishes disordered people from those who are simply criminal or anti-social…the criminal's actions are planned, motivated and controlled; they are fully voluntary," it is chillingly true that even the pathologically violent psychopath's behavior can be equally planned, motivated, and controlled but take places within a meaning system that allows the performance of cruel actions that are not often psychologically possible for the normal person of conscience. All personality traits, normal or disordered, shape and constrain subsequent voluntary actions, so the voluntary versus involuntary distinction cannot be what generally discriminates personality disorder from nondisordered personality.

With regard to paraphilias such as pedophilia, there may in general be a range of degrees of voluntariness and involuntariness in responding to one's sexual desires, but the diagnosis of paraphilias depends on the paraphilic nature of the content of one's desire and whether harm results, not on anything having to do with voluntariness or involuntariness. There is nothing necessarily more or less voluntary about attraction to and desire for sex with an adult versus attraction to and desire for sex with a child. It is the paraphilic content of the desire in pedophilia and the harm that results that indicates disorder. Just as normal sexual desire varies in many ways as to the content that is found arousing but the voluntariness level can remain the same across normal sexual preferences, so across the disorder/nondisorder divide the voluntariness level can also remain the same. Indeed, the widened scope for instrumental action beyond the normal range of inhibiting processes might be part of the reason why the pedophile is seen as having a dysfunction.

There are also compelling reasons why Cooper's "involuntariness" analysis is not sufficient for disorder. Many normal psychological processes involve the movement of initially voluntary deliberative processing into a background of learned skills that are no longer within routine voluntary control. Think of learned skills such as playing a piano or speaking a second language. One starts out with entirely deliberative voluntary actions, but as one becomes skilled or fluent, the choice process disappears into the background and action becomes automatic to the point that one becomes totally unaware of the process. Such biologically designed capacities to decrease the degree of voluntariness of behavior are integral to normal psychological functioning. Beyond these sorts of examples, there are many areas of life in which emotional reactions to an object ranging from love to disgust create increasingly involuntary reactions to the object (e.g., when a lover becomes increasingly "simply irresistible"), but such reductions in voluntary responses are not necessarily disorders.

It is also worth noting that a serious consequence of defining mental dysfunctions as pathologies of voluntary control is that this approach defeats one of the central purposes of the analysis of "mental disorder," which is to explain how psychiatry can be a legitimate subdiscipline of medicine and thus how mental disorders are medical disorders. The voluntary/involuntary distinction does not apply to most physical disorders, so the "involuntariness" account cannot serve as a general analysis of the concept of medical disorder, although it can certainly be a theory of the specific type of problem in some mental disorders. To explain what unites medical disorders across mental and physical domains, one needs something like the HDA that proposes a feature, dysfunction, that applies to both domains. With that in hand, one could then test the involuntariness account as a specific theory of some mental dysfunctions.

Why, one might ask, does Cooper feel the need to propose such an obviously inadequate account of disorder? After all, the HDA offers a clear answer to the question with which she starts, "How can we distinguish between disorders and normal criminal or antisocial behavior that harms others?" The HDA explains this sort of distinction in terms of dysfunction. That is, disorder always involves the failure of some mechanism to perform its biologically designed function, where biological design is interpreted in evolutionary terms. It is a plausible hypothesis that a dysfunction occurs in severe antisocial conditions, but there are other more plausible explanations for routine criminality. However, Cooper ignores this feature of the HDA because elsewhere (Cooper 2007b), she has rejected the HDA's evolutionary dysfunction component and argued against its validity. Though Cooper does not herself mount this argument here, De Vreese leverages it in the course of her chapter in this volume, and I examine it in some detail in a supplement following this reply to Cooper.

In sum, dysfunctions that cause harm are disorders whether the functions that they interfere with involve voluntary or involuntary responses. Voluntary control is one domain of natural functions and thus one domain for potential dysfunctions, but it is not defining of mental disorder. Involuntary behavior is a disorder when and only when it is a harmful dysfunction.

DSM-5 and Harm

Toward the end of her paper, Cooper considers "harm in practice" as it relates to *DSM* diagnosis and specifically "how the idea that disorders are necessarily harmful has a crucial role to play in ensuring that classifications of disorders, such as the influential *DSM*, do not medicalize normal oddities." The harm criterion prevents harmless biologically normal (nondysfunction) states from being classified as disorders, but those conditions are already eliminated from disorder status by the lack of a dysfunction. Thus, the primary impact of the harm criterion is to eliminate *dysfunctions* that are not harmful from disorder status, where there might be a temptation to pathologize the dysfunction despite it doing no harm.

Cooper's statement that the harm requirement prevents pathologization of "normal oddities" is subtly misleading because "nondisordered" does not imply "normal." Nonharmful dysfunctions include anomalous biological design failures, ranging from harmless genetic mutations to fused toes, and inhabit an ample middle ground between disorder and normality. Consequently, for example, the common inference from depathologization of homosexuality to the conclusion that homosexuality is a normal variation of sexual desire is problematic because of the possibility that homosexuality in some forms could still turn out to be due to a dysfunction even if not a disorder (e.g., De Block and Sholl, this volume; Powell and Scarffe 2019).

Cooper tends to emphasize the distress or impairment requirement in the definition of mental disorder and the parallel distress-or-impairment clinical significance criterion (CSC) in diagnostic criteria sets as *the* harm criterion. However, distress and role impairment are not the only kinds of harms in which people can suffer from dysfunctions, and most disorders' symptom-based diagnostic criteria include harmful symptoms of various kinds. So, in many cases, the clinical significance criterion is unnecessary to ensure harm (Spitzer and Wakefield 1999). It is intended as a backup criterion to ensure harm reaches a certain level and to provide suggestive evidence that there is indeed a dysfunction in cases when symptoms are mild.

Given her view of the importance of the harm requirement in protecting against invalid pathologization, Cooper's primary concern is that *DSM-5*'s (2013) definition of disorder says that the dysfunction "usually" (rather than always) causes distress or disability: "Mental disorders are *usually* associated with significant distress or disability" (20, emphasis added). This, Cooper argues, weakens the conceptual link between disorder and harm and so could open the door to classifying harmless conditions as disorders or even to eliminating the harm requirement entirely as superfluous. I think there is no such danger and that Cooper's apprehension is based on a misinterpretation of the point of *DSM-5*'s "usually" qualifier.

Cooper interprets the "usually" qualifier as an attempt to coordinate with the goal of the *International Classification of Diseases* (ICD) to separate diagnosis from role impairment due to the cross-cultural possibilities for spurious diagnosis based on differences in social roles. However, despite that goal, the recent *ICD-11* incorporates virtually the same definition of mental disorder as *DSM-5*, including the "usually" qualifier, so this cannot be the heart of the story.

The "usually" qualifier is intended to allow diagnosis under unusual circumstances in which a type of dysfunction is linked to harm but is either not harmful at the time of diagnosis in the present patient for one reason or another or causes harm that does not fit into the distress-or-role-impairment category. This preserves the link between disorder and harm rather than challenges it. Moreover, Cooper's notion that this is a misconceived novelty introduced into *DSM-5* is factually mistaken. *DSM-III* (1980), the edition that inaugurated the modern *DSM* system of operationalized diagnostic criteria and the first edition to include a definition of mental disorder, defined a mental disorder as "a clinically significant behavioral or psychological syndrome or pattern that occurs in an individual and that is *typically* associated with" harms such as distress or role impairment (Spitzer 1980, 6, emphasis added). So, *DSM-5* simply returns to the earlier *DSM-III* approach on this matter.

Indeed, this sort of qualifier was included in definitions long before *DSM-III*. For example, in defining "medical disorder" in a paper that presented a lengthier forerunner of the *DSM-III* definition of mental disorder, Spitzer and Endicott (1978) state that the condition "in the fully developed or extreme form" (18) is associated with certain harms, including distress, disability, or certain forms of disadvantage. They explain, "The phrase *in the fully developed or extreme form* is used because in medicine many conditions are recognizable in an early form, frequently with the aid of laboratory tests, before they have any undesirable consequences" (1978, 19). Thus, they imply that disorders are not always at the time of diagnosis associated with harm. In a still earlier attempt at defining mental disorder, Spitzer and Wilson (1975) propose the following criterion: "The condition *in its full blown state* is *regularly* and intrinsically associated with" (829, emphasis added) various harms. They explain,

> The phrase "full blown" acknowledges that some psychiatric conditions in an early stage of development may not be associated with subjective distress or impairment, just as many nonpsychiatric medical illnesses may be initially asymptomatic. Similarly, the phrase "regularly…associated with" recognizes that, just as some highly unusual cases of carcinoma may remain totally asymptomatic, so it is possible that some rare persons with even a psychotic illness may not evidence subjective distress or impairment in social effectiveness. These criteria are for defining conditions that are mental disorders, not for defining persons who are overtly ill. (829)

So, Cooper is wrong to portray the introduction of the qualifier "usually" as a break with the past that threatens the integrity of diagnosis. Spitzer and Wilson's comment that "these criteria are for defining conditions that are mental disorders, not for defining persons who are overtly ill," is particularly enlightening in understanding the dispositional nature of the harmfulness criterion.

What, then, happened in between *DSM-III* and *DSM-5*, when no such qualifier was included? In its place, Spitzer introduced a new set of potential "harms" in the form of risks of harm. Consequently, a disorder was now defined as a dysfunction "that is associated with present distress (a painful symptom) or disability (impairment in one or more important areas of functioning) *or with significantly increased risk of suffering death, pain, disability, or an important loss of freedom*" (American Psychiatric Association 1987, xxii, emphasis added). The risk clause was in effect a replacement for the "typically" qualifier because the cases that the qualifier was designed to address were all cases with a risk of harm. These include prodromal conditions at an early stage before actual harm has occurred—for example, in *DSM-5*, mild neurocognitive disorder prior to overtly harmful dementia—and instances of full-blown dysfunction in which usual harms are for some idiosyncratic reason not yet expressed at the time of diagnosis even though the condition is disposed to cause harm. The "risk" criteria had their own validity problems (e.g., they encouraged risk of disorder to be confused with actual disorder) and have been eliminated in *DSM-5*. And so, the "usually" qualifier has returned.

In sum, Cooper is incorrect to portray the introduction of the qualifier "usually" as a major break with the past that threatens the integrity of diagnosis. At no point from the earliest *DSM*-related attempts to define mental disorder in 1975 to the latest *DSM-5* definition was there a definition that required actual harm in every instance of diagnosed disorder. Despite this, clear examples of false positives due to ignoring or misattributing the harm component are hard to find given the manifest harmfulness of most *DSM* symptom criteria and the clinical significance requirement. Indeed, Cooper's paper contains not one clear instance of a current *DSM* false positive due to lack of harm. Of her two past examples, eliminating homosexuality from the *DSM* was a relatively unique situation, and *DSM-III* stereotypic movement disorder was quickly recognized as not harmful and corrected in *DSM-III-R*. In contrast, in my opinion,

DSM abounds with false positives due to ignoring the dysfunction requirement. It thus remains to be demonstrated that attention to the harm requirement is in fact important in safeguarding the validity of *DSM* psychiatric diagnosis in the way that attention to the dysfunction criterion is manifestly critical. Caution is warranted because there is a danger that premature attempts to impose a culturally transcendent harm criterion to "provide a barrier against medicalization" without any systematic account of harm can lead to tendentious diagnostic constraints that block treatment of culturally specific direct *pro tanto* harms (Powell and Scarffe 2019; Wakefield and Conrad 2019).

References

American Psychiatric Association. 1980. *Diagnostic and Statistical Manual of Mental Disorders*. 3rd ed. American Psychiatric Association.

American Psychiatric Association. 1987. *Diagnostic and Statistical Manual of Mental Disorders*. 3rd rev. ed. American Psychiatric Association.

American Psychiatric Association. 2013. *Diagnostic and Statistical Manual of Mental Disorders*. 5th ed. American Psychiatric Association.

Bergner, R. M. 1997. What is psychopathology? And so what? *Clinical Psychology Science and Practice* 4(3): 235–248.

Cooper, R. 2007a. Can it be a good thing to be deaf? *Journal of Medicine and Philosophy* 32: 563–583.

Cooper, R. 2007b. *Psychiatry and Philosophy of Science*. Routledge.

Feit, N. 2017. Harm and the concept of medical disorder. *Theoretical Medicine and Bioethics* 38(5): 1–19.

First, M. B., and J. C. Wakefield. 2010. Defining "mental disorder" in *DSM-V*. *Psychological Medicine* 40(11): 1779–1782.

First, M. B., and J. C. Wakefield. 2013. Diagnostic criteria as dysfunction indicators: Bridging the chasm between the definition of mental disorder and diagnostic criteria for specific disorders. *Canadian Journal of Psychiatry* 58(12): 663–669.

Limbaugh, D. G. 2019. The harm of medical disorder as harm in the damage sense. *Theoretical Medicine and Bioethics* 40(1): 1–19.

Muckler, D. S., and J. S. Taylor. 2020. The irrelevance of harm for a theory of disease. *Journal of Medicine and Philosophy* 45(3): 332–349.

Ossorio, P. G. 1985. Pathology. *Advances in Descriptive Psychology* 4: 151–201.

Powell, R., and E. Scarffe. 2019. Rethinking "disease": A fresh diagnosis and a new philosophical treatment. *Journal of Medical Ethics* 45(9): 579–588.

Schwartz, P. H. 2007. Decision and discovery in defining "disease." In *Establishing Medical Reality: Essays in the Metaphysics and Epistemology of Biomedical Science*, H. Kincaid and J. McKitrick (eds.), 47–63. Springer.

Spitzer, R. L. 1980. Introduction. In *Diagnostic and Statistical Manual of Mental Disorders*, 1–12. 3rd ed. American Psychiatric Association.

Spitzer, R. L. 1997. Brief comments from a psychiatric nosologist weary from his own attempts to define mental disorder: Why Ossorio's definition muddles and Wakefield's "harmful dysfunction" illuminates the issues. *Clinical Psychology: Science and Practice* 4(3): 259–261.

Spitzer, R. L. 1998. Diagnosis and need for treatment are not the same. *Archives of General Psychiatry* 55: 120.

Spitzer, R. L. 1999. Harmful dysfunction and the *DSM* definition of mental disorder. *Journal of Abnormal Psychology* 108(3): 430–432.

Spitzer, R. L., and J. Endicott. 1978. Medical and mental disorder: Proposed definition and criteria. In *Critical Issues in Psychiatric Diagnosis*, D. F. Klein and R. L. Spitzer (eds.), 15–40. Raven Press.

Spitzer, R. L., and J. C. Wakefield. 1999. *DSM-IV* diagnostic criterion for clinical significance: Does it help solve the false positives problem? *American Journal of Psychiatry* 156: 1856–1864.

Spitzer, R. L., and P. T. Wilson. 1975. Nosology and the official psychiatric nomenclature. In *Comprehensive Textbook of Psychiatry*, A. M. Freedman, H. I. Kaplan, and B. J. Sadock (eds.), 826–845. Vol. 2. Williams & Wilkins.

Wakefield, J. C. 1992a. The concept of mental disorder: On the boundary between biological facts and social values. *American Psychologist* 47: 373–388.

Wakefield, J. C. 1992b. Disorder as harmful dysfunction: A conceptual critique of *DSM-III-R*'s definition of mental disorder. *Psychological Review* 99: 232–247.

Wakefield, J. C. 1993. Limits of operationalization: A critique of Spitzer and Endicott's (1978) proposed operational criteria of mental disorder. *Journal of Abnormal Psychology* 102: 160–172.

Wakefield, J. C. 1995. Dysfunction as a value-free concept: A reply to Sadler and Agich. *Philosophy, Psychiatry, and Psychology* 2: 233–46.

Wakefield, J. C. 1997a. Diagnosing *DSM-IV*, part 1: *DSM-IV* and the concept of mental disorder. *Behaviour Research and Therapy* 35: 633–650.

Wakefield, J. C. 1997b. Diagnosing *DSM-IV*, part 2: Eysenck (1986) and the essentialist fallacy. *Behaviour Research and Therapy*: 35: 651–666.

Wakefield, J. C. 1997c. Normal inability versus pathological disability: Why Ossorio's (1985) definition of mental disorder is not sufficient. *Clinical Psychology: Science and Practice* 4: 249–258.

Wakefield, J. C. 1997d. When is development disordered? Developmental psychopathology and the harmful dysfunction analysis of mental disorder. *Development and Psychopathology* 9: 269–290.

Wakefield, J. C. 1998. The *DSM*'s theory-neutral nosology is scientifically progressive: Response to Follette and Houts. *Journal of Consulting and Clinical Psychology* 66: 846–852.

Wakefield, J. C. 1999a. Evolutionary versus prototype analyses of the concept of disorder. *Journal of Abnormal Psychology* 108: 374–399.

Wakefield, J. C. 1999b. Mental disorder as a black box essentialist concept. *Journal of Abnormal Psychology* 108: 465–472.

Wakefield, J. C. 2000a. Aristotle as sociobiologist: The "function of a human being" argument, black box essentialism, and the concept of mental disorder. *Philosophy, Psychiatry, and Psychology* 7: 17–44.

Wakefield, J. C. 2000b. Spandrels, vestigial organs, and such: Reply to Murphy and Woolfolk's "The harmful dysfunction analysis of mental disorder." *Philosophy, Psychiatry, and Psychology* 7: 253–269.

Wakefield, J. C. 2001. Evolutionary history versus current causal role in the definition of disorder: Reply to McNally. *Behaviour Research and Therapy* 39: 347–366.

Wakefield, J. C. 2006. What makes a mental disorder mental? *Philosophy, Psychiatry, and Psychology* 13: 123–131.

Wakefield, J. C. 2007. The concept of mental disorder: Diagnostic implications of the harmful dysfunction analysis. *World Psychiatry* 6: 149–156.

Wakefield, J. C. 2009. Mental disorder and moral responsibility: Disorders of personhood as harmful dysfunctions, with special reference to alcoholism. *Philosophy, Psychiatry, and Psychology* 16: 91–99.

Wakefield, J. C. 2011. Darwin, functional explanation, and the philosophy of psychiatry. In *Maladapting Minds: Philosophy, Psychiatry, and Evolutionary Theory*, P. R. Andriaens and A. De Block (eds.), 143–172. Oxford University Press.

Wakefield, J. C. 2013. Addiction, the concept of disorder, and pathways to harm: Comment on Levy. *Frontiers in Addictive Disorders & Behavioral Dyscontrol* 4(34): 1–2.

Wakefield, J. C. 2014. The biostatistical theory versus the harmful dysfunction analysis, part 1: Is part-dysfunction a sufficient condition for medical disorder? *Journal of Medicine and Philosophy* 39: 648–682.

Wakefield, J. C. 2016a. The concepts of biological function and dysfunction: Toward a conceptual foundation for evolutionary psychopathology. In *Handbook of Evolutionary Psychology*, D. Buss (ed.), 2nd ed., vol. 2, 988–1006. Oxford University Press.

Wakefield, J. C. 2016b. Diagnostic issues and controversies in *DSM-5*: Return of the false positives problem. *Annual Review of Clinical Psychology* 12: 105–132.

Wakefield, J. C., and J. A. Conrad. 2019. Does the harm component of the harmful dysfunction analysis need rethinking? Reply to Powell and Scarffe. *Journal of Medical Ethics* 45(9): 594–596.

Wakefield, J. C., and M. B. First. 2003. Clarifying the distinction between disorder and nondisorder: Confronting the overdiagnosis ("false positives") problem in *DSM-V*. In *Advancing DSM: Dilemmas in Psychiatric Diagnosis*, K. A. Phillips, M. B. First, and H. A. Pincus (eds.), 23–56. American Psychiatric Press.

Wakefield, J. C., and M. B. First. 2012. Placing symptoms in context: The role of contextual criteria in reducing false positives in *DSM* diagnosis. *Comprehensive Psychiatry* 53: 130–139.

Wakefield, J. C., and M. B. First. 2013. The importance and limits of harm in identifying mental disorder. *Canadian Journal of Psychiatry* 58(11): 618–621.

Widiger, T. A., and L. M. Sankis. 2000. Adult psychopathology: Issues and controversies. *Annual Review of Psychology* 51: 377–404.

Wakefield, J. C., and M. B. First. 2003. Clarifying the distinction between disorder and nondisorder: Confronting the overdiagnosis (false positives) problem in DSM-V. In *Advancing the DSM: Dilemmas in Psychiatric Diagnosis*, K. A. Phillips, M. B. First, and H. A. Pincus (eds.), 23–56. American Psychiatric Press.

Wakefield, J. C., and M. B. First. 2012. Placing symptoms in context: The role of contextual criteria in reducing false positives in DSM diagnosis. *Comprehensive Psychiatry* 53: 130–139.

Watson, D., L. C., and J. L. Blais. 2011. The importance and limits of a team in identifying mental disorder. *Canadian Journal of Psychiatry* 56(11): 618–625.

Widiger, T. A., and L. M. Smith. 2008. Adult psychopathology and personality disorders. *Annual Review of Psychology* 51: 172–104.

29 Are There Naturally Selected Disorders? Supplementary Reply to Rachel Cooper

Jerome Wakefield

In this supplement to my reply to Rachel Cooper, I leave the topic of harm on which her chapter focuses and turn to another area of Cooper's critique of the harmful dysfunction analysis (HDA; see my main reply to Cooper in this volume for references) that is not addressed in Cooper's chapter but is prominently cited by another critic in this volume. Some critics, rather than presenting claimed counterarguments directly themselves, "outsource" crucial arguments by simply referring to others' writings as having established that there are counterexamples to the HDA. One such critic is Leen De Vreese, who in her chapter in this volume proclaims that "it cannot be denied that Wakefield's approach has also been refuted in the literature on the basis of counterexamples demonstrating that people's intuitions are not always in accordance with the HDA....These can be found in the literature (see, e.g., Cooper 2007; Schwartz 2007)." I do deny that there is any such refutation of the HDA in Cooper's writings. Thus, although Cooper's paper in this volume does not address the dysfunction component of the HDA, I now consider Cooper's arguments against the dysfunction component that are referred to by De Vreese. For good measure, I will also address the proposed counterexamples to the HDA's evolutionary dysfunction component in the passage De Vreese cites from Schwartz.

In the relevant passage, Cooper (2007), after arguing that evolutionary dysfunction is not by itself sufficient for disorder (I agree; there has to be harm as well), then turns her attention to the HDA and asks, "Could we claim that a condition is only a disorder if it is a *harmful* dysfunction?" (33). She answers that "such an account of disorder cannot be accepted either, as it is not even necessary that a condition be a biological dysfunction for it to be a disorder" (33). She argues for this claim as follows:

> This is because in some cases the genetic bases of disorders may confer a biological advantage and thus be selected. In such a situation, from a biological point of view, there is maybe no dysfunction when cases of the disorder occur. This may well be the case with several types of mental disorder. Conditions including manic-depression, sociopathy, obsessive-compulsivity, anxiety, drug abuse and some personality disorders seem to have a genetic basis and yet occur at prevalence rates that are too high to be solely the result of mutations. This has led

evolutionary psychologists to suggest that the genetic bases of these mental disorders must be adaptive in some way or other. (33)

This is a manifestly invalid argument based on a common fallacy. From the premise that certain elements of the genetic basis of a disorder were naturally selected, it does not follow that the disorder itself was selected. For example, in the case of genetic disorders such as sickle cell anemia and cystic fibrosis, it is thought that having one copy of certain genes was selected to protect against certain pathogens, but when an individual by chance inherits two doses of that gene, that constitutes a dysfunction and a disorder. Neither the resulting disorder nor its specific genetic basis of two doses of the gene was naturally selected. However, the fact that one dose of the gene confers advantages and was selected for explains the higher-than-expected rate of the disorder. Some have theorized that schizophrenia or bipolar disorder may similarly be partly the result of inheriting combinations of genes that when present individually, in lower frequencies, or in other combinations confer some advantage such as more fluid or creative thought. However, even if some genes underlying a disorder were naturally selected individually or in certain configurations and when they appear in those configurations confer advantages and are not dysfunctions, it may still be the case that there is a specific configuration of the same genes that is a dysfunction and was selected against.

For example, a recent study of the genetics of autism (Polimanti and Gelernter 2017) found that individual genes that confer a risk for autism are associated with cognitive advantages and were positively selected: "Using genome-wide data, we observed that common alleles associated with increased risk for ASD present a signature of positive selection. ... ASD risk alleles could positively affect these [cognitive] mechanisms, causing better cognitive ability in carriers as a consequence" (4, 8). However, certain polygenic combinations to the contrary yielded autism: "However, an excessive burden of these risk variants is correlated with the onset of the developmental disorders included in the autism spectrum as the evolutionary cost" (8). Thus, "According to our interpretation of our data, such small-effect alleles were accumulated across the genome (polygenic adaptation) to the benefit of most but to the detriment of some" (9). Cooper's objection is based on a simple misunderstanding of the difference between, for example, single-gene function versus polygenic dysfunction.

Cooper then proceeds to offer some examples that, based on the existence of genetic components, are supposed to show that naturally selected conditions can be disorders:

The genetic basis of pathological conditions may be selected for a number of reasons. Most obviously, a condition may be selected because it enhances sufferers' biological fitness in some present environment. Linda Mealey (1995a) suggests that the genes for sociopathy are selected for this reason. Sociopaths tend to be more violent and promiscuous than other males, and in tough environments these traits may be adaptive. Other conditions might be of no benefit at present but have been biologically beneficial in earlier times. Agoraphobia and other anxiety disorders, for example, may be of no benefit now, but could have been adaptive when human beings lived in more hazardous environments. (Cooper 2007, 33)

Psychopathy, the counterexample Cooper singles out for mention, is one of the most regularly cited proposed counterexamples to the HDA due to Mealey's theory. Psychopathy has long been generally considered a disorder, ever since its distant origins in the concept of "moral insanity," yet here it is being claimed to be naturally selected. So, I will examine in some depth this prototypical example of what critics like Cooper think is wrong with the HDA. (I will address Cooper's other example of anxiety disorders later.)

In response to proposed claims of selected disorders, like Cooper's example of psychopathy, the HDA implies the following counterclaim: because the judgments that a condition is a disorder and that the condition is a biologically designed naturally selected adaptation are incompatible, as one comes to believe that a condition currently considered a disorder is in fact biologically designed, one will also abandon one's belief that it is a disorder. The HDA's prediction of changed disorder intuitions surely qualifies as a bold, novel, and unexpected prediction that has a very low independent prior probability and does not generally follow from other extant accounts of disorder. Consequently, if the prediction is confirmed, it provides strong evidence for the HDA. That is, Cooper's example of Mealey's theory of psychopathy, rather than being a counterexample to the HDA, is a powerful test case for the HDA's counterclaim. (The psychopathy example is also a congenial topic for me to consider because I have examined the related issue of the diagnostic status of youth antisocial behavior [Kirk et al. 1999; Wakefield et al. 1999; Wakefield et al. 2002; Wakefield et al. 2006].)

The story starts a bit before Mealey. In her seminal work on youth antisocial behavior diagnosed as conduct disordered by the *Diagnostic and Statistical Manual of Mental Disorders* (*DSM*), Terrie Moffitt (1993), although not applying an evolutionary perspective, drew a distinction between a pathological form due to brain dysfunction and a nonpathological form that was a strategic response to modern environmental circumstances in which there is a lengthy gap between physical maturity and social independence:

Life-Course-Persistent Antisocial Behavior as Psychopathology. The life-course-persistent antisocial syndrome, as described here, has many characteristics that, taken together, suggest psychopathology....The syndrome of life-course-persistent antisocial behavior described here has a biological basis in subtle dysfunctions of the nervous system. (Moffitt 1993, 685)

Adolescence-Limited Antisocial Behavior Is Not Pathological Behavior....Instead of a biological basis in the nervous system, the origins of adolescence-limited delinquency lie in youngsters' best efforts to cope with the widening gap between biological and social maturity. (Moffitt 1993, 692)

Moffitt's analysis illustrated that even a condition long considered a disorder (namely, adolescent conduct disorder as measured by *DSM* antisocial behavioral criteria) is no longer seen as a disorder once no internal dysfunction is inferred.

A couple of years later, Linda Mealey (1995a) published a watershed analysis distinguishing two types of adult psychopathy or sociopathy, one of which consists of largely genetically determined personality traits and the other of which is more environmentally responsive and strategic. She argued, against standard wisdom, that the former "primary" genetic form is in fact a naturally selected adaptation that confers advantages when the psychopath is among mostly nonpsychopathic community members. She thus hypothesized it to be a "frequency-dependent adaptation" that has a potentially successful niche only when it is relatively rare and occurs in the context of a population in which the majority are other naturally selected variants that are not sociopathic. In this case, unlike the cases of cystic fibrosis, sickle cell anemia, and schizophrenia, natural selection is hypothesized to act directly on the condition that has been considered a disorder rather than on a partial genetic basis of the condition that was selected for independent reasons. Thus, this is indeed an ideal test case for Cooper's claim that disorders can be naturally selected adaptations.

The result of this test is that neither Mealey's views nor the views of her colleagues support Cooper's claims. Rather, they confirm the HDA's prediction that disorder and natural section are antithetical hypotheses. Cooper fails to report the fact that Mealey, in her response to comments on the very paper cited by Cooper, dichotomously titles a section "Adaptation or Abnormality?" and poses the straightforward either/or question, "Is sociopathy an adaptation or an abnormality?" (Mealey 1995b, 58). Like Moffitt, Mealey predictably hypothesizes that her category of secondary sociopaths, whose behavior is a strategic response to social circumstances and who are not a genetically shaped personality type, is prima facie a nondisorder. More surprising is what Mealey says about primary sociopaths, who share largely genetically determined personality features and that she recognizes is the condition most likely to be labeled as disordered by others:

> Sociopaths…clearly have both social and psychophysiological "deficits" if the standard we use is the nonsociopath. But in some ways, if sociopathy is indeed a type, using a nonsociopathic standard would be like using a male standard to assess the "normal functioning" of a female, or an adult standard to assess the "normal functioning" of an infant. If sociopaths are not a type designed by natural selection to fill a particular niche, then we could probably agree that they do not function normally; but if they are a type, then…the medical model is no longer appropriate. (Mealey 1995b, 584)

Thus, Mealey, the author Cooper cites to support her claim that a disorder can be an adaptation, in fact directly contradicts Cooper's claim. Instead, consistent with the HDA, Mealey sees the two hypotheses that psychopathy is a medical disorder and that psychopathy is a naturally selected niche adaptation as conflicting hypotheses on conceptual grounds, such that once one believes primary psychopathy is a naturally selected variation, then despite the history of considering the condition a pathology, "the medical model is no longer appropriate." She pointedly suggests that the distinction between psychopaths and other people is best conceptualized not as psychopathological deviation from normality but as analogous to the often dramatic distinctions between naturally selected variants of normal human beings, such as male versus female and adult versus child.

This reaction is not distinctive to Mealey. Richard Machalek (1995), commenting on Mealey (1995a), similarly expresses the incompatibility between a condition being a medical disorder and being naturally selected:

> As the term itself suggests, the medical model attributes sociopathy to a "pathogen," in this case an emotional deficit that may be genetically rooted and physiologically expressed....Evolutionary theory takes us beyond mere diagnostic descriptors and prompts us to ask whether such antisocial behaviors may, in some fundamental sense, be advantageous to those who express them....Framing sociopathy in evolutionary terms accordingly frees us from the explanatory constraints imposed by the medical model that would have us attribute its causes to some "pathogen," when it is not at all clear that the sorts of genetic and physiological processes attributed to sociopathy are necessarily pathological. Rather, we can explore an alternative explanatory possibility. (Machalek 1995, 564)

Here, "pathogen" is a stand-in for "dysfunction." The intuition that the medical disorder hypothesis and the naturally selected adaptation hypothesis are mutually exclusive is widely shared and has been expressed by researchers in subsequent publications on this topic. For example, Kinner (2003) says, "From an evolutionary perspective psychopathy seems to be an adaptation rather than a disease" (67).

Similarly, Lalumière et al. (2001) rely on this basic distinction in formulating their empirical study of developmental trajectories aimed at testing which of the two hypotheses is more likely to be true:

> Psychopaths are manipulative, impulsive, and callous individuals with long histories of antisocial behavior. Two models have guided the study of psychopathy. One suggests that psychopathy is a psychopathology, i.e., the outcome of defective or perturbed development. A second suggests that psychopathy is a life-history strategy of social defection and aggression that was reproductively viable in the environment of evolutionary adaptedness (EEA). These two models make different predictions....These results provide no support for psychopathological models of psychopathy and partial support for life-history strategy models. (Lalumière et al. 2001, 75)

Reimer (2008) echoed this view: "On any such 'selectionist' model, psychopaths are certainly different than the rest of us, biologically speaking. However, they are not, in any biological sense, disordered" (187). Here, "disordered in a biological sense" is presumably a stand-in for biological dysfunction.

Krupp et al. (2012) further illustrate the way that researchers reconsidered and questioned the pathological status of psychopathy in light of the natural selection analysis and transformed the distinction between selected and disordered into researchable hypotheses:

> Psychopaths routinely disregard social norms by engaging in selfish, antisocial, often violent behavior. Commonly characterized as mentally disordered, recent evidence suggests that psychopaths are executing a well-functioning, if unscrupulous, strategy that historically increased reproductive success at the expense of others. Natural selection ought to have favored strategies that spared close kin from harm, however, because actions affecting the fitness of genetic relatives contribute to an individual's inclusive fitness. Conversely, there is evidence that mental disorders can disrupt psychological mechanisms designed to protect relatives. Thus, mental disorder and adaptation accounts of psychopathy generate opposing hypotheses: psychopathy should be associated with an increase in the victimization of kin in the former account but not in the latter.... These results stand in contrast to models positing psychopathy as a pathology, and provide support for the hypothesis that psychopathy reflects an evolutionary strategy. (1)

The Lalumière et al. (2001) and Krupp et al. (2012) papers illustrate that the HDA allows for the hypothesis of disorder versus natural selection to give rise to testable empirical hypotheses.

In a response to Krupp et al. (2012), Leedom and Almas (2012), although accepting the same overall conceptual distinctions, argued that psychopathy is in fact a disorder after all because it is a spandrel (i.e., a side effect of adaptation) rather than an adaptation per se that was specifically selected for: "Psychopathy may persist because it represents a dominance-related spandrel." The fact that spandrels are not strictly speaking adaptations but side effects of adaptations allows Leedom and Almas to pathologize psychopathy, for they agree that natural selection implies nondisorder.

Krupp et al. (2013), in a paper responding to critics, insisted that their surprising finding of a negative association between psychopathy and violence against genetic relatives "failed to support the hypothesis that psychopathy is a mental disorder, suggesting instead that it supports the hypothesis that psychopathy is an evolved life history strategy" (1), again expressing the assumed opposition between the naturally selected and the disordered. In addition, Krupp et al. lucidly explain why, if psychopathy is a personality type due to an adaptation, then even if brain differences are found between psychopaths and others, the condition should not be pathologized:

> We take it as given that the brains of psychopaths differ from those of nonpsychopaths in systematic ways. Without such differences, psychopaths could not be reliably set apart in their cognition and behavior from nonpsychopaths. But difference is not isomorphic with dysfunction. For instance, although the brains of men and women have much in common, they must also be different on average, as must the brains of young and old, married and single, androphile and gynephile, Anglophone and Francophone, and so on, even if these brain differences are solely the result of differences of experience. While the life sciences have begun

to recognize that such differences do not inherently reflect disorder, the relationship between difference and disorder nevertheless continues to bedevil the study of mental health.

An argument for dysfunction must marshal supporting evidence, and this must be distinguishable from evidence of difference. (2013, 1)

I conclude from this review that Cooper's own cited counterexample to the HDA not only fails to support her claim that evolutionary dysfunction is not a necessary condition for disorder but, given the unusual occurrence of a major shift in classificatory intuitions by expert researchers, strongly supports the HDA. The literature on psychopathy confirms what I have previously argued primarily on the basis of the history of classificatory judgments about fever, namely, that the HDA correctly predicts that no matter how firmly a condition is initially located within the category of disorder, if it comes to be believed that the condition is biologically designed, then the belief that the condition is a disorder will be challenged and will undergo revision. Of course, such alterations of firm beliefs due to anomalies are likely to be resisted and take place gradually. On the other hand, the examples of fever, adolescent antisocial behavior, and psychopathy illustrate that the change in a condition's disorder status can occur rather rapidly in a research community where new theories of etiology rapidly become known and accepted.

I now consider a further argument in which Cooper adds kin selection to the list of natural-selection evolutionary processes that supposedly can yield disorder:

Or a condition might be selected through kin-selection processes. As individuals are genetically similar to their kin, an individual can increase the number of copies of their genes by helping their relatives to breed successfully. Thus, through kin selection, a condition that is of no direct benefit to an individual may be selected because it benefits the individual's relatives. (33–34)

Before getting to Cooper's specific example of a possible kin-selected disorder, it is worth pointing out that, consistent with the HDA, it is generally assumed that showing that a feature is due to kin selection demonstrates that it is part of normal variation and not pathological. An example is the ongoing attempt to empirically demonstrate E. O. Wilson's (1975) hypothesis that the prevalence of homosexuality, despite obvious reproductive disadvantages, is due to kin selection. The hypothesis is that although homosexual individuals have not themselves reproduced as much as others, they expended the time liberated from caring for their own children to take care of the children of their kin and thus, by increasing their kin's reproductive success, indirectly caused their own genes to be reproduced. A primary and explicit motive behind this research program is to prove that homosexuality is, via kin selection, a naturally selected normal variant of sexuality and thus, it is inferred, not a disorder.

Cooper's proposed example of a disorder that might be due to kin selection is generalized anxiety disorder (GAD):

The genetic basis of generalized anxiety disorder might be promoted for this reason. Generalized anxiety disorder causes sufferers to worry a lot, about, among other things, the welfare of
their families. While worrying may be of no direct benefit to people with generalized anxiety
disorder, it might help their relatives to have someone looking out for them. (34)

The problem with this example is that GAD as defined by recent *DSMs* covers a wide
range of conditions, some of which are disputable as instances of disorder, and so the
question is whether the solid intuitions about disorder and the plausible explanation
of kin selection line up and apply to the same conditions. Often, claims that a category
of conditions is both a disorder and naturally selected are due to a failure to distinguish
between mild and severe subsets within a category, with the more severe intuitively
being disorders while the milder seemingly might be selected but are not persuasive
cases of disorder. The argument thus seems to work only because it is based on a subtle
equivocation between the two subsets of cases, in which one subset pulls intuitions
toward "disorder" while the other subset seems plausibly explainable by natural selection, and both intuitions are then carelessly attributed to the entire category based on
a generic label.

GAD offers a good illustration of this fallacy. Anyone who has experienced or treated
genuine GAD—I've done both—would scoff at Cooper's argument. When Sigmund Freud
initially defined anxiety neurosis (the early name for GAD) as a distinct disorder, separating it off from the wastebasket somatic distress category of neurasthenia, it consisted of
continual intense free-floating anxiety not directed at any particular object. If the patient
experienced specific worries, they were often primarily inner-directed anxieties about
health in reaction to the experience of chronic somatic arousal. There is no imaginable
way that this debilitating disorder of undirected anxiety arousal would yield increased
safety for kin due to threat monitoring, any more than it would make you safer from fire
for your smoke detector to be going off all day even when there is no smoke at all.

However, over time and under the influence of cognitive theoreticians, *DSM* revisions to the diagnostic criteria have expanded the GAD category and refashioned classic GAD to be more "cognitive," requiring that the anxiety take the form of unrealistic
but directed worry about multiple concerns such as one's family's welfare. This "worry
disorder" category (in fact, an attempt was made during the *DSM-5* revision to rename
the category "worry disorder" because it had come so far from the original undirected-
anxiety intention) encompasses conditions that are close to normal-range anxieties in
our highly vigilant species and are not persuasive cases of disorder, and those are the
ones that one might speculate with Cooper might have been a product of kin selection.
If this explanation was to be accepted, no doubt these conditions would come to be
seen more firmly as nondisorders. In contrast, GAD strictly construed in terms of the
kinds of severe anxiety conditions that prompted the formation of the category in the
first place confers no conceivable benefit and lacks any plausible kin-related adaptive
advantage.

This sort of equivocation is also observed in arguments claiming that depression is a naturally selected disorder. Of course, it is plausible that sadness—even intense sadness, of the kind that occurs in grief—is a naturally selected feature of human life, and the circumstantial evidence is clear cut in favor of natural selection for some range of depressions. However, carefully examined, none of the extant theories of the natural selection of depressive symptoms—whether, for example, that people withdraw to process complex social dilemmas, or withdraw after loss of status to avoid additional harm analogous to primates withdrawing after losing a dominance hierarchy dispute, or withdraw after loss because reduced resources portend danger, or withdraw after a failure to process a redirection of one's actions toward more achievable goals— account for the severe conditions that led to the formation of the category. Depression started as "melancholia" in Greek medicine and was redefined by Kraepelin, and the conditions that fell under the disorder were typically extremely immobilizing, often psychotic, enduring, or recurring over time with no necessary relationship to environmental events such as losses or failures and often involved suicidality. So, while the claim that depressive disorder is naturally selected may seem on first glance to be plausible and in conflict with the HDA, if one is willing to "go into the details," one finds it is generally based on an equivocation between the subset of depression that is nondisordered and naturally selected and the subset of depression that is at this time beyond the explanatory power of any plausible natural selection hypothesis and has always been generally judged as clearly disordered, consistent with the HDA.

A philosopher might attempt to do an end run around the scientific and nosological details and ask: Whatever the actual facts, isn't it *conceivable* that we could tomorrow discover that a prototype mental disorder is in fact a naturally selected condition? This is Cooper's ultimate point, made explicit in her summary statement: "In any event, that it is *conceivable* that some disorders might be biologically adaptive is enough to show that it is not *necessary* for a condition to be a biological dysfunction for it to be a disease. It makes sense to think that some disorders may be evolutionarily beneficial, and this shows that biological dysfunction is not a necessary component of our concept of disorder" (Cooper 2007, 34).

However, Cooper's argument from conceivability is invalid because it is based on an incorrect suppressed premise about what is conceivable. She assumes that a prototype mental disorder must remain a mental disorder no matter what we discover about it (this is the same assumption made by Garson; see his chapter and my reply in this volume)—that is, she assumes that it is inconceivable that there are empirical discoveries that would imply that what we currently consider a prototype disorder is in fact a nondisorder. This, combined with the reasonable claim that it is conceivable that almost any organismic feature could be discovered to be naturally selected, yields her conclusion that it is conceivable that a disorder could be naturally selected. These presuppositions to her thought experiment, in which disorder status necessarily remains constant while biological design status is allowed to vary, bias its outcome.

However, the thought experiment imagined by Cooper has occurred multiple times as an actual natural experiment, and the results disconfirm her claim. Fever was once considered a prototypical toxin-induced physical disorder until it was discovered to be a biologically designed response to infection, and then it was no longer considered a disorder. Psychopathy was considered a prototypical mental disorder when it was thought to be a failure of biologically designed moral, empathic, impulse-control, or other evolved mechanisms, but experts who became convinced that psychopathy is a naturally selected variant revised their classification and consider psychopathy a nondisorder. Attention-deficit/hyperactivity disorder (ADHD) has been considered a prototype childhood neurodevelopmental disorder, but, despite the fact that in our social environment, ADHD-like behaviors are indisputably harmful in terms of school performance, those who believe that some variants are due to naturally selected novelty-seeking genes that were adaptive in some past environment also have tended to reclassify those variants as nondisorders. That is, the evidence suggests that it is *not conceptually conceivable* that a genuine medical disorder is itself a naturally selected biological adaptation. Yes, we could discover tomorrow that a condition *that we currently consider a clear case of disorder* is in fact is a biologically designed variant. However, we would then question whether it is a disorder. Cooper argues that, because some disorders are biologically selected and therefore not evolutionary dysfunctions, the HDA is thus refuted. However, in every case Cooper cites, the loss of the dysfunction label tracks the loss of the disorder attribution. The results of multiple natural experiments that are actual empirical versions of Cooper's thought experiment strongly support the HDA's account and falsify Cooper's armchair claim.

Reply to Peter Schwartz's Proposed Counterexamples to the HDA's Dysfunction Requirement

I noted that De Vreese, in addition to citing Cooper's objections to the HDA's dysfunction requirement, also asserts that Peter Schwartz's (2007) proposed counterexamples undeniably refute the HDA. Schwartz himself is confident that he has an endless supply of knock-down counterexamples to the HDA, comparing any attempt by me to defend such an analysis to "the scene in the movie Fantasia where the sorcerer's apprentice is trying to eliminate the magical brooms: crush one, and two spring up" (2007, 56). Recall, however, that the brooms' threatening multiplication was due to the apprentice's ineptitude and his shameful hubris. When the experienced sorcerer returned, the brooms were easily subdued and turned out to pose no real threat at all. Thus encouraged, I consider the objections Schwartz conjures up and examine whether the claimed threat to the HDA is real or illusory.

Schwartz, like Cooper, argues that the HDA fails to adequately explicate "disorder" because it mistakenly requires dysfunction as a necessary condition of disorder. In the passage cited by De Vreese, Schwartz offers two proposed counterexamples that, he claims, are disorders without dysfunctions, which I consider below. (He also presents some concerns regarding the HDA's harm component that I discuss elsewhere in this volume.)

Schwartz's first counterexample to the dysfunction requirement is female anorgasmia: "Female anorgasmia will still not count as disease if orgasm has no function in women" (Schwartz 2007, 56). At another point, when critiquing Boorse's account of disorder, he elaborates,

> For example, it may be that female orgasm makes no specific contribution to survival or reproduction, and thus the mechanisms that bring it about have no biological function. But at the same time, a woman's inability to orgasm may be a serious problem for her, and one which physicians should treat as a disease. (2007, 54)

One must of course agree with Schwartz that when lack of orgasm is a problem for a woman, a physician should try to help. But where does Schwartz get the conclusion that it should be treated "as a disease"? He appears to assume without argument that treatment of a condition must imply that the condition is a disorder. This makes no sense. Physicians treat many nondisorders, from the pain of childbirth to normal grief, and both the *DSM* and the *International Classification of Diseases* (*ICD*) have lengthy lists of "Z Code" categories for commonly treated conditions that are not disorders (*DSM-5* states that these conditions "may be encountered in clinical practice" but "are not mental disorders" [American Psychiatric Association 2013, 715]). As Schwartz himself says, "Doctors have long been involved in inducing sterility and fixing ugly noses, but they do so without claiming that fertility or ugliness are diseases" (2007, 54). As Robert Spitzer, the leading expert on psychiatric diagnosis of the past century, put it in the title to a commentary, "Diagnosis and the need for treatment are not the same" (Spitzer 1998).

In fact, the diagnostic status of anorgasmia—especially during intercourse—is a much disputed question. It is very common for women to have difficulties reaching orgasm during intercourse without some additional clitoral stimulation. Scholarly analyses of the relevant evidence, ranging from Donald Symons's (1979) classic book on the evolution of human sexuality to Elizabeth Lloyd's (2005) recent review, have concluded that female orgasm is likely not a biologically designed feature of female sexuality but rather a variable side effect of other design features, and this is generally taken to imply that orgasm difficulties are not disorders but normal variation.

The psychiatric consensus at this time is represented by *DSM*'s official ambivalence about this diagnosis due to the ambiguity of whether there is a dysfunction. Despite our culture's valuing of the experience of orgasm during intercourse, the evidence has led most experts to conclude that lack of orgasm is not necessarily a disorder and is instead normal female variation. *DSM-IV* expressed this in the cautionary note to the orgasmic dysfunction criteria that "women exhibit wide variability in the type or intensity of stimulation that triggers orgasm" (1994, 505). *DSM-5* is considerably more explicit: "Many women require clitoral stimulation to reach orgasm, and a relatively small proportion of women report that they always experience orgasm during penile-vaginal intercourse. Thus, a woman's experiencing orgasm through clitoral stimulation but not during intercourse does not meet criteria for a clinical diagnosis of female orgasmic disorder" (2013, 430). Thus, contrary to Schwartz's claims, there is no shared intuition that anorgasmia is a medical disorder even when treated. The example of female anorgasmia shows that even culturally highly undesirable conditions that are often treated are not considered disorders if there is not thought to be a dysfunction.

Note that even if orgasm itself is not a selected function but virtually all women are capable, say, of masturbatory orgasm as a side effect of biological design, then if some dysfunction, such as an inhibition resulting from a psychological trauma, prevents the successful exercise of that capacity in a culture that values sexual pleasure, that would be a harmful dysfunction and a disorder despite the fact that orgasm itself is not a biologically designed effect. This is analogous to reading disorder being a genuine disorder when the harm of inability to be able to learn to read results from some neurological dysfunction, even though reading itself is not a biologically designed function.

Schwartz next argues that a mild case of pneumonia can be a disorder that lacks dysfunction. Before getting to Schwartz's example, it is worth observing that mild cases that fall close to a fuzzy boundary area between disorder and nondisorder are likely to raise perplexing challenges for almost any account of disorder. They may be considered disorders only because, as Spitzer and Endicott (1978) put it, in their "fully developed or extreme form" (18), they are clear disorders. However, Schwartz's "mild pneumonia" example raises issues of a different kind than those raised by boundary fuzziness or early stages of pathology.

Schwartz imagines a case of pneumonia in which the patient "has the bad cough and fever but no problem with his breathing" because there is fluid in only some alveoli so "he has preserved lung function" despite the infection. Schwartz argues that this is a counterexample to the HDA:

> Assume that his doctor properly diagnoses and treats him, and he gets better. But then…it's not clear where the dysfunction was. The lungs were able to carry out their function of gas exchange, and the immune system carried out its function of fighting the infection. Although the cough and fever were unpleasant, they were also important components of the body's response to the microbe.…
>
> So although a serious case of pneumonia involves biological dysfunction, it's not clear that a mild case does too. And we can come up with many cases like this. (55)

Schwartz relies here on the fact that some infectious diseases—such as common colds, the flu, and perhaps in some very mild instances pneumonia—have as their primary symptoms the results of biologically designed defensive mechanisms (e.g., cough, runny nose, fever) that are involved in fighting an infection. Thus, it could conceivably be the case that none of the typically cited symptoms of a specific infectious disease are themselves dysfunctions but rather biologically designed defenses.

Both Christopher Boorse and I have addressed this objection and offered the same response. The symptoms are the result of fighting an infection, and the underlying infection and its effects on the cells and organs—which is what both the body's defenses and the doctor's treatment aim to end—constitute a clear dysfunction of cellular and other processes. Indeed, without certain bodily defenses putting a stop to an infection's advance, even the common cold's destruction of cells could advance deep into the body and pose a threat to the individual's life. So, there is certainly a threatening dysfunction in the form of the infection taking place, and it is that dysfunction to which the various defenses are reacting. The fact that one fends off a serious attack does not mean that no attack took place.

Responding to this reply to the proposed cold- and flu-type counterexamples to the HDA, Schwartz says,

> But this makes the necessary condition so easy to satisfy that it verges on triviality. During menstruation, after all, there is massive cell death as the uterine lining is shed. And during the third-trimester of pregnancy the large uterus interferes with the normal function of the bladder storing urine and of the veins carrying blood back from the legs. But menstruation and pregnancy are normal, healthy conditions. (55)

Taking Schwartz's examples seriously, one might ask: if in both colds and menstruation there is underlying cell death and overt symptoms, and in both cases we treat the condition (yes, Schwartz here contradicts his earlier position on anorgasmia that anything treated is a disorder), yet we consider one and not the other a disorder, what then is the difference that changes our classificatory intuitions? The answer is that menstruation, including the shedding of the uterine lining and the consequent cell deaths that the shedding inevitably entails, is considered an inevitable part of a biologically designed process, whereas the death of mucosal cells due to viral invasion that triggers the symptoms of flu or pneumonia is not. The symptoms of infection pointed to by Schwartz are also biologically designed responses, but they are responses to a nondesigned assault by an infectious pathogen.

Having made a clean sweep of Schwartz's as well as Cooper's supposed counterexamples, I conclude that there is no successful objection to the HDA's dysfunction requirement in the passages cited by De Vreese, and her argument based on the presupposition that such counterexamples are available is left without foundation. More important, the claim by Cooper that the HDA is refuted by the fact that there are or can be prototypical disorders that are naturally selected is falsified by the evidence.

References

American Psychiatric Association. 1994. *Diagnostic and Statistical Manual of Mental Disorders*. 4th ed. American Psychiatric Association.

American Psychiatric Association. 2013. *Diagnostic and Statistical Manual of Mental Disorders*. 5th ed. American Psychiatric Association.

Cooper, R. 2007. *Psychiatry and Philosophy of Science*. Routledge.

Kingma, E. 2013. Naturalist accounts of mental disorder. In *The Oxford Handbook of Philosophy and Psychiatry*, K. W. M. Fulford, M. Davies, R. G. T. Gipps, G. Graham, J. Z. Sadler, G. Stanghellini, and T. Thornton (eds.), 363–384. Oxford University Press.

Kinner, S. A. 2003. Psychopathy as an adaptation: Implications for society and social policy. In *Evolutionary Psychology and Violence*, R. Bloom and N. Dess (eds.), 57–81. Praeger.

Kirk, S. A., J. C. Wakefield, D. Hsieh, and K. Pottick. 1999. Social context and social workers' judgment of mental disorder. *Social Service Review* 73: 82–104.

Krupp, D. B., L. A. Sewall, M. L. Lalumière, C. Sheriff, and G. T. Harris. 2012. Nepotistic patterns of violent psychopathy: Evidence for adaptation? *Frontiers in Psychology* 3: 305.

Krupp, D. B., L. A. Sewall, M. L. Lalumière, C. Sheriff, and G. T. Harris. 2013. Psychopathy, adaptation, and disorder. *Frontiers in Psychology* 27: 139.

Lalumière, M. L., G. T. Harris, and M. E. Rice. 2001. Psychopathy and developmental instability. *Evolution and Human Behavior* 22(2): 75–92.

Leedom, L. J., and L. H. Almas. 2012. Is psychopathy a disorder or an adaptation? *Frontiers in Psychology* 3: 549.

Lloyd, E. 2005. *The Case of the Female Orgasm: Bias in the Science of Evolution*. Harvard University Press.

Machalek, R. 1995. Sociobiology, sociopathy, and social policy. *Behavioral and Brain Sciences* 18(3): 564.

Mealey, L. 1995a. The sociobiology of sociopathy: An integrated evolutionary model. *Behavioral and Brain Sciences* 18(3): 523–541.

Mealey, L. 1995b. Primary sociopathy (psychopathy) is a type, secondary is not. *Behavioral and Brain Sciences* 18(3): 579–599.

Moffitt, T. E. 1993. Adolescence-limited and life-course-persistent antisocial behavior: A developmental taxonomy. *Psychological Review* 100(4): 674–701.

Polimanti, R., and J. Gelernter. 2017. Widespread signatures of positive selection in common risk alleles associated to autism spectrum disorder. *PLoS Genetics* 13(2): e1006618.

Reimer, M. 2008. Psychopathy without (the language of) disorder. *Neuroethics* 1(3): 185–198.

Schwartz, P. H. 2007. Decision and discovery in defining "disease." In *Establishing Medical Reality: Essays in the Metaphysics and Epistemology of Biomedical Science*, H. Kincaid and J. McKitrick (eds.), 47–63. Springer.

Spitzer, R. L. 1998. Diagnosis and need for treatment are not the same. *Archives of General Psychiatry* 55: 120.

Spitzer, R. L., and J. Endicott. 1978. Medical and mental disorder: Proposed definition and criteria. In *Critical Issues in Psychiatric Diagnosis*, D. F. Klein and R. L. Spitzer (eds.), 15–40. Raven Press.

Symons, D. 1979. *The Evolution of Human Sexuality*. Oxford University Press.

Wakefield, J. C., S. A. Kirk, K. Pottick, and D. Hsieh. 1999. Disorder attribution and clinical judgment in the assessment of adolescent antisocial behavior. *Social Work Research* 23: 227–241.

Wakefield, J. C., S. A. Kirk, K. Pottick, X. Tian, and D. K. Hsieh. 2006. The lay concept of conduct disorder: Do non-professionals use syndromal symptoms or internal dysfunction to distinguish disorder from delinquency? *Canadian Journal of Psychiatry* 51: 210–217.

Wakefield, J. C., K. J. Pottick, and S. A. Kirk. 2002. Should the *DSM-IV* diagnostic criteria for conduct disorder consider social context? *American Journal of Psychiatry* 159: 380–386.

Wilson, E. O. 1975. *Sociobiology: The New Synthesis*. Harvard University Press.

Contributors

Rachel Cooper, Professor of Philosophy, University of Lancaster

Andreas De Block, Professor of Philosophy, KU Leuven

Steeves Demazeux, Professor of Philosophy, Université de Bordeaux Montaigne

Leen De Vreese, Post-Doc, Department of Philosophy and Moral Sciences, Ghent University

Luc Faucher, Professor of Philosophy, Université du Québec à Montréal

Denis Forest, Professor of Philosophy, Université Paris 1 Panthéon-Sorbonne

Justin Garson, Associate Professor of Philosophy, Hunter College–City University of New York

Philip Gerrans, Professor of Philosophy, University of Adelaide

Harold Kincaid, Professor, School of Economics, and Director, Research Unit in Behavioural Economics and Neuroeconomics, University of Cape Town

Maël Lemoine, Professor of Philosophy, Université de Bordeaux Montaigne

Dominic Murphy, Associate Professor of Philosophy, University of Sydney

Jonathan Sholl, Assistant Professor of Philosophy, School of Culture and Society, Aarhus University

Tim Thornton, Professor of Philosophy and Mental Health, University of Central Lancashire

Jerome Wakefield, Professor of Social Work, New York University–Silver School of Social Work; Professor of the Conceptual Foundations of Psychiatry, School of Medicine (2007–2019); and Associate Faculty, Center for Bioethics, College of Global Public Health–New York University

Peter Zachar, Professor, Department of Psychology, Auburn University–Montgomery

Index

Autism (cont.)
  as a disorder, 89, 398, 421, 433, 434, 438,
    441, 449–453, 455, 457, 459, 578
  as the effect of a dysfunction, 421, 435, 436,
    437, 439, 444, 452
  explanation of, 397, 434–436, 438, 450,
    460
  forms of, 442, 443, 453, 454, 458
  genes for, 149, 454, 578
  high-functioning, 433, 438, 440, 443–445,
    450, 453–457, 459
  mindblindness theory of, 435, 450
  neurodiversity account of, 421, 442, 450
  as a normal variation, 89, 433, 434, 440,
    442–444, 449, 452, 453, 459
  research on, 433, 434, 437, 450, 451
  severe, 441, 443, 456
  spectrum disorder (ASD), 116, 136, 188,
    276, 444
  symptoms of, 436, 464
  theory of mind account of, 421
  treatment, 451
  weak coherence theory of, 435, 438, 439,
    440, 441, 450, 459, 460

Belief fixation, 398, 401–403, 418, 422–424
Bias, 84, 202, 419, 444, 540, 541, 586
  adaptive, 405, 406
  anticonceptual, 135
  behavioral, 405
  cognitive, 162
  essentialist, 162
  judgment, 320
  negative, 433
  positive, 399
  sampling, 54, 78, 81
  sexual, 4
Biological design, 331, 415, 416, 451
  analysis, 416, 417
  assumptions about, 328
  belief about, 421
  explanation of, 327
  evolutionary perspective on, 418

evolved, 205, 209, 216
failure of, 89, 165, 191, 218, 267, 278, 293,
  360, 451, 565, 569, 587
functional, 238, 239, 241–243
historical, 264, 275
history of, 453
human, 92, 107, 135, 144, 145, 181, 353,
  458, 504, 515
intuitions about, 327
limits, 529
natural, 5, 38, 39
of neurobiological systems, 418
obviousness of, 60, 92
theory of, 421, 451
trade-off, 459, 460
Biologically designed
  adaptation, 226, 579
  behavior, 160, 181, 568
  causal role, 269
  condition, 144, 579, 583
  development, 137, 183, 224, 460
  disorder, 144, 146, 148, 150
  effect, 245, 588
  evolutionary processes, 71
  feature, 215, 234, 243, 245, 587
  function (see Function: biologically
    designed)
  functioning (see Functioning: biologically
    designed)
  mechanism, 144, 217, 567, 587, 589
  mental modules, 286
  organism, 328
  pregnancy, 529
  processes, 223
  reaction (see Biologically designed: response)
  response, 144, 146, 234, 360, 586, 589
  sleep capacity, 328
  system, 88, 90, 143, 285
  traits, 281 (see also Biologically designed:
    feature)
Biology, 213, 226, 259, 261, 263, 289, 291,
  329, 488, 540, 541
  causal relations in, 263